THE VETERINARY WORKBOOK OF SMALL ANIMAL CLINICAL CASES

T0206629

THE VETERINARY WORKBOOK OF SMALL ANIMAL CLINICAL CASES

Ryane E. Englar, DVM, DABVP (Canine and Feline Practice)

Associate Professor
Director, Veterinary Skills Development
University of Arizona College of Veterinary Medicine
Oro Valley, AZ

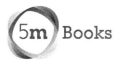 Books

First published 2021

Published by
5M Books Ltd,
Lings, Great Easton,
Essex CM6 2HH, UK,
Tel: +44 (0)330 1333 580
www.5mbooks.com

A Catalogue record for this book is available from the British Library

ISBN 9781789181296
eISBN 9781789181586
DOI 10.52517.9781789181586

Book layout by KSPM, 8 Wood Road, Codsall, Wolverhampton, WV8 1DB
Printed by CPI Group (UK) Ltd, Croydon CR0 4YY
Photos by the author unless otherwise indicated

Contents

PART I

Making Clinical Medicine Come Alive: An Introduction to Case-Based Decision Making   1

PART II

Common Cases in Pediatric Canine/Feline Medicine   25

PART III

Common Cases in Adult and Geriatric Canine and Feline Medicine 207

NEUROMUSCULAR CHIEF COMPLAINTS

REPRODUCTIVE CHIEF COMPLAINTS

END-OF-LIFE

About the Author

Ryane E. Englar, DVM, DABVP (Canine and Feline Practice) graduated from Cornell University College of Veterinary Medicine in 2008. She practiced as an associate veterinarian in companion animal practice before transitioning into the educational circuit as an advocate for pre-clinical training in primary care. She debuted in academia as a Clinical Instructor of the Community Practice Service at Cornell University's Hospital for Animals. She then transitioned into the role of Assistant Professor as founding faculty at Midwestern University College of Veterinary Medicine. While at Midwestern University, she had the opportunity to teach the inaugural Class of 2018, the Class of 2019, and the Class of 2020. While training these remarkable young professionals, Dr. Englar became a Diplomate of the American Board of Veterinary Practitioners (ABVP). She then joined the faculty at Kansas State University between May 2017 and January 2020 to launch the Clinical Skills curriculum.

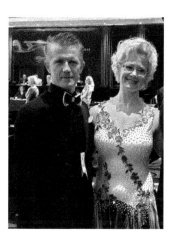

In February 2020, Dr. Englar reprised her role of founding faculty when she returned "home" to Tucson to join the University of Arizona College of Veterinary Medicine. As a dual appointment Associate Professor and the Director of Veterinary Skills Development, Dr. Englar currently leads the Clinical and Professional Skills curriculum. In her current role, she has developed a series of standardized client encounters for student training in clinical communication. She is also committed to furthering her research as to how clinical communication drives relationship-centered care.

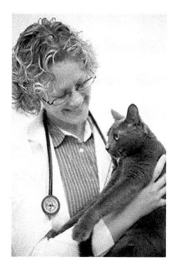

Dr. Englar is passionate about advancing education for generalists by thinking outside of the box to develop new course materials for the hands-on learner. This labor of love is preceded by four texts that collectively provide students and clinicians alike with functional, relatable, and practice-friendly tools for success:

- *Performing the Small Animal Physical Examination* (John Wiley & Sons, 2017)
- *Writing Skills for Veterinarians* (5M Publishing, 2019)
- *Common Clinical Presentations in Dogs and Cats* (John Wiley & Sons, 2019)
- *A Guide to Oral Communication in Veterinary Medicine* (5M Publishing, 2020)

Dr. Englar's students fuel her desire to create. They inspire her to develop the tools that they need to succeed in clinical practice. If the goal of educators, as they are tasked by the accrediting bodies, is to create "Day-One," "Practice-Ready" veterinarians, then this text and her others complement the mission.

When Dr. Englar is not teaching or advancing primary care, she trains in the art of ballroom dancing and competes nationally with her instructor, Lowell E. Fox.

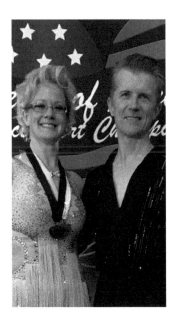

Preface

"What do I need to know?"

It's a question that greets me at the start of every semester. At least once. Like clockwork. And often, multiple times over, like the chorus of a showtune set on repeat.

It's a fair question and if I'm honest, it's one I asked when I myself stood in my students' shoes. Back then, when I phrased it, I had only one endpoint in mind: the exam.

In the pre-clinical years, "What do I need to know?" was code for "How do I survive the test?"

In the clinical year, "What do I need to know?" was code for "How do I pass this rotation?"

In those years, there was always a seemingly insurmountable bar to leap over and we lived in perpetual fear of falling short.

We compensated by memorizing. Everything. All the time. Everywhere. We lulled ourselves into believing that if we just crammed enough factual content into our reserves, it would ooze out of us on command when we needed it most.

Learning was a race. And we believed that we made it one step closer to the finish line with each fact we committed to memory.

What we didn't realize then was that there would come a day when we would graduate from tests yet still face the ultimate test: clinical practice.

Practice, as it turned out, was less about facts and more about the *approach*.

Suddenly, it didn't matter if you could recite what was on page 1252 of Ettinger's *Textbook of Veterinary Internal Medicine*. You could always, simply, go look it up.

What mattered more was your ability to see the clinical picture unfold before you, in slow motion, like a dream, as you sifted through fluff to find the relevance and complete the portrait, often with time constraints and limited funds.

You leveled up in this Game of Life not by spitting out facts, but by creating connections. Connections between content and patients that all too often didn't read the textbook. Connections between past mistakes and present chances at "take 2"s. Connections between what you had learned in school and what actually happened in Real Life. Connections between what you thought you knew and everything you still had left to learn.

Practice was hard and it was humbling. I learned how much I didn't know. I learned to question what I thought I did.

And I learned, most importantly of all, that learning the art and science of veterinary medicine was less like competing in a race with a certifiable end and more like peeling back an onion, one layer at a time. An onion with endless layers and incredible depth.

The more layers you peel, the more there are to greet you. It feels like forever because it is. But despite what it may sound like or feel like in the moment, *forever* is actually a good thing.

That there is no end to veterinary education means that we are *forever* on a trajectory of growth.

We are *forever* learning how to practice in a world where clinical practice is *forever* changing.

With each step we take, we forge a new and uncharted course for ourselves as practitioners. Our growth transforms us into *forever* learners.

We are not static, as we once assumed our graduate selves would be. Instead, we grow, we change, we blossom, we adapt into stronger, better, more defined, more refined doctors. Doctors who are skilled at approaches, not facts.

To get there, to wrap our heads around the idea that we are and have always been *enough*, that our willingness to evolve as clinicians is in fact our strongest suit, we must rethink the way we approach learning.

We need to forget about learning as a means to the end and reconsider learning as a means to new beginnings.

Each clinical case that crosses our path is an opportunity to begin again. To put what we've learned to the test and stretch ourselves one step further to problem-solve and critically think our way into a viable solution.

What this means for our learners is that they learn best by doing, by being introduced to casework rather than having it held captive under lock and key until they are deemed "ready."

One is never ready *enough*, skilled *enough*, brilliant *enough* to know it all. Yet we are all *more than enough* to start *somewhere*.

This text represents that starting point, that *somewhere*, that beginning step in a revamped curricular effort to introduce casework early and often.

This text is intentionally learner-centered. It teaches patterns, not facts, as a backdrop to exploring the world of clinical practice that awaits. A world that you all belong in, in your own way. You just have to find your own path there and trust in it.

Let this text be a guide to set you on course when you find yourself in need of a compass.

Dedication

Life is about the journey: where we start, where the path leads, and all the rabbit holes we end up finding along the way, some of which take us way off course, while other roads less traveled lead us unknowingly to our destiny.

Life is also about those in our lives and in our hearts: those who set out on the trail with us, those who join us along the way and inspire us to go in search of more, and those who are waiting for us when we circle back to where we were always meant to be. This text is dedicated to these three spheres of influence, all of whom have shaped my journey and strengthened my path.

In honor of the one who shared my journey for nearly 16 years – I dedicate this text to the late Nina Englar, my Platinum mink Tonkinese cat – the one who could only join me in spirit for the final leg of my journey "home," from Kansas to Arizona.

(April 21, 2004–January 6, 2020)

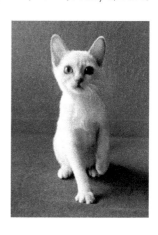

From the moment that my family and I met Nina in kitten form, she was a fruitcake. She leapt at me from across the room like a flying squirrel, then clung to my head like a mini koala. She was a bit loopy and not quite all there. But she was ours and we loved her more than I could ever imagine.

She had these big bug-eyes, and when her pupils dilated, she looked like a creature from another planet. Like ET. Only plusher. She was in trouble more times than I can count, but no amount of scolding squelched her spirit. She had a thirst for life and the gift of gab. There was never a conversation that she wasn't a part of, and she had a guttural wail that could curl your toes.

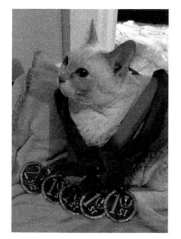

Nina may not have understood anything about my passion for dance other than that she loved to shoulder-ride when I practiced foxtrot in the living room. She also loved dance bling. Unlike her housemate, Bailey, who only "tolerated" one medal around her neck, Nina wanted them *all* . . . three, four, five medals, it didn't matter. They were hers. And she wore them proudly.

As much as she drove me crazy; she also made me whole.

My little "snow leopard" had the most empathy of any cat I ever knew. If you had a bad day, she was there. If you started to cry, she stopped what she was doing to console you. She waited for me at the front door every night. She was the ultimate greeter. She was always in my way and underfoot, but she brought a welcome sort of chaos to life that will be forever missed. She reminded me always to go with the flow and to live life fully, without regret. Nina made our house into a home.

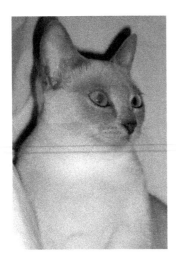 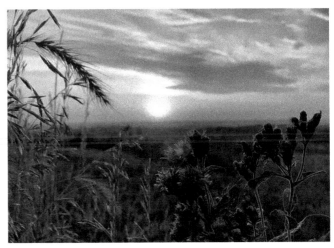

Courtesy of Anna Kucera

In honor of those who gave me the courage to carve out a new journey for myself – I dedicate this text to the Doctor of Veterinary Medicine (DVM) Classes of 2021, 2022, and 2023 at Kansas State University.

You were my raison d'etre in Manhattan, Kansas. You welcomed me into your lives and hearts. You gave me a sense of belonging in a place where a "fit" was hard to come by. You trusted me with reshaping your curriculum and allowed me a voice in your education. You gave me a reason to shine.

You also reminded me to follow my own advice.

I once told you that a favorite quote of mine was this: "You cannot discover new oceans unless you have the courage to lose sight of the shore." Each day, every day you were courageous.

You taught me that I, too, could spread my wings and fly, to find the path that would lead me "home."

In honor of the one who managed to infuse Kansas with enough memories of Arizona to teleport me "home" to Arrowhead Arthur Murray – I dedicate this text to my dance instructor and life coach, Lowell E. Fox.

Lowell came into my life when I was just discovering my role in academia and my place on the dance floor. At that time, I saw the studio as an outlet, a harmless approach to coaxed socialization that could get me out of my shell so I could experience the world outside of the office. That was a time in my life when I didn't think I could be good at anything other than science. Had you asked me then how I defined myself, a "dancer" would never have been on my radar. I had yet to realize that being a vet was just one sliver of me and that as much as I loved my profession, I could be equally passionate about other pursuits. I didn't realize then, as I do now, that dance could and would provide the fuel I needed to sustain my love for and commitment to veterinary medicine.

Fast forward to the present, 7 years later. My sense of self and how I choose to define myself have broadened immensely. In addition to my two loving and supportive parents, I have Lowell to thank for my metamorphosis.

Lowell may have been tasked with training me in American Smooth, Standard, American Rhythm, and Latin dance, but over the years, he's grown to be so much more. Lowell is my sounding board, both on and off the dance floor. It is not uncommon for me to write chapters in my head as we waltz, or work through a research proposal aloud as we tango.

His energy and thirst for knowledge collectively inspire my creativity. His faith in me has pushed me to believe in myself more. He is a true coach. He saw potential in me and ignited the spark that lit my world ablaze.

That I can translate my aspirations into action items is because he showed me the way. He may teach me dance, but our choreography is life.

Every day that I grow in dance is a day that I feel inspired and whole, peaceful and calm, supported and free.

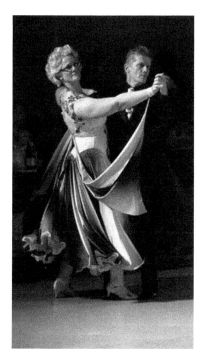
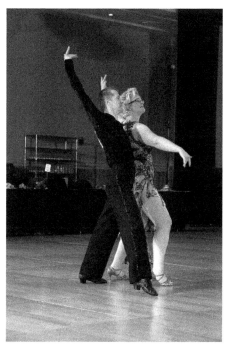

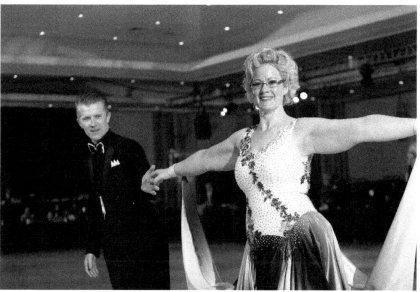

Acknowledgements

I have been fortunate to find support in every walk of life, including those journeys that took me far from home. My years in Kansas were challenging because I found myself in a world that I was constantly trying to understand. In many ways, I felt like a fish out of water. I knew my purpose; I knew why I was there. It took time to find a sense of belonging amidst those who didn't always get me.

I didn't realize just how important a sense of community was until I struggled to find one of my own. For starters, there was no Arthur Murray studio in Manhattan, Kansas – and let's face it, dance had become the world that knew me best.

It took time and perseverance to test the waters and find my people, and in so doing, discover a group of loved ones who weren't afraid to grow right alongside of me.

One of my favorite proverbs is:

"If you want to go fast, go alone. If you want to go far, go together."

The individuals whom I would like to acknowledge at this time epitomize this culture of togetherness. Their presence brought support, kindness, and understanding at a time in my life when I needed it most.

To Keleigh Schettler

You not only walked the walk in Kansas, you journeyed with me abroad. Some of my favorite moments teaching were with you by my side at the China Agricultural University Veterinary Teaching Hospital (Beijing) and Huazhong Agricultural University (Wuhan). You taught me to stretch outside of my comfort zone. You were my courage when I had none. You gifted me friendship and a lifelong connection that no geographical distance can ever come between.

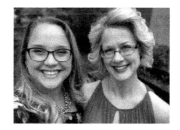

To Richard Foveaux DC, MS, DACBSP, RMSK, and his wife, Jennifer

You were the family that I needed in Kansas, and Joint Fit Chiropractic & Sports Medicine became my oasis. Over the years, you patched my body up more times than I can count, yet your true gift of healing came from the heart. You shared my passion for teaching and dreamed of making a difference to the community. I am living proof that you did. You became my community.

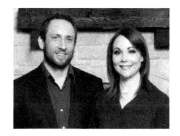

To Cathryn Stevens-Sparks and her husband, James

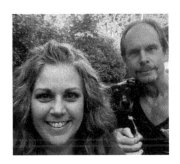

To paraphrase one of my favorite songs from the *Greatest Showman*, you were the ones who reminded me to "live a little, finally laugh a little" and you gave me "the freedom to dream." True to the lyrics, you showed me the Other Side of life. You reminded me that time is a gift and that we need to make the most of life, with those we love most. Thank you for telling me to take that leap of faith when I needed the extra push to step out of the nest and into the unknown.

To Steph Rivera and her partner, Tim Gregory, of Ballroom Dance School Manhattan (KS)

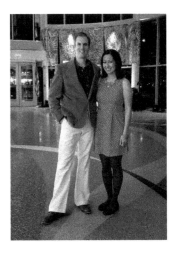

You introduced a world I knew (dance) to a world I didn't. You bridged my past to my future by creating a safe and supportive present tense. You brought perspective, familiarity, and comfort to our time together. We may have met because of our mutual love of dance, but dance was the impetus for friendship that survived a cross-country move. Thank you for opening your studio, your home, and your hearts to me. You made me a better version of myself by inspiring authenticity.

Abbreviations

AAFCO	Association of American Feed Control Officials
AAFP	American Association of Feline Practitioners
AAHA	American Association of Hospitals for Animals
ABCD	Advisory Board on Cat Diseases
ACE	angiotensin-converting enzyme
ADH	antidiuretic hormone
AIDS	acquired immunodeficiency syndrome
AKI	acute kidney injury
ALP	alkaline phosphatase
ANNPE	acute non-compressive nucleus pulposus extrusion
ARF	acute renal failure
ARVC	arrhythmogenic right ventricular cardiomyopathy
ASA	American Society of Anaesthesiologists
ASPCA	American Society for Prevention of Cruelty to Animals
AVMA	American Veterinary Medical Association
BAR	bright, alert, and responsive
BCS	body condition score
BG	blood glucose
BP	blood pressure
BPH	benign prostatic hyperplasia
BSAVA	British Small Animal Veterinary Association
BUN	blood urea nitrogen
CAV-2	canine adenovirus
CBC	complete blood count
cc	chief complaint
CDI	central diabetes insipidus
CDV	canine distemper virus
CHF	congestive heart failure
CI	cephalic index
CIRD	canine infectious respiratory disease
CIRDC	canine infectious respiratory disease complex
CK	creatine kinase
CKD	chronic kidney disease
CLO	Campylobacter-like organism
CN	cranial nerve
CNS	central nervous system
CPR	cardiopulmonary resuscitation
CRF	corticotropin-releasing factor
CRI	continuous rate infusion
CRT	capillary refill time
CT	computed tomography

DEXA	dual-energy X-ray absorptiometry
DexSP	dexamethasone sodium phosphate
DIC	disseminated intravascular coagulation
DLH	domestic long-haired
DMH	domestic medium-haired
DSH	domestic short-haired
DTM	dermatophyte test medium
ED	equilibrium dialysis
ELISA	enzyme-linked immunosorbent assay
EPI	exocrine pancreatic insufficiency
FAS	fear, anxiety, or stress
FeLV	feline leukemia virus
FHO	femoral head ostectomy
FIC	feline interstitial cystitis
FIV	feline immunodeficiency virus
FLUTD	feline lower urinary tract disease
FNA	fine-needle aspirate
FS	female spayed
FSH	follicle-stimulating hormone
FUS	feline urologic syndrome
FVR	feline viral rhinotracheitis
FVRCP	feline viral rhinotracheitis-calicivirus-panleukopenia
GABA	gamma-aminobutyric acid
GDV	gastric dilatation and volvulus
GFR	glomerular filtration rate
HARD	heartworm-associated respiratory disease
HE	hepatic encephalopathy
HIV	human immunodeficiency virus
HR	heart rate
HSV	herpes simplex virus
IBD	inflammatory bowel disease
IBE	International Bureau for Epilepsy
ICA	iridocorneal angle
ILAE	International League Against Epilepsy
IOP	intraocular pressure
IRIS	International Renal Interest Society
IVDD	intervertebral disc disease
LH	luteinizing hormone
LMN	lower motor neuron
MA	megestrol acetate
MER	maintenance energy requirement
MLV	modified live virus
MN	male neutered
MR	mitral regurgitation
MRI	magnetic resonance imaging
NAVC	North American Veterinary Conference
NDI	nephrogenic diabetes insipidus
NI	neonatal isoerythrolysis
NOAH	National Office of Animal Health
NPO	nil per os
NSAID	non-steroidal anti-inflammatory drugs
OCD	obsessive–compulsive disorder

ORS	ovarian remnant syndrome
PAF	platelet activating factor
PCR	polymerase chain reaction
PCV	packed cell volume
PDA	patent ductus arteriosus
PLE	protein-losing enteropathy
PLR	pupillary light reflex
PMI	point of maximal intensity
PNS	peripheral nervous system
PO	per os
PPE	personal protective equipment
PRAA	persistent right aortic arch
PS	pulmonic stenosis
PT	prothrombin time
PU	perineal urethrostomy
QAR	quiet, alert, and responsive
QATS	quick assessment tests
ROS	reactive oxygen species
RR	respiratory rate
RSM	rapid sporulating media
SARDS	sudden acquired retinal degeneration syndrome
SCC	squamous cell carcinoma
SCFE	slipped capital femoral epiphysis
SI	small intestinal
SIBO	small intestinal bacterial overgrowth
SLO	symmetrical lupoid onychodystrophy
SSI	surgical site infection
TCC	transitional cell carcinoma
TP	total protein
TPR	temperature, pulse (beats per minute), and respiration (breaths per minute)
TSH	thyroid-stimulating hormone
UMN	upper motor neuron
UPR	unconditional positive regard
URI	upper respiratory infection
USG	urine specific gravity
UTI	urinary tract infection
UTO	urinary tract obstruction
VPC	ventricular premature complex
WSAVA	World Small Animal Veterinary Association

Part 1

Making Clinical Medicine Come Alive

An Introduction to Case-Based Decision Making

Chapter 1

Rethinking How We Ask Students to Problem-Solve in Clinical Medicine

Traditional veterinary curricula cram knowledge into the pre-clinical years at the expense of active learning.(1, 2) Most programs in the United States require doctors of veterinary medicine to graduate with over 160 semester credits. This is the equivalent of five-and-a-half academic calendar years compressed into four.(2)

Lectures distance students from the clinic floor. Patients historically have been gifted to students at the finish line rather than the starting gate, and students are expected to make the leap overnight, from reciting abstract classroom concepts to doctoring real world cases.

The separation between scientific disciplines in many programs has contributed to the challenges that students face during this transition period. Many universities classify team members as pre-clinical or clinical faculty, and do not initiate dialogue between the two. Students are handed over like batons in a relay race, from the so-called Basic Sciences faculty to university teaching hospital faculty and staff.

Clinicians depend upon pre-clinical faculty to deliver students to rotations with an adequate foundation in medical knowledge. The Basic Sciences faculty depend upon the clinicians to make medicine come to life. Neither really knows fully what students have been or will be exposed to, and when gaps in knowledge occur, as they are bound to do, each side may be quick to cast blame upon the other.

In the absence of horizontal and vertical integration of coursework, students are expected to form their own connections between related content areas.(3) Some students struggle with the autonomy of this approach to education: are they on target or are they way off base?

As educators, we often worry if our students are actually learning.

If we do not provide them with a clear road map, then how do we expect them to know where to begin in their quest to acquire a working knowledge of veterinary medicine that extends into clinical acumen?

Many students struggle with the passivity of lecture-based education. They may have difficulty motivating themselves to find relevance in material that is being presented in an abstract fashion.(4) It is difficult to practice the application of material to clinical scenarios when all that is being asked of you is that you commit course content to memory.

Students memorize at the expense of learning all the time. In many circumstances, our educational methods are set up in such a way as to encourage this behavior. Courses in which students' entire grade rests upon one or two examinations support cramming. Facts are retained only as long as is necessary, that is, for students to survive the next assessment.(5)

When content load is manageable, students make it work. They perform well and believe that their assessment scores reflect true learning. Students may be lulled into the misconception that good doctors are walking encyclopedias. This may be reinforced by faculty who appreciate when students parrot what they have read in texts or heard from the chief of service on the clinic floor.

Many of my own students have shared a seemingly universal belief that they would be more successful in their studies and beyond if they just crammed "more" because at a certain point, then they would "just know it all."

Yet advances in science and, in particular, biotechnology have outpaced our students' ability to master one entire facet of veterinary medicine, let alone the entire profession.(1) As educators, we fail our students if we lead them to believe that the convoluted road to patient diagnosis, treatment, and recovery is smoothed out by committing to memory every muscle origin, insertion, biochemical pathway, or clinicopathologic anomaly.

The world of doctoring is rarely one of certainty, made complete by textbook patients with classic presentations and predictable outcomes, and clinical facts should not be cataloged at the expense of problem-solving, critical thinking, and the practical application of theory to real life.

Knowledge alone does not make clinical diagnosis and patient outcomes unambiguous. The thought that it might is an impractical perspective on an imperfect science.

The truth is that medicine is strikingly human.

Sir William Osler captured it best when he wrote that, "[Medicine is the] practice of an art which consists largely in balancing possibilities."(6) "It is a science of uncertainty and an art of probability."(7)

Doctoring requires clinicians to make educated guesses in the face of uncertainty. Practitioners are often called upon to consider complex problems that may not be well-defined and may even contradict one another.(8, 9) These tasks are not designed for the faint-hearted or for those who thrive in a world of absolutes.

The practice of medicine requires a unique approach to clinical problems. Successful clinicians are effective at clinical reasoning. Clinical reasoning is set apart from scientific reasoning:

> Science starts with the hypothetical answer and works backward, in a process of hypothetico-deductive logic, to check that all the elements present are as predicted. In contrast, much of clinical reasoning starts with the problem and works forward, probabilistically, through a process of inductive logic to the likely answer. (10)

Clinicians work in terms of probabilities every day. Patient interventions and outcomes are often guided by the most likely diagnosis. Likewise, treatments may be selected less so because they are the perfect fit and more often because they are the best option.

It is not always about making the right call, and more so about making the best call.

As a healthcare profession, veterinary medicine embodies the art of probabilities every day. Veterinarians are called upon to make best guesses all the time, based upon true uncertainties as well as those instances where we cannot obtain the answers we need to solve our patients' problems because our hands are tied. Like all other healthcare industries, we rely upon informed consent to proceed with diagnostic testing and therapeutic trials. Without consent, we cannot proceed with delivery of care.

Cost is often the limiting factor in veterinary practice. Oftentimes we know what we want to do to diagnose, or what we want to prescribe to treat, but we are unable to deliver the gold standard to our patient because of financial constraints. Consider, for example, a patient that presents with acute kidney injury (AKI). We know that patient survival and renal recovery are improved when hemodialysis is initiated early in the course of disease, before the development of hyperkalemia and metabolic acidosis. Yet, how many veterinary clients can afford this level of care?

Cost aside, how many veterinary facilities can offer this service as a viable treatment option?

In veterinary practice, we are taught to offer gold standard care to all our patients – and to the best of our abilities, we do. Yet, the reality is that most of our day-to-day recommendations stem from answers to the following two questions:

1. Is diagnostic test "X" or treatment "Y" available?
2. Is diagnostic text "X" or treatment "Y" affordable?

- How often do we stray from the gold standard? How often are we tasked with providing a Plan B approach, or even a Plan C, or a Plan D?
- How often do we treat diarrhea empirically, that is, without a true diagnosis?
- How often do we initiate conservative treatment in the absence of complete or perfect information?
- How often do we initiate care based upon clinical educated guesses?

The practice of veterinary medicine – and for that matter, any form of healthcare – is rarely ever black and white. To be successful practitioners, students must learn to navigate the shades of grey. Students must learn how to interact with and ultimately make sense of an incomplete data set.

Students must learn how to accept the unknown and to make choices in spite of uncertainty.

- How do you teach students these nuances of medicine and these realities of clinical practice in a classroom setting?
- How do you teach students to make choices, particularly when they might not have access to all the information they need?
- How do you teach decision making in a way that models those behaviors that are essential for student doctors to be successful in clinical practice?

We can lecture to students all we want, but very little of what we say, if anything, will feel real to them unless they themselves experience it.

Students must be given the opportunity to actively engage in casework in a safe, supportive environment that allows them to explore, confront, and make decisions about the very situations that they will face in practice.

Students must be allowed to consider a clinical problem, obtain data, consider that which is known against that which is not, make a decision, witness the consequences of that decision, reflect upon their actions, and consider next steps in the case moving forward.

In working through this process, students may take three steps forward and two steps back or two steps forward and three steps back.

Students may recognize that decision "X" led to unexpected consequences that now require intervention "Y."

Students may recognize that they failed to ask the right question, or that they went about the problem in the wrong way. Maybe they focused on problem "Z," but problem "Z" was a red herring. In so doing, they failed to adequately address the root of the presenting complaint, which, in turn, persisted.

These actions are not unique to students. Practitioners work through the same process throughout their careers. As educators, we need to highlight and embrace the similarities in the journeys that both students and clinicians share.

We need to demystify the practice of medicine by showing students that their footprints in the sand are matched by the doctors who walk the path beside them. Both sets of pupils require lifelong learning. One never truly reaches the pinnacle because there will always be another peak to climb.

Learning is best achieved by doing. And practicing medicine is, just that, practice.

Students need to be gifted the opportunity to practice well before their clinical year. Students need to be introduced to casework early on and often. Students need to be able to formulate decision trees, make clinical decisions, and receive feedback so that they can see firsthand and follow-up on the consequences of their actions. Students need to be able to make mistakes in low stakes settings so that they can learn from them.

Every action is an opportunity for reflection and growth.

Pre-clinical students are capable beings. They are our future colleagues. They are also our profession's future. As such, they can and should be coaxed to critically think and problem-solve outside of the traditional classroom mode.

Pre-clinical students need to be taught how to process clinical cases as an expert would.(5) This type of learning is complex. It requires three stages:(5, 11)

1. The accumulation of knowledge.
2. The ability to sift through knowledge to find that which is essential for and can be applied to specific procedures.
3. The development of routines that automate procedures, such that procedures become hardwired.

Students do not become experts overnight, although traditional curricula have often asked them to.

Students are novices. They do not necessarily see connections between related content areas because their understanding of the fluidity of topics is incomplete.(5) They need lists and algorithms in the initial stages of learning because they cannot default to pattern recognition. They have yet to learn the patterns that make solutions to problems seem obvious to experts.

As educators, we must give students a starting point. We must set them up for success by providing them with foundational knowledge. Knowledge, after all, provides the basis for evidence-based medicine and best practice.(10)

For any subject, educators must decide where to begin. In other words, which knowledge captures the essentials? Which knowledge is most critical to have at our fingertips in the consultation room? Which knowledge is necessary and why? Which knowledge is enough?

The reality is that knowledge evolves over time.(2) Knowledge is transformative. It reshapes what was once unimaginable into something attainable. It makes the impossible possible. New medical products and services are developed and marketed each day, every day. How does one make sense of this ever-changing face of medicine? How does one even attempt to stay current?

The successful student – and, ultimately, the successful practitioner – breaks away from the temptations of rote memorization because, simply put, you can never know it all.

To be successful in the practice of medicine is to learn how to sift through, compare, contrast, analyze, and interpret data.

Practicing medicine is not about accumulating knowledge just for the sake of it. It is about putting knowledge into context to give it meaning.(5, 12–14)

Context provides structure. Structure provides the framework for students to link facts to cases in a way that helps them to conceptualize the bigger picture.(5, 12–14) Learning that is conceptualized is meaningful because it helps students to see scientific disciplines as interrelated units rather than separate entities.

The successful practice of medicine requires deliberate integration of content areas. For instance, anatomy and physiology must be considered together when planning patient care and health outcomes because structure without function or function without structure gets us nowhere.

Note that clinical reasoning is both a process and a skill:

> Learning this skill is more akin to learning how to play the piano or training for an athletic event than preparing for prerequisite courses. None of us has ever observed a concert pianist or an Olympic athlete cramming for a competition.(5)

Clinical reasoning takes time to develop and refine. For this reason, we must introduce this skill to students during the pre-clinical years. Ideally, this would involve exposure to real patients and real clients in an authentic teaching hospital.

This is not always possible or pragmatic. There are time and spatial constraints as well as concerns for patient/client/student safety and wellbeing. Students and doctors alike will make mistakes. That is a given. However, mistakes have the potential to become the best learning opportunities when they are made in a safe, supportive learning environment, one in which neither patient nor client are harmed.

Simulated cases provide the next most authentic opportunity for learning. Simulated cases offer a built-in safety factor while still providing rich, effective context in the form of a patient/client narrative.(5) Consider, for instance, the clinical condition of hypertrophic cardiomyopathy (HCM). When presented in the format of a lecture, HCM may seem like a distant concept to students who lack any real connection to it. This disease may seem like just another one in a long list of conditions to commit to memory. In other words, the condition lacks context.

But what if HCM were instead crafted into a case vignette, with a named client and named patient that presented with clinical signs "X," "Y," and "Z"?

Better yet, what if students were presented with audiovisual material that depicted the case as it unfolded?

Maybe students were shown a video recording that demonstrated the patient's posterior paralysis on initial presentation, following presumptive aortic thromboembolism as a known sequela of HCM. Maybe students were shown a photograph that demonstrated paw pad and nailbed cyanosis of both distal pelvic limbs.

Maybe students had to take it to the next level and formulate a treatment plan for the patient in question. Maybe they had to engage in a discussion about the patient's prognosis with a simulated client.

Any of the aforementioned scenarios managed to effectively transform HCM from a generic disease that, out-of-context, held very little meaning, to a "real life" case that impacts a patient that students now feel somewhat tied to.

Furthermore, the case vignette about HCM requires students to actively engage – to interpret case history or physical exam findings; to design a treatment plan; to consider prognosis; and to role-play clinical conversations. Active learning crystallizes key concepts for students and in this way makes learning most effective.(5, 12, 15, 16)

Active learning also creates connections in a way that lectures do not. By actively involving themselves in the learning process, students learn to connect the dots for themselves. In the process, students recognize that scientific knowledge is not linear, but web-like.(17) Disciplines are bridged together by interwoven threads of silk that sprawl out only to twist and turn and double back on themselves.

As educators, it is not our responsibility to provide students with all the answers. It is not our responsibility to spoon feed students.

Our role is less to be the "sage on the stage" as it is to be the "guide on the side".

We are tasked with providing students with the tools they need to identify, define, make sense of, untangle, unravel, and refine connections so that they can see the forest for the trees.

Recognizing this, we need to change our approach to the delivery of medical content. We need to halt the delivery of mountains of facts that are too tall to scale.

We need to replace meaningless mountains with meaningful molehills that are not insurmountable, that are within students' grasp, yet require students to work at them to discover their own solutions, and that are strategically placed in the curriculum to inspire discussion and debate.

After all, students need to be able to observe, touch, handle, manipulate, and transform knowledge into learning that can be applied to procedural tasks and casework. This learning is essential to their success in clinical practice because it is retained and can be refined as needed, not memorized and purged the day after a final examination.

This text represents an effort to create opportunities for students to discover linkages between course content. There is no reason that a pre-clinical student cannot practice thinking like a clinician well before his/her clinical year. Let this text offer a new mindset, in which the student leads the charge, discovers a world of clinical applications in these pages, and learns how to translate concepts into real-world every day clinical practice.

Students, as the journey unfolds, enjoy the ride. Explore. Dive in. Skip around. Free yourself from the belief that you will ever know it all. The truth is that none of us do.

Accept where you are at right here and now as your starting point. Where you are at and who you are today will be uniquely different from where you will be and who you will be tomorrow. And the next day. And the day after that. Isn't that remarkably true for all of us as people, first, and as clinicians, second?

Just like knowledge, our professional journey is not static. As you evolve as a clinician, so, too, will your way of thinking. The novice of today becomes tomorrow's leader. Tomorrow's leader becomes the future's expert.

References

1. Lane EA. Problem-based learning in veterinary education. J Vet Med Educ 2008;35(4):631–6.
2. Fletcher OJ, Hooper BE, Schoenfeld-Tacher R. Instruction and curriculum in veterinary medical education: A 50-year perspective. J Vet Med Educ 2015;42(5):489–500.
3. Malher X, Bareille N, Noordhuizen JP, Seegers H. A case-based learning approach for teaching undergraduate veterinary students about dairy herd health consultancy issues. J Vet Med Educ 2009;36(1):22–9.
4. Nandi PL, Chan JN, Chan CP, Chan P, Chan LP. Undergraduate medical education: comparison of problem-based learning and conventional teaching. HK Med J 2000;6(3):301–6.
5. Bender HS, Lockee BB, Danielson JA, Mills EM, Boon GD, Burton JK, et al. Mechanism-based diagnostic reasoning: thoughts on teaching introductory clinical pathology. Vet Clin Pathol 2000;29(3):77–83.
6. Olser W. Chapter 3: Teacher and student. Aequanimitas, with other addresses to medical students, nurses and practitioners of medicine. Philadelphia, PA: P. Blakiston; 1910. p. 40.
7. Bean WB. Sir William Osler: Aphorisms from his bedside teachings and writings. 3rd ed. Springfield, IL: Charles C. Thomas; 1968.
8. Spencer J. Learning and teaching in the clinical environment. BMJ 2003;326(7389):591–4.
9. Tomlin JL, Pead MJ, May SA. Veterinary students' attitudes toward the assessment of clinical reasoning using extended matching questions. J Vet Med Educ 2008;35(4):612–21.
10. May SA. Clinical reasoning and case-based decision making: the fundamental challenge to veterinary educators. J Vet Med Educ 2013;40(3):200–9.
11. Norman DA. Learning and memory. San Francisco: WH Freeman; 1982.
12. Collins A, Brown JS, Newman SE. Cognitive apprenticeship: teaching the crafts of reading, writing, and mathematics. In: Resnick LB, editor. Knowing, learning, and instruction: essays in honor of Robert Glaser. Hillsdale, NJ: Lawrence Erlbaum Associates; 1989. p. 453–94.
13. Vanderbilt CaTGa. Anchored instruction and situated cognition revisited. Educ Technol 1993;33:52–70.
14. Vanderbilt CaTGa. Anchored instruction and its relationship to situated cognition. Educ Res. 1990;19:2–10.
15. Brown JS, Collins A, Duguid P. Situated cognition and the culture of learning. Educ Res 1989;18(1):32–42.
16. Burton JK, Moore DM, Magliaro SG. Behaviorism and instructional technology. In: Jonassen DH, editor. Handbook of research for educational communications and technology. New York: Simon and Schuster; 1996. p. 46–73.
17. Khosa DK, Volet SE, Bolton JR. Making clinical case-based learning in veterinary medicine visible: analysis of collaborative concept-mapping processes and reflections. J Vet Med Educ 2014;41(4):406–17.

Chapter 2

Building a Relationship

The Veterinary Client's Role in Healthcare

In most healthcare professions, the patient is the client. Although healthcare decisions may impact the patient's support system, it is ultimately a team of two that determines how best to proceed with the delivery of care. Patient education and informed consent are driving forces that contribute to decision making. At the end of the day, the patient is the one who is planted firmly in the driver's seat, not the doctor. The physician makes recommendations. It is up to the patient to decide whether to act upon them.

The veterinary profession represents a unique segment of the healthcare industry because its patients are furred and inarticulate. Although our patients do speak to us, it is not always in a way that we can understand, and while a dog or cat cannot consent to treatment, its owner can.

Our patients are therefore wholly dependent upon their owners to make healthcare decisions on their behalf. A pet's lifestyle "choices" are determined for them. Consider the breadth and depth of decision making that rests upon the shoulders of each companion animal-owning veterinary client.

Should the pet:

- be purchased or adopted?
- undergo serological or genetic testing?
- receive core and elective vaccinations?
- be fed meals or ad libitum?
- consume kibble or canned food, commercial or homemade diets, branded food or generic?
- live with other pets of the same or different species?
- socialize outside of the home with conspecifics, either informally, at dog parks, or in structured gatherings such as doggie day care?
- frequent grooming salons?
- board at kennels or veterinary clinics?
- travel out of state or out of the country?
- be bred or not, and if not, whether the pet should undergo elective sterilization surgery?
- maintain an indoor-only versus indoor–outdoor versus outdoor-only lifestyle?
- receive monthly, year-round prophylaxis against ecto- and endoparasites?
- be enrolled in preventative health care plans and pet insurance?

Appreciate that these decisions about wellness only begin to scrape the surface of what we ask owners to decide for pets that dabble in the murky waters between health and disease. Consider the weight of being tasked with decisions surrounding illness.

Should the pet:

- be taken to an emergency clinic overnight or be seen by its primary care clinician first thing in the morning?

- undergo baseline diagnostic testing (i.e. complete blood count, biochemistry profile, and urinalysis)?
- undergo diagnostic imaging (i.e. thoracic or abdominal radiography versus ultrasound)?
- undergo exploratory surgery (i.e. laparotomy to rule out a foreign body obstruction)?
- undergo incisional or excisional biopsies?
- be hospitalized or receive outpatient care?
- receive a prescription diet?
- wear an Elizabethan collar?
- be prescribed topical therapies?
- be given injectable medication(s) or oral treatment(s)?
- receive follow-up care and, if so, what does that imply in terms of timeline (when is the next visit?) and affordability of care (how much will the next visit cost?)?
- be referred to a specialty practice for advanced care?
- receive lifelong treatment for a condition that can be medically managed?
- receive palliative treatment for an incurable condition?
- be euthanized?

In weighing these decisions, clients must also consider the following factors:

- the patient's tractability.
- their ability to provide at-home care.
- their ability to administer medications the correct way.
- their schedule and whether it can be flexible in providing care around the clock as needed.
- the bond between the individual patient and client.
- the availability of care (i.e. is there an emergency practice nearby? Is specialty care within reach?).
- the cost of care (i.e. if care is available, is it affordable?).

As veterinarians, we have dual responsibilities. Our primary oath is to our patient, but in order to manage our patient's healthcare effectively and efficiently, we need buy-in from the client.(1) Buy-in requires us to connect with clients on a deeper level, through effective, transparent communication. (1–4) Clients need to see that we are providing healthcare recommendations that are truly in the best interest of their pet. Clients need to see that we are customizing care.

How do we as professionals outline best practices without defaulting to a 'one-size-fits-all' approach?

How do we as professionals take what we know and tailor it to promote the wellbeing of the individual patient?

Our past experiences as practitioners, both in the classroom and on the clinic floor, shape our understanding of what is best for the patient. We may also approach cases, for right or wrong, with the one question that clients never fail to ask of us, front and center, on our minds: what would we do if the patient were ours, in terms of choices that we would make?

2.1 The Client Determines If and How Healthcare Delivery Proceeds

Despite our best intentions to provide for the patient, at the end of the day it is the veterinary client, rather than the patient, that drives care forward, if at all.

The veterinary client is the ultimate caregiver, much like a parent to a child.(5, 6) Both client and parent are patient advocates.(5, 6) Both are responsible for relaying patient history, initiating dialogue about patient health concerns, and making informed decisions about the patient's wellness.(5–9)

Informed decision making requires an active exchange of ideas between veterinarians and clients in the examination room. Clients seek us out, as veterinary professionals, for advice and answers.

As veterinarians, we are assets to healthcare because we come into the consultation armed with knowledge. We have both advice and answers. But we are not omniscient. We can never possibly know it all.

There are gaps in our understanding of the individual patient, missing details that only our clients can provide.

The client is, in fact, an expert when it comes to what is normal for his or her pet versus that which is clearly abnormal. We don't know, for example, what a typical day in the life of Bailey Englar looks like, but Bailey's "mom" does.

As veterinarians, we must come to see the client as a wealth of patient-specific data. The client is a resource in the consultation room, not a hindrance. The client is our partner in healthcare, not our adversary.

We may have advice and answers to share with the client who has sought our wisdom. Yet our advice and answers are only useful when placed in the immediate context of the case.

As veterinarians, we need to open our ears before our mouths, so that we can invite and ultimately hear the client's perspective. We need to know the backstory if we are ever to gain a complete picture of the patient in sickness and in health.

To obtain the backstory, we must be willing to gather information from the client with an open mind. Gathering information is often referred to as establishing the database. Consider the database as a collection of details specific to the patient that will help to guide decision making.

2.2 The Comprehensive Patient History

As the technology in healthcare has evolved to support new methods of testing for disease, it may be tempting to forego data mining through history-taking. However, the history remains one of the most important diagnostic tools in clinical medicine.(10) In fact, it has been suggested that approximately two-thirds of diagnoses in human healthcare can be made based upon the patient's history alone.(11)

History-taking is likely to play an even greater role in veterinary medicine because our patients cannot communicate with us through their own language. Their health must be relayed to us through observant clients who may get it wrong, but also oftentimes get it right.

Taking a comprehensive health history is an extensive task in clinical practice. It requires patience and persistence to learn how to gather large amounts of patient data efficiently. Whole references have been prepared to guide you through this process. For more information, consult *A Guide to Oral Communication in Veterinary Medicine* and *Writing Skills for Veterinarians*. These partnered reference texts walk readers through these so-called soft skills in veterinary practice.

How to take a history is beyond the scope of this text; however, for the purpose of getting readers on the same page, let us review briefly those features that a comprehensive health history should include:(12–16)

- demographic data or signalment

  - patient's age
  - patient's sex
  - patient's sexual status
  - patient's breed
  - patient's species

- presenting complaint or chief complaint (cc)

  - a concise summary statement that identifies the reason for the consultation

- client expectations for the patient

  - the patient is expected to be a companion
  - the patient is expected to be a therapy dog
  - the patient is expected to be a service dog
  - the patient is expected to be a working dog

- lifestyle
  - indoor-only
  - indoor–outdoor
  - outdoor-only
- activity level
- travel history
  - in state
  - out of state
  - out of country
- serological status
  - feline leukemia virus (FeLV)/feline immunodeficiency virus (FIV) status [cats]
  - heartworm (HW), lyme (L), ehrlichia (E), and anaplasma (A) status [dogs]
- diet history
  - meals
    - contents
    - frequency
    - volume
  - treats and table scraps
- current medications
  - over-the-counter products
  - prescriptions
  - vitamins
  - supplements
- history of preventative care, including vaccinations
- past familial, medical, surgical, and reproductive history
- past pertinent diagnostic tests and test results, including laboratory and imaging
- past pertinent therapeutic trials and outcomes.

2.3 How Consultation Questions are Phrased Influences History-taking

History-taking is like a treasure hunt. Your job as the clinician is to find buried treasure. This requires you to dig deep. You must probe the client's memory for details that you require to formulate a diagnosis.

Clients do not always know what to share. They are often in the dark concerning what is and is not significant. Unless we guide them in our quest for answers, they may choose to hold back key content that we need access to if we are going to be successful.

Successful clinicians understand how to solicit information, the right information, from their clients. They recognize that sometimes the same question will elicit different answers, depending upon the way in which the question is phrased. Moreover, they understand how to strategically place questions in the line-up so as to yield productive answers, with efficiency.

2.3.1 Open-Ended Inquiries

Successful consultations often begin with an open-ended question or statement. This line of questioning opens the door to dialogue by asking the client to share more than a yes/no, numerical, or one-word response. Open-ended questions and statements invite the client to verbalize thoughts, ideas, concerns, and emotions using their own words, shared in the context of their own unique perspective.(1) This is the client's first opportunity in the consultation to share freely, and they must be allowed to speak without interruption, to complete their thought.

Open-ended statements often begin with the following.(17–20)

- Tell me . . .
- Help me . . .
- Show me . . .
- Give me . . .
- Share with me . . .
- Describe . . .
- List . . .
- Demonstrate for me . . .
- Take me through . . .
- Walk me through . . .

For example:

- Walk me through a day in the life of your cat.
- Take me through your thought process: what's it like for you to have to be his sole caregiver?
- Demonstrate what his posture looks like just before you say that he is having trouble breathing.
- List the concerns that you would like to discuss at today's visit.
- Describe how he was acting before this episode.
- Share with me what was going through your head when you witnessed his seizure.
- Give me an example of what he does at home that makes you think he is disoriented.
- Show me how Benny postured when he threw up.
- Help me to understand which aspect of his care is most stressful for you.
- Tell me what you saw your dog do that frightened you.

Some students have expressed their concern that open-ended statements as written above may sound forced or stilted. To improve upon their usability, these statements may be rephrased by inserting "can you," "please," or "it would help" if in front of the verb to soften the request and make it seem more inviting.

- Please walk me through a day in the life of your cat.
- Can you take me through your thought process: what is it like for you to have to be his sole caregiver?
- Can you demonstrate what his posture looks like just before you say that he is having trouble breathing?
- Please list the concerns that you would like to discuss at today's visit.
- It would help if you could describe how he was acting before this episode.
- Please share with me what was going through your head when you witnessed his seizure.
- Can you give me an example of what he does at home that makes you think he is disoriented?
- Please show me how Benny postured when he threw up.
- Can you help me to understand which aspect of his care is most stressful for you?
- It would help if you could tell me what you saw your dog do that frightened you.

Open-ended inquiries may also take the form of questions. Open-ended questions often lead with "How." Consider the following examples of what this might look like in clinical conversations.

- How do you feel about putting Tilly under anesthesia to clean her teeth?
- How would you feel if I asked you to switch out some of Marlow's high-calorie treats for healthier alternatives?
- How would it be if you tried to trim Pickles' nails at home?
- How concerned are you about having London spayed?

Open-ended questions may also lead with "What."

- What are your thoughts about having Tilly's teeth cleaned professionally under general anesthesia?
- What would you say if I asked you to switch out some of Marlow's high-calorie treats for healthier alternatives?
- What would you say if I asked you to work on trimming Pickles' nails at home?
- What concerns you most about having London spayed?

Open-ended questions may also lead with the interogative, "Why."

- Why do you think that housetraining is so difficult for Beta?
- Why are you so concerned about anesthetizing Florence today?
- Why are you hesitant to neuter Earl Grey?
- Why don't you want to schedule Milton's dental cleaning?
- Why do you want to hold off on vaccinating Roo?

This last set of questions invites the client to share. However, be aware that the use of "why" as well as the tone in which it is voiced may trigger defensiveness from the client.(20) Tread lightly when leading with "why," so as not to come across as being judgmental or condescending. Open-ended questions promote dialogue, but only when clients feel safe and supported.

2.3.2 Closed-Ended Questions

Open-ended questions provide a valuable starting point when taking a patient history. Clients will often provide the bulk of the information that you need to know about the patient and its presenting complaint up front if offered this initial opportunity to speak. However, there are times when you need to clarify what has been shared or fill in the gaps with missing information. This is made possible through the use of closed-ended questions.(21)

Closed-ended questions are intended for use in history-taking as follow-up. They collect data that is easy to capture in few words. For example, closed-ended questions are asked when you need a client to commit to a definitive yes/no answer.

- Has Pepper had diarrhea?
- Has Cinnamon been sneezing?
- Has Paprika vomited?
- Is Cilantro peeing outside of his pan?
- Is Spice defecating in the house?
- Did Herb's stool look bloody?
- Was his stool black and tarry?

Closed-ended questions may also ask the client to respond with a number.

- How many times did Thyme vomit?
- How many piles of diarrhea did you see?
- How many times a day do you clean the litter box?
- How many times has Ginger wet the bed?

In addition, closed-ended questions may yield answers that come in the form of short phrases.

- Question: What does Pumpkin eat?
- Answer: Dry food.
- Question: Which kind of dry food?
- Answer: Science Diet.
- Question: Which formulation of Science Diet?
- Answer: Senior.

2.3.3 Determining Which Line of Questioning Is Most Appropriate

Both open- and closed-ended questions have their place in the consultation.(17, 19, 20) Successful clinicians decide which kind of information they need from the client, then phrase their questions accordingly.

For instance, in an emergency, closed-ended questions are likely to predominate to speed patient stabilization and expedite care.

- Can we initiate CPR?
- Did he eat rat poison?
- How long has he been seizing?
- When was he hit by a car?
- How long has he been unresponsive?
- After you administered peroxide at home at the recommendation of the Pet Poison Control Helpline, did he throw up?

By contrast, first impressions are essential during a wellness visit, when meeting a new client and new patient for the first time. Consider, for example, the following lead-in statements to a wellness consultation.

- Tell me how Finnick came to be a part of your life.
- Share with me what sparked your interest in this particular breed of cat.
- Describe what it was that made you decide to take Connor home with you.
- What was it about Connie that made you decide to foster her?
- What made you decide to purchase a Ragdoll cat?
- What is the meaning behind her name?

These lead-ins offer opportunities for sharing. They set the foundation for a professional working relationship that is mutually beneficial and is built on mutual understanding. It is not just small talk. It is essential. These sharing moments in the consultation room provide us with insight that helps to facilitate the delivery of healthcare. We are better able to make recommendations when we understand the relationships that are involved, as well as their intricacies.

Open-ended questions build trust and partnership. This questioning style also allows the veterinarian to elicit the client's perspective. Because the client has been asked to share insight with the veterinary team, s/he feels heard. In this respect, open-ended questions act as relationship-builders. When genuinely delivered, they set the stage for a lifelong relationship of longitudinal care.

2.4   How This Text Incorporates Clinical Communication

Case-based decision making is a challenging skill to master. It is difficult for novices to engage in pattern recognition and to be tasked with clinical decisions that they have never thought about, let alone encountered in the real world.

Students' foundational knowledge is still likely to be in the early stages, so asking them to apply that knowledge to a clinical case may be quite a stretch. Students may stress that they don't "know it all" or that they don't "know enough" to work their way through the material. Yet educators need to reinforce that clinical cases are a necessary part of learning.

> To study the phenomenon of disease without books is to sail an uncharted sea, while to study books without patients is not to go to sea at all. (22)

It is important that educators reference patients, even if students do not fully understand every aspect of the medicine that underlies each case. Patients are a vehicle for the study of medicine because they motivate learning. They are what make medicine come alive.

Because casework is essential, it may be tempting to focus solely on the patient and abandon thought of how to incorporate the client into the clinical picture. However, it is important to remind students that the practice of veterinary medicine does not involve patients in isolation. Veterinary healthcare requires a unique tripartite relationship that connects the veterinarian to the client as much as the patient, if not more so.(5, 6, 9) Case decisions cannot be made without consideration for and conversations with the client.

The practice of clinical medicine is largely interpersonal. Whether a case proceeds, how, when, and why all hinge upon clinical conversations. Successful clinicians know what they need to convey and how they need to convey that information to pave the way for mutual understanding. Successful clinicians know that to move forward, they must gain the trust and the perspective of the client.

Because client communication is critical to the practice of medicine, it cannot be overlooked. Although this text cannot replicate the experience of simulated client encounters, this guide will reinforce the principles of client interactions throughout cases, when and where applicable.

Students are also encouraged to reflect upon all cases as opportunities to consider the following.

- How might you introduce yourself to your client?
- How might you engage in relationship-building?
- How might you build trust with your client (and patient)?
- How would you initiate history-taking?
- Which details of the case history will you prioritize?
- Which clarifying questions are most important for you to ask and why?
- How might the case history details change if you phrased history-taking questions in a different manner?
- How would you explain physical exam findings to your client?
- How might you explain your list of differentials?
- How would you develop and communicate your diagnostic plan?
- How might you explain diagnostic test results?
- How would you explain the patient's diagnosis?
- How might you explain the patient's prognosis?
- How would you develop and communicate your treatment plan?
- How might you engage in follow-up to determine the patient's response to treatment?

References

1. Englar RE, Williams M, Weingand K. Applicability of the Calgary-Cambridge guide to dog and cat owners for teaching veterinary clinical communications. J Vet Med Educ. 2016;43(2):143–69.
2. Case DB. Survey of expectations among clients of three small animal clinics. J Am Vet Med Assoc. 1988;192(4):498–502.
3. Antelyes J. Client hopes, client expectations. J Am Vet Med Assoc. 1990;197(12):1596–7.
4. Antelyes J. Difficult clients in the next decade. J Am Vet Med Assoc. 1991;198(4):550–2.
5. Englar RE. Common clinical presentations in dogs and cats. Hoboken, NJ: Wiley/Blackwell; 2019.
6. Shaw JR, Adams CL, Bonnett BN, Larson S, Roter DL. Use of the Roter interaction analysis system to analyse veterinarian–client–patient communication in companion animal practice. J Am Vet Med Assoc. 2004;225(2):222–9.
7. Gillis J. The history of the patient history since 1850. Bull Hist Med. 2006;80(3):490–512.
8. Gillis J. Taking a medical history in childhood illness: representations of parents in pediatric texts since 1850. Bull Hist Med. 2005;79(3):393–429.
9. Murphy SA. Consumer health information for pet owners. J Med Libr Assoc. 2006;94(2):151–8.
10. Rich EC, Crowson TW, Harris IB. The diagnostic value of the medical history. Perceptions of internal medicine physicians. Arch Intern Med. 1987;147(11):1957–60.

11. Lichstein PR. The Medical Interview. In: Walker HK, Hall WD, Hurst JW, editors. Clinical Methods: The History, Physical, and Laboratory Examinations. Boston: Butterworths; 1990.

12. Cameron S, Turtle-song I. Learning to write case notes using the SOAP format. J Couns Dev. 2002;80(3):286–92.

13. Rockett J, Lattanzio C, Christensen C. The Veterinary Technician's Guide to Writing SOAPS: A Workbook for Critical Thinking. Heyburn, ID: Rockett House Publishing LLC; 2013.

14. Borcherding S. Documentation manual for writing SOAP notes in occupational therapy. 2nd ed. Thorofare, NJ: SLACK Incorporated; 2005.

15. Kettenbach G, Kettenbach G. Writing patient/client notes: ensuring accuracy in documentation. 4th ed. Philadelphia, PA: F.A. Davis; 2004. 248 p. p.

16. Kettenbach G. Writing SOAP notes: With patient/client management formats. 3rd ed. Philadelphia, PA: F.A. Davis Company; 2004.

17. Kurtz SM, Silverman JD, Draper J. Teaching and learning communication skills in medicine. Grand Rapids, MI: Radcliffe; 2004.

18. Adams CL, Kurtz SM. Skills for communicating in veterinary medicine. Oxford: Otmoor Publishing and Dewpoint Publishing; 2017.

19. Silverman J, Kurtz S, Draper J. Skills for communicating with patients. Oxford: Radcliffe; 2008.

20. Shaw JR. Four core communication skills of highly effective practitioners. Vet Clin North Am Small Anim Pract 2006;36(2):385–96.

21. Hunter L, Shaw JR. What's in Your communication toolbox? Exceptional Veterinary Team 2012(November/December):12–17. Available from: http://csu-cvmbs.colostate.edu/Documents/vcpe-whats-in-your-communication-toolbox.pdf.

22. Olser W. Chapter 12: Books and men. Aequanimitas, with other addresses to medical students, nurses and practitioners or medicine. Philadelphia, PA: P. Blakiston; 1910.

Chapter 3

Approaching the Clinical Cases That Appear in Parts II and III

Reading through cases is different than reading through most medical textbooks. The latter are most often outlined by clinical presentation, as is true of the author's *Common Clinical Presentations in Dogs and Cats*, or by clinical disease, as is true of Ettinger's *Textbook of Veterinary Internal Medicine*.

In either case, readers know with certainty which symptom or diagnosis they are researching. There is no mystery in terms of what they expect to find in the pages assigned to each chapter.

Consider, for example, Chapter 16 – Hyphema – in the author's *Common Clinical Presentations in Dogs and Cats*. The chapter begins with a description of the clinical sign as it is likely to present in general practice. This written description is matched with photographic displays of hyphema as a quick and easy guide to clinical presentation. Photographs are followed by a list of the primary causes of hyphema: trauma, bleeding disorders, systemic hypertension, anterior uveitis, and neoplasia. The reader is then led to consider potential sequelae to hyphema as well as important considerations for history-taking.

Common Clinical Presentations in Dogs and Cats is composed of 78 chapters. Although the specific content of each chapter varies, the formatting is similar across the board. Each chapter begins with an overview of the clinical problem, followed by a tidy approach to the diagnostic work-up, which includes everything from gross description of the lesion to differentials that might have caused the lesion, followed by how to make the diagnosis. The text is, in a sense, the Cliff Notes version of clinical medicine, with each chapter serving as a summary of the most important take-aways of a symptom.

This is precisely the kind of reading that most of us are familiar with when it comes to our quest to study. For many learners, studying has become synonymous with passively reviewing one or more sets of notes that must be committed to memory and recalled for assessment purposes.

Yet recall is, at best, a low-order cognitive skill.[1, 2] The ability to recite facts does not demonstrate that one truly understands them.[3]

Academic success that is based solely on what learners remember does not in fact reflect the outcome that interests educators.[1] Educators wish to measure what learners can do with knowledge rather than what facts they can regurgitate on final exams.[1]

It is essential that postgraduate professional studies learners learn how to apply content. Successful doctors are competent not because they know a lot, but because they can do a lot with what they know.

Application and critical thinking are higher order cognitive skills.[1, 2] It does not come as a surprise that learners often struggle to master this skillset. Despite our best efforts as educators, we infrequently ask learners to act on knowledge that they have received.

Reading textbooks to memorize content does not motivate learners to make use of the material. Reading textbooks to study for tests does not build bridges between theory and practice. Reading through cases does.[4, 5]

Case-based learning requires learners to start with what they know, then proceed up the ladder through a hierarchy of cognitive skills that increase in difficulty. In the process, learners make a giant leap away from a state of declarative knowledge, that is, descriptions of information stored in memory.(5, 6) Learners move towards procedural knowledge, descriptions of how to perform, how to reason, how to make decisions, and how to problem-solve.(5, 6)

Case-based learning improves student engagement with course content and performance outcomes.(5, 7, 8) Learners are motivated to learn if the content is delivered in a way that makes it meaningful. Content is meaningful when it is both applicable and relevant to their professional journey.

Learners need to experience cases as they present in real life, if they are to be successful at managing real patients on the clinic floor.

- Most veterinary patients do not present the way that many textbook chapters unfold.
- Most veterinary patients do present with ambiguous symptoms that could mean one of many ailments. This explains the nebulous patient descriptor that appears, for better or worse, throughout so many of our patient files – "ADR" – ain't doing right.
- Most veterinary patients do not present with a clear diagnosis.
- Most veterinary patients do present with a presumptive diagnosis (by their owners) that is often incorrect.

We often do not know the diagnosis before we enter the consultation room. If we did, imagine what our appointment roster might look like for the morning:

8:00AM	Bailey Englar	Chronic kidney disease
8:30AM	Bliss Englar	Colitis
9:00AM	Mr. Tuffy Symonds	Diabetes mellitus
9:30AM	Wicket Gregory	Hemorrhagic gastroenteritis
10:00AM	Zoolander Gregory	Flea allergy dermatitis
10:30AM	Buddy Pearsall	Leptospirosis
11:00AM	Honey Murphy	Phenol Toxicosis

It would be nice if patients arrived at our clinics pre-labeled. It would certainly make decision making about diagnostic and treatment plans that much easier.

Unfortunately, patients do not read the textbook and they rarely present to us with diagnosis in hand. Instead, most of our patients arrive as medical mysteries. Most of our patients find their way to us as problems for us to solve.

Case-based learning mimics real life veterinary practice because the patients in the pages also present as unknowns. It is up to the student to investigate and deliberate as to the underlying disease process and its related pathophysiology. The student must make decisions about diagnostic and therapeutic plans, and then consider patient outcome.

In order to be successful with case management, in real life or on paper, learners must be able to:

- recall knowledge
- demonstrate an understanding of that knowledge
- be able to apply that knowledge to the case at hand
- analyze key findings that are pertinent to the case
- synthesize new material (e.g. treatment plan) from old data (e.g. patient history)
- evaluate the plan.

This taxonomy of learning objectives was first proposed in 1956 as a classification scheme for cognitive skills.(9) This collection, referred to as Bloom's taxonomy, ranges from low to high-order cognitive processing and reflects the transformation of the student from novice, through the advanced beginner stage, towards competent and proficient practitioner. In effect, these steps walk the learners toward completing milestones in their professional journey.

Each step in the hierarchy is associated with multiple tasks that are required for effective and efficient case management.

- Recall knowledge:

  - Review the clinical vignette.
  - Identify the patient's signalment.
  - Define the problem as the patient's chief (presenting) complaint.
  - Review the patient-specific data that has been gathered through history-taking.
  - Classify historical data into groups based upon similar themes.
  - Paraphrase physical examination findings.
  - Describe what is being asked of you.

- Demonstrate an understanding of that knowledge:

  - Discuss physical examination findings with the client.
  - Summarize the facts that are known.
  - Recognize which facts remain to be determined.
  - Tell the client what you still need to know.
  - Suggest next steps.

- Be able to apply that knowledge to the case at hand:

  - Interpret history and physical exam findings.
  - Organize a plan for how to proceed with case management.

- Analyze key findings that are pertinent to the case:

  - Perform diagnostic tests to gain answers to patient-specific ailments.
  - Analyze diagnostic test results.
  - Categorize diagnostic data.
  - Determine which diagnoses are more likely based upon diagnostic test results.
  - Determine which diagnoses are less likely based upon diagnostic test results.
  - Differentiate primary from secondary disease processes.
  - Debate any lingering uncertainties regarding the case, for instance, ambiguous diagnostic test results.

- Synthesize new material (e.g. treatment plan) from old data (e.g. patient history):

  - Formulate a plan for additional diagnostic testing.
  - Collect additional data.
  - Propose a working diagnosis.
  - Design a treatment plan.
  - Prepare for hospitalization or transfer to at-home care.

- Evaluate the plan:

  - Decide if treatment plan is effective.
  - If treatment plan is deemed ineffective, then revise the treatment plan.

These tasks are a daily part of clinical practice. Successful veterinarians perform these tasks with competence and proficiency in order to expedite diagnosis and delivery of healthcare.

For learners who are just beginning the process, it is often a steep upward climb. Even tasks that are considered low-order skills, meaning that they require less cognition, may present quite a challenge to the novice.

Each learner is also unique in his/her journey. Each may experience different stumbling blocks along the way.

3.1 Where to Begin?

To facilitate case-based learning, my recommendation is to read the clinical vignette twice.

Consider the first read to be an overview. Absorb generalities. Think big picture. Ask yourself what kind of pet is presenting in the context of what kind of problem.

Next, read through the Guiding Questions. These are intended to provide a clear sense of direction.

Reading with a purpose should facilitate retention of case details during the next read. As you read through the clinical vignette for the second time, keep the end goals of case management in mind.

- What is your target?
- What is being asked of you?
- How will you go about finding a solution?

Questions are likely to recur throughout Part II (Case Studies) and may assist you in reaching your end goals of case management.

- What information about the patient/case do you know?
- What information about the patient/case do you still lack?
- How will you obtain the missing information about the patient/case?
- What questions do you still need to ask the client about the patient?
- What is your next step in case management?
- What is Plan B in terms of next steps if you cannot move forward with Gold Standard care?
- What is the most likely diagnosis?
- How will you confirm this diagnosis?
- How will you rule out other diagnoses?
- What is likely to have caused this condition?
- What are potential complications of this condition?
- What is the best treatment for this condition?
- How do you evaluate the success of treating for this condition?
- What are potential complications of treatment for this condition?
- What is the patient's prognosis with treatment?
- What is the patient's prognosis without treatment?
- Is this condition curable? If not, what can you do to palliate?
- Is this condition transient or is it lifelong?
- Is this condition painful?
- Is this condition debilitating?
- How does this condition impact the patient's lifestyle?
- How does this condition impact the client?
- How does this condition impact the human–animal bond?
- What can you and your team do to support the client and patient during this time?

3.2 Clinical Pearls

Every case that is presented here has relevance to the learner who wishes to graduate into companion animal practice. Each case and the comprehension questions that have been paired with it open the door to a vast world of knowledge that provides the framework for evidence-based medicine.

Learners are encouraged to stretch themselves in their approach to clinical cases and reach for content that may seem beyond the initial scope of the case presentation. However, the sheer breadth and depth of knowledge that is out there may be, at times, overwhelming.

Sometimes it is helpful for key take-aways to be shared with learners so that they focus their energy on the most important concepts rather than losing the forest for the trees. When these free-standing pieces of clinically relevant material are deemed necessary, they will be provided in the form of a clinical pearl.

3.3 Variability in Answers

Comprehension questions for each clinical case will be paired with answer sets whenever possible as a way for learners to assess their performance. Answer sets provide a means of self-check, so that learners can be sure that they are on course and meeting expectations.

When learners find themselves way off course, answer sets provide a way to rein them in by gently tugging in the right direction. Answer sets may jog learners' memories so that they recall why the solution is correct. Answer sets may also facilitate self-reflection by prompting learners to consider where they went astray.

Keep in mind, however, that very little in the practice of veterinary medicine is black and white. Most decisions, procedures, and best practices involve shades of grey. Therefore, learners' answers may not in some cases match the author's, yet they may still be correct. It may be that the learner is looking at things from a different perspective in a way that is commendable.

Just because the learners' answers are not identical does not by default make them wrong.

In cases where the validity of answers is questionable, please seek counsel from your faculty and support staff. They are your best resource to guide you through your professional journey because they know precisely where you are at in your studies and how best to measure your progress against yourself and your peers.

3.4 Opportunities for Growth

At times, learners will answer questions incorrectly. You may think that you have a solid grasp of the material only to find that there are holes, conceptually, with your thought process, either in terms of basic understanding or your ability to apply what you thought you understood from theory into practice.

Recall that the practice of veterinary medicine is just that, practice. You will answer questions and you will misdiagnose patients throughout life.

The difference between an average clinician and an extraordinary one is the way in which s/he comes to view his/her mistakes. The average clinician accepts mistakes but takes no measures to investigate them. The extraordinary clinician sees mistakes as opportunities for growth.

When you make a mistake, own it.

Use mistakes to your benefit. Listen to them. Learn from them. Understand why you made them so that you do not replicate them in subsequent cases on subsequent patients.

None of us will ever know it all.

We all have strengths and weaknesses. We all have content area that we excel in and content area that we abhor.

We all rely upon a network of experts to strengthen our reserve on cases where a second opinion is handy. We are each other's colleagues. We all have had to, at some point, lean on someone when times got tough.

So, don't be reluctant to reach out to a classmate or colleague, or open a reference guide.

Investigate all areas of uncertainty, as often as is needed. I still find myself having to look up acid-base principles and practical applications after all this time.

Each case has its own reference list. This list is not intended to be all-inclusive. It is simply a starting point.

If you work through and successfully understand the case, then the references are not essential. Consider them, in this instance, to be supplementary, and refer to them only as time or interest permits.

If, on the other hand, a case asks you to reach beyond your comfort zone, to a disease, process, prognosis, or plan that you feel ill-equipped to handle, then, dive into the references. Consider the case to be opportunity for growth and self-discovery. Frequent the reference list as much as you need, gain insight, and then return to the case to try again.

Not knowing something should never be shameful.
It is only a shame when we fail to learn from it.

CLINICAL PEARLS

- Clinical pearls will be separated from the text in a box format, like so, to highlight that they are stand-alone bits of information that will hopefully help the learner to stay on track.

References

1. Crowe A, Dirks C, Wenderoth MP. Biology in bloom: implementing Bloom's Taxonomy to enhance student learning in biology. CBE Life Sci Educ 2008;7(4):368–81.
2. Zoller U. Are lecture and learning compatible? Maybe for LOCS: unlikely for HOCS. J Chem Educ 1993;70(3):195–7.
3. Adams NE. Bloom's taxonomy of cognitive learning objectives. J Med Libr Assoc 2015;103(3):152–3.
4. Thistlethwaite JE, Davies D, Ekeocha S, Kidd JM, MacDougall C, Matthews P, et al. The effectiveness of case-based learning in health professional education. A BEME systematic review: BEME Guide No. 23. Med Teach 2012;34(6):e421–44.
5. Turk B, Ertl S, Wong G, Wadowski PP, Löffler-Stastka H. Does case-based blended-learning expedite the transfer of declarative knowledge to procedural knowledge in practice? BMC Med Educ 2019;19(1):447.
6. Frenk J, Chen L, Bhutta ZA, Cohen J, Crisp N, Evans T, et al. Health professionals for a new century: transforming education to strengthen health systems in an interdependent world. Lancet 2010;376(9756):1923–58.
7. Mohyuddin GR, Isom N, Thomas L. Applying the principles of bloom's taxonomy to managing tachyarrhythmia: results of a tachyarrhythmia workshop. Cureus 2019;11(2):e4037.
8. Rodriguez Muñoz D, Alonso Salinas G, Franco Diez E, Moreno J, Matía Francés R, Hernández-Madrid A, Zamorano J. Training in management of arrhythmias for medical residents: a case-based learning strategy. Int J Med Educ 2016;7:322–3.
9. Bloom BS, ed. Taxonomy of educational objectives: the classification of educational goals. New York: Longmans, Green; 1956.

Part 2

Common Cases in Pediatric Canine/Feline Medicine

Case 1

The Unexpected Litter of Pups

A Good Samaritan presents an intact female mongrel of unknown age and background for postnatal examination of an unexpected litter of puppies that was delivered overnight. The bitch was found approximately a week ago wandering the streets without identification.

The client, Miss Albright, took the bitch into her home reluctantly. She describes herself as more of a "cat person" but could not bear to see an animal go hungry. Miss Albright lives alone, with no other pets in the household. She reports that the bitch settled in quite well and appears to be well-socialized to the home environment. The bitch eats well, and her appetite has been ravenous. Miss Albright had planned on getting the bitch evaluated next week because she had a surprisingly round belly for being so skeletal. Waking up this morning to a litter of four pups certainly explains a lot!

The bitch has accepted the pups and is allowing them to nurse. She also tolerates handling of the pups by Miss Albright without complaint. The client is confident that the bitch can rear the pups successfully, but Miss Albright has no experience owning dogs, let alone newborns, and has concerns about what to expect. She brings a list to today's visit that outlines the following questions about the pups.

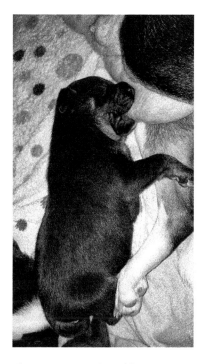

Figure 1.1 One-day-old puppies. Courtesy of Tara Beugel.

1. The puppies seem to sleep a lot. Is that normal?
2. Are the puppies warm enough? They don't seem to be shivering.
3. I haven't seen the puppies eliminate. Is that expected?
4. What are critical indicators of neonatal health? What should I be measuring at home?
5. What are signs of illness in newborn pups?
6. When will the pups' eyes and ears open?
7. I read somewhere that handling puppies helps with their development. Is this true?
8. How long should the pups stay with each other and their mom?
9. I've heard that pups need to be exposed to lots of new things early in life. Is that correct?

Answers to Case 1: The Unexpected Litter of Pups

1. A healthy newborn is usually either nursing or asleep. In fact, 80 to 90% of the day in the life of a newborn is spent sleeping.(1–4) Well-fed pups tend to rest often and quietly, vocalizing only when hunger strikes or if their sleep has been disturbed.(4, 5) It is not unusual to see pups falling asleep while nursing.(2)

2. Newborn puppies tend to huddle together for warmth. They are not very good at maintaining their core body temperature, which is already quite a bit lower than their mother's. A normal rectal temperature of a 1-week-old or less pup is 95–99°F (35–37.2°C).(2, 3, 6) **QUESTION FOR YOU:** *Do you recall what the normal body temperature is for an adult dog?*

    When pups get chilled, they aren't as easily able to raise their core body temperature through shivering, as we do.(6) In response to cold climates, our blood vessels also vasoconstrict – that is, the diameter of blood vessels that supply our skin shrinks down to reduce blood flow to the surface, to retain heat. Newborn puppies are limited in their ability to thermoregulate in this manner.(6) This means that neonates are extraordinarily susceptible to hypothermia.(6) To protect against hypothermia, the client can maintain a clean, dry nesting area or whelping box.(7) Soiled blankets or towels should be removed and washed; soiled newspaper should be tossed out and replaced with new.

    Ambient temperatures of the nest should be maintained to reduce morbidity.(7) Reports vary somewhat as to the ideal thermal conditions of the whelping box for the first 24 hours after birth, but ambient temperature should typically range between 86–91.4°F(30–33°C).(4) Be cautious about using electric heating pads to warm the nest because puppies are susceptible to scalding. (4) They will not relocate themselves to prevent being burned until neuromuscular reflexes have been established at or about 7 days of age.(3, 7) If a heat source for the nest is indicated, then warm-water heating blankets or infrared lamps are preferred.(3, 4) Ambient temperature may be adjusted to 75–80°F as pups make the transition to 1-week old (24–26.7°C).(7)

3. When puppies nurse for the first time, they are stimulated to expel meconium from their bowels. (6) Meconium is a thick brown material that has been accumulating in the digestive tract during fetal life. It is essentially the first fecal matter that is passed, provided that the pups have a present and patent anus.(6) The client probably did not witness the passage of meconium because the pups were born overnight, and mothering behavior is such that the bitch would have ingested it during routine cleaning of the nest.

    After meconium has been passed, defecation is stimulated by the bitch, as is micturition.(4) Pups less than 3 weeks of age cannot exert voluntary control over either the urinary bladder or the bowels.(4) Therefore, newborns are entirely dependent upon the bitch to stimulate elimination by licking at the perineum.(4)

    If the bitch is a fastidious cleaner and ingests the waste products, the client may not actually see urine or fecal matter produced by the pups and may question whether or not they are eliminating. If there is any concern, the client can imitate the actions of the bitch by applying a moist, warm towel to the perineal region and rubbing gently. This should stimulate elimination. The urine of newborns is typically very pale to clear.(2) Any sign of hematuria should trigger concern. **QUESTION FOR YOU:** *What is hematuria?*

4. Body weight is a critical measurement of neonatal health that is easy to keep track of at home. Simply put, a healthy puppy should feel hefty or solid in your hands.

    Low birthweight pups are at greater risk of succumbing to hypothermia and infection.(4) Pups that are significantly underweight at birth are also less likely to survive.(4, 6) Because weight gain shortly after birth is linked to survival, it is important to assess how much each pup weighs daily to track trends in gains and losses.(8)

    Measurement of weight at birth provides a baseline.(6) Thereafter, pups should be weighed twice daily using an appropriate scale.(6) Digital and gram scales provide greater accuracy.(6) Body weight at birth depends largely upon breed. Toy breeds tend to weigh, on average, between 100–200 grams. Small to medium breeds typically weigh between 200–400 grams as compared to 400–500 grams for large breeds and 700 grams or more for giant breeds.(2)

    Within the first 24 hours of life, it is not unusual for pups to lose less than 10% of their birthweight.(2) This is primarily due to water loss.(6) Any pup that loses more than 10% of its birthweight during the first 24 hours of life should be watched closely as this could indicate failure to thrive.(2, 6)

Beyond day one, weight should only climb, not decline.(6) It is expected that each pup should increase in body weight by 5 to 10% of birthweight each day.(6) This means that pups should gain anywhere from one to three grams per day per pound of anticipated adult weight.(6) **QUESTION FOR YOU: *What is the conversion factor for pounds to kilograms? If an adult dog's anticipated body weight was 25 pounds, how many kilograms would that be?***

By 7 to 10 days old, each pup is expected to have doubled its birthweight.(6) If weight trends are not as anticipated, then the affected pup(s) may benefit from supplemental feeding.

Rectal temperature is a second valuable indicator of neonatal health.(4)

Respiratory rate is less easily detected at home by the novice but can provide insight concerning the neonate's wellbeing. At birth, breaths are irregular.(4) Respiratory rate is typically slow, ranging from 10 to 20 breaths per minutes.(4) This rate rises by 1 week of age to 15 to 40 breaths per minute.(4) Small and toy breeds are more likely to have a respiratory rate at the higher end of the normal range.(4) Respiratory rates that are significantly higher than what has been reported here are likely indicative of neonatal distress. Breathing should not appear labored.(3)

5. Sick newborns are often exceptionally vocal.(2) Other signs suggestive of illness in neonates include:(2, 9, 10)

- failure to suckle after latching onto the teat
- failure to latch onto the teat
- disinterest in nursing altogether
- separating from littermates, rather than huddling
- no longer twitching while asleep
- becoming increasingly bony in feel or appearance
- feeling limp to the touch
- developing an unthrifty coat
- developing a slack, rather than rounded, abdomen
- feeling cold to the touch – and confirmed by a rectal temperature that is below 94°F (34.4°C)
- feeling warm to the touch – and confirmed by a rectal temperature that exceeds 98°F (36.7°C)
- developing nasal discharge or audible airway congestion
- developing respiratory distress (e.g. gasping, panting)
- developing diarrhea
- developing omphalitis **QUESTION FOR YOU: *What does this mean, in layman's terms?***
- sloughing toes or tail tips.

Any of these clinical signs should prompt veterinary investigation urgently.

Neonatal loss, sometimes referred to as fading puppy syndrome, is not uncommon in veterinary practice.(2) Neonatal mortality is typically greatest during the first week of life.(10) Mortality rates ranging from 5 to 40% have been reported in the veterinary literature as being considered "normal."(2)

Reasons for neonatal loss are numerous and include, but are not limited to, the following factors:(6, 10)

- poor condition of the bitch
- fetal distress secondary to dystocia
- low birthweight
- poor weight gain
- insufficient colostrum or another nutritional deficit
- hypothermia
- hypoglycemia
- hypoxemia

- dehydration
- aspiration pneumonia:
    - secondary to meconium
    - potential complication of assisted (tube) feeding
- endoparasitism
- ectoparasitism
- bacterial and/or viral infection.

Subtle signs may be missed. Familiarizing yourself with what is normal is of significant aid when trying to determine if something is not quite right with a puppy or a litter. Trends are also helpful. For instance, a puppy that is historically very active, yet now is limp, with decreased muscle tone, is ill until proven otherwise.

6. At birth, puppies cannot see because their upper and lower eyelids have yet to separate.(4) This separation typically occurs in pups between 5 to 14 days after birth and gives way to blue-grey irises that change in color over the next few weeks of life.(3) Pups develop pupillary light reflexes (PLRs) within 24 hours of eyelid separation; however, vision is relatively poor until three to four weeks of age.(3)

    At birth, puppies' sense of hearing is muffled, at best, because their external ear canals are closed.(2, 4) These structures open, on average, between 14 and 16 days after birth.(4) A waxy discharge may be appreciated from both ear canals for up to 1 week after they open.(2) This is due to the sloughing of cells that were obstructing the canals.(4)

7. It is true that early handling from birth to 5 weeks of age makes pups more confident and more likely to explore their surroundings.(11, 12) Early handling also speeds maturation of both motor and nervous system development.(12) Eyes open sooner in pups that have been handled.(12) Handled pups are also more likely to gain weight.(12) Handling pups is thought to improve their sociability. It may encourage and expedite learning as well as help pups to develop emotional stability.(12) Well-handled pups are thought to develop more effective coping strategies so that they can more readily adapt to stress in adulthood.(13)

8. It is important for pups to remain with their mom and littermates until 6–8 weeks of age.(12) This is critical so that puppies can develop appropriate species-specific behavior and learn how to have healthy interactions with other dogs.(12)

9. Socialization is an important developmental phase for all species because it the process by which an individual connects to other animals, including conspecifics.(12) Each species has a unique timeframe for socialization. For dogs, the primary period falls between 3 and 13 weeks of age.(14) What this means is that new objects, environments, conspecifics, and other species, including humans, should be encountered by pups before 13 weeks of age.(12) This provides pups with the opportunity to explore new items and surroundings, and to engage with other animals to develop comfort and confidence.(12) Positive reinforcement can promote healthy interactions with novel objects, animals, and people.(12) Exposure is not a one-time experience, but should be reinforced through six to eight months of age so that pups continue to build healthy relationships.(12) Lack of socialization can lead to undesirable fears and phobias that will perpetuate into adulthood if they are not addressed.(12)

Approaching the Neonatal Exam

Now that you have answered Miss Albright's questions, you are ready to examine the litter.

> **Q:** *What key structures do you observe and/or palpate when you perform a physical examination of each neonate?*

> **A:** *When you examine puppies as soon after birth as possible, you should evaluate each individual patient for the following:(3, 6, 7, 15)*

- body weight
- rectal temperature
- posture
- muscle tone
- activity level
- reflexes:
    - righting **QUESTION FOR YOU:** *Which action does this reflex describe?*
    - rooting **QUESTION FOR YOU:** *Which action does this reflex describe?*
    - suckling
- presence of a large, domed skull
- evidence of open fontanelle **QUESTION FOR YOU:** *Define this condition and consider potential risks to the patient if this structure remains open.*
- presence of fluid at one or both nostrils
- presence of discharge seeping from beneath the eyelids of one or both eyes
- coat coverage and quality
- hydration status **QUESTION FOR YOU:** *How do you assess this in a neonate?*
- check for any wounds
- check for congenital defects:
    - cleft lip
    - cleft palate
    - assess patency of anus **QUESTION FOR YOU:** *What is the appropriate medical terminology that refers to the condition by which the anal opening is not patent?*
    - sternal or spinal abnormalities
- assess mucous membrane color associated with the oral cavity:
    - mucous membranes should not be cyanotic
- evidence of ectoparasitism
- thorax:
    - symmetry of right and left halves
    - rib fractures
    - heart rate (requires auscultation)
    - check for murmurs
    - breathing quality
    - respiratory rate
    - auscultation of lungs:
        - should be clear
        - should be free of fluid

- abdomen:
  - shape should be rounded with a supple feel
  - abdominal palpation should be non-painful
  - umbilicus should be dry and not inflamed
  - check for umbilical hernia

- perineum:
  - determine sex
  - check for anal or genital redness and/or swelling
  - stimulate urination using a warm, moist towel and use urine color as an indicator of hydration status.

The Neonatal Exam

Now that you know what you are looking at and/or feeling for, you proceed with your exam of the litter. The following items crop up along the way:

1. You notice how Pup #1 is laying. This shape or posture is characteristic of the rest of the litter. Is this positioning age-appropriate? Explain your answer.

2. You examine the muzzle of Pup #2. What is this pup's condition called?

3. You examine the oral cavity of Pup #3. What is this pup's condition called? What are the consequences of having this condition?

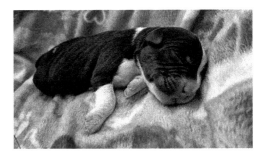

Figure 1.2 One-day-old puppy. Courtesy of Tara Beugel.

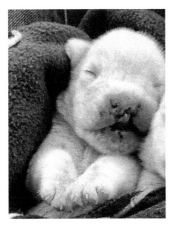

Figure 1.3 One-day-old puppy. Courtesy of Rachel Luhan, Fuzzy Texan Animal Rescue.

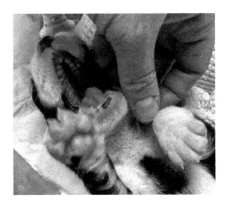

Figure 1.4 One-day-old puppy. Courtesy of Rachel Luhan, Fuzzy Texan Animal Rescue.

4.   Pup #4 weighs 180 grams, the least among his littermates, who average 250 grams apiece.

   a.   How many kilograms does Pup #4 weigh?
   b.   How many pounds does Pup #4 weigh?

Answers to the Neonatal Exam

1.   Yes, this pup's classic comma shape is characteristic of newborns. It is attributed to flexor tone, which predominates for the first few days of life.(15) By the time the pup reaches four or five days old, extensor dominance will take over and last for a little under a month.(15) By one month old, the pup's posture will mirror an adult's in that trunk, neck, and head are held upright, with right and left-sided symmetry, and no evidence of any unilateral tilt.(15)

2.   This pup has a cleft of the primary palate, which is the first stage of developmental separation between the nasal and oral cavities. It involves migration of maxillary and nasal processes towards midline, to form the nose and upper lip.(16) This pup's cleft of the primary palate involves only the lip, so it is primarily cosmetic. However, clefts of the primary palate may also affect nostril formation and air passage through the nose.(16)

3.   This pup has a cleft of the secondary palate. This condition refers to an abnormal opening along the roof of the mouth, causing abnormal communication between the oral and nasal cavities. This is a congenital malformation that occurs, on average, once out of every thousand canine births.(16) This defect is diagnosed when you assess the oral cavity of newborns. However, it may be suspected when the affected pup develops unusual nasal discharge. Inexperienced breeders who have not examined the neonate's mouth may report that milk drips out of the nose during nursing.(16) Cleft palates can be surgically repaired.(17)

4.   Pup #4 weighs 0.18 kg because 1 kg equals 1000 g.
   Pup #4 weighs 0.40 lb because 1 kg equals 2.2 lb.

Approach to the Bitch

Miss Albright thanks you for being so informative and she feels much more settled about what to watch for in the coming days and weeks. Although she plans on rehoming the pups, she has decided to keep the bitch, which she has named "Olivia."

   Miss Albright does not want Olivia to experience any subsequent litters and would like to spay her straight away. She asks you if spaying Olivia now will dry up her milk production? She does not wish to do anything that will adversely impact the health or wellbeing of the pups.

   Q: *What do you tell her?*

   A: *Even bitches that are spayed during C-sections will still lactate, so there is no reason to believe that elective ovariectomy or ovariohysterectomy at any time will dry up Olivia's milk production.*

Some bitches will dry up after being spayed; however, that is the exception to the general rule. As long as the pups continue to nurse, Olivia should be capable of producing milk. However, her current state of mammary engorgement may give us pause. Her mammary glands are highly vascular during this physiologic stage. Waiting to spay Olivia until after her mammary glands have reduced in size at or around the time of weaning will make the procedure easier for surgeon and patient alike if the intended surgical approach is via a midline incision. If, on the other hand, the surgeon intended to perform a flank ovariectomy, then s/he would avoid incising the mammary chain altogether.(18) This alternate approach would also avoid having to surgically handle the extraordinarily friable postpartum uterus.

CLINICAL PEARLS

- Newborn pups are inefficient at thermoregulation: their core body temperature is lower than their mother's and they have difficulty maintaining homeostasis. Management of ambient temperature is an essential part of newborn care to reduce neonatal losses.

- Rectal temperature and body weight are vital measurements that allow you to track neonatal health and flag neonates that are at increased risk of morbidity and mortality.

- An important part of any neonatal exam is to evaluate the oral cavity to look for a cleft palate. A history of unusual nasal discharge should also prompt this investigation.

References

1. Casal ML. Management and critical care of the neonate. In: England GCW, von Heimendahl A, editors. BSAVA manual of canine and feline reproduction and neonatology. 2nd ed. Gloucester: British Small Animal Veterinary Association (BSAVA); 2010.
2. Greer ML. Neonatal and pediatric care. In: Greer ML, editor. Canine reproduction and neonatology. Jackson, WY: Teton New Media; 2015. p. 140–215.
3. Hoskins JD, Partington BP. Physical examination and diagnostic imaging procedures. In: Hoskins JD, editor. Veterinary pediatrics: dogs and cats from birth to six months. 3rd ed. Philadelphia, PA: Saunders; 2001. p. 1–21.
4. Moxon R, England G. Care of puppies during the neonatal period: Part 1 Care and artificial rearing. Veterinary Nursing Journal 2012;27(1):10–3.
5. Davidson AP. Approaches to reducing neonatal mortality in dogs. Recent Advances in Small Animal Reproduction. Ithaca, NY: International Veterinary Information Service; 2003.
6. Rickard V. Birth and the first 24 hours. In: Peterson ME, Kutzler MA, editors. Small animal pediatrics: The first 12 months of life. Philadelphia, PA: Saunders; 2011. p. 11–19.
7. Casal ML. Pediatric care during the postpartum period. In: Ettinger SJ, Feldman EC, Cote E, editors. Textbook of veterinary internal medicine. 8th ed. St. Louis, MO: Elsevier; 2017. p. 1901–3.
8. Wilsman NJ, Van Sickle DC. Weight change patterns as a basis for predicting survival of newborn Pointer pups. J Am Vet Med Assoc 1973;163(8):971–5.
9. Moxon R, England G. Care of puppies during the neonatal period: Part 2 Care of the sick neonate. Veterinary Nursing Journal 2012;27(2):57–61.
10. Rickard V. Neonatal losses. In: Kutzler MA, editor. Cote's clinical veterinary advisor: dogs and cats. 4th ed. St. Louis, MO: Elsevier; 2020. p. 687–9.
11. Fox MW. Socialization, environmental factors, and abnormal behavior development in animals. In: Fox MW, editor. Abnormal behavior in animals. Philadelphia, PA: W.B. Saunders; 1968. p. 332.
12. Landsberg G. Behavior development and preventive management. In: Hoskins JD, editor. Veterinary pediatrics: dogs and cats from birth to six months. 3rd ed. Philadelphia, PA: Saunders; 2001. p. 22–34.
13. Levine S. Maternal and environmental influences on the adrenocortical response to stress in weanling rats. Science 1967;156(3772):258–60.
14. Freedman DG, King JA, Elliot O. Critical period in the social development of dogs. Science 1961;133(3457):1016–17.
15. Englar RE. Performing the small animal physical examination. Hoboken, NJ: Wiley/Blackwell; 2017.
16. Englar RE. Common clinical presentations in dogs and cats. Hoboken, NJ: Wiley-Blackwell; 2019.
17. Fiani N, Verstraete FJ, Arzi B. Reconstruction of congenital nose, cleft primary palate, and lip disorders. Veterinary Clinics of North America. Small Animal Practice 2016;46(4):663–75.
18. Janssens LAA, Janssens GHRR. Bilateral flank ovariectomy in the dog – surgical technique and sequelae in 72 animals. Journal of Small Animal Practice 1991;32(5):249–52.

Case 2

The Orphan Kittens

A Good Samaritan presents four orphan kittens of unknown age and background for evaluation. The kittens were found underneath a shrub at the perimeter of the client's yard when she went outside to mow the lawn. They appear, to the client, to be very young. Based upon a cursory glance at the kittens, which are huddled at the bottom of a laundry tote, you agree. Their eyes and ears are still closed, and they are curled around one another in characteristic comma shapes that are suggestive of flexor tone. They are a few days old, at most. They appear to be of the domestic short-haired (DSH) variety; that is, moggies.

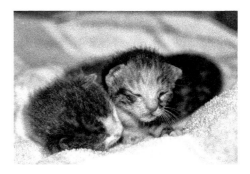

Figure 2.1 One-day-old kittens. Courtesy of Laura Polerecky.

The kittens are mewing loudly. You ask the client, Mrs. Whitney Carson, if the kittens have been fed. She answers in the negative. Never having cared for cats, let alone newborns, she drove to the clinic as soon as she found the litter. She is eager to try her hand at rearing the orphan litter but needs significant guidance. She has brought a list with her of the following questions.

1.   How much do newborn kittens typically weigh and how fast should they grow?
2.   What do I feed them? Do I have to purchase a commercial formula, or can I make my own?
3.   What are some challenges that are associated with homemade diets?
4.   Are there any ingredients that I should not include in homemade formulations?
5.   How often should the kittens nurse?
6.   How do I feed newborn kittens?
7.   I read online that many newborns die of some sort of blood cell incompatibility. Can you explain what that means? Is it a disease? Why does it happen?
8.   When are kittens old enough to wean?

Answers to Case 2: The Orphan Kittens

1.   Newborn kittens typically weigh, on average, 100 grams (3.5 ounces) apiece.(1, 2) Birthweight typically doubles by the time each kitten reaches 7 to 10 days of age.(1) After that point, weight gain tends to be linear in cats, with kittens weighing approximately 1 pound for every month old they are, up through 6 months.(1) So, for example, a 1-month-old kitten typically weighs 1 pound; a 2-month-old weighs 2 pounds; a 3-month-old weighs 3 pounds; and so forth, all the way up to 6 pounds at 6 months of age.(1)
     Like pups, it is not unusual for kittens to lose less than 10% of their birthweight in the first 24 hours of life.(1, 3) This is primarily due to water loss (dehydration) and elimination of fecal matter in the form of meconium.(1, 4) Any kitten that loses more than 10% of its birthweight during the first 24 hours of life should be watched closely as this could indicate failure to thrive.(1, 3, 4)

Because weight is linked to survival, it is important to weigh neonatal kittens twice daily to track trends in gains and losses.(1, 5) Use digital gram scales to improve accuracy.(4)

2.   Commercially prepared kitten formula is the preferred food of choice for feline neonates because it is nutritionally balanced for the species and lifestage.(5, 6) In the United States, kitten milk replacer is commercially available over-the-counter in most pet stores in the common formulations KMR®, PetLac, and Just Born. Most are available for purchase as either an already prepared liquid formulation or as a powder that can be reconstituted. In the United Kingdom, a popular kitten milk replacer is sold under the brand name Lactol, produced by the company Beaphar.

There are many other brand names as well as generic formulations that are available for purchase. Each contains its own guidelines in terms of how to constitute (when the formulation is in powder form) and how much to feed as a liquid. It is important that clients read the instruction label that matches their brand of formula so that caloric intake is appropriate. Powdered formulations that require reconstitution are not advised for the novice because of the potential for mixing errors.(5) When mixing errors lead to overly concentrated formula, neonates are likely to experience gastrointestinal distress, either in the form of emesis or diarrhea.(5) When mixing errors lead to overly dilute formula, then neonates are not actually taking in the caloric density that is required per feeding to sustain growth.(5)

It is possible to prepare homemade diets and several recipes have been proposed, both in print and online.(5, 7) Recipes for home-prepared kitten formula often include egg yolk, yogurt, water, and condensed milk.(5)

3.   It is challenging to ensure consistency and quality of home-prepared diets.(5) It is also difficult to replicate the nutritional composition of queen's milk.(5) Cow's milk, for instance, does not have an appropriate calcium–phosphorus ratio for kittens.(7) Cow's milk is also much too high in lactose and much too low in terms of energy content, protein, and fat.(7) Excess lactose in the diet risks the development of diarrhea.(5) Neonatal diarrhea is a significant concern because the renal immaturity of our patients at this age increases their susceptibility to dehydration.(4)

4.   It is not advised to incorporate cottage cheese or egg white into the neonate's diet.(5, 7) The former clots in the stomach and may obstruct the digestive tract.(5) The latter contains a protein that binds biotin, an essential vitamin that then becomes unavailable to the neonate.(7)

Human infant milk replacer is also not a valid substitute for queen's milk because it provides insufficient protein and fat.(8)

5.   During the first week of life, neonates require approximately 133 calories per kilogram of body weight per day.(4) This caloric requirement is usually divided between six and eight feedings per day.(2, 5) Kittens typically nurse once every 2–3 hours.(5) Protein is the primary energy source for neonatal kittens as compared to pups, which rely heavily on fat during the first week of life.(4)

6.   There are two approaches to feeding newborn kittens:(2, 5)

*   bottle feeding
*   tube feeding.

As long as the kittens in this litter have a strong suckle reflex, bottle feeding is the preferred method for providing nourishment because they will suckle until full.(2, 5) Bottle feeding also allows the feeder to monitor the kitten's suckle reflex and gauge its strength as an overall indicator of health.(2) A kitten that started out strong, but is now latching on with less vigor, will be identified more rapidly when it is bottle-fed. The change in suckle strength is quite apparent and should allow for medical intervention before the patient's heath becomes critical.(2)

Kittens are too small to suckle from human baby bottles.(5) There are, however, commercially available neonatal bottles with smaller nipples that are marketed for kittens.(2, 5) Most of these do not come with premade openings, so clients need to be instructed to pierce the tip of the bottle with a hot needle to melt through the plastic to create an opening.(5) Otherwise, kittens may attempt to nurse, but not actually receive any nourishment!

Avoid creating an opening in a commercial bottle that is over-sized. Large is not always better and will increase the risk of aspiration because the formula is flowing too rapidly.(5) By contrast, an opening that is too small makes the kitten work too hard to obtain nourishment.(5) An appropriate sized hole will allow milk to slowly drip from the bottle when the bottle is inverted.(5)

When bottle feeding neonates, you want to be sure that you are allowing them to suckle. You do not want to ever squeeze the bottle.(5) This increases the risk of aspiration.

Neonates that are nursing from a bottle should be placed in sternal recumbency with front legs outstretched as they would be positioned when nursing from the queen (see Figure 2.2).

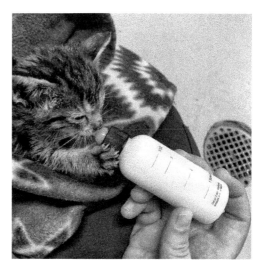

Figure 2.2 Appropriate positioning of the kitten in sternal recumbency during bottle feeding. Courtesy of Rachel Sahrbeck.

During bottle feeding, kittens should also be able to reach the nipple of the bottle without having to overextend their head and neck.(5) Doing so will increase the risk of aspiration.

The nipple should also be aligned such that it inserts straight into the mouth as opposed to at an angle.(5) If the nipple is angled relative to the mouth, then the kitten cannot create a seal around the nipple with its tongue.(5) This causes the neonate to take in an excess of air during its attempts to suckle.(5) This intake may precipitate colic.(5)

Tube feeding is an appropriate alternative to bottle feeding. It can be advantageous, particularly when there are many mouths to feed. Tube feeding, when done well, is much more efficient than bottle feeding.(5)

However, tube feeding can be challenging for the novice to perform. Tube size and length are important considerations. A tube that is too long may flex back on itself and kink.(5) To guard against this, tubes should be measured against the side of the patient. The tube is placed against the body wall, from the neonate's last rib to the end of the nose when the head is extended.(5) The tube should be marked at 75% of this distance.(4) This will ensure that the end of the tube lands in the stomach, assuming that the tube has been properly placed.

It takes time to learn the appropriate technique for tube placement so that the tube does not inadvertently insert into the lungs. An important checkmark for this is to listen for the neonate to vocalize after tube placement. If the neonate is able to vocalize clearly, then the tube is correctly seated in the stomach and not the lower respiratory tract. If the neonate coughs after tube placement, then the tube may have accidentally been inserted into the airway.(4)

Once tube placement has been confirmed, formula can be delivered. Formula should be pulled into a syringe so that the tube is kept full of milk rather than air.(5) Neonates should receive the formula in an upright position with head flexed.(5) Milk should be delivered to the stomach via tube slowly, over 1–2 minutes.(5) This lessens the likelihood that the neonate will vomit.

Prior to pulling the tube, the tube should be kinked.(4) This prevents milk from dripping into the patient as the tube is removed, thereby lessening the chance that fluid will be aspirated into the lungs.(4)

Tube feeding is not without risk. It is possible to rupture the esophagus or stomach when placing the tube.(2) Kittens are also much better at self-regulating intake than we are at "guestimating" how much volume to deliver to the stomach directly.(2)

Other concerns about tube feeding when it is not essential are that it denies the kitten of its innate behavior to suck.(2) It has been suggested that kittens that lack the opportunity to exhibit suckling are more likely to mutilate themselves or littermates through overgrooming.(2, 9)

Regardless of whether neonates are bottle-fed or tube fed, the formula should be warmed to maternal body temperature (101.5°F/38.6°C) prior to administration.(5) You can test that the milk is warmer than your skin by dripping formula onto the back of your hand.(5) This is a good test to ensure that the milk is in fact warm.

If formula is fed chilled or even at room temperature, then absorption of the nutrients may be impaired due to slowing of peristalsis.(5) Formula that has not been warmed also may contribute to neonatal hypothermia.(5)

At the same time, care should be taken that formula is not overheated. Oral, esophageal, and gastric ulceration is possible secondary to milk scald.(5)

Just as it is important to be sure that the formula has been warmed, kittens should also be warm at the time of feedings. If the rectal temperature of the neonate is below 96°F (35.5°C), then the patient is at risk of developing ileus.(4) When neonates experience ileus, ingested formula does not digest. Instead, it ferments.(4) This leads to bloat and gastrointestinal distress.(4)

After any meal, kittens will need to be coaxed to eliminate. Elimination is stimulated by rubbing the perineum and preputial areas with a warm wash cloth or cotton ball.(4) This simulates the queen's licking actions of the tongue that occur during grooming.

If patients do not urinate after stimulation or if their urine is darker than pale or clear, then they may be dehydrated. If patients do not have bowel movements, then they may be constipated.(4) In either situation, medical attention is indicated.

7. The condition that the client is referring to is neonatal isoerythrolysis (NI). NI is not unique to cats. It has also been observed in people as well as other domesticated animals such as horses. (10, 11) The primary difference between NI in people as compared to animals is the onset of disease. In humans, NI develops during embryogenesis, but NI develops postpartum in non-human animals.(10) NI is a disease state in which the immune system initiates widespread hemolysis. (12) The trigger for such hemolysis is the presence of naturally occurring alloantibodies against cells of a blood type that the patient lacks.(10)

Cats are characterized by blood type based upon the AB group system. There are two main blood types in cats, A and B. These are inherited as a simple autosomal Mendelian trait.(10) Type A is dominant over type B.(10)

Based upon this inheritance pattern, possible genotypes and phenotypes include:

- type A cats (AA or Ab)
- homozygous recessive Type B cats (bb).

There is a rarer blood type among cats, AB; however, this is beyond the scope of this discussion.

Type A cats may or may not have measurable anti-B alloantibodies – that is, naturally occurring antibodies against type B blood cells or products.(10) Of those cats that do, anti-B alloantibodies tend to be weak.(10)

However, type B cats have strong anti-A alloantibodies, meaning that when they encounter type A blood cells or products, they incite hemolysis.(10) In mild cases, hemolysis may precipitate anemia.(10, 13, 14) In severe cases, affected cats may succumb to disseminated intravascular coagulation and/or death.(10, 13, 14) Veterinarians experience this clinically as a certain type of transfusion reaction.

How does this relate to neonatal care and neonatal loss? When neonates first nurse from the queen, they ingest colostrum. Naturally occurring alloantibodies from the queen are passed onto progeny through this "first milk."(10) Once in circulation within the neonates, these maternal alloantibodies recognize surface proteins on neonatal erythrocytes.(10)

When type B queens mate with type A toms, their offspring may be of mixed blood types (Ab and bb). The erythrocytes of type A kittens will be targeted by the strong anti-A alloantibodies from the type B queen. (10, 12, 13, 15) These kittens will be healthy at birth, but will exhibit "fading kitten syndrome" after ingesting colostrum.(10) They develop signs of illness within hours or days. These include: (10, 11, 13)

- decreased, if any, interest in nursing
- decreased activity
- depressed mental state
- weakness
- pallor
- collapse
- tachypnea
- respiratory distress
- icterus
- dark red-brown urine
- sudden death.

Without treatment, affected kittens experience high mortality rates.(10) If kittens do survive, they often exhibit necrosis of the tail tip.(10, 16) This is because the IgM cold agglutinin binds to erythrocytes only in regions of the body where the temperature is low enough to be in the thermal range of the antibody. In the adult cat, affected sites would include the ears, paws, nose, and scrotum in addition to the tail tip.(10) However, these sites are more or less protected in kittens due to close contact with the queen and the fact that the ears, at this point in development, are folded against the head.(10)

In this clinical scenario, we do not know anything about the queen, but we suspect that the kittens are moggies, that is, unpedigreed. Based upon what we know about the prevalence of feline blood types in the UK, 87.1% of non-pedigree cats are type A.(17) By contrast, the majority of type B cats in the UK are pedigreed, with overrepresentation from the British shorthair breed.(17)

Within the US, there is also an abundance of type A cats, representing 97.2% of DSH and domestic long-haired cats (DLH) that were tested in a study by Giger et al.(18) Siamese cats as well as American Shorthair and Norwegian Forest cats exclusively tested as type A.(10, 18) Type B blood was overrepresented among purebred cats, particularly Abyssinians, Birmans, British Shorthair, Devon Rex, Himalayan, Persian, Scottish Fold, and Somali.(18)

To avoid NI, experienced breeders will blood type breeding pairs prior to mating so that B-type queens are only bred to B-type toms.(4) In the event that an accidental mating happens between a B-type queen and a type A tom, then the resultant newborns should be removed from the queen for the 24 hours that follow parturition to prevent ingestion of colostrum.(4) Thereafter, the kittens may be returned to the queen for rearing.(4)

This case represents a common scenario in clinical practice. Given that the kittens appear to be moggies, they are likely to be type A. If they were born to a type A mom, then there is no reason for concern. If they were born to a type B mom, then all type A kittens are at risk. It is too late to prevent NI from occurring because the kittens either ingested their mother's colostrum or didn't. If they ingested colostrum with anti-A alloantibodies, then the risk for NI is real. At this point, all the client can do is monitor for signs of NI. However, the likelihood is low given that most moggies are blood type A.

If queens are allowed to determine when to wean their litter, kittens often continue to nurse until at or around nine weeks of age.(2) In this case, the queen is not present so the client must make the determination. By week three of bottle feeding, the time in between feedings can increase to every eight hours.(2) As early as week five, the client may offer a slurry of solid food soaked in the formula that the kittens have been receiving.(2, 5) Some kittens may show immediate interest; others take time to warm up to its texture.(5) Kittens may be encouraged to sample the gruel-like consistency by offering a taste via syringe (see Figure 2.3).

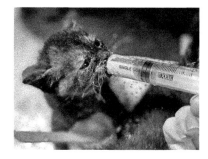

Figure 2.3 Offering a slurry of gruel to an orphan kitten. Courtesy of Kaitlyn Thomas Foster, Coordinator, Maryland SPCA.

Kittens should not be force-fed in this manner. It is meant to be a positive experience. Once kittens see other kittens eating, they are likely to latch on and follow suit. Kittens are rarely still on the bottle of their own accord by 9 weeks old.(2)

Some individuals advocate for forced early weaning between 3 and 5 weeks old. However, there is some concern that this may hinder normal behavioral development.(2, 19) Early weaned kittens are more likely to exhibit predatory behavior.(19) This behavior may be misdirected towards people.

Revisiting the Orphan Kittens

Mrs. Carson is appreciative of your guidance, particularly your team's willingness to walk her through bottle feeding for the very first time. She departs from the practice with the essential supplies that she needs to get started on this new adventure. You telephone her daily to check in and troubleshoot any concerns. All four kittens are reportedly "doing well" – nursing vigorously and gaining weight on schedule – until the bedtime feeding on the third day. Kitten #3 was less eager to latch onto the bottle and stopped drinking formula long before his littermates had finished. Mrs. Carson was concerned that he didn't get enough to eat, but was relieved when he fell into a sound sleep without a fuss.

On the morning of day five, Kitten #3 was less responsive than his siblings at his breakfast feeding. He felt limp when Mrs. Carson picked him up, and this time he refused the bottle altogether. When you pull into the clinic parking lot this morning, Mrs. Carson is already there, waiting for you.

Work through the following questions as you manage this case.

1. One of the first questions that you ask the client when she hands over Kitten #3 is whether she has witnessed any seizures. Why do you ask this?
2. You would like to draw some blood to run in-house diagnostic tests to get some answers for Mrs. Carson straight away. Your technician is concerned about exsanguinating the patient. What do you tell her is the estimated blood volume of kittens in terms of milliliter per pound of body weight? What is a safe volume to collect from Kitten #3 today?
3. What is considered to be a minimum database for ill neonates?
4. What is the site of choice for blood collection in a neonatal kitten?
5. When performing venipuncture on a neonatal kitten, what can you do to minimize heat loss?
6. How does a complete blood count (CBC) for a healthy neonate differ from that of a healthy adult?
7. How does a chemistry profile for a healthy neonate differ from that of a healthy adult?
8. Which parameter on a chemistry profile is considered a more accurate indicator of renal function (or dysfunction) in a neonate?
9. How does a urinalysis for a healthy neonate differ from that of a healthy adult?
10. Where do you expect this patient's blood glucose to fall relative to what is considered the norm for a neonate?
11. If the patient's blood glucose is as you suspect, how will you respond? Include drug name and route of administration. Drug dose is not required but will be provided in the answer.
12. What is the best way to assess hydration in a neonate?
13. What is the maintenance fluid rate in neonates?
14. How would you administer fluid therapy to the neonate if you are unable to place an IV catheter?
15. How do you assess for overhydration secondary to overzealous fluid therapy?

Answers to: Revisiting the Orphan Kittens

1. Kitten #3 has not consumed any nutrients since bedtime feeding last night – and by the client's own admission, he did not consume much. Hypoglycemia is a significant concern in neonates because they have limited glycogen reserves.(4) Gluconeogenesis cannot occur for very long without depleting hepatic stores.(4) If nursing does not occur at the frequency that it should,

neonates may develop clinical signs reflective of an underlying hypoglycemic state. These include abnormal mentation, apparent weakness, lethargy, inconsolable crying, tremors, and seizures.(4) If the client has witnessed a seizure since you last spoke with her, then hypoglycemia is even more likely. Therefore, it is important to ask the client to describe changes in the patient, if any.

2. Total blood volume approximates 5–10% of a patient's body weight. This means that a 100 gram kitten has an approximate blood volume of only 6 mL!

    Another way to estimate blood volume in kittens is to calculate 25.4 mL/lb of body weight. (1) When calculated this way, a 100 gram kitten is estimated to have a blood volume of only 5.5 mL!

    This means that your technician's concern is valid!

    As a rule, a maximum of one percent of an animal's body weight can be removed safely without fluid supplementation.(20) So, for instance, it is safe to remove 1.0 mL from a 100 gram kitten. This amount represents one-sixth of the kitten's total blood volume, so it is essential to keep track of blood collection so as not to inadvertently exsanguinate the patient.

3. Because the extent of diagnostic hematology is limited greatly by the volume that can be safely collected from your patient, you need to consider a minimum database for ill neonates. This database is compiled of the essential baseline tests that are indicated when a neonatal patient presents acutely sick. Essential blood tests for sick neonates include: (1)

    *   hematocrit
    *   total protein (TP)
    *   blood glucose (BG)
    *   blood urea nitrogen (BUN)

4. The site of choice for blood collection in a neonatal kitten is the external jugular vein.(1) This is because peripheral vasculature is too small to access at this life stage.(1)

5. When performing venipuncture on a neonatal kitten, you can minimize heat loss by moistening the area over the vein with water rather than alcohol.(1, 20) This lessens evaporative cooling.

6. As compared to a healthy adult cat, a healthy neonatal kitten's CBC is characterized by:(1, 21)

    *   a lower hematocrit**
    *   nucleated erythrocytes
    *   Heinz bodies **QUESTIONS FOR READER: *Can you identify these on a blood smear? What are these structures and what do they represent?***
    *   increased polychromasia **QUESTION FOR READER: *What does this term mean?***

    **Unless hematocrit is measured at time of birth. At time of birth, the hematocrit is quite high. (21) This value drops significantly through the first month of age as the patient accommodates to an oxygen-rich environment.(21) At 4–6 weeks of age, the hematocrit experiences its nadir of 27%.(21)*

7. As compared to a healthy adult cat, a healthy neonatal kitten's chemistry profile is characterized by:(1, 21)

    *   decreased alanine aminotransferase (ALT)
    *   decreased TP
    *   decreased albumin
    *   decreased creatinine
    *   decreased BUN
    *   decreased cholesterol
    *   elevated alkaline phosphatase (ALP)
    *   elevated phosphorus.

    Neonates have poor muscle mass, which explains why creatinine is lower than in adults.(21) Neonates also have immature hepatic function, which explains the depressed values for both BUN and cholesterol.(21)

8. BUN is considered to be a more accurate indicator of renal function (or dysfunction) than creatinine in a neonate.(1)

9. As compared to a healthy adult cat, a neonatal kitten's urinalysis may demonstrate:(1, 21)

   • proteinuria, secondary to excretion of colostral antibodies during the first few days of life
   • glucosuria, due to immature renal function
   • low urine specific gravity (USG): 1.006–1.017, due to age-related inability to concentrate urine.

   Proteinuria and glucosuria should resolve by 3 weeks of age. (1) Kittens should be able to concentrate their urine, thereby achieving a USG that is comparable to that in adults, by eight weeks of age.(1)

10. Because Kitten #3 exhibited reduced appetite last night and has refused to nurse this morning, I would expect that his BG is below the normal reference range for a neonatal kitten (76–129 mg/dL).(1) Clinical signs are likely to develop when BG drops below 40 mg/dL.(4)

11. If the patient's BG is registering low enough to warrant emergency intervention (i.e. below 40 mg/dL), particularly if the patient is exhibiting clinical signs of hypoglycemia, then I will need to administer dextrose via either the intravenous (IV) or intraosseous (IO) route.(4) If I have access to 10% dextrose solution, then I will administer 2–4 mL/kg.(4) It would be inappropriate to administer a solution of 50% dextrose IV because the concentration is such that it could cause phlebitis.(4) I would also avoid administering a solution of 50% dextrose subcutaneously (SQ) because it could result in sloughing of the skin.(4)

    In a non-emergent situation (i.e. the neonate is still trying to nurse and perhaps only exhibiting signs of weakness), then I might initially apply 50% dextrose solution to the gums.(4) It is questionable how much of this will truly be absorbed into circulation; however, it may be all that is needed to perk up the neonate.

12. It is not very effective to assess skin turgor in neonates because they have less subcutaneous fat. (1, 21) The preferred method of checking for hydration is to assess the neonate's mucous membranes for moisture.(1, 4) However, this is not foolproof: some neonates will still exhibit moist mucous membranes even in the face of severe dehydration.(21)

    Dehydration may also cause the skin at the neonate's muzzle and along the ventral abdomen to darken up so that it appears to be a shade of darker red.(4) However, this is a subjective measure and can be challenging for the novice to appreciate because in health, neonatal kittens and puppies of light pigmentation already have a striking pink muzzle.(1) (See **Plate 1**.)

    Another measure of hydration status in the neonate is to assess the color of urine. When a well-hydrated neonate is stimulated to urinate, its urine should be very pale to clear.(1) If the urine has any depth of yellow coloring to it, then the neonate is said to be dehydrated.(1)

    In an adult patient, packed cell volume (PCV) would be used as an indicator of hydration in combination with other details outlined here. However, PCV is challenging to interpret in neonates because it varies neonate-to-neonate how many erythrocytes passed through the placenta and umbilicus at birth.(1) PCV also decreases with age until about 16 weeks of age.

13. The maintenance fluid rate in neonates is 3–6 mL/kg/hour.(4) This does not account for fluid deficits, which should be corrected over 12–24 hours. Recall that hypothermia is a very real concern for neonates. Therefore, IV fluids should be warmed prior to delivery.(21)

14. If you are unable to place an IV catheter, then the next best plan is to pass a spinal needle through the trochanteric fossa of the femur or the greater tubercle of the humerus.(4) By inserting the needle into the intramedullary canal, you can administer sterile fluids through the intraosseous route.(4) The same rate of fluid administration applies as if the fluid were being given IV.(4)

15. It is easy to overhydrate neonates through overzealous efforts to administer IV fluid therapy because the kidneys are immature during this life stage and therefore they have difficulty ridding the body of excess water.(21) When neonates are receiving IV fluid therapy, they should be weighed three to four times a day on a gram scale to track trends in weight.(21) It is easier to determine volume overload through repeated measurements of weight than thoracic radiographs unless serial images are taken.(21) A single thoracic radiograph is of little assistance because neonatal lungs will appear to be more radiopaque due to increased interstitial fluid.(21)

CLINICAL PEARLS

- Orphaned kittens will require bottle feeding or tube feeding.

- Feed a species-specific commercial formulation when possible: cow's milk does not match the nutritional composition of a queen's milk, and homemade formulations, while possible, are more prone to error, especially if in the hands of a novice.

- Neonatal kittens are inefficient at thermoregulation and hypothermia is a significant concern. To reduce the risk of hypothermia, intravenous fluids should be warmed prior to administration.

- The intraosseous route is an acceptable alternative to the administration of fluid therapy if placement of an intravenous catheter is not possible.

- Fluid therapy must be monitored carefully: it is easy to volume overload a neonatal kitten!

- Neonatal kittens that exhibit reduced appetite or become anorexic are at risk of developing hypoglycemia. Clinical signs associated with hypoglycemia include weakness and lethargy. Neurologic signs (e.g. seizures, abnormal mentation) will develop if hypoglycemia is severe.

References

1. Root Kustritz MV. History and physical examination of the neonate. In: Peterson ME, Kutzler MA, editors. Small animal pediatrics: The first 12 months of life. St. Louis, MO: Saunders; 2011. p. 20–7.
2. Snook SS, Riedesel EA. Feline neonatal medicine. Iowa State Univ Vet 1987;49(2).
3. Greer ML. Neonatal and pediatric care. In: Greer ML, editor. Canine reproduction and neonatology. Jackson, WY: Teton New Media; 2015. p. 140–215.
4. Rickard V. Birth and the first 24 hours. In: Peterson ME, Kutzler MA, editors. Small animal pediatrics: The first 12 months of life. St. Louis, MO: Saunders; 2011. p. 11–9.
5. Peterson ME. Care of the orphaned puppy and kitten. In: Peterson ME, Kutzler MA, editors. Small animal pediatrics: The first 12 months of life. St. Louis, MO: Saunders; 2011. p. 67–72.
6. Casal ML. Pediatric care during the postpartum period. In: Ettinger SJ, Feldman EC, Cote E, editors. Textbook of veterinary internal medicine. 8th ed. St. Louis, MO: Elsevier; 2017. p. 1901–3.
7. Baines FM. Milk substitutes and the hand rearing of orphan puppies and kittens. J Small Anim Pract 1981;22(9):555–78.
8. Bush JE. Neonatal kitten care: Alley cat allies. Available from: https://www.animalsheltering.org/sites/default/files/documents/neonatal-kitten-care.pdf.
9. Hart BL. Maternal behavior II – The nursing sucking relationship and the effects of maternal deprivation. Feline Pract 1972;2:6–8.
10. Silvestre-Ferreira AC, Pastor J. Feline neonatal isoerythrolysis and the importance of feline blood types. Vet Med Int 2010;2010:753726.

11. Hubler M, Kaelin S, Hagen A, Fairburn A, Canfield P, Ruesch P. Feline neonatal isoerythrolysis in two litters. J Small Anim Pract 1987;28(9):833–8.
12. Cain GR, Suzuki Y. Presumptive neonatal isoerythrolysis in cats. J Am Vet Med Assoc 1985;187(1):46–8.
13. Bücheler J. Fading kitten syndrome and neonatal isoerythrolysis. Vet Clin North Am Small Anim Pract 1999;29(4):853–70.
14. Giger U, Casal ML. Feline colostrum – friend or foe: Maternal antibodies in queens and kittens. J Reprod Fertil Suppl 1997;51:313–6.
15. Casal ML, Jezyk PF, Giger U. Transfer of colostral antibodies from queens to their kittens. Am J Vet Res 1996;57(11):1653–8.
16. Bridle KH, Littlewood JD. Tail tip necrosis in two litters of Birman kittens. J Small Anim Pract 1998;39(2):88–9.
17. Knottenbelt CM, Addie DD, Day MJ, Mackin AJ. Determination of the prevalence of feline blood types in the UK. J Small Anim Pract 1999;40(3):115–8.
18. Giger U, Bucheler J, Patterson DF. Frequency and inheritance of A and B blood types in feline breeds of the United States. J Hered 1991;82(1):15–20.
19. Landsberg G. Behavior development and preventive management. In: Hoskins JD, editor. Veterinary pediatrics: Dogs and cats from birth to six months. 3rd ed. Philadelphia, PA: Saunders; 2001. p. 22–34.
20. Bassert JM, Thomas J. Workbook for McCurnin's clinical textbook for veterinary technicians. St. Louis, MO: Elsevier, Inc.; 2018.
21. McMichael MA. Emergency and critical care issues. In: Peterson ME, Kutzler MA, editors. Small animal pediatrics: The first 12 months of life. St. Louis, MO: Saunders; 2011. p. 73–81.

Case 3

The New Puppy Wellness Examination

A full consultation room greets you at your next appointment. The Everest family of four is excited to introduce you to their four-legged addition to the family, Brooklyn. Brooklyn is a 10-week-old intact female Corgi puppy that joined the family last night. She was purchased from a local breeder, who reported that she was the only female of six healthy pups. Her brothers had all been sold the previous week, so she was getting a bit antsy as the "only child" without any playmates. When she met the Everest family, it was love at first sight. Brooklyn was so enthusiastic with her rump wiggle that she nearly toppled over.

Brooklyn was purchased primarily as a companion for 5-year-old Jennifer and 10-year-old Aiden. Brooklyn's adult owners, Jason and Tiffany, have no other pets at home and no prior dog-owning experience to lean on, so everything about puppyhood is new to them. They are eager to do right by their new addition, but they feel overwhelmed by the amount of care that is needed, and it has not even been a full 24 hours since Brooklyn arrived! Help them to prioritize Brooklyn's care by answering the list of questions that they brought to today's visit.

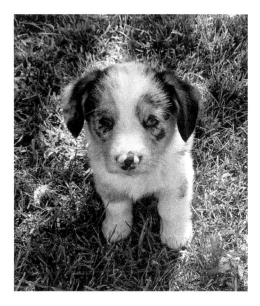

Figure 3.1 Your patient, 10-week-old Corgi puppy, Brooklyn. Courtesy of Jason Paine.

1. Brooklyn feels a bit bony to us. Is that normal? What should a healthy weight be?
2. Talk to me about feeding my puppy. What should I feed and how much?
3. Brooklyn really likes people food. Is it okay to feed her table scraps?
4. The breeder said that Brooklyn was already dewormed, so is a stool sample really necessary?
5. I read somewhere that kids can go blind if they handle dog poop. Is that true? We want Aiden and Jennifer to help with chores, including cleaning up after Brooklyn in the yard.
6. Are worms really an issue? Our yard is clean and we live in a good neighborhood.
7. We don't see ticks where we live. Do we still need to give Brooklyn monthly preventative? I really hate the idea of her taking medication that she doesn't need.
8. Is heartworm disease something to worry about? We don't have spare money to spend.
9. Does Brooklyn need any shots while she's here? The breeder says she's up to date, and it's not like she's going to be hanging out with other dogs. Where do we go from here?
10. What is typical puppy behavior? Is there anything that I need to watch out for?

Answers to Case 3: The New Puppy Wellness Examination

1. It is typical for pups to go through growth spurts. They often have rounded, doughy bellies, yet feel lean and lanky during this stage of life. Weighing Brooklyn is a good place to begin because it provides us with actual numbers that we can track as she grows. However, no two Corgis are identical, so there is no magic number that she ought to weigh today or tomorrow or the next day. Weight will continue to be a very individual measurement throughout her life, just as it is in people.

   A helpful at-home measurement tool to share with Brooklyn's owners is body condition score (BCS), using either a 5-point or 9-point scale (1–3). Visible and palpable landmarks are identified and assessed, taking into account both lateral and aerial views of the patient.(3)

   BCS approximates percentage of body fat in dogs using a sliding scale in which end-of-scale values denote extremes.(3) A score of 1/5 or 1/9 confers that a patient is emaciated, whereas a score of 5/5 or 9/9 confers that a patient is morbidly obese.(3)

   Our primary task when it comes to nutrition is to avoid the extremes. We want to work with Brooklyn's owners to help her attain and maintain an ideal BCS throughout her life. Ideal BCS is 3/5 or 4–5/9, depending upon which scale is used. My training in veterinary college referenced the Purina 9-point system of body condition scoring (see Figure 3.2)

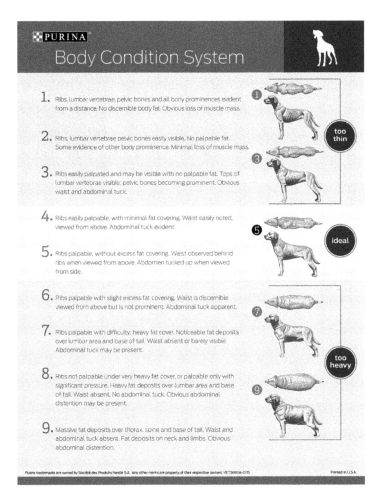

Figure 3.2 Assessing Canine BCS using the Purina 9-point system. Courtesy of Nestlé-Purina PetCare.

Brooklyn's owners can be taught how to use this scale appropriately to assess where she falls on the scale relative to what is considered "ideal." Keep in mind that there are breed-specific differences and individual variability when it comes to body composition.(4) Some dogs will score a BCS of 6/9 for their whole lives. They will always be, simply put, "big dogs." Other dogs will score a BCS of 3/9 and will always be "skinny."

Brooklyn's breed presents an additional challenge because of her plush, weather-proof, double coat. It is challenging to see through her fur to visually assess her ribs, lumbar vertebrae, and pelvic bones. Brooklyn's coat may make her seem stocky even if she is ideal in terms of BCS. It is therefore critical to show Brooklyn's parents where to feel on her body to assess palpable landmarks.

Let's now walk Brooklyn's owners through the Purina 9-point system of body condition scoring so that they understand what they are using to make their determination about BCS.

Dogs are considered underweight if they score a BCS of 1/9, 2/9, or 3/9 on the Purina 9-point system of body condition scoring.(3)

- A dog that has a BCS of 1/9 is emaciated. These dogs have prominent ribs, lumbar vertebrae, and pelvic bones that are visible without palpation. There is no palpable body fat and muscle mass is poor. The waist is exaggerated. The patient looks skeletal.
- A dog that has a BCS of 2/9 is moderately underweight. Ribs, lumbar vertebrae, and pelvic bones are easily visible. The abdominal tuck is pronounced, and there is no palpable fat. However, these dogs have adequate muscle mass.
- A dog that has a BCS of 3/9 is mildly underweight. The ribs may or may not be visible, but they are easy to feel, without overlying fat. The wings of the ilia are prominent, and the tips of the spinous processes of the lumbar vertebrae are visible. There is minimal body fat. The waistline is obvious.

Dogs with a BCS of 4/9 are considered "lean normal."(3) Some might say that these patients have "athletic build." Ribs are easily palpable, but not visible. There is a prominent abdominal tuck. These patients are ideal, as are dogs that are scored as having a BCS of 5/9. These patients are also well-proportioned, with a visible waist and palpable ribs.

For every BCS value that is above a 5/9, the patient is considered to be an additional 10% overweight. A dog that has a BCS of 6/9 is 10% overweight; a dog that has a BCS of 7/9 is 20% overweight; a dog that has a BCS of 8/9 is 30% overweight; and a dog that has a BCS of 9/9 is 40% overweight. Scoring systems for BCS have been validated for use in patients with <45% body fat.(2, 5) When the percentage of body fat in veterinary patients exceeds 45%, the 9-point scale falls short of accurately predicting body composition. At that point, body composition could only be accurately determined in the laboratory by means of dual-energy x-ray absorptiometry (DEXA).(5)

Returning to the Purina 9-point system of body condition scoring, dogs are considered slightly overweight if they score a BCS of 6/9.(3) There is slight fat coverage of otherwise palpable ribs. The waist is present, but not prominent.

Dogs are increasingly over-conditioned if they score a BCS of 7/9, 8/9, or 9/9.(3)

- A dog that has a BCS of 7/9 is mildly overweight. The ribs are difficult to feel due to heavy fat coverage, and fat deposits may have started to accumulate over the lumbar region and tail base. The waist is absent. So is the abdominal tuck.
- A dog that has a BCS of 8/9 is moderately overweight. It is not possible to feel the ribcage due to heavy fat coverage, and there is no waistline. Fat deposits are present and palpable in the lumbar region and at the tail base. The abdomen appears rounded due to fat deposition.
- A dog that has a BCS of 9/9 is morbidly obese. Fat deposits are diffuse. In addition to lumbar "love handles," fat is present over the neck, thorax, spine, tail, and limbs.

BCS is an important screening tool that is often underutilized (6). Brooklyn's parents can be trained to score her on a regular basis so that they are better equipped to identify trends. Changes in body size or shape may alert clients to present their pets for veterinary consultation sooner rather than later. This may lead to early detection of otherwise subclinical disease.(3)

Obesity is a growing problem among canine populations throughout the world.(7–15). Clients are more likely to underestimate body weight than members of the veterinary team(13, 14, 16–18), so it is critical that we introduce clients to BCS as a measurement tool as early as Brooklyn's first wellness visit.

It is also important that clinicians go out of their way to describe what constitutes healthy body structure so that when clients hear the opposite from friends and family, they know how to respond. Because obesity is rampant throughout companion animal practice, it is rare to examine dogs that have waistlines. Friends and family members who see dogs with waists often comment that they are "too thin" when in fact the patients are ideal. We need to continuously remind clients that it is ideal to see a waist (in a short-coated dog) and to feel, but not see ribs. This is a mark of health, rather than disease.

2. Clients should start by selecting a food that is appropriate for the pet's life stage. Puppy formulations are not a gimmick. They are specifically formulated by pet food manufacturers to meet nutritional standards. In the United States, these standards are set by the Association of American Feed Control Officials (AAFCO).(19)

AAFCO defines nutritional adequacy based upon life stage: (19)

- adult maintenance
- growth and reproduction.

Brooklyn should be fed a diet that is marketed for growth and reproduction. Dog food that is marketed for "all life stages" is also an appropriate choice.

Certain breeds have additional requirements for nutritional adequacy. Large and giant breeds, for instance, benefit from slow, controlled growth. Excess calcium in the diet adversely impacts maturation of the skeleton and predisposes to orthopedic maladies.(19–22)

As a Corgi, Brooklyn will not require a large-breed formulation. However, she will benefit from a food that has been carefully formulated to meet the needs for growth. In general, puppies have higher requirements for protein, fat, and minerals (particularly calcium and phosphorus) than adults.(19)

Brooklyn's owners may ask you to recommend a brand of food or they may ask you to critique her current diet. Oftentimes, clients will feed a brand that I have never heard of! There are just too many brands for veterinarians to keep track of. We each have our own individual preferences for certain companies. Many of these preferences are based upon the following stipulations, which help to ensure that a diet is nutritionally balanced and safe.

- The company has veterinarians on staff, including nutritionists.
- The company conducts feedings trials to test their products prior to going to market.
- The company has quality control measures and checkpoints during production.
- The company operates its own manufacturing plants.

Breeders may also have influenced clients by sharing their own preferences, both in terms of brand and ingredients. Encourage open dialogue between clients and the veterinary team and speak to breeders, whenever possible, so that everyone can be on the same page.

Rarely is a food "bad." More likely, there are "adequate" choices and then there are "preferred" options. Help clients and breeders to understand why a certain food is or is not recommended – and do what you can to both acknowledge and understand the breeders' perspective.

- Is the breeder's perspective valid?
- Is the breeder's recommendation safe?
- Is the breeder's recommendation evidence-based?

If the answers are yes, then the breeder's perspective is worthy of consideration. We will get further working as a team if we do not alienate team members. After all, we are all in this together. We may not always agree with the breeder – for example, a current hot button topic is whether to feed raw diets. It is our responsibility as veterinarians to explain our reasoning – and any safety concerns. We must provide the facts and do what we can to help our clients make an educated decision, one that is best for their pet and best for their family.

Clients often continue to feed what the breeder has recommended until they run out of it – then they find themselves making decisions about whether to re-purchase the diet or transition to a new one.

Transitions should be gradual, over the course of a week, in order to reduce the chance of gastrointestinal upset. Every few days, clients may be encouraged to replace more of the old food with the new. For instance, on days one and two of the transition, the pup can consume 75% of the old diet and 25% of the new. By days three and four of the transition, the pup can consume 50% of the old diet and 50% of the new. By days 5 and 6 of the transition, the pup can eat 25% of the old diet and 75% of the new. By day 7, the pup is exclusively eating the new food.

Once clients decide upon a brand of food to feed, their attention quickly turns to how much to feed. What I always tell my clients as a starting point is that it is critical to watch the dog, not the dish. Each breed and each dog within a given breed is unique. Individuals vary in terms of body type and metabolism. Portion size should be correlated with body condition.

Read the label on the bag to determine the specific feeding instructions for the diet of interest. Each diet typically reports how much to feed (in cups) based upon the dog's weight (in kilograms or pounds). Keep in mind that these are generic recommendations and that the instructions for feeding that are listed on the bag are often overly generous. Many pups benefit from eating less than this estimated amount. Therefore, use this measure of food per day as a starting point and adjust as needed based upon changes that you see and feel in terms of BCS.

3. Treats are fun to give, and they are effective positive reinforcement tools during training, but they must be given in moderation. Small portions add up! For example, one ounce of cheese may not seem like a lot to us, but its calorie count contributes to well over 15% of a 25–30 lb dog's daily intake.

It is easy to overfeed, particularly when snacks are energy dense. Deli meats, hotdogs, peanut butter, and cheese are frequently shared, but they add empty calories. Encourage clients who want to feed snacks to follow the 90/10 rule. Roughly 90% of Brooklyn's daily calories should come from her balanced diet, and 10% may come from treats.

Another important consideration when feeding table scraps is the potential for Brooklyn to ingest something toxic. Many foods that are safe for people to consume are dangerous for dogs to ingest.(23–26) The following list of human foods could endanger Brooklyn, even in small quantities:(23–26)

- chocolate (dark chocolate, semi-sweet chocolate, milk chocolate)
- cocoa (cocoa beans, cocoa powder)
- currants
- garlic
- grapes
- macadamia nuts
- onions
- raisins
- uncooked bread and pizza dough
- xylitol.

Clients should be given a list of food items that are unfit for canine consumption as well as what to do in the event of an emergency. Not all veterinary clinics offer after-hours services, yet treatment of toxicosis cannot always be delayed so it is critical that Brooklyn's owners know how to troubleshoot emergencies before they happen.

In the United States, clients are most often directed to the following organizations for assistance with presumptive toxicosis.

American Society for Prevention of Cruelty to Animals (ASPCA) Animal Poison Control Center (https://www.aspca.org/pet-care/animal-poison-control; telephone: (888) 426–4435).

Pet Poison Helpline (https://www.petpoisonhelpline.com/; telephone: (855) 764–7661).

In the United Kingdom, clients may be directed to:

Animal Poison Line (https://www.animalpoisonline.co.uk/; telephone: 01202 509000).

Many clients are already aware that chocolate is dangerous and may adversely impact the digestive tract, causing vomiting and diarrhea.(23, 24) However, they should be informed that the danger extends beyond the gut and there is potential for cardiac and neurologic issues:(23, 24)

* tachycardia, arrhythmias, hypertension, premature ventricular contractions
* panting, restlessness/hyperactivity, ataxia, tremors, seizures.

Clients may not be aware of other household toxins. Consider, for example, plants that belong to genus *Allium*. These include onions, leeks, garlic, and chives.(27–29) All of these plants contain organosulfoxides that are metabolized into compounds that cause oxidative hemolysis.(27–29) Affected patients will develop anemia, methemoglobinemia, impaired oxygen transport, Heinz body formation, and red blood cell fragility.(27, 28) Affected patients may become icteric.(27, 28) Clients may report weakness, lethargy, respiratory effort, and/or respiratory distress. They may notice pale pink, brown, cyanotic, or yellowed gums in a patient that is panting.

Cats are especially susceptible, but ingesting 15–30 g/kg will induce toxicity in dogs.(27, 28) Cooking *Allium* does not make it less toxic.(27, 28) Owners may not directly feed *Allium* spp. to dogs; however, certain foods contain it as an ingredient. Consider, for example, commercially prepared rotisserie chickens, powdered soup mix, and jars of baby food.(29) It is important to teach clients to review ingredient labels before feeding any people food to pets.

Another example of a lesser known toxin in dogs is ethanol, as from the ingestion of rotten apples or uncooked dough.(23, 30–33) The yeast in dough, *Saccharomyces cerevisiae*, breaks down carbohydrates into ethanol and carbon dioxide.(34) The former is absorbed from the gut and crosses the blood-brain barrier to cause significant changes in mentation.(23, 35) Affected patients may present with stupor or obtundation.

The field of veterinary toxicology is immense. It is easy to overwhelm our clients with details. Rather than provide the mechanism of action for every toxic agent, focus on the big picture.

* Which household foods should not be given to dogs?
* What do you do and whom do you contact if there is an accidental ingestion?

Brief client handouts or refrigerator magnets can be helpful items to send home after an initial wellness visit as reminders of pet poison hotlines that offer round-the-clock guidance.

4. It is considered standard practice for breeders to deworm puppies. Puppies are routinely administered deworming medications, such as pyrantel pamoate, to protect against roundworms (ascarids) and hookworms. Some formulations include febantel and praziquantel for additional coverage against other types of helminths, including whipworms and tapeworms.

   Toxocara canis, the primary canine roundworm, infects all pups prenatally. Larvae that had been dormant in the pregnant bitch activate during the second half of pregnancy.(36) The fetuses become infected when nematodes migrate to the uterus.(36) Infection is also transmitted through the milk during nursing.(36)

   To counter infection, pups are often dewormed as early as 2 weeks of age.(36) Doses are repeated every 2 weeks for typically four treatments.(36)

   Infection can be prevented in canine fetuses if the bitches are given daily fenbendazole, beginning at day 40 of gestation.(36) This daily regime continues through parturition and into neonatal life, until the pups are 2 weeks of age.(36)

Prophylactic deworming is considered good practice but does not guarantee that all worms have been targeted and eliminated. For example, pyrantel is ineffective against whipworms and tapeworms.

In addition, puppies can be re-infected. The primary source for roundworms is contaminated soil.(36) Puppies ingest roundworm eggs when they eat dirt, repeating the cycle of infection.

It is important to perform a fecal test on all puppies, even if they have been dewormed, because we need to screen for parasites that may still be present. Of particular interest are those parasites that can be transmitted to people. Fecal testing is an important safety measure for public health.

5. Some, but not all, endoparasites are zoonotic. Roundworms and hookworms are the two most common types that come to mind, and we can diagnose both in puppies.

    When Brooklyn's owners express concern that there is a link between blindness and the handling of fecal matter, they are probably referring to what they have read about toxocariasis. Toxocariasis is the name for the infection that occurs in people when parasitic roundworms from animals are transmitted to humans. Dogs or cats that are infected with roundworms shed eggs in their feces. People become infected when they inadvertently ingest eggs. For instance, if good hand hygiene is not followed, then handling food with contaminated hands will set the stage for infection. Children who play in dirt or sandboxes are particularly at risk.(37)

    When humans contract toxocariasis, they may be asymptomatic or they may develop one of two conditions:(29, 37–42)

- ocular toxocariasis
- visceral toxocariasis.

Ocular manifestations of disease occur more frequently in people than visceral presentations. (29) Ocular toxocariasis occurs when roundworm larvae migrate to the eye. Typically, this presentation results in severe unilateral disease. In the United States alone, there are at least 750 reported cases annually involving uveitis, vision loss, and blindness in people secondary to toxocariasis.(37, 40, 42)

By contrast, visceral toxocariasis is characterized by migration of larvae to other parts of the body, typically the liver or central nervous system. Clinical signs are linked to the organ(s) that are under attack. Fever and non-specific malaise are common. Abdominal pain is typical if the liver is involved.

Yes, it is true that Brooklyn increases the household risk for contracting roundworms. However, we can significantly lessen the risk for zoonotic transmission by deworming her monthly.(29) In addition, Jennifer and Aidan can be taught good hand hygiene practice. Washing hands after handling fecal matter is an essential means of preventing toxocariasis.(43)

Hookworms have also been implicated in zoonotic disease transmission.(29, 37, 38) Infected dogs and cats shed hookworm eggs in their feces. Humans become infected when larvae penetrate the skin, causing cutaneous larval migrans. Those who travel to tropical and subtropical regions of the world are most at risk, although zoonotic hookworms are also present in the United States. Walking barefoot or sitting on soil or sand that has been contaminated with hookworms increases the likelihood of disease transmission.(37) Clinical signs include pruritus and red, raised lines that mark the parasites' migratory path. Secondary bacterial infection is possible if skin surfaces are damaged because of severe itch. When the skin is compromised, it can no longer serve as an effective barrier to opportunistic invaders. Visceral disease is also possible if larvae migrate beneath the skin. Typically this results in enteritis.(37, 38)

Hookworm exposure can be minimized by regularly deworming Brooklyn. In addition, disposing of Brooklyn's feces immediately will help to prevent eggs from contaminating the soil. Walking barefoot can be discouraged to further lessen risk of transmission.

It is important to acknowledge the potential for zoonotic disease transmission so that clients can make educated decisions about preventative care. Clients need to know what the risks are so that they can plan accordingly. As veterinarians, we will encounter high-risk individuals every day in clinical practice. One in five people who reside in North America are immunocompromized.(44) Consider those who are: (43)

- battling chronic, systemic disease, such as diabetes mellitus; infectious disease, such as human immunodeficiency virus (HIV); or neoplasia
- living without a spleen (after having the organ surgically excised)
- taking immunosuppressive drugs to manage illness or organ transplantation.

It is our responsibility to engage in thoughtful discussion with clients about risk management. We also need to encourage clients to share their immune status with us so that we can advocate for those who are immunosuppressed and keep them healthy as pet owners.(43)

6. Endoparasitism is common. However, when a pet contracts intestinal parasites, it does not mean that the pet came from an unclean environment. Eggs contaminate the soil. This promotes recurrent infections when pets do not receive routine prophylaxis against endoparasites.

7. Brooklyn's owners may not be seeing ticks, but that doesn't mean they aren't present in the environment. Ticks are adaptable and widespread. They thrive in many regions of the US and UK, year-round.
    Ticks cause several serious diseases in companion animals, including, but not limited to:(45, 46)

- anaplasmosis
- coxiellosis (Q fever)
- ehrlichiosis
- Lyme disease
- Rocky Mountain spotted fever (RMSF)

Ticks are also the primary source of vector-borne illness in people.(47) Some of these illnesses cause substantial morbidity and mortality.(47)
    In addition, exotic ticks present a global concern as people and their pets engage in travel worldwide. In the UK alone, the Tick Surveillance Scheme (TSS) confirmed that at least 399 ticks from 15 different countries have accidentally been imported since 2005.(48) This means that exotic tickborne diseases are more likely to develop in regions of the world that previously had not encountered them.
    We also know that the risk of being bitten by a tick is 1.5× greater if you own a pet than if you don't, so year-round administration of tick preventative is protective of both animal and public health.(49)
    So, yes, it pays for Brooklyn's owners to be vigilant and take proactive measures to prevent tick infestation. No one wants to use unnecessary medication; however, I would rather exercise caution to prevent potentially fatal disease.
    Many clients prefer to administer seasonal preventative.(50) However, climate change is creating favorable conditions for ticks to survive year-round.(51)

8. Yes, heartworm disease really does occur, although geography and climate both play a large role in transmission.(52) The heartworm, *Dirofilaria immitis*, requires relatively warm temperatures for the ingested microfilariae to mature within the insect vector, the mosquito.(52) Maturation cannot occur if the temperature is below 57.2°F (14°C).(52) Because of this, seasonal use of heartworm prophylaxis is common practice within some geographical zones. In a 2010 study by Gates et al., owner compliance with heartworm prophylaxis was greatest from May through November among canine patients that presented to an East Coast US college of veterinary medicine.(50)
    However, the perceived seasonal trend in heartworm transmission is not necessarily accurate.(53) When the US is examined as a whole, dogs are in fact at greatest risk during the autumn and winter months, particularly when weather is mild.(54) Yet on average, only half of companion animals that present for examinations in winter are receiving monthly heartworm

prevention. This is a concern because poor owner compliance, compounded by ineffective communication between veterinarians and clients, is allowing transmission of heartworm disease to occur during temperate months.

Not administering heartworm preventative to Brooklyn is much like gambling. Will the odds be in your favor? At the end of the day, her health is not worth betting on. It is true that dogs can survive heartworm disease. However, they do not come out of the battle without scars. Heartworm disease is associated with the following cardiopulmonary lesions:(52)

- caval syndrome:
    - intravascular hemolysis
    - right-sided heart failure:
        - ascites
        - hepatomegaly
        - jugular distension
- immune-mediated glomerular disease
- pulmonary fibrosis
- pulmonary hypertension
- pulmonary thromboembolism
- tricuspid valve incompetence.

Many of these sequelae will resolve with adulticidal and microfilaricidal treatments, but there is no guarantee. Some of these complications will persist. Treatment for heartworm disease is also not benign. It is easier to prevent disease than to medically or surgically manage it. Therefore, it is well worth the expense and peace of mind to administer prophylaxis to Brooklyn.

9. Vaccinations are a critical component of every patient's preventative healthcare plan. By preventing disease in the individual, they effectively manage population health.(55)

Vaccination plans should be tailored to the individual. That is, Brooklyn's risk factors should be taken into consideration when deciding if the pros outweigh the cons for any given vaccine. Vaccines themselves are not without risk. It is our role as veterinarians to partner with clients to decide which approach to vaccinology constitutes the best fit for the patient and its lifestyle.

To assist decision making, many veterinary organizations provide vaccination guidelines for both core and elective vaccines. Core vaccines are considered essential for all members of the population, regardless of lifestyle or where they reside.(55)

Core canine pediatric vaccines protect against diseases that have high morbidity and mortality, are easy to transmit, are ubiquitous in the environment, or pose a threat to human health. (55) These include:(55)

- rabies
- canine distemper virus (CDV)
- canine adenovirus (CAV-2)
- canine parvovirus.

The rabies vaccination is typically administered as early as 12 weeks of age. Brooklyn is not old enough to receive this vaccination. Based upon her current age (10 weeks), she will need to wait at least 2 additional weeks in order for the administration of the vaccine to match its label and intended use.

CDV, CAV-2, and canine parvovirus are often packaged together as a modified live vaccine. This combination vaccine is usually administered between 6–8 weeks of age and is then followed up with a booster every 2–4 weeks until the puppy reaches 16 weeks of age. This schedule will need to be worked out for Brooklyn. If she has already started this series, then her next booster needs to be planned so that it falls within the 2–4 week window. If she has not yet started the series, then she is age-appropriate to begin today. She will require additional boosters based upon the schedule outlined above.

Core vaccines are the easiest to plan because they are considered standard. In addition, decisions must be made surrounding non-core or elective vaccines. Non-core canine pediatric vaccines include:(55)

- bordetella bronchiseptica
- canine coronavirus
- canine influenza
- leptospirosis
- Lyme disease
- parainfluenza virus
- rattlesnake vaccine.

Elective vaccines are tailored to the individual based upon risk factors and lifestyle. Geography also plays a role.

Each country (and, within the US, each state) may also have different guidelines (including patient age) for vaccine administration. It is important to reference the most current resources when developing evidence-based vaccination plans for the individual patient. The following resources may serve as guidelines in helping you to take these initial steps in planning vaccine schedules for puppies such as Brooklyn.

Global Resources for Vaccination Guidelines:

- World Small Animal Veterinary Association (WSAVA) Vaccination Guidelines – https://wsava.org/global-guidelines/vaccination-guidelines/

Resources for Vaccination Guidelines in the UK:

- British Small Animal Veterinary Association – https://www.bsava.com/Resources/Veterinary-resources/Position-statements/Vaccination
- National Office of Animal Health (NOAH) Dog Vaccination Summary – https://www.noah.co.uk/briefingdocument/dog-vaccination/
- VMD position paper on authorized vaccination schedules for dogs, November 2015: www.gov.uk/government/uploads/system/uploads/attachment_data/file/485325/Vaccines_VMDPositionPapaer.pdf
- UK government pet travel requirements for rabies vaccination guide – www.gov.uk/take-pet-abroad/rabies-vaccination-boosters-and-blood-tests

Resources for Vaccination Guidelines in the US

- American Animal Hospital Association (AAHA) Canine Vaccination Guidelines – https://www.aaha.org/aaha-guidelines/vaccination-canine-configuration/vaccination-recommendations-for-general-practice/

Keep in mind also the importance of referencing product guides because manufacturers provide specific instructions concerning dosing, reconstitution, and route of administration.(55) Vaccine efficacy depends upon our ability to follow instructions. Breaches in immunity are likely to occur when products are administered in a way that was not intended. For example, it is medically inappropriate to administer a half-dose of a vaccine to a dog because it is a toy breed.

10. Behavioral concerns are a leading cause of relinquishment to the shelter and euthanasia.(56) It is therefore important to devote some of the initial consultation time to discussing normal puppy behavior and how to manage problems as they arise before they become ingrained and risk a permanent break in the human–animal bond.(56)

Undesirable behaviors that may be reported at puppy visits include:(56)

- aggressive behavior
    - directed at other dogs
    - directed at people
- begging for food

- excessive play
- house-soiling
- mounting
- mouthing of people.

Opening the door to dialogue at that first puppy visit is an important step in the right direction to acknowledging "problem" behavior and taking measures towards resolution. Sometimes what presents itself as a "problem" is normal puppy behavior. On other occasions, behavior truly is inappropriate and requires correction. If we don't take the time to ask, then we may never find out that a problem existed until it is too late.

Although most primary care veterinarians are not board-certified behaviorists, they are responsible for (and capable of) educating clients in basic canine ethology and training techniques. Clients benefit from learning how to read and interpret canine body language, including posture, gestures, ear and tail carriage.(56) Clients need to understand how to facilitate key interactions during the socialization period that will influence the puppy's future experiences in life. Clients also need to learn how to initiate interactions; reinforce positive behaviors; and extinguish negative behaviors.(56) These lessons provide clients with a solid foundation for recognizing problem behaviors early and intervening in a constructive manner. When they are unable to resolve the issue, clients may feel more comfortable circling back to discuss the problem with us because we made it clear at the first visit that behavior is a key component of individualized healthcare.

CLINICAL PEARLS

- Clients should be trained to assess BCS so that they can identify concerning trends that may lead to early detection of subclinical disease.

- Teach clients that it is a sign of health to be able to palpate their dog's ribs!

- Maintain an open dialogue with clients (and breeders!) regarding what type of puppy food is being fed (and why!). Encourage discussion rather than dictation. Sit with the views on the other side of the table and take the time to understand them before commenting about what your clients should or shouldn't do. If there is something that they are doing wrong, take the time to explain "why."

- In terms of how much to feed, start with the label on the bag (or can) of food. Then watch the dog, not the dish.

- Treats are an important part of the human–animal bond but be cautious about portion size.

- Warn clients of potential dangers of household foods that are safe for people, but not for dogs.

- Individualize preventative care (flea/tick/heartworm/endoparasites/vaccines) to maximize the benefit to the patient (and to the client!).

- Address concerns about zoonotic disease because that opens the door to discussion about whether there are high-risk individuals in the household and, if so, what can be done to keep them safe.

- Include behavior as part of every consultation. It may be time-intensive up front, but it may save the pet from relinquishment later.

References

1. Laflamme D. Development and validation of a body condition score system for dogs. Canine Practice 1997;22(4):10–5.

2. Toll PW, Yamka RM, Schoenherr WD, et al. Obesity. In: Hand MS, Thatcher CD, Remillard RL, et al., editors. Small animal clinical nutrition. Topeka, KS: Mark Morris Institute; 2010. p. 501–42.
3. Englar RE. Performing the small animal physical examination. Hoboken, NJ: Wiley/Blackwell; 2017.
4. Jeusette I, Greco D, Aquino F, Detilleux J, Peterson M, Romano V, Torre C. Effect of breed on body composition and comparison between various methods to estimate body composition in dogs. Research in Veterinary Science 2010;88(2):227–32.
5. Witzel AL, Kirk CA, Henry GA, Toll PW, Brejda JJ, Paetau-Robinson I. Use of a novel morphometric method and body fat index system for estimation of body composition in overweight and obese dogs. J Am Vet M Assoc 2014;244(11):1279–84.
6. Burkholder WJ. Use of body condition scores in clinical assessment of the provision of optimal nutrition. J Am Vet Med Assoc 2000;217(5):650–4.
7. Robertson ID. The association of exercise, diet and other factors with owner-perceived obesity in privately owned dogs from metropolitan Perth, WA. Preventive Veterinary Medicine 2003;58(1–2):75–83.
8. Anderson RS. Obesity in the dog and cat. Vet Ann 1973;1441:82–186.
9. Crane SW. Occurrence and management of obesity in companion animals. J Small Anim Pract 1991;32(6):275–82.
10. Sloth C. Practical management of obesity in dogs and cats. J Small Anim Pract 1992;33(4):178–82.
11. Wolfsheimer KJ. Obesity in dogs. Compendium on Continuing Education for the Practicing Veterinarian 1994;16(8):981-and.
12. Colliard L, Ancel J, Benet JJ, Paragon BM, Blanchard G. Risk factors for obesity in dogs in France. Journal of Nutrition 2006;136(7);Suppl:1951S–4S.
13. McGreevy PD, Thomson PC, Pride C, Fawcett A, Grassi T, Jones B. Prevalence of obesity in dogs examined by Australian veterinary practices and the risk factors involved. Vet Rec 2005;156(22):695–702+.
14. Robertson ID. The association of exercise, diet and other factors with owner-perceived obesity in privately owned dogs from metropolitan Perth, WA. Preventive Veterinary Medicine 2003;58(1–2):75–83.
15. Holmes KL, Morris PJ, Abdulla Z, Hackett RM, Rawlings JM. Risk factors associated with excess body weight in dogs in the UK. Journal of Animal Physiology and Animal Nutrition 2007;91:166–7.
16. Scarlett JM, Donoghue S, Saidla J, Wills J. Overweight cats: Prevalence and risk factors. International Journal of Obesity and Related Metabolic Disorders: Journal of the International Association for the Study of Obesity 1994;18;Suppl 1:S22–8.
17. Courcier EA, Mellor DJ, Thomson RM, Yam PS. A cross sectional study of the prevalence and risk factors for owner misperception of canine body shape in first opinion practice in Glasgow. Preventive Veterinary Medicine 2011;102(1):66–74.
18. White GA, Hobson-West P, Cobb K, Craigon J, Hammond R, Millar KM. Canine obesity: Is there a difference between veterinarian and owner perception? J Small Anim Pract 2011;52(12):622–6.
19. AAFCO. Methods for substantiating nutritional adequacy of dog and cat Foods 2014. Available from: https://www.aafco.org/Portals/0/SiteContent/Regulatory/Committees/Pet-Food/Reports/Pet_Food_Report_2013_Midyear-Proposed_Revisions_to_AAFCO_Nutrient_Profiles.pdf.
20. Hedhammer AF, Wu F, Krook L, Schryver HF, deLahunta A, Whalen JP, et al. Overnutrition and skeletal disease: An experimental study in growing Great Dane dogs. Cornell Veterinarian 1974;64:9–160.
21. Goedegebuure SA, Hazewinkel HA. Morphological findings in young dogs chronically fed a diet containing excess calcium. Vet Pathol 1986;23(5):594–605.
22. Laflamme D. Effect of breed size on calcium requirements for puppies. Comp Contin Educ Pract Vet 2001;23(9):66–9.
23. Cortinovis C, Caloni F. Household food items toxic to dogs and cats. Front Vet Sci 2016;3:26.
24. Bates N, Rawson-Harris P, Edwards N. Common questions in veterinary toxicology. J Small Anim Prac. 2015;56(5):298–306.
25. Mahdi A, Van der Merwe D. Dog and cat exposures to hazardous substances reported to the Kansas State Veterinary Diagnostic Laboratory: 2009–2012. J Med Toxicol 2013;9(2):207–11.
26. Plumlee KH. Clinical veterinary toxicology. St. Louis, MO: Mosby, Inc.; 2004.
27. Cope RB; 2005. Toxicology Brief: Allium species poisoning in dogs and cats. DVM. Available from: http://veterinarymedicine.dvm360.com/toxicology-brief-allium-species-poisoning-dogs-and-cats.

28. Cope RB. Allium species poisoning in dogs and cats. Vetmed-US 2005;100(8):562.

29. Englar RE. Common clinical presentations in dogs and cats. Hoboken, NJ: Wiley/Blackwell; 2019.

30. Kammerer M, Sachot E, Blanchot D. Ethanol toxicosis from the ingestion of rotten apples by a dog. Vet Hum Toxicol 2001;43(6):349–50.

31. Suter RJ. Presumed ethanol intoxication in sheep dogs fed uncooked pizza dough. Aust Vet J 1992;69(1):20.

32. Thrall MA, Freemyer FG, Hamar DW, Jones RL. Ethanol toxicosis secondary to sourdough ingestion in a dog. J Am Vet Med Assoc 1984;184(12):1513–4.

33. Means C. Bread dough toxicosis in dogs. J Vet Emerg Crit Care 2003;13(1):39–41.

34. Thrall MA, Hamar DW. Alcohols and glycols. In: Gupta RC, editor. Veterinary toxicology: Basic and clinical principles. San Diego, CA: Elsevier, Inc.; 2012. p. 735–44.

35. Richardson JA. Ethanol. In: Peterson ME, Talcott PA, editors. Small animal toxicology. St. Louis, MO: Saunders; 2013. p. 547–9.

36. Datz C. Parasitic and protozoal diseases. In: Peterson ME, Kutzler MA, editors. Small animal pediatrics: The first 12 months of life. St. Louis, MO: Saunders; 2011. p. 154–60.

37. Schantz PM; 2007. Zoonotic parasitic infections contracted from dogs and cats: How frequent are they? DVM. Available from: http://veterinarymedicine.dvm360.com/zoonotic-parasitic-infections-contracted-dogs-and-cats-how-frequent-are-they.

38. Guidelines for veterinarians: Prevention of zoonotic transmission of ascarids and hookworms. Available from: https://www.cdc.gov/parasites/zoonotichookworm/resources/prevention.pdf.

39. Bowman DD, Georgi JR. Georgis' parasitology for veterinarians. 9th ed. St. Louis, MO: Saunders/Elsevier, 451 p. p.; 2009.

40. Schantz PM. Larva migrans syndromes caused by Toxocara species and other helminths. In: Gorbach SL, Bartlett JG, Blacklow NR, editors. Infectious diseases. Philadelphia, PA: W. B. Saunders; 2004. p. 1529–35.

41. Glickman LT, Schantz PM. Epidemiology and pathogenesis of zoonotic toxocariasis. Epidemiologic Reviews 1981;3:230–50.

42. Schantz PM. Toxocara larva migrans now. Am J Trop Med Hyg 1989;41(3);Suppl:21–34.

43. Stull JW, Stevenson KB. Zoonotic disease risks for immunocompromised and other high-risk clients and staff: Promoting safe pet ownership and contact. Vet Clin North Am. Small Anim. Pract 2015;45(2):377–92.

44. Trevejo RT, Barr MC, Robinson RA. Important emerging bacterial zoonotic infections affecting the immuno-compromised. Vet Res 2005;36(3):493–506.

45. Kidd LB, Breitschwerdt EB. Diseases formerly known as rickettsial. In: Peterson ME, Kutzler MA, editors. Small animal pediatrics: The first 12 months of life. St. Louis, MO: Saunders; 2011. p. 143–53.

46. Tulloch JSP. What is the risk of tickborne diseases to UK pets? Vet Rec 2018;182(18):511–3.

47. Jones TF, Garman RL, LaFleur B, Stephan SJ, Schaffner W. Risk factors for tick exposure and suboptimal adherence to preventive recommendations. Am J Prev Med 2002;23(1):47–50.

48. Hansford KM, Pietzsch ME, Cull B, Gillingham EL, Medlock JM. Potential risk posed by the importation of ticks into the UK on animals: Records from the Tick Surveillance Scheme. Vet Rec 2018;182(4):107.

49. Jones EH, Hinckley AF, Hook SA, Meek JI, Backenson B, Kugeler KJ, Feldman KA. Pet ownership increases human risk of encountering ticks. Zoonoses Public Health 2018;65(1):74–9.

50. Gates MC, Nolan TJ. Factors influencing heartworm, flea, and tick preventative use in patients presenting to a veterinary teaching hospital. Prev Vet Med 2010;93(2–3):193–200.

51. Medlock JM, Leach SA. Effect of climate change on vector-borne disease risk in the UK. Lancet Infect Dis 2015;15(6):721–30.

52. Ferasin L. Disease risks for the travelling pet: Heartworm disease. In Practice 2004;26(7) (July/August):350–7.

53. Nolan TJ, Smith G. Time series analysis of the prevalence of endoparasitic infections in cats and dogs presented to a veterinary teaching hospital. Vet Parasitol 1995;59(2):87–96.

54. Mohamed AS, Moore GE, Glickman LT. Prevalence of intestinal nematode parasitism among pet dogs in the United States (2003–2006). J Am Vet Med Assoc 2009;234(5):631–7.

55. Davis-Wurzler GM. 2013 Update on current vaccination strategies in puppies and kittens. Vet Clin North Am Small Anim Pract 2014;44(2):235–63.

56. Gazzano A, Mariti C, Alvares S, Cozzi A, Tognetti R, Sighieri C. The prevention of undesirable behaviors in dogs: Effectiveness of veterinary behaviorists' advice given to puppy owners. J of Vet Behavior 2008;3(3):125–33.

Case 4

The New Kitten Wellness Examination

Cynthia Ferguson was not expecting to add to her household of two. Having recently graduated from college and moved out of her parents' home into her own one-bedroom apartment, Cynthia is just barely making ends meet. She has an entry-level office job that puts food on the table, but at the end of the day, there is very little money left over for extras. Sharing the apartment is her ten-year-old spayed female Labrador retriever, Jamie. Jamie was the family dog that Cynthia could not take with her to the university. Cynthia was ecstatic when her parents entrusted her with Jamie's care now that she was living on her own. Cynthia envisioned a quiet few months, just the two of them, adjusting to the "new normal." That was before one of her friend's barn cats had an unexpected litter of kittens and she held Tux in her hands for the very first time.

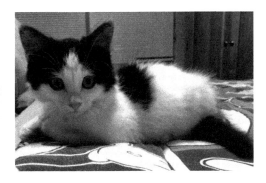

Figure 4.1 Your patient, 9-week-old DMH kitten, Tux. Courtesy of Sarah Greenway.

Cynthia first met Tux during a visit to Julie's ranch. They had planned an afternoon of horseback riding and were just getting back to the barn to unload the horses' tack when Cynthia heard a mew. She turned around and there was Tux. He was one of three kittens, but the only one that gravitated towards people. When she bent down to offer her hand, he came racing over. Julie asked if Cynthia was in the market for a cat. The rest was history.

Tux came home with Cynthia last weekend. He is currently a 9-week-old domestic medium haired (DMH) kitten of unknown background. Julie provided his mom with food, water, and shelter, but that is the extent of her veterinary care. The way Julie sees it, she receives free room and board in exchange for keeping the rodent population in check.

Since arriving at his new home, Tux has adjusted well. Tux wasn't initially thrilled to cross paths with a dog for the very first time, but Jamie was persistently inquisitive, and it wasn't long before they became instant friends.

Cynthia's only experience owning pets relates to Jamie. She has never lived with a cat before and is eager to hear your insight with regards to Tux's health, his needs, and his lifestyle. She apologizes in advance for the laundry list of questions, but she wants to be sure that he is getting all that he needs.

1. It was a fight to get Tux here. He doesn't seem to do well with confinement. I had to shove him into the carrier, and he wailed the whole ride here. Is it going to be like this every time?
2. Tux sometimes sucks on things. I don't mind if it's my shirt sleeve, but I do mind if it's me. Is he going to grow out of this?

3. It's not often, but every now and then he makes this face, often after smelling something – like last night, for example, he did this after sniffing socks in the laundry bin. What is he doing? Is this normal? She shows you a photograph of a cat online that is replicating the same action (see Figure 4.2).

4. I bought kitten chow and Tux has access to it all the time, but he often snacks on Jamie's food. Is it bad for him to eat dog food?

5. Julia said that cats can get herpes. What should I be looking for and can I catch it?

6. I noticed that Tux has fleas. Jamie receives a product every month that I put on the back of her neck, so I know that she's safe, but I would rather not have the house infested. I tried to purchase some over-the-counter product, but the salesperson warned me that cats can be very sensitive to flea medication and advised me to check with you first.

7. My parents sent me a bouquet of flowers for my birthday, but I'm concerned that some of them might be harmful to Tux. Can you look at this photo and tell me if I need to be careful? (See Figure 4.3.)

8. I read online that cats need to be tested for leukemia and acquired immunodeficiency syndrome (AIDS). What does that involve? And if he tests positive, what does that mean?

9. I know that Tux has not received any vaccines, but my plan is for him to be indoor-only. Are vaccines really necessary?

10. I would rather hold off on any shots for now because I've heard that they cause cancer in cats. Is that true?

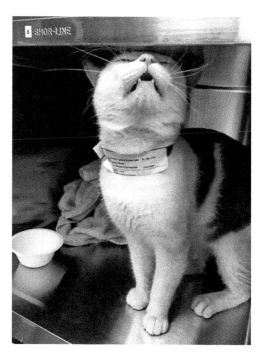

Figure 4.2 Unique facial expression in a cat

Answers to Case 4: The New Kitten Wellness Examination

1. I would tell Cynthia that she is not alone. The number of owned cats in the United States exceeds the number of owned dogs by millions, yet cats are by far less likely to present for veterinary care.(1–4) According to the Bayer Veterinary Care Usage Study, only 37% of veterinary clients bring cats to the clinic for annual wellness examinations.(2) A primary reason for their no-show status, as a species, is that clinic visits are perceived as stressful ordeals that take a toll

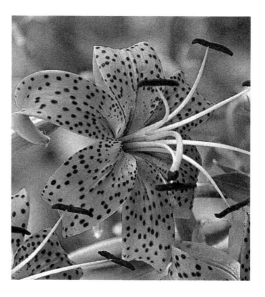

Figure 4.3 Client's photograph of a flower that is representative of the sample that comprises her bouquet.

on both client and cat long before either set foot in the clinic.(2, 5, 6) As a rule, cats do not like to be captured and confined to carriers, and less than one out of every five clients has been instructed by the veterinary team how to acclimate cats to the transportation process.(2, 6) By the time cats arrive at the clinic, most are sufficiently stressed and their tolerance for examination may have reached its limit.(5, 6) Clients witness this process from beginning to end and the less-than-pleasant experience takes a toll on them, too. More than half of cat owners who were surveyed in the Bayer Veterinary Care Usage Study described their cats as hating veterinary visits. (7) That will never change unless we are proactive in our approach to acclimating cats early in life to travel and handling.

Tux is young, but Cynthia will need to invest time and energy to alter his behavior surrounding confinement and transportation. The socialization period for kittens typically ranges from 2 to 7 weeks of age.(8) Tux is currently 9 weeks old. It is safe to say, given his upbringing as a semi-feral cat, that he likely did not experience daily or even frequent handling. And although he was likely exposed to a variety of stimuli based upon his living arrangement in the barn, he did not encounter cat carriers, the interior of cars, waiting areas of veterinary clinics, or consultation rooms. Lack of exposure to these stimuli has likely contributed to Tux's fear response.(8)

The good news is that there are measures that Cynthia can take at home to hopefully improve Tux's experience at future visits. For starters, Cynthia can acclimate Tux to the cat carrier. Too often, the carrier is only taken out on the eve of or day of the vet visit. This does not afford the cat the opportunity to associate the carrier with the home environment and positive experiences. By making the carrier a fixture in the home, much like furniture, Tux can explore it at his own pace. This gives him some degree of control: he can choose whether to enter or not.(9)

Cynthia can further encourage Tux to engage with the carrier by tossing in items with which he has a positive association, such as favorite toys or catnip. Cynthia can even offer treats or feed meals in the carrier to make it a positive experience.

Teach Cynthia to read feline body language to recognize signs of stress or fear. A crouched body posture and tail flicks are easy indicators to observe from a distance and are suggestive of anxiety.(9) Flattened ear position (what I like to refer to as 'airplane ears'), a tightened jaw, and dilated pupils also clue Cynthia in to a developing fear response.(9) These are all body language cues that we hope to minimize by giving Tux the opportunity to investigate the carrier on his own, before he is required to use it as transportation.

Other ways to entice Tux into the carrier include the use of synthetic feline facial pheromone. (9) Cats possess five pheromones in their facial secretions: F1–F5 (10). Cats preferentially deposit the F3 fraction onto familiar objects.(6) It is thought that F3 fraction denotes security and comfort. (6) The F3 fraction also contributes positively to cats exploring their environment.(10) Because of its role in inspiring calm and safety, F3 has been commercially produced and marketed as Feliway (Ceva Santé Animale).(6) Feliway diffusers are often plugged into consultation rooms in feline-friendly practices to reduce stress. Cynthia can take advantage of the over-the-counter wipes or spray to make the carrier feel more secure. Because the spray has an alcohol base, Cynthia will need to spritz the carrier 30 minutes ahead of transportation.(9) This will allow time for the odor of alcohol to disperse. Alcohol is aversive to cats.(6, 11)

Certain carriers are preferred over others to improve the feline experience. In general, cardboard carriers are not recommended because they do not provide an easy way to extract a resistant patient other than dumping the cat onto the exam room table.(6) As you can imagine, that does not make the cat any more excited to return to the clinic for the next visit.

Encourage Cynthia to invest in an easy-to-disassemble carrier, such as those with a removable top or ones that unzip.(6, 9) That way, if Tux decides not to come out of the carrier on his own at the clinic, he can be examined while remaining in the bottom half.

If visual cues tend to startle Tux, a towel can be placed over the carrier during transportation.(9) This can keep Tux feeling as if he is hidden from the rest of the world. The towel may be sprayed in advance with Feliway for the added calming effect.

When it comes to transportation, encourage Cynthia to remain calm even if Tux is not. She can use a soft, indoor voice, and turn the radio off unless choice of music is soothing.(9) Background music has been studied more extensively in dogs than cats, but it has been found that in both shelter and kennel environments, hard rock and heavy metal music is stressful, as opposed to classical music, which is calming.(12, 13)

Discourage Cynthia from shushing Tux in an attempt to quiet him. To a cat, shushing sounds remarkably similar to hissing.(6, 14) Shushing may intensify fear, rather than resolve it.

Finally, the American Association of Feline Practitioners (AAFP) has published a consensus statement with tips for travel. This may serve as an additional client education brochure or pamphlet: https://catvets.com/public/PDFs/PositionStatements/2010-Transport-of-Cats.pdf.

2. Tux's sucking behavior is likely residual from nursing. This is not commonly seen, but when it occurs, it usually resolves on its own by 6 to 12 months of age.(8) Nonproductive sucking is more likely to occur in kittens who have been weaned early or in certain breeds, such as Siamese.(8) The latter does not apply to Tux, but we do not know much about his weaning history, so that may have been a contributing factor.

Sucking may be benign; however, Cynthia needs to watch for any evidence of self-trauma. For instance, kittens who suckle on others may also start to suckle on themselves. This may result in hypotrichosis or patches of alopecia. If fur loss becomes extensive or if the underlying skin becomes traumatized, then intervention is necessary.

Sometimes sucking involves inanimate objects, such as clothing or blankets. If this transpires with Tux, then Cynthia needs to pay attention to ensure that sucking does not progress to ingestion. Otherwise, foreign bodies in the digestive tract could become a real concern.

Cynthia may provide more acceptable substrates for Tux to suck on, with the hopes of lessening the chance of foreign body ingestion. For instance, she may offer cat grass or treats of varying textures. Chewy snacks, such as beef jerky, may be of interest.

Keep in mind that sucking may evolve into a compulsive behavior if it is reinforced, so redirecting the behavior is ideal.(8) Maintaining a highly stimulating environment will keep Tux occupied and may direct his focus elsewhere.

Cynthia should avoid punishment of this behavior through words or actions, even if Tux is sucking on her skin. Sucking can be anxiety-based and punishment is likely to contribute to anxiety.(8) If Tux is sucking on Cynthia, then an acceptable option is to displace the kitten from the situation, that is, she can pick Tux up and put him on the floor.(8) He will soon learn that his mouth on Cynthia results in immediate loss of the privilege of being able to contact her skin.

3. What Cynthia is describing – and what she has demonstrated by way of photograph – is flehmen behavior or the gape response. When Tux makes this facial expression, he is participating in an unusual form of communication through chemicals called pheromones. Pheromones are chemical messengers that trigger a specific response in the recipient. They may communicate alarm or attraction. Sometimes they are used to identify territories or colonies. They help cats learn about other cats and may promote familiarity or bonding.

Cats are not the only species that exhibit this behavior. It is also displayed by hoofstock, particularly as a means of communicating sexual status after investigating voided urine.(15) When horses exhibit this behavior, they curl their upper lip up and back, exposing the front teeth.(15) Cats do a variation of this behavior. They do not quite curl the lip back. Instead, they elevate the upper lip and hold their mouth ajar; hence the description that they are gaping.(15) They hold this position for, on average, 10 to 15 seconds, as they inhale air through an open mouth.(15) It is thought that this grimace makes accessible the nasopalatine (incisive) duct, which is located behind the cat's incisors. Saliva is a solvent for the pheromones, which are transported from the mouth, through this incisive duct, and into the vomeronasal organ, where they can be processed.(15)

Both males and females display flehmen behavior, and it occurs commonly in response to voided urine.(15–17) Males appear to rely upon it more and exhibit it with greater frequency to assess compatibility of females and their phase of the estrous cycle.(16, 17) However, non-sexual, yet unfamiliar stimuli may also elicit the gape response. I have seen it in response to clothing that has been in contact with other conspecifics. Dirty laundry, particularly socks, may also pique Tux's interest and cause him to make this unusual sneer.

I might suggest to Cynthia that the gape response is a bit like smelling and tasting at the same time. It is a perfectly normal way for Tux to explore and experience his new environment.

4. It is not unusual for Tux to mimic feeding behavior within the household. If he sees Jamie eating, then he is likely to investigate that food source and try it out for himself. In my experience, dogs tend to prefer kitten chow much more so than cats tend to prefer dog chow so it is unlikely that Tux will abandon his food altogether. However, it is important to share with Cynthia that Tux cannot exclusively consume dog food. He may snack on it, but he cannot rely upon it as his sole source of nutrition. This is because kittens and cats have distinct nutritional challenges that puppies and dogs do not face. Perhaps the largest of these challenges is cats' need to consume pre-formed amino acid taurine in the diet.(18) Most other species, including dogs, can synthesize it from two other dietary amino acids, methionine and cysteine.(19, 20) Cats cannot.(21) Cats ingest taurine when they consume animal tissues.(19) In particular, muscle, viscera, and brain tissue contain high levels of this essential amino acid, whereas plant-based diets contain very little, if any.(19, 20, 22)

Because taurine is not an essential amino acid in the dog, dog food does not contain the amount of taurine that is required by cats.(21) If Tux exclusively consumes dog food, then he will not ingest adequate levels of taurine for growth, development, and maintenance. The consequences of ingesting insufficient taurine are deleterious to both the cardiovascular and special senses systems.

Taurine deficiency causes a heart condition called dilated cardiomyopathy (DCM) in cats. (23–29) This condition is best described as having an enlarged, flaccid left ventricle that is no longer an effective pump.(21) Because the heart is no longer able to contract efficiently, blood is pumped into systemic circulation at reduced volumes and velocity.(21) Ultimately, there is a back-up of blood into the left atrium, and from the left atrium into the pulmonary tree.(21) Left-sided congestive heart failure (CHF) is a common sequela.(21)

Taurine deficiency also causes degeneration of the retina as soon as taurine levels drop below 50% of that which is considered normal.(21, 22, 30–33) Clinically, this presents as acute vision loss and blindness.(21) Fundic examination is diagnostic. Although lesions are variable between patients, a band-shaped hyperreflective lesion can be identified on fundoscopy.(21) This band worsens as disease progresses and will ultimately extend from the nasal to temporal quadrants.(22)

Although both cardiomyopathy and retinopathy can be reversed if taurine deficiency is identified early in the disease processes, they are preventable conditions. Therefore, Cynthia can allow Tux to snack on Jamie's kibble, but it should never become his main source of nutrition.

5. Tell Cynthia that, yes, cats can get herpesvirus, but they cannot transmit it to people because the virus is species-specific.(21)

Feline herpesvirus-1 (FHV-1) is in fact quite common.(34–40) It is sometimes called feline viral rhinotracheitis (FVR).(41) This virus typically results in clinical presentations of conjunctivitis.(42–44) Kittens and cats often present with weepy eyes. Initial infection is typically bilateral. Affected eyes may exhibit blepharospasm and photophobia. Clients will often report that their cat is "squinting" or "winking." This is easy to observe from across the room and will be quite apparent on physical examination.

In addition to conjunctivitis, affected kittens and cats often develop a concurrent upper respiratory infection (URI).(34, 43) Clients may observe sneezing and nasal discharge. Cats' appetites are enticed by scent, so when cats develop snotty noses, they may not want to eat. Decreased appetite may be compounded by fever. Cats breathe through their noses, so nasal congestion may also complicate respiration. Affected kittens and cats may be depressed and lethargic, particularly if they are febrile.(34, 35, 38, 41, 45–47)

Cats with FHV-1 may also develop corneal ulcers.(43, 48–50) Classic FHV-1 ulcers are dendritic, meaning that they are linear and branching.(41, 43) These can be identified in the examination room using fluorescein stain to check for corneal uptake. This is a quick and easy test that is diagnostic for corneal ulceration.

Clinical disease typically resolves on its own; however, secondary bacterial infection is possible.(43) An important consideration and a unique feature of FHV-1 is that the virus is able to persist within the trigeminal ganglion for the life of the host.(34, 43, 51, 52) This so-called latency allows FHV-1 to reactivate, particularly during times of stress.(34, 39, 40, 49, 51) Rehoming a kitten or cat is a very stressful time in its life. If Tux has been exposed to FHV-1, then his adoption may precipitate a bout of clinical disease. Cynthia should keep a close watch on him for signs of developing oculonasal discharge.

Clinical signs will recur in the host during reactivation, although they are usually mild.(43) During this period of time, transmission of FHV-1 to other naïve cats is likely to occur.(43) The good news is that Cynthia will not have to worry about contracting FHV-1 herself. FHV-1 targets only cats.

6. Share with Cynthia that the salesperson was correct. Cats can be extremely sensitive to insecticides. Some of these over-the-counter products can even be fatal, particularly when used off-label in cats.

Cats are extraordinarily sensitive to a class of compounds called pyrethroids. Pyrethroids, such as permethrin, are synthetic versions of pyrethrins, which occur naturally in the flowers of chrysanthemums.(53–56) Pyrethrins can be absorbed orally or through the skin (of mammals) or exoskeleton (of arthropods), and they are fat soluble.(55) Once inside their target, they act as neurotoxicants.(53, 54) They disable the nervous system of arthropods by altering conductance of ions through sodium channels, but tend to have low toxicity profiles for mammals, which is why they are marketed as effective insecticides.(53–55)

Pyrethrins can be strengthened in terms of potency by being combined with a synergist. Piperonyl butoxide (PBO) and n-octyl bicycloheptane dicarboximide are often added to pyrethrin in commercial products to increase efficacy of the active ingredient, which ultimately causes repetitive nerve firing.(53, 54) This is demonstrated clinically as muscle fasciculations, tremors, hyperesthesia, seizures, and ataxia.(53–55)

Clinical signs are related to the concentration of pyrethrin or pyrethroid that has been absorbed.(53) Canine spot-on insecticides often contain exceptionally high concentrations of permethrin, which, while safe when used in dogs, is inappropriate for administration in cats. (54, 55) Cat products may contain 0.05–0.1% permethrin without adverse effect, as compared to 45–65% permethrin in canine formulations.(54, 55) The latter has the potential to kill cats, even in the smallest of doses.(57)

Cats are exquisitely sensitive to pyrethrins and pyrethroids because both compounds are metabolized through the liver after absorption or ingestion. Hepatic metabolism requires hydroxylation and conjugation of these compounds, but cats lack efficiency with the latter pathway. (53, 54) Cats are restricted in their ability to generate glucuronides as metabolites because cats are deficient in the necessary enzyme, glucuronyl transferase.(21, 53, 54, 58) This means that pyrethrin and pyrethroid concentrations build up in tissue at a rate faster than they can be eliminated, precipitating toxicity.

Most cats are presented within a few hours of exposure for intense muscle twitches, if not generalized seizure activity.(53–55) Affected cats are often disoriented and may exhibit transient blindness.(54) In addition to neurologic manifestations of toxicity, affected cats may present with the following signs:(53–55)

- anorexia
- ptyalism
- vomiting
- collapse
- hyperthermia
- dyspnea.

Prognosis for these patients is guarded, and sudden death is possible. For this reason, advise Cynthia to only use prescription products on Tux that have been recommended for use by the veterinary team.

7. The plant that Cynthia has described by way of photograph is a tiger lily. This plant, as well as others within the genera *Lilium* and *Hemerocallis* are nephrotoxic, including:(21, 59, 60)

- asiatic lilies
- day lilies
- easter lilies
- stargazer lilies.

Lily of the Valley has not been listed here because it is cardiotoxic, not nephrotoxic.(59) The peace lily and the rubrum lily are both non-toxic.(60)

Lily toxicosis is unique to cats.(59–65) All parts of the plant are toxic, including the pollen. (59) The toxic agent is unknown, yet must be water-soluble because even just drinking from a vase that contains lily pollen has the potential to induce nephropathy.(21, 59) The toxic agent causes AKI that is characterized by renal tubular cell death.(59) Patients are polyuric until dehydration sets in. Thereafter, they develop oliguria that progresses to anuria.(59)

Patients present with swollen, painful kidneys.(59, 60) They are dehydrated and recumbent. (59) As azotemia progresses, they develop uremic syndrome. This is characterized by one or more of the following signs:(21)

- anorexia
- depression
- oral ulceration
- vomiting
- melena
- muscle tremors
- seizure activity.

Patients can recover; however, prognosis is guarded and many cats are euthanized due to complications of lily toxicosis.(21)

8. Cynthia is partially right. Cats can be infected with feline leukemia virus (FeLV). Cats can also be infected with feline immunodeficiency virus (FIV), which is similar, but not the same as AIDS, a sequela of HIV. Both FeLV and FIV are relatively common infectious diseases of cats with worldwide distribution.(66) Neither virus is transmissible to humans, but both can be spread to other cats.

For detailed information on etiology, pathogenesis, and outcomes of infection, please refer to a comprehensive resource in infectious disease, such as *Infectious Diseases of the Dog and Cat* by Jane E. Sykes and Craig E. Greene.

To summarize for the purpose of educating Cynthia, the following talking points are beneficial to share in the consultation room regarding FeLV.

- The prevalence of FeLV varies based upon geographical residence (country and state); however, in most parts of the world, less than 5% of cats test positive for FeLV antigen.(66–70)
- Young cats are most susceptible to infection.(66)
- FeLV requires close contact for disease transmission through body fluids.(66) Saliva, nasal secretions, and milk are most often implicated, which is why viral transmission occurs primarily between queens and nursing kittens as well as among cats that live in proximity to one another.(66)
- FeLV has historically been called "the nice cat disease" because virus can be shed through mutual grooming; however, FeLV can also be transmitted through bite wounds.(66)
- Patient outcomes following exposure are diverse and largely depend upon the cat's immune system.(66) Some cats will clear the infection straight away. Some will develop transient infection. Others will develop latent infection. Some will experience persistent viremia, meaning that the virus is not contained, and viral replication occurs throughout the body. Persistently viremic cats have shortened lifespans and are likely to succumb to FeLV-linked diseases, such as certain types of lymphoma.(66, 71, 72)

The following talking points are beneficial to share in the consultation room regarding FIV.

- The prevalence of FIV varies based upon geographical residence (country and state); however, in most parts of the world, less than 5% of cats test positive for FIV antibody.(66–70)
- FIV is most often spread when infected saliva contaminates bite wounds.(66) Because of this, FIV has historically been called "the mean cat disease" because virus is shed through fighting; however, there are other mechanisms for transmission.(66)
- It is possible for FIV to be transmitted between queens and their kittens, but this occurs less frequently than in cases of FeLV.(66)
- Unlike HIV, FIV is infrequently spread through mating, even though semen contains viral particles and the mating process itself often involves the tom nipping at the nape of the queen's neck. (66, 73)
- Patients that contract FIV are typically asymptomatic for years.
- FIV(+) patients' immune systems progressively malfunction. This predisposes them to chronic and recurrent infections.(66) FIV(+) cats are also 5× more likely to develop neoplasia than FIV(-) cats.(66)

In accordance with recommendations from the AAFP, all newly acquired cats and kittens should be screened for FeLV/FIV infection.(66) These screening tests should be repeated if there is a history of a cat fight and/or any other exposure to cats of unknown serological status.(66)

Point-of-care testing can be performed on Tux today while Cynthia waits for the results. Most point-of-care tests screen for FeLV antigen and FIV antibody.(66) These tests tend to be highly sensitive, meaning that negative test results are generally reliable.(66) Because false positives are possible, a single (+) test result requires confirmatory testing.(66)

An additional consideration for FIV is that antibody-based tests may report a false positive for any kitten that nursed on a naturally infected queen.(66) Likewise, some regions of the world vaccinated against FIV. If vaccinated, the queen will also pass FIV-antibodies onto her offspring, which will then test (+) despite the fact that the kittens are not actually infected.(66) Therefore, a kitten who tests (+) should be retested at or after six months of age, at which point all maternal antibodies will have waned.(66)

Cats can also be vaccinated against FeLV. Because FeLV preferentially targets kittens and young cats, the AAFP recommends that all kittens up to and including 1-year-olds – as well as all at risk cats – be vaccinated.(66) Vaccination recommendations are then tailored to the patient at and after 2 years of age.(66)

If Tux is positive for either or both FeLV and FIV, and this is confirmed through follow-up testing, then he can still lead a good quality life, provided that he receives adequate husbandry and veterinary care.

9. Vaccinations are an important part of every patient's preventative healthcare plan. They not only prevent disease in the individual, they effectively manage population health.(74, 75)

Many veterinary organizations provide vaccination guidelines for both core and elective vaccines.

Core feline pediatric vaccines protect against diseases that have high morbidity and mortality, are easy to transmit, are ubiquitous in the environment, or pose a threat to human health.(74) These include:(74)

- rabies
- FHV-1
- calicivirus
- panleukopenia
- +/– FeLV

The rabies vaccination is typically administered as early as 12 weeks of age. Tux is not old enough to receive this vaccination. Based upon his current age (9 weeks), he will need to wait at least three additional weeks for the administration of the vaccine to match its label and intended use.

Although Cynthia plans to maintain Tux as an indoor-only cat, it is still advised that he be vaccinated against rabies. Rabies presents a public health risk. In addition, he can still contract rabies even if he never sets foot aside. For example, bats can become infected with and transmit rabies – and clients often report in certain parts of the country and world that bats obtain access to the house! In addition, what if Tux were to escape outdoors? We will not know what he encounters during his escape. It is not worth the risk of having him unprotected, particularly when the only definitive diagnosis for rabies at this time requires postmortem examination.

FHV-1, calicivirus, and panleukopenia are often packaged together as a modified live vaccine, feline viral rhinotracheitis-calicivirus-panleukopenia (FVRCP). This combination vaccine is usually administered between 6 and 8 weeks of age and is then followed up with a booster every 2–4 weeks until the kitten reaches 16 weeks of age. Tux has never received this vaccination and would be on schedule to receive this today; however, Cynthia's concerns need to be addressed before we can proceed.

Although it is true that Tux will be minimally exposed to infectious agents as an indoor-only cat, some clients will elect to allow supervised activity outside, as through walks on harnesses/leash.(75) Cats may also potentially encounter other cats when family members and friends visit; if Cynthia decides to foster or adopt other cats into the household; and/or if Tux must be boarded at an animal care or veterinary facility.(75) All of these represent opportunities when Tux may be exposed to infectious agents.(75) In addition, some pathogens may be inadvertently and indirectly transmitted to Tux through Cynthia's clothing and shoes after she herself has spent time outdoors and/or has encountered other cats.(75) All of these variables make a reasonable case as to why FVRCP is still considered to be a core vaccination, even in an indoor-only cat such as Tux.

One final consideration is that each country (and, within the US, each state) may also have different guidelines (including patient age) for vaccine administration. It is important to reference the most current resources when developing evidence-based vaccination plans for the individual patient. The following resources may serve as guidelines in helping you to take these initial steps in planning vaccine schedules for kittens such as Tux.

Global Resources for Vaccination Guidelines:

- World Small Animal Veterinary Association (WSAVA) Vaccination Guidelines – https://wsava.org/global-guidelines/vaccination-guidelines/

Resources for Vaccination Guidelines in the UK:

- British Small Animal Veterinary Association – https://www.bsava.com/Resources/Veterinary-resources/Position-statements/Vaccination
- National Office of Animal Health (NOAH) Cat Vaccination Summary – https://www.noah.co.uk/briefingdocument/cat-vaccination/

Resources for Vaccination Guidelines in the US:

- Scherk MA, Ford RB, Gaskell RM, Hartmann K, Hurley KF, Lappin MR, et al. 2013 AAFP Feline Vaccination Advisory Panel Report. J Feline Med Surg. 2013;15(9):785–808.

Keep in mind also the importance of referencing product guides because manufacturers provide specific instructions concerning dosing, reconstitution, and route of administration.(74) Vaccine efficacy depends upon our ability to follow instructions. Breaches in immunity are likely to occur when products are administered in a way that was not intended.

10. Cynthia is most likely referring to injection-site sarcomas. Historically, these were referred to as rabies or FeLV vaccine-induced or vaccine-associated sarcomas until it was discovered that injectables other than vaccines could also set the stage for tumor development.(76) These tumors primarily occur in cats, but isolated cases have been reported in ferrets and dogs.(76–78)

Injection-site sarcomas most often arise in the subcutis as firm, well-circumscribed masses that are not freely moveable.(76) They are locally invasive and spread aggressively along fascial planes.(76)

The timeframe with which these tumors arise is extremely variable, on the order of months to years.(76)

It is estimated that feline injection-site sarcomas occur in 1 to 4 out of every 10,000 vaccinated cats within the US.(76, 79, 80) In the UK, the rate has been reportedly lower, with feline injection-site sarcomas reported in one out of every 10,000–20,000 feline consultations in veterinary practice.(81) Although these tumors are relatively uncommon, they are devastating to both patient and client alike when they occur.

Cynthia's concern is commonly voiced by our cat-owning clients, which is why it is essential that we communicate risks and benefits at the time of vaccination and tailor the plan to the individual patient.

Yes, injection-site sarcomas are a real phenomenon. We do not completely understand why they occur.

It is thought that inflammation at the site of the reaction sets the stage for neoplasia, but the exact process by which this happens remains a mystery.(76) A common adjuvant, aluminum, has been identified on histopathologic examination of injection-site sarcomas, leading some experts to conclude that adjuvanted vaccines carry greater risk for malignant transformation.(76) It is true that adjuvanted vaccines intentionally create more intense inflammation at the site of injection to stimulate the immune system's response to vaccination. So if the inflammation hypothesis is accurate, then it makes sense that adjuvanted vaccines present a greater risk.

Non-adjuvanted vaccines have been developed and marketed with the hope of eliminating injection-site sarcomas. These are preferred over inactivated vaccines that contain adjuvant; however, injection-site sarcomas still occur.(76) Therefore, other factors must be at play that we do not fully understand.

It does appear that temperature of the vaccine is an influencer: cold vaccines are associated with sarcomas more so than room temperature vaccines.(76) If we take vaccinations out of storage from the refrigerator 15 minutes before injection, then we can potentially reduce the risk of sarcoma development without impacting vaccinal efficacy.(76)

Needle size, syringe size, and how fast we administer the vaccination do not seem to make a difference.(76)

If an injection-site sarcoma does develop, we can control where it forms by standardizing where to administer injectables, including vaccines.(76) When injectables are administered in the interscapular region, it is challenging to resect tissue to the extent that is necessary to control and eradicate disease.(76) To be effective, surgical resection of injection-site sarcomas must be extensive.(76) Margins of 3 to 5 cm are recommended for the patient's best chance at long-term survival. The interscapular region does not afford this degree of space in three-dimensions for surgical resection. The vertebral column prohibits how much tissue can be resected if a sarcoma were to develop.

By contrast, limbs can be amputated while still maintaining quality of life in the affected patient. This has stimulated discussion among experts about preferred sites of administration for injectables. The distal limb (i.e. distal to the elbow in the forelimb, and distal to the stifle in the pelvic limb) and tail have been proposed as optimal locations.(76) The AAFP is supportive of these recommendations and has recommended the following guidelines for vaccine administration.(75, 76)

- FVRCP vaccines are to be administered below the right elbow.
- FeLV vaccines are to be administered below the left stifle.
- Rabies vaccinations are to be administered below the right stifle.

The tail has not yet been incorporated into the AAFP guidelines; however, a recent study demonstrated that vaccinating the tail was well-tolerated by patients in a clinical setting.(82)

If an injection-site swelling develops, we can also be proactive in our response to expedite early diagnosis.(82) We can share the 3–2–1 rule with Cynthia so that she can monitor injection site following vaccination. According to the 3–2–1 rule, biopsies should be performed if:(76)

- a site swelling persists at/after three months of vaccination
- a site swelling exceeds 2 cm in diameter
- a site swelling continues to grow at/after one month of vaccination.

These are important considerations that require an open dialogue between veterinarians and their clients. All too often, these discussions do not occur during the consultation or, if they are, client concerns about vaccines are glossed over, rather than acknowledged, validated, and addressed.

Most of the time, adverse reactions to vaccinations do not occur, so lack of client education in this content area is a non-issue. But if an injection-site sarcoma does form and we never discussed at time of vaccination that this development was a possibility, albeit rare, then we have fractured our relationship with the client. That broken trust may not be easy to recover from.

Cynthia's concern about the link between vaccines and neoplasia needs to be addressed openly so that she has a clear understanding about what Tux needs and why, what the potential risks are, and how we manage those risks appropriately.

CLINICAL PEARLS

- The veterinary visit begins long before the consultation room. Clients play a major part in acclimating kittens and cats to the carrier and can make significant strides at home and during transport to improve the travel experience.

- Teach clients to read body language so that they recognize signs of stress, fear, and anxiety before those signs intensify.

- Cats are likely to feel less anxious when they maintain some degree of control over a situation. Educate clients regarding carrier selection so that they ultimately pick a design that works for the patient and the clinic. For example, carriers that can be disassembled with ease in the consultation room facilitate examinations by allowing reserved cats to "hide" in the bottom half of the carrier.

- Teach clients what constitutes normal behavior (such as the gape response) versus what can evolve into compulsive behaviors, such as nonproductive sucking.

- Educate clients how to curb unwanted behaviors without punishment; also share the importance of not inadvertently reinforcing behaviors that are undesirable.

- Cats are not "little dogs." Maintain an open dialogue with clients who lack cat-owning experience to be sure they understand cat-specific pathology and risks (i.e. FHV-1, taurine deficiency, pyrethrin and permethrin toxicity, lily toxicosis, injection-site sarcomas).

- Elicit clients' perspective to hear their concerns and be transparent when addressing them. Doing so builds trust.

- Tailor vaccination protocols to the patient, based upon lifestyle and individual risk factors, but rely upon guidance from organizations such as the American Association of Feline Practitioners (AAFP).

- Be proactive: explain the potential for adverse reactions and give the client a role in keeping an eye out for them. For example, teach the 3–2–1 rule for injection-site swellings so that clients know what to watch for and when to seek medical attention.

References

1. American Veterinary Medical Association. 2017–2018 U.S. pet ownership & demographics sourcebook. Schaumburg, IL: American Veterinary Medical Association; 2012.
2. Volk JO, Thomas JG, Colleran EJ, Siren CW. Executive summary of phase 3 of the Bayer veterinary care usage study. J Am Vet Med Assoc 2014;244(7):799–802.
3. Nolen RS. Feline-friendly handling guidelines aim for perfect veterinary visits. Veterinary team, pet owner have a hand in limiting stress in cat patients. J Am Vet Med Assoc 2011;239(1):26–7.
4. Vogt AH, Rodan I, Brown M, Brown S, Buffington CAT, Forman MJL, et al. AAFP-AAHA: feline life stage guidelines. J Am Anim Hosp Assoc 2010;46(1):70–85.
5. Volk JO, Felsted KE, Thomas JG, Siren CW. Executive summary of the Bayer veterinary care usage study. J Am Vet Med Assoc 2011;238(10):1275–82.
6. Englar RE. Performing the small animal physical examination. Hoboken, NJ: Wiley/Blackwell; 2017.
7. Volk JO, Felsted KE, Thomas JG, Siren CW. Executive summary of phase 2 of the Bayer veterinary care usage study. J Am Vet Med Assoc 2011;239(10):1311–6.
8. Radosta L. Feline behavioral development. In: Peterson ME, Kutzler MA, editors. Small animal pediatrics: The first 12 months of life. St. Louis, MO: Saunders; 2011. p. 88–96.
9. Rodan I, Sundahl E, Carney H, Gagnon AC, Heath S, Landsberg G, et al. AAFP and ISFM feline-friendly handling guidelines. J Feline Med Surg 2011;13(5):364–75.
10. Pereira JS, Fragoso S, Beck A, Lavigne S, Varejão AS, da Graça Pereira G. Improving the feline veterinary consultation: the usefulness of Feliway spray in reducing cats' stress. J Feline Med Surg 2016;18(12):959–64.
11. Herron ME, Shreyer T. The pet-friendly veterinary practice: A guide for practitioners. Vet Clin N am. Small 2014;44(3):451.
12. Wells DL, Graham L, Hepper PG. The influence of auditory stimulation on the behaviour of dogs housed in a rescue shelter. Anim Welf 2002;11(4):385–93.
13. Kogan LR, Schoenfeld-Tacher R, Simon AA. Behavioral effects of auditory stimulation on kenneled dogs. J Vet Behav 2012;7(5):268–75.
14. Scherk M. The cat-friendly practice. In: Harvey A, Tasker S, editors. BSAVA manual of feline practice: A foundation manual. Gloucester: British Small Animal Veterinary Association; 2013.
15. Hart BL, Leedy MG. Stimulus and hormonal determinants of flehmen behavior in cats. Horm Behav 1987;21(1):44–52.
16. Verberne G. Chemocommunication among domestic cats, mediated by the olfactory and vomeronasal senses. II. The relation between the function of Jacobson's organ (vomeronasal organ) and Flehmen behaviour). Z Tierpsychol 1976;42(2):113–28.
17. Verberne G, de Boer J. Chemocommunication among domestic cats, mediated by the olfactory and vomeronasal senses. I. Chemocommunication. Z Tierpsychol 1976;42(1):86–109.
18. H.P. Nutritional requirements and feeding of growing puppies and kittens. In: Peterson ME, Kutzler MA, editors. Small animal pediatrics: The first 12 months of life. St. Louis, MO: Saunders; 2011. p. 58–66.
19. Spitze AR, Wong DL, Rogers QR, Fascetti AJ. Taurine concentrations in animal feed ingredients; cooking influences taurine content. J Anim Physiol Anim Nutr (Berl) 2003;87(7–8):251–62.
20. Hayes KC. Nutritional problems in cats: taurine deficiency and vitamin A excess. Can Vet J 1982;23(1):2–5.
21. Englar RE. Common clinical presentations in dogs and cats. Hoboken, NJ: Wiley/Blackwell; 2019. pages cm p.
22. Aguirre GD. Retinal degeneration associated with the feeding of dog foods to cats. J Am Vet Med Assoc 1978;172(7):791–6.
23. Novotny MJ, Hogan PM, Flannigan G. Echocardiographic evidence for myocardial failure induced by taurine deficiency in domestic cats. Can J Vet Res 1994;58(1):6–12.
24. Sisson DD, Knight DH, Helinski C, Fox PR, Bond BR, Harpster NK, et al. Plasma taurine concentrations and M-mode echocardiographic measures in healthy cats and in cats with dilated cardiomyopathy. J Vet Intern Med 1991;5(4):232–8.
25. Pion PD, Kittleson MD, Rogers QR, Morris JG. Myocardial failure in cats associated with low plasma taurine: a reversible cardiomyopathy. Science 1987;237(4816):764–8.

26. Pion PD, Kittleson MD, Rogers QR, Morris JG. Taurine deficiency myocardial failure in the domestic cat. Prog Clin Biol Res 1990;351:423–30.

27. Pion PD, Kittleson MD, Thomas WP, Skiles ML, Rogers QR. Clinical findings in cats with dilated cardiomyopathy and relationship of findings to taurine deficiency. J Am Vet Med Assoc 1992;201(2):267–74.

28. Ferasin L. Feline myocardial disease. 1: Classification, pathophysiology and clinical presentation. J Feline Med Surg 2009;11(1):3–13.

29. Ferasin L. Feline myocardial disease 2: diagnosis, prognosis and clinical management. J Feline Med Surg 2009;11(3):183–94.

30. Schmidt SY, Berson EL, Hayes KC. Retinal degeneration in cats fed casein. I. Taurine deficiency. Invest Ophthalmol 1976;15(1):47–52.

31. Schmidt SY, Berson EL, Watson G, Huang C. Retinal degeneration in cats fed casein. III. Taurine deficiency and ERG amplitudes. Invest Ophthalmol Vis Sci 1977;16(7):673–8.

32. Berson EL, Hayes KC, Rabin AR, Schmidt SY, Watson G. Retinal degeneration in cats fed casein. II. Supplementation with methionine, cysteine, or taurine. Invest Ophthalmol 1976;15(1):52–8.

33. Hayes KC. A review on the biological function of taurine. Nutr Rev 1976;34(6):161–5.

34. Ofri R. Conjunctivitis in cats. NAVC Clin's Brief 2017 (April):95–100.

35. Stiles J. Feline ophthalmology. In: Gelatt KN, Gilger BC, Kern TJ, editors. Veterinary ophthalmology. Ames, IA: Wiley/Blackwell; 2013. p. 1477–559.

36. Stiles J. Ocular manifestations of feline viral diseases. Vet J 2014;201(2):166–73.

37. Stiles J, Pogranichniy R. Detection of virulent feline herpesvirus-1 in the corneas of clinically normal cats. J Feline Med Surg 2008;10(2):154–9.

38. Maggs DJ. Update on pathogenesis, diagnosis, and treatment of feline herpesvirus type 1. Clin Tech Small Anim Pract 2005;20(2):94–101.

39. Gould D. Feline herpesvirus-1: ocular manifestations, diagnosis and treatment options. J Feline Med Surg 2011;13(5):333–46.

40. Westermeyer HD, Thomasy SM, Kado-Fong H, Maggs DJ. Assessment of viremia associated with experimental primary feline herpesvirus infection or presumed herpetic recrudescence in cats. Am J Vet Res 2009;70(1):99–104.

41. Smith RIE. The cat with ocular discharge or changed conjunctival appearance. In: Rand J, editor. Problem-Based Feline Medicine. Edinburgh. New York: Saunders; 2006. p. 1207–32.

42. Chandler EA, Gaskell RM, Gaskell CJ. Feline medicine and therapeutics. Chichester: John Wiley & Sons; 2008.

43. Lim CC, Maggs DJ. Ophthalmology. In: Little SE, editor. The cat: Clinical medicine and management. St. Louis, MO: Saunders Elsevier; 2012. p. 807–45.

44. Reinstein S, editor. The squinting cat: Herpes until proven otherwise. Michigan VMA. MI; 2017.

45. Maggs DJ. Conjunctiva. In: Maggs DJ, Miller PE, Ofri R, editors. Slatter's fundamentals of veterinary opthalmology. St. Louis, MO: Elsevier; 2013. p. 140–58.

46. Aroch I, Ofri R, Sutton G. Ocular manifestations of systemic diseases. In: Maggs DJ, Miller PE, Ofri R, editors. Slatter's fundamentals of veterinary ophthalmology. St. Louis, MO: Elsevier; 2013. p. 184–219.

47. Nasisse MP, Guy JS, Stevens JB, English RV, Davidson MG. Clinical and laboratory findings in chronic conjunctivitis in cats: 91 cases (1983–1991). J Am Vet Med Assoc 1993;203(6):834–7.

48. Mitchell N. Feline ophthalmology Part 2: Clinical presentation and aetiology of common ocular conditions. Ir Vet J 2006;59(4):223–+.

49. Plummer CE. Herpetic keratoconjunctivitis in a cat. NAVC Clin's Brief 2012 (January):26–8.

50. Smith L. The dos and don'ts of treating ocular disease in cats (Proceedings). DVM 360. 2011. Available from: http://veterinarycalendar.dvm360.com/dos-and-donts-treating-ocular-disease-cats-proceedings.

51. Grahn BH, Sandmeyer LS. Diagnostic ophthalmology. Can Vet J 2010;51(3):327.

52. Nasisse MP, Davis BJ, Guy JS, Davidson MG, Sussman W. Isolation of feline herpesvirus 1 from the trigeminal ganglia of acutely and chronically infected cats. J Vet Intern Med 1992;6(2):102–3.

53. Dymond NL, Swift IM. Permethrin toxicity in cats: a retrospective study of 20 cases. Aust Vet J 2008;86(6):219–23.

54. Linnett PJ. Permethrin toxicosis in cats. Aust Vet J 2008;86(1–2):32–5.

55. Richardson JA. Permethrin spot-on toxicoses in cats. J Vet Emerg Crit Care 2000;10(2):103–6.

56. Valentine WM. Toxicology of selected pesticides, drugs, and chemicals. Pyrethrin and pyrethroid insecticides. Vet Clin North Am Small Anim Pract 1990;20(2):375–82.

57. Hansen SR, Villar D, Buck WB. Pyrethrins and pyrethroids in dogs and cats. Comp Cont Educ Pract 1994;16:707–12.

58. Allen AL. The diagnosis of acetaminophen toxicosis in a cat. Can Vet J 2003;44(6):509–10.

59. Fitzgerald KT. Lily toxicity in the cat. Top Companion Anim Med 2010;25(4):213–7.

60. Stokes JE, Forrester SD. New and unusual causes of acute renal failure in dogs and cats. Vet Clin North Am Small Anim Pract 2004;34(4):909–22.

61. Gulledge L, Boos D, Wachsstock R. Acute renal failure in a cat secondary to tiger lily (Lilium tigrinum) toxicity. Feline Pract 1997;25(5–6):38–9.

62. Hadley RM, Richardson JA, Gwaltney-Brant SM. A retrospective study of daylily toxicosis in cats. Vet Hum Toxicol 2003;45(1):38–9.

63. Langston CE. Acute renal failure caused by lily ingestion in six cats. J Am Vet Med Assoc 2002;220(1):49–52.

64. Brady MA, Janovitz EB. Nephrotoxicosis in a cat following ingestion of Asiatic hybrid lily (Lilium sp). J Vet Diagn Invest 2000;12(6):566–8.

65. Hall JO. Lily nephrotoxicity. In: August JR, editor. Consultations in Feline Internal Medicine. Philadelphia, PA: W. B. Saunders; 2001.

66. Little S, Levy J, Hartmann K, Hofmann-Lehmann R, Hosie M, Olah G, Denis KS. 2020 AAFP feline retrovirus testing and management guidelines. J Feline Med Surg 2020;22(1):5–30.

67. Studer N, Lutz H, Saegerman C, Gönczi E, Meli ML, Boo G, et al. Pan-European study on the prevalence of the feline leukaemia virus infection – reported by the European Advisory Board on Cat Diseases (ABCD Europe). Viruses 2019;11(11).

68. Burling AN, Levy JK, Scott HM, Crandall MM, Tucker SJ, Wood EG, Foster JD. Seroprevalences of feline leukemia virus and feline immunodeficiency virus infection in cats in the United States and Canada and risk factors for seropositivity. J Am Vet Med Assoc 2017;251(2):187–94.

69. Levy JK, Scott HM, Lachtara JL, Crawford PC. Seroprevalence of feline leukemia virus and feline immunode-ficiency virus infection among cats in North America and risk factors for seropositivity. J Am Vet Med Assoc 2006;228(3):371–6.

70. Little S, Sears W, Lachtara J, Bienzle D. Seroprevalence of feline leukemia virus and feline immunodeficiency virus infection among cats in Canada. Can Vet J 2009;50(6):644–8.

71. Hofmann-Lehmann R, Cattori V, Tandon R, Boretti FS, Meli ML, Riond B, et al. Vaccination against the feline leukaemia virus: outcome and response categories and long-term follow-up. Vaccine 2007;25(30):5531–9.

72. Helfer-Hungerbuehler AK, Widmer S, Kessler Y, Riond B, Boretti FS, Grest P, et al. Long-term follow up of feline leukemia virus infection and characterization of viral RNA loads using molecular methods in tissues of cats with different infection outcomes. Virus Res 2015;197:137–50.

73. Jordan HL, Howard J, Barr MC, Kennedy-Stoskopf S, Levy JK, Tompkins WA. Feline immunodeficiency virus is shed in semen from experimentally and naturally infected cats. AIDS Res Hum Retrovir 1998;14(12):1087–92.

74. Davis-Wurzler GM. 2013 Update on current vaccination strategies in puppies and kittens. Vet Clin North Am Small Anim Pract 2014;44(2):235–63.

75. Scherk MA, Ford RB, Gaskell RM, Hartmann K, Hurley KF, Lappin MR, et al. 2013 AAFP Feline Vaccination Advisory Panel Report. J Feline Med Surg 2013;15(9):785–808.

76. Hartmann K, Day MJ, Thiry E, Lloret A, Frymus T, Addie D, et al. Feline injection-site sarcoma: ABCD guidelines on prevention and management. J Feline Med Surg 2015;17(7):606–13.

77. Munday JS, Stedman NL, Richey LJ. Histology and immunohistochemistry of seven ferret vaccination-site fibrosarcomas. Vet Pathol 2003;40(3):288–93.

78. Vascellari M, Melchiotti E, Bozza MA, Mutinelli F. Fibrosarcomas at presumed sites of injection in dogs: characteristics and comparison with non-vaccination site fibrosarcomas and feline post-vaccinal fibrosarcomas. J Vet Med A Physiol Pathol Clin Med 2003;50(6):286–91.

79. Coyne MJ, Reeves NC, Rosen DK. Estimated prevalence of injection-site sarcomas in cats during 1992. J Am Vet Med Assoc 1997;210(2):249–51.

80. Gobar GM, Kass PH. World Wide Web-based survey of vaccination practices, postvaccinal reactions, and vaccine site-associated sarcomas in cats. J Am Vet Med Assoc 2002;220(10):1477–82.

81. Dean RS, Pfeiffer DU, Adams VJ. The incidence of feline injection site sarcomas in the United Kingdom. BMC Vet Res 2013;9:17.
82. Hendricks CG, Levy JK, Tucker SJ, Olmstead SM, Crawford PC, Dubovi EJ, Hanlon CA. Tail vaccination in cats: a pilot study. J Feline Med Surg 2014;16(4):275–80.

Case 5

The Snotty, Squinty Kitten

Johnny Castle was not expecting to adopt anything when he walked through the doors of the local humane society 9 days ago. He was there as moral support only, at the request of his friend, Penny, who had been searching high and low for the perfect four-legged addition to her household. She liked a certain look in a cat – preferably a Siamese – but so far, all that had turned up were moggies. Cute, but not the kind of chatty that she envisioned coming home to, at the end of a long workday. Her quest to find the "right" cat led her to the Catskills Shelter for Feline Friends. Johnny was simply along for the ride . . . until his eyes locked with Mambo.

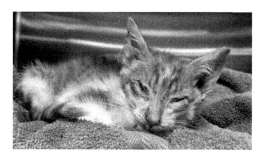

Figure 5.1 Your patient, 10-week-old DSH kitten, Mambo. Courtesy of Genevieve LaFerriere, DVM.

Mambo was the only sign of life in the shelter. The other temporary residents were either sound asleep or quietly disinterested in their surroundings. Most were older cats, waiting for their forever homes, but watching life pass them by. It made Johnny sad to see. They all deserved a family that he was not prepared to offer. Johnny was thinking this through when the sound of a clatter broke through his thoughts and captured his attention.

Just over his left shoulder, in a cage near the corner, his eye caught movement. There was a flash of orange and white engaged in a spinning action against the static, austere sheen of stainless steel. In the absence of a playmate, Mambo had invented his own game of chase the tail. He spun again and again until dizziness took over, tossing him on his rump. There he sat for a bit, bewildered, with his tail in his mouth, as if to say, "Okay, now what?"

That's precisely when Johnny came into view. Mambo's ears perked first in Johnny's direction and then his whole body as he whisked himself up and off to the cage front to investigate this new visitor. Mambo was unafraid and eager for contact. He reached out a paw through the opening between cage bars to swat Johnny playfully with half unsheathed claws. The kitten's antics caught Johnny's attention. Before he knew what was happening, Mambo was taken out of the cage by the attendant and handed over. Mambo spent the rest of the visit on Johnny's shoulder, where he stayed until after the adoption paperwork was signed.

Johnny wasn't at all ready for a kitten. Penny set him up with the household essentials that Mambo would need and walked him through how to "kitten-proof" his home in brief ("Good luck!" were her final words to him!). She also suggested that Johnny telephone your clinic to schedule a consult. Johnny had every intention of making contact, but Mambo seemed to be settling into the bachelor pad like a pro, so much so that there seemed to be no need until three days ago.

Mambo developed a bit of a sniffle. At first, it was just a dry sneeze now and again. Then the sneezes became more frequent. As they did, Mambo developed nasal discharge. When the discharge was copious, but clear, it was easy to overlook. Johnny chalked it up to allergies. After all, it was the season for it and his nose had been running, too. But when, two days later, the discharge had transformed into plugs of yellow-green snot, it was evident to Johnny that this was far more than just ragweed. This morning, Mambo's eyes were crusted over and he sounded audibly congested. When he refused to eat breakfast, Johnny scheduled an appointment for this afternoon.

Your technician greets Johnny in the waiting area and directs him and Mambo into an examination room. She takes the kitten's vital signs and reports them to you as follows:

Your technician also wants you to double-check Mambo's sex because she is not convinced that Mambo is in fact a male cat.

Mentation: Depressed

TEMPERATURE, PULSE, AND RESPIRATION (TPR)

T: 103.6°F (39.8°C)
P: 220 beats per minute
R: 52 breaths per minute

Round One of Questions

1. Mambo's mentation has been described above. How is mentation defined in veterinary medicine? Walk us through the sliding scale of mentation in terms of how our patients are characterized.
2. Mambo's temperature was taken rectally. What is the reference range for rectal temperature in a cat? Is his temperature considered normal?
3. The pulse should match the heart rate. What is the reference range for heart rate in an adult cat?
4. Is Mambo's respiratory rate considered normal? What is the reference range for respiratory rate in an adult cat?
5. Mambo is reportedly a 10-week-old neutered male DSH kitten. Which image of the feline perineum below best represents his alleged sex and sexual status? (See Figure 5.2)

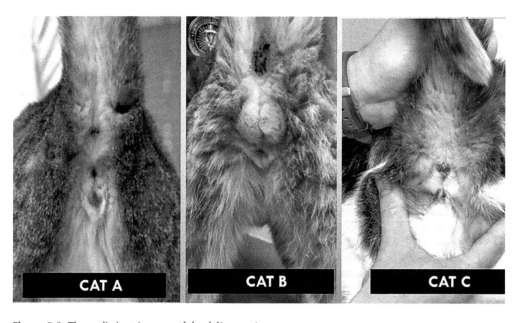

CAT A   CAT B   CAT C

Figure 5.2 Three distinct images of the feline perineum.

Answers to Round One of Questions for Case 5: The Snotty, Squinty Kitten

1. Mentation is an important aspect of assessing each patient during a clinical consultation. It refers to how the patient interacts with and responds to external stimuli.(1, 2) A patient that exhibits normal mentation may be described as bright, alert, and responsive (BAR) or quiet, alert, and responsive (QAR). Mentation is often confused with the patient's behavior; however, mentation is distinct. Mentation signifies the patient's level of alertness as opposed to the patient's temperament.(2)

   Abnormal mentation is described along a sliding scale because rarely is alertness "all" or "none."(3–6) In this regard, mentation can be thought of as a dimmer switch rather than a light that is either "off" or "on."

   Depressed patients exhibit the mildest form of abnormal mentation. A depressed patient is aware of yet less responsive towards its surroundings. Some clinicians might describe the patient's behavior as being lethargic. The patient appears less active.

   The classic example of a neurologically normal, yet depressed patient is one that is febrile. However, depression can also result from non-infectious diseases, such as a lesion within the central nervous system (CNS).(4) Both the cerebrum and the ascending reticular activating system (ARAS), a collection of neurons that extend from the medulla of the brainstem to the thalamus, contribute to mentation.(2) When there is a space-occupying mass in one or both of these pathways or when there is vascular compromise to one or both areas of the brain, then the patient's mental state can be compromised.(2)

   Patients that exhibit progressively intense abnormalities in mentation are described as being: (5–7)

   * obtunded
   * stuporous
   * comatose.

   An obtunded patient is more than just depressed. Being obtunded denotes mental dullness.(1) The patient's response to external stimuli is markedly decreased. Many patients who present in hypovolemic shock are obtunded. Other examples of obtunded patients include cats that are significantly hypothermic.

   A patient that is stuporous is even less responsive than one that is obtunded. A stuporous patient only responds to noxious stimuli.(1) Calling its name will not rouse the patient. Petting the cat will not rouse it, but a pinch between the toes will.

   Comatose patients lose all responsiveness to external stimuli, even those that are noxious. Nothing, not even pain, provokes a response. These patients act as if they are in the deepest possible plane of anesthesia. They are wholly unaware of their surroundings.(3–5, 8)

   So what? Why does mentation matter? When a cat or dog is a long-term patient it is helpful to track mentation at each visit so that you are aware of trends. For instance, it is a concern if the patient that has always been hypervigilant in the examination room is suddenly sleeping during a consultation. This is inappropriate given the patient's typical response to the environment. This abnormal awareness (or lack thereof) should clue us in to something being out of sorts with the patient.

   Because this is our first-time meeting Mambo, we must rely upon Johnny to share details about their interactions at home. It is important to take a comprehensive patient history to elicit what constitutes "normal" for the kitten, keeping in mind that they are only just getting to know one another.

2. The normal reference range for feline rectal temperature is 100.5–102.5°F, although this range varies somewhat depending upon your choice of reference text.(1, 9) Given Mambo's current activity level and his depressed state of mind, his rectal temperature is abnormal and is considered elevated.

3. Heart rate for a cat is largely dependent upon sympathetic tone. The resting heart rate of an adult cat in its home environment is 120–140 beats per minute.(10) The heart rate of an adult cat in a clinic setting tends to be much greater, averaging 180–220 beats per minute. Stress activates the sympathetic nervous system, causing the heart to beat faster and with greater force. This pathway is particularly accentuated in cats. Stress elicits tachycardia and hypertension. Collectively, this is referred to as "white coat syndrome."(1)

    If Mambo were stressed to the point that would be necessary to elicit this degree of tachycardia, then we would expect him to present with bilateral mydriasis, that is, dilated pupils. Cats' pupils dilate when the sympathetic nervous system is activated during "fight or flight."(1) This transforms the vertical slit shape of the pupil into saucers.

    If Mambo were stressed, then we might also expect to see a change in his ear carriage. Feline ears are an important part of their body language because they are quite dynamic and expressive. (11) Ears tend to be asymmetrically positioned in cats that are uncertain or uncomfortable with their environment, meaning that one or both ears swivel to the side.(1) Stressed cats may also present with what I like to refer to as "airplane ears," that is, they are flattened or pinned down, denoting that the patient is on guard and high alert.

    None of these descriptions fit Mambo's presentation. He is depressed, meaning that he is less aware of his surroundings, rather than exhibiting heightened awareness.

    His elevation in heart rate is therefore more consistent with his age and/or elevation in temperature.

4. The normal reference range for respiratory rate of a kitten should match an adult's as soon as that kitten reaches four weeks of age.(12) This range is 20–40 breaths per minute.(13, 14) An increased respiratory rate in a cat may indicate airway or cardiac disease.(1) A cat that is breathing faster may also simply be stressed.(1)

    Given Mambo's mentation as well as his history of nasal discharge, it is likely that upper airway disease is complicating respiration. If his upper airways are narrowed by copious nasal discharge and/or inflammation of the nasal mucosa, then he may feel like he is breathing through a straw. His body will respond with tachypnea to take in more air for gas exchange so that tissues can remain oxygenated.(1)

    Cats do not typically breathe through their mouth, so their response to nasal congestion is to breathe faster rather than change the route of air flow.

Returning to Case 5: The Snotty, Squinty Kitten

You proceed to examine Mambo. In addition to Mambo's abnormal values for TPR, you identify the following abnormalities:

- photophobia
- blepharospasm, OD>OS
- chemosis OU
- conjunctivitis OU
- prominent nictitans OU
- green-yellow ocular discharge OU
- green-yellow nasal discharge
- decreased airflow through both nostrils
- audible upper airway congestion.

By the way, your technician is correct. You lift the tail to find that Mambo is female, so her perineum matches the image of cat C in Figure 5.2.

Round Two of Questions for Case 5: The Snotty, Squinty Kitten

1. Define the following terms:

    a. photophobia   b. blepharospasm   c. chemosis

2. What is the nictitans?
3. What do the following abbreviations stand for?

    a. OD   b. OS   c. OU

4. Where within the SOAP note format of medical documentation do you record pertinent physical exam findings?

Answers to Round Two of Questions for Case 5: The Snotty, Squinty Kitten

1. Photophobia is light sensitivity. Patients with photophobia often exhibit blepharospasm, that is, they squint. Squinting may be unilateral or bilateral.

    The conjunctiva of a healthy cat is thin, smooth, and relatively transparent.(15, 16) When the conjunctiva becomes swollen from inflammation, it takes on a "puffy" appearance.(15, 17) This is quite pronounced in cats. The appropriate medical terminology to describe this clinical appearance is chemosis. Chemosis indicates that there is some degree of conjunctival edema. (18)

2. The nictitans, sometimes referred to as the nictitating membrane, is a normal structure that is associated with the canine and feline eye. In non-medical terms, it is the third eyelid.(19, 20) Decades ago, this structure was called the haw and it was erroneously thought to be vestigial, like the appendix or wisdom teeth.(21)

    The nictitans plays an important role in ocular health. Seated in the ventro-medial orbit, it consists of a T-shaped hyaline cartilage that acts like a windshield wiper.(20) Every time the patient blinks, the nictitans glides across the surface of the cornea to spread tears across the surface of the eye.(20) This maintains ocular moisture and a smooth refractive surface for the cornea. In addition, the nictitans protects the globe from external stimuli.(20) When something such as particulate matter from the surroundings comes at the eye suddenly, the nictitans pops up like a catcher in a game of baseball to block entry to the eye.

    Barring foreign objects that come flying at the globe, the nictitans remains hidden, out of sight, tucked into a pocket within the orbit. The sympathetic tone of the orbital smooth muscles maintains this hidden position such that, in health, the veterinarian must manipulate the soft tissue over each orbit in order to elevate the nictitans for visual inspection.(19)

    The nictitans often becomes prominent in cases of ocular disease. It is thought that this is a protective function. When a patient presents to me with a prominent nictitans, then I must rule out ocular pain and injury, as might be caused by a corneal ulcer.(17)

3. These terms are conventional abbreviations that stem from the Latin names for certain body parts as outlined here: (22)

    OD   *Oculus dexter*, right eye
    OS   *Oculus sinister*, left eye
    OU   *Oculus uterque*, both eyes

4. By convention, physical exam findings are listed in the "O" or objective section of the SOAP note. The SOAP note is a standard form in medical documentation. Its purpose is to provide a written summary of every consultation. Whereas the "S" section of the SOAP note contains historical data, the "O" section reports patient-specific, measurable data.(22) For more information about how to create proper medical documentation, refer to my manual, *Writing Skills for Veterinarians*.

Returning to Case 5: The Snotty, Squinty Kitten

You review key physical exam findings with Mambo's owner. You express concern that Mambo has contracted an upper respiratory infection (URI) and bilateral conjunctivitis. Based upon her age, her history (unknown past, acquired recently from the shelter; acclimating to a new home), your primarily differential diagnosis is feline herpesvirus (FHV-1). You propose additional diagnostic tests to guide your treatment plan.

Round Three of Questions for Case 5: The Snotty, Squinty Kitten

1. Other than conjunctivitis, which ocular malady has been linked to FHV-1?
2. Which diagnostic test do you recommend to evaluate Mambo for the condition that you identified in the previous question? Walk me through how you perform this test. If Mambo tests (+) for the condition of interest, what will you expect to see?
3. How will you manage Mambo's ocular condition?
4. Are there any contraindications to treatment for Mambo's ocular condition?
5. What is your recommended diagnostic plan for Mambo's presumptive URI?
6. What is your recommendation for treating Mambo's presumptive URI?
7. Your client asks if administering the nutraceutical, lysine, will improve Mambo's recovery. How do you respond?
8. What are other potential causes of infectious conjunctivitis in cats? What are other potential causes of URI in cats?
9. If you had identified one or more lingual ulcerations on examination of Mambo's oral cavity, which infectious agent might you have prioritized?

Answers to Round Three of Questions for Case 5: The Snotty, Squinty Kitten

1. FHV-1 has been associated with viral keratitis.(2) Keratitis means inflammation of the cornea. Inflammation may be diffuse or focal. Focal areas of inflammation may cause a corneal ulcer to form. Corneal ulcers are essentially damaged regions of the cornea. When they occur, they disrupt the corneal epithelium. This creates pain because an ulcer is essentially a raw and open sore. This may contribute to some of the clinical signs that Mambo has presented with today, including photophobia, blepharospasm, ocular discharge, and elevated nictitating membranes bilaterally.

   Not all cats that succumb to FHV-1 develop corneal ulcers. However, those that do often present with classic so-called dendritic ulcers.(23–26) These are linear and branching. (See **Plate 2**)

2. Corneal ulcers are most easily detected using fluorescein as a diagnostic test.(27) Fluorescein is a water-soluble stain that is applied to the cornea. It is marketed either as a pre-made solution or impregnated onto a commercial strip where in high concentration it appears orange.(27–29)
   When diluted with sterile saline, it appears green.

Most practices purchase the strips for longer shelf life and to avoid risk of contaminating the stock bottle of fluorescein. There are two ways to make use of the strip. I prefer to use the strip to make my own solution. This solution is created easily in-house by inserting the fluorescein strip into the barrel of a 3 cc or 6 cc syringe, then filling the syringe up with sterile 0.9% saline. (27) The mixture is then squirted onto the surface of the cornea without attaching a needle to the syringe. I find that most patients tolerate this well.

Alternatively, some clinicians touch the dry fluorescein strip itself to the dorsal bulbar conjunctiva.(27). The clinician then gently closes and opens the patient's eyelids a few times to force them to blink. This allows the fluorescein to spread across the surface of the globe. Finally, sterile saline is flushed over the eye to wash off any extra stain.

Fluorescein cannot bind to or stain intact corneal epithelium. However, where there is a break in the epithelium, the stain can and will adhere to the hydrophilic stroma. When the cornea is then illuminated by an intense cobalt blue light, the stained cornea will fluoresce a brilliant green color.(15, 27, 29, 30) This is diagnostic for a corneal ulcer.

Note that even if a patient presents with unilateral clinical signs, it is standard practice to stain both eyes. It is possible that the patient's presentation involves both eyes, but one eye is not as advanced in terms of outward clinical signs and visible progression of disease.

3. Superficial corneal ulcers, such as those caused by FHV-1, typically heal rapidly without scarring.(27) Even so, it is advisable to prescribe topical antibiotic therapy to protect against secondary bacterial infection as might occur due to opportunistic invaders during the healing phase.(27, 31–33)

It is also important to address the patient's discomfort. Corneal ulcers are quite painful. Pain that is associated with the open sore is often exacerbated by ciliary muscle spasms. These can be effectively managed by prescribing the mydriatic agent, atropine.(27) This maintains the pupil in a dilated state. Dilation of the pupil of the affected eye blocks ciliary muscle action.

Backing up for a moment to consider the big picture, it is important to prepare clients that complete clearance of FHV-1 is not possible. This virus is uniquely able to persist within the trigeminal ganglion for the life of the host.(23, 34–36) This latency allows FHV-1 to reactivate. It is important to prepare the client that Mambo could experience relapse or recurrence of clinical signs.(23)

Anti-viral therapy may be considered for patients who continue to have severe clinical signs. Topical therapy with 0.1% idoxuridine OU every 4 to 6 hours is purported to slow replication of FHV-1. However, not all cats are tolerant of topical therapy, especially at that frequency and long-term. In these situations, the anti-viral agent famciclovir may be prescribed at 62.5 mg/cat per os (PO) every 8 to 12 hours or 125 mg/cat once per day. Kittens receive a fraction of a dose at 15.625–31.25 mg/kitten PO once per day.(37)

4. Corticosteroids are contraindicated for use in the management of corneal ulcers.(38) At best, they delay or halt healing of the cornea. At worst, they may deepen the ulcer. It is imperative that you adhere to this critical aspect of management of ocular disease because it is essential for providing gold standard care.

You must be extra cautious when prescribing combination products for ocular disease because there are several combination products ("triple antibiotic" preps, for instance, such as Neo-Poly Bac), some of which contain corticosteroids while others do not. Medical errors happen in clinical practice. Double-check what you have prescribed and what you have dispensed to avoid an unnecessarily poor patient outcome.

You also may be tempted to include a corticosteroid to reduce chemosis. It is true that corticosteroids are often prescribed to manage conjunctivitis. When conjunctivitis is not paired with a corneal ulcer, this is an appropriate treatment plan. But when there is a concurrent ulcer, prescription of a corticosteroid could be considered malpractice.

5. There are many possible causes of nasal discharge. Although in theory every differential diagnosis should be explored in every patient, that is often not the reality of clinical practice. Clients often prefer to treat what is most likely and seek diagnostic testing when patient response to therapy is poor. Client communication is an essential aspect of the diagnostic and therapeutic plan. It is important to partner with clients and elicit their perspective to see if their expectations align with yours.

    When a patient such as Mambo presents with clinical signs that are suggestive of URI and it is a first-time offense, then patient signalment and history appreciably narrow the list of differential diagnoses into those that are most versus least likely. Most likely, Mambo has developed a bacterial URI secondary to FHV-1.

    Oropharyngeal swabs may be used for viral isolation to confirm and/or rule out FHV-1, or FHV-1 may be detected by polymerase chain reaction (PCR) using conjunctival swabs.(34, 39–41) However, the reality is that FHV-1 is ubiquitous: eighty-percent of cats worldwide are thought to be carriers and 95% have been exposed.(36, 41–47) Therefore, we typically assume FHV-1 infection until proven otherwise.

    Concerning Mambo's presumptive bacterial infection, we could in theory culture her nasal discharge. However, the sample is likely to be contaminated by resident flora.(48) Therefore, more often than not for a first-time offense in a kitten, we skip airway diagnostics in favor of treatment.

    One exception to this tendency to treat presumptive illness without further defining it is the standard point-of-care combination feline leukemia (FeLV) and feline immunodeficiency virus (FIV) test. This diagnostic tool is advised for use in all new household additions as well as in any sick kitten or cat that presents to the clinic.(49) Feline serological status is essential because of the implications that FeLV or FIV have on the patient's systemic health. Kittens or cats with FeLV/FIV can lead good quality, productive lives; however, they are at greater risk for relapses and may require additional treatment considerations.

6. The treatment plan for Mambo's presumptive URI is by and large supportive. Critical aims of therapy include monitoring appetite and hydration.

    Cats are scent-driven when it comes to appetite. Cats with upper airway congestion are likely to experience a dulled sense of olfaction, that is, if they can smell at all. This is likely to result in a sharp decline in appetite or even anorexia.

    To improve appetite, you might consider canned food because it tends to carry a stronger odor than kibble. As a bonus, warm the food. This will enhance its aroma and may improve its palatability. Exercise caution, though, if instructing the client to warm food through the microwave. This can lead to uneven pockets of heat throughout the food, which could result in oral erosions and burns. To guard against this inherent danger, stir food well after heating. As an extra precaution, dab a sample of food onto your wrist in the same way that you might check the temperature of milk from a baby bottle. If the sample of food can comfortably sit on your wrist without scalding, then it is safe for consumption by the patient.

    Note that Mambo's pyrexia may contribute to inappetence. Systemic non-steroidal anti-inflammatory drugs (NSAIDs) can be prescribed to reduce fever, provided that the patient is adequately hydrated. Use of NSAIDs in the face of dehydration is medically unsound.

    Hydration must be assessed at the initial visit, prior to initiating NSAID therapy. To assess hydration, several parameters can be evaluated:(1, 50, 51)

    - skin turgor
    - moisture associated with the mucous membranes
    - eye position within the orbits
    - heart rate
    - peripheral pulse quality
    - capillary refill time.

Skin turgor is widely used as a baseline measure of hydration on the physical exam. Skin turgor is a means by which we can assess skin elasticity. To evaluate this aspect of patient health, gently but securely grasp a fold of skin at the nape of the neck or between the shoulder blades. Hold this fold of skin between your thumb and fingers. Lift it up and twist it to one side using a flick of the wrist. This process is called "tenting the skin." You then release the skin fold. One of two outcomes is possible.(1)

- If the patient is hydrated, then the fold of skin returns to its normal position almost instantaneously. In other words, there is skin elasticity, which means that the patient lacks a persistent "skin tent."
- If the patient is dehydrated, there is a variable degree in the loss of skin elasticity that causes the skin to be slow to bounce back to its normal position. As dehydration progresses, the skin remains "tented."

Dehydrated patients should not receive NSAIDs. Instead, dehydrated patients benefit from fluid therapy. The degree to which the patient is dehydrated dictates route of fluid administration, that is, whether fluid should be given intravenously or can be administered subcutaneously, with slower uptake and absorption.

Broad-spectrum antibiotic therapy is often given at the discretion of the clinician, provided that they are able to penetrate the respiratory tract. First-line drugs of choice include oral administration of amoxicillin or doxycycline. Alternatively, the combination product, amoxicillin/clavulanic acid (Clavamox), is a popular choice. The liquid formulation is most appropriate for dosing kittens and is administered PO every 12 hours. Such liquid formulations require reconstitution. Follow instructions carefully and instruct owners to do the same. Failure to reconstitute as directed and/or failure to refrigerate the product after reconstituting will adversely impact drug efficacy.

7. The recommendation that cats with FHV-1 be given L-lysine orally was originally borrowed from human medicine.(52–55) L-lysine in people appears to reduce outbreaks of herpes simplex virus (HSV) and/or their severity because it antagonizes arginine, an amino acid that is essential for viral replication.(52–55)

   Veterinary medical reports offer mixed reviews as to the efficacy of L-lysine administration in cats with FHV-1.(56–58) Although the majority of feline practitioners recommend that it be given as an interventional therapy for FHV-1, a systemic review of the literature in 2015 did not back up this recommendation.(59) Moreover, there is concern that lysine supplementation in some cases may even increase frequency of FHV-1 flare-ups and/or severity of clinical signs.(59)

8. Mambo was diagnosed with presumptive URI and conjunctivitis.
   In cats, the most common causes of infectious conjunctivitis are:(24, 41, 60)

- feline herpesvirus type-1 (FHV-1)
- *chlamydophila felis*
- *mycoplasma* spp.
- feline calicivirus
- *bordetella bronchiseptica.*

All of these infectious agents can also induce URI. However, the severity of clinical signs of URI in all is not the same. For example, *Chlamydophila felis* is characterized as having mild respiratory signs, if any.(23)

9. Of the infectious agents listed in the answer to question #8 (above), only two cause oral lesions: FHV-1 and calicivirus. Of these, feline calicivirus is much more likely than FHV-1 to cause ulcerations of the oral, lingual, and oropharyngeal mucosa.(23, 41) For this reason, oral ulceration and/or stomatitis are considered hallmark signs for feline calicivirus rather than FHV-1.(41)

CLINICAL PEARLS

- There are several infectious agents that cause URI and conjunctivitis in kittens and cats. Of these, FHV-1 is commonly implicated.

- FHV-1 is a unique virus in that it takes up residence in the host's trigeminal ganglion, where it will persist for life.

- Cats that have been infected with FHV-1 are likely to experience viral recrudescence during times of stress.

- Stressful situations, such as relinquishment to a shelter, relocation from one residence to another, unanticipated travel or stay within a boarding facility, and/or additions/subtractions to the household (i.e. new cat, new dog, new baby) can cause FHV-1 to come out of latency.

- When kittens or cats present with clinical signs that are related to one or both eyes (i.e. presence of ocular discharge; change in amount/color/consistency/frequency of ocular discharge, photophobia, blepharospasm, chemosis, so-called "red eye," pawing at the eye, and/or conjunctivitis), it is important to perform the fluorescein stain test.

- Staining both eyes (even if only one appears to be clinically affected!) with fluorescein will confirm or rule out corneal ulcers.

- The classic type of corneal ulcer that is caused by FHV-1 is a dendritic (branching or linear) ulcer. This is a superficial ulcer that tends to respond well to supportive care.

- Never prescribe topical corticosteroids for conjunctivitis in the presence of a corneal ulcer as this may delay healing and/or deepen the ulcer, risking corneal melting and/or rupture of the globe.

- Secondary bacterial URIs are common in kittens or cats that are afflicted with FHV-1. Antibiotics are prescribed at the clinician's discretion. If antibiotics are prescribed, they should be broad-spectrum with good penetration of the respiratory tract.

- Appetite is important to monitor in cats with URI. Upper airway congestion can decrease appetite or inhibit altogether.

- Offering canned food or warming food may help to intensify its aroma and penetrate the upper airway congestion.

References

1. Englar RE. Performing the small animal physical examination. Hoboken, NJ: Wiley/Blackwell; 2017.
2. Englar RE. Common clinical presentations in dogs and cats. Hoboken, NJ: Wiley/Blackwell; 2019.
3. van Nes JJ, Meij BP, van Ham L. Nervous system. In: Rijnberk A, van Sluijs FJ, editors. Medical history and physical examination in companion animals. 2nd ed. St. Louis, MO: Saunders Elsevier; 2009. p. 160–74.
4. Thomas WB. Initial assessment of patients with neurologic dysfunction. Vet Clin North Am Small Anim Pract 2000;30(1):1–24, v, v.
5. Garosi L. Neurological examination of the cat. How to get started. J Feline Med Surg 2009;11(5):340–8.
6. Englar RE. Performing the small animal physical examination. Hoboken, NJ: Wiley; 2017.
7. Thomas WB, Dewey CW. Performing the neurologic examination. In: Dewey CW, editor. A practical guide to canine and feline neurology. 2nd ed. Ames, IA: Wiley/Blackwell; 2008. p. 53–74.
8. Averill DR, Jr. The neurologic examination. Vet Clin North Am Small Anim Pract 1981;11(3):511–21.

9. Rijnberk A, Stokhof AA. General examination. In: Rijnberk A, van Sluijs FJ, editors. Medical history and physical examination in companion animals. New York, NY: Elsevier Limited; 2009.

10. Merck Vet Man. Whitehouse Station, NJ: Merck & Co., Inc. 2016.

11. Overall KL. Clinical behavioral medicine for small animals. St. Louis: Mosby. 544 p; 1997.

12. Root Kustritz MV. History and physical examination of the neonate. In: Peterson ME, Kutzler MA, editors. Small animal pediatrics: the first 12 months of life. St. Louis, MO: Saunders; 2011. p. 20–7.

13. Rijnberk A, van Sluijs FS. Medical history and physical examination in companion animals. The Netherlands: Elsevier Limited. 333 p; 2009.

14. Cote E, MacDonald KA, Meurs KM, Sleeper MM. Feline cardiology. Ames, IA: Wiley/Blackwell; 2011.

15. Englar RE. Performing the small animal physical examination. Hoboken, NJ: Wiley; 2017. pages cm p.

16. Dyce KM, Sack WO, Wensing CJG. Textbook of veterinary anatomy. 4th ed. St. Louis, MO: Saunders/Elsevier, 2010.

17. Lim CC. Small animal ophthalmic atlas and guide. xiii, 151 pages p.

18. Smith RIE. The cat with ocular discharge or changed conjunctival appearance. In: Rand J, editor. Problem-based feline medicine. Edinburgh. New York: Saunders; 2006. p. 1207–32.

19. Maggs DJ. Third eyelid. In: Maggs DJ, Miller PE, Ofri R, Slatter DH, editors. Slatter's fundamentals of veterinary ophthalmology. 5th ed. St. Louis, MO: Elsevier; 2013. p. 151–6.

20. Brooks DE. Removal of the third eyelid. NAVC Clin's Brief 2005(January):47–9.

21. Miller P. Why do cats have an inner eyelid as well as outer ones? Scientific American [Internet]; 2006. Available from: https://www.scientificamerican.com/article/why-do-cats-have-an-inner/.

22. Englar R. Writing skills for veterinarians. Sheffield: 5m Publishing; 2019.

23. Lim CC, Maggs DJ. Ophthalmology. In: Little SE, editor. The cat: clinical medicine and management. St. Louis, MO: Saunders Elsevier; 2012. p. 807–45.

24. Mitchell N. Feline ophthalmology Part 2: Clinical presentation and aetiology of common ocular conditions. Ir Vet J 2006;59(4):223.

25. Plummer CE. Herpetic keratoconjunctivitis in a cat. NAVC Clin's Brief 2012 (January):26–8.

26. Smith L. The dos and don'ts of treating ocular disease in cats (Proceedings). DVM. 360 [Internet]; 2011. Available from: http://veterinarycalendar.dvm360.com/dos-and-donts-treating-ocular-disease-cats-proceedings.

27. Ollivier FJ. Bacterial corneal diseases in dogs and cats. Clin Tech Small Anim Pract 2003;18(3):193–8.

28. Moore CP, Nasisse MP. Clinical microbiology. In: Gelatt KN, editor. Veterinary ophthalmology. Philadelphia, PA: Lippincott Williams & Wilkins; 1999. p. 259–90.

29. Strubbe TD, Gelatt KN. Ophthalmic examination and diagnostic procedures. In: Gelatt KN, editor. Veterinary ophthalmology. Philadelphia, PA: Lippincott Williams & Wilkins; 1999. p. 427–66.

30. Slatter D. Fundamentals of veterinary ophthalmology. Philadelphia, PA: Saunders; 1990.

31. Whitley RD. Canine and feline primary ocular bacterial infections. Vet Clin North Am Small Anim Pract 2000;30(5):1151–67.

32. Slatter DH, Dietrich U. Cornea and sclera. In: Slatter DH, editor. Textbook of small animal surgery. Philadelphia, PA: W. B. Saunders; 1985. p. 1368–9.

33. Regnier A. Antimicrobials, anti-inflammatory agents, and antiglaucoma drugs. In: Gelatt KN, editor. Veterinary ophthalmology. Philadelphia, PA: Lippincott Williams & Wilkins; 1999. p. 297–336.

34. Grahn BH, Sandmeyer LS. Diagnostic ophthalmology. Can Vet J 2010;51(3):327–.

35. Nasisse MP, Davis BJ, Guy JS, Davidson MG, Sussman W. Isolation of feline herpesvirus 1 from the trigeminal ganglia of acutely and chronically infected cats. J Vet Intern Med 1992;6(2):102–3.

36. Ofri R. Conjunctivitis in cats. NAVC Clin's Brief 2017 (April):95–100.

37. Plummer CE. Herpetic keratoconjunctivitis in a cat. NAVC Clin's Brief 2012; January:26–8.

38. Hildebrand D. The use of corticosteroids in ocular disease of small animals. Iowa State Univ Vet 1969; 31(2).

39. Tilley LP, Smith FWK. The 5-minute veterinary consult: canine and feline. 3rd ed. Baltimore, MD: Lippincott Williams & Wilkins, 1487 p. p.; 2004.

40. Côté E. Clinical veterinary advisor. Dogs and cats. 3rd ed.. ed. St. Louis, MO: Elsevier Mosby; 2015.

41. Heinrich C. Assessing conjunctivitis in cats. Vet Times [Internet]; 2015. Available from: https://www.vettimes.co.uk/app/uploads/wp-post-to-pdf-enhanced-cache/1/assessing-conjunctivitis-in-cats.pdf.

42. Stiles J. Feline ophthalmology. In: Gelatt KN, Gilger BC, Kern TJ, editors. Veterinary ophthalmology. Ames, IA: Wiley/Blackwell; 2013. p. 1477–559.
43. Stiles J. Ocular manifestations of feline viral diseases. Vet J 2014;201(2):166–73.
44. Stiles J, Pogranichniy R. Detection of virulent feline herpesvirus-1 in the corneas of clinically normal cats. J Feline Med Surg 2008;10(2):154–9.
45. Maggs DJ. Update on pathogenesis, diagnosis, and treatment of feline herpesvirus type 1. Clin Tech Small Anim Pract 2005;20(2):94–101.
46. Gould D. Feline herpesvirus-1: ocular manifestations, diagnosis and treatment options. J Feline Med Surg 2011;13(5):333–46.
47. Westermeyer HD, Thomasy SM, Kado-Fong H, Maggs DJ. Assessment of viremia associated with experimental primary feline herpesvirus infection or presumed herpetic recrudescence in cats. Am J Vet Res 2009;70(1):99–104.
48. Burrow RD, editor. Approach to investigation of nasal disease. British Small Animal Veterinary Congress; 2008.
49. Little S, Levy J, Hartmann K, Hofmann-Lehmann R, Hosie M, Olah G, Denis KS. 2020 AAFP feline retrovirus testing and management guidelines. J Feline Med Surg 2020;22(1):5–30.
50. DiBartola SP, Bateman S. Introduction to fluid therapy. In: DiBartola SP, editor. Fluid, electrolyte, and acid–base disorders in small animal practice. 3rd ed. St. Louis, MO: Saunders/Elsevier; 2006. p. 325–44.
51. DiBartola SP, Bateman S. Introduction to fluid therapy. In: DiBartola SP, editor. Fluid, electrolyte, and acid–base disorders in small animal practice. 4th ed. St. Louis, MO: Saunders/Elsevier; 2006.
52. Griffith RS, Norins AL, Kagan C. A multicentered study of lysine therapy in Herpes simplex infection. Dermatologica 1978;156(5):257–67.
53. Griffith RS, Walsh DE, Myrmel KH, Thompson RW, Behforooz A. Success of L-lysine therapy in frequently recurrent herpes simplex infection. Treatment and prophylaxis. Dermatologica 1987;175(4):183–90.
54. McCune MA, Perry HO, Muller SA, O'Fallon WM. Treatment of recurrent herpes simplex infections with L-lysine monohydrochloride. Cutis 1984;34(4):366–73.
55. Thein DJ, Hurt WC. Lysine as a prophylactic agent in the treatment of recurrent herpes simplex labialis. Oral Surg Oral Med Oral Pathol 1984;58(6):659–66.
56. Stiles J, Townsend WM, Rogers QR, Krohne SG. Effect of oral administration of L-lysine on conjunctivitis caused by feline herpesvirus in cats. Am J Vet Res 2002;63(1):99–103.
57. Maggs DJ, Nasisse MP, Kass PH. Efficacy of oral supplementation with L-lysine in cats latently infected with feline herpesvirus. Am J Vet Res 2003;64(1):37–42.
58. Drazenovich TL, Fascetti AJ, Westermeyer HD, Sykes JE, Bannasch MJ, Kass PH, et al. Effects of dietary lysine supplementation on upper respiratory and ocular disease and detection of infectious organisms in cats within an animal shelter. Am J Vet Res 2009;70(11):1391–400.
59. Bol S, Bunnik EM. Lysine supplementation is not effective for the prevention or treatment of feline herpesvirus 1 infection in cats: a systematic review. BMC Vet Res 2015;11:284.
60. Millichamp NJ. Ocular diseases unique to the feline patient. DVM. 360 [Internet]; 2010. Available from: http://veterinarycalendar.dvm360.com/ocular-diseases-unique-feline-patient-proceedings.

Case 6

The Coughing Puppy

Joshua Marlowe and his fiancé Sabrina had more than enough on their plates without adding to their family. Their fur baby, Titan the Golden Retriever, was a 6-year-old neutered male bundle of energy that never grew out of puppyhood. He constantly kept them on the move. They often joked that he'd missed the memo that weekends were for rest and relaxation.

Titan was not so much into R&R. He was more of a weekend warrior. From dawn to dusk, he wanted to be on the move. No amount of activity was too great. This family of three could hike for five miles or ten, it didn't matter. Titan was as exuberant on the final leg as he was at the start, to the point that he was starting to wear out the couple. Josh and Sabrina got to thinking that perhaps he could use a four-legged companion. It would give Titan something to do while allowing them the freedom to get back to wedding planning. The big day was just three months away and there was a ton of work to be done in preparation.

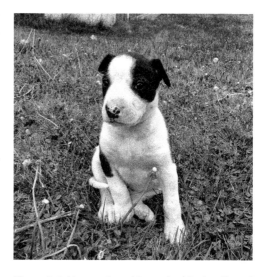

Figure 6.1 Your patient, 12-week-old mixed breed dog, Samba. Courtesy of Riley County Humane Society (RCHS)

Friends thought they were crazy to consider adding a puppy to the mix, but Josh's response was, "How hard can a puppy be?" Sabrina agreed. If couples they knew could raise infants and work full time – and make it seem easy, then a puppy should be a breeze. Besides, what could possibly go wrong?

So it was that this Saturday found the pair trading hiking shoes for a walk down the aisle at the local shelter. The shelter had posted online that several pups were available for adoption and their descriptions matched the couple's wish list. They didn't care so much about breed. They just wanted a rough-and-tumble companion who could give Titan a run for his money.

They fell in love with Samba instantly. His Oreo cookie coloring and mottled nose made Sabrina smile. He reminded her of the Holsteins that filled childhood memories of her parents' dairy farm. His name came from Josh's favorite Latin dance. As a top-level instructor for the Arrowhead Arthur Murray franchise, he was constantly perfecting his sport – and thought a name such as Samba might inspire his students to work on their voltas.

Samba came home with them that afternoon and instantly bonded with Titan. Titan never let Samba out of his sight. He was just the kind of big brother that Josh and Sabrina had hoped for – curious, yet welcoming; gentle yet playful. In fact, that first night home, the two played so hard that they nearly forgot to eat dinner! Josh had to separate them to get them to settle long enough to gulp their kibble before they were back at it in the living room.

Life seemed to be working out for the best until a cough developed 2 days after Samba became a member of the Marlowe household. The cough was slight and only Samba exhibited it. At first,

Sabrina chalked it up to Samba tugging on the collar – he was still acclimating to a leash and often pulled so hard that he would choke himself. Then the cough happened indoors, at rest. It was an isolated cough initially. Then it persisted into the next day. By that night, it was clear that the cough wasn't going away. It was more frequent, and it seemed to be getting worse. Activity intensified the cough, which Josh describes as "harsh." Samba sounded like a "goose." He would cough so loudly and so hard that he appeared to gag. It was common now to see him spit up a bit of phlegm at the end of each coughing fit. Samba was still active and playful. If he felt bad, he certainly didn't show it. Samba continued to eat and drink and act like an otherwise normal pup.

Josh telephoned the shelter and spoke with the manager, who advised him to seek veterinary medical care. Although the manager said that colds were common in pups, she expressed concern that if left untreated, it could turn into pneumonia, so it was best that Samba be evaluated right away.

Samba presented to you just now as a 12-week-old castrated male mixed breed dog. Your technician recorded his vital signs as follows:

On physical exam, you identify the following abnormalities:

- serous ocular discharge bilaterally
- clear nasal discharge from both nostrils
- paroxysmal dry cough elicited on tracheal palpation
- retching at the end of coughing fits
- frothy sputum
- bilaterally symmetrical, palpably enlarged submandibular lymph nodes.

Mentation: BAR

TEMPERATURE, PULSE, AND RESPIRATION (TPR)

T: 100.8°F (38.2°C)
P: 98 beats per minute
R: 20 breaths per minute

Round One of Questions: Medical Documentation

1. What is Samba's signalment?
2. What is the patient's chief complaint (cc)? Sometimes this is referred to as the presenting complaint.
3. In which section of the medical record will you record Samba's patient history?
4. How would you summarize Samba's history in his medical record?
5. The clinical vignette (above) represents an incomplete patient history. What additional data should be gathered during history-taking and documented in the medical record?
6. How might you abbreviate the phrase, castrated male, as listed in Samba's signalment?
7. In which section of the medical record do you record Samba's physical examination findings?
8. Based upon Samba's history and physical examination findings, which differential diagnoses will you prioritize?
9. Identify risk factors for the differential diagnoses that you have considered.
10. In broad terms, describe the morbidity and/or mortality of the differential diagnoses that you have considered.
11. In broad terms, consider the incubation period for most infections that result in canine infectious respiratory disease (CIRD).
12. In which section of the medical record will you outline these differentials?
13. Why is it important not to have tunnel vision when compiling your list of differentials?
14. What tools may help new graduates to compile their list of differentials?
15. In which section of the medical record will you outline next steps for diagnostic testing and/or therapeutic recommendations?

Answers to Round One of Questions for Case 6: The Coughing Puppy

1. The signalment refers to the patient's age, sex, sexual status, breed, and species.(1) Samba's signalment is: 12-week-old castrated male mixed breed dog or 12-week-old castrated male mixed breed puppy. Either is correct. Puppy simply clarifies Samba's life stage.

2. The patient's chief complaint is a progressive cough.

3. By convention, historical data is listed in the "S" or subjective section of the SOAP note.(1) The SOAP note is a standard form in medical documentation.(1) Its purpose is to provide a written summary of every consultation.(1)

4. Based upon the information that can be gleaned from the clinical vignette, I would document the following case details in the subjective section of Samba's SOAP note for today's visit.

   - Signalment: 12-week-old castrated male mixed breed puppy.
   - Adopted this past Saturday from shelter.
   - Co-owned by Josh and Sabrina.
   - One other pet in household: 6-year-old castrated male Golden Retriever, Titan.
   - Cough developed 2 days post-adopted. Slight. Initially related to tugging on the collar?
   - Progressed to cough at rest.
   - By the next day, coughing by day and night with frequency; harsh sounding "goose" honk.
   - Cough exacerbated by activity.
   - Cough progresses to retching, phlegm produced.
   - Still eating/drinking.
   - No sneezing/vomiting/diarrhea.
   - Playful, good attitude.
   - Housemate is asymptomatic.

5. In order to be complete, the subjective portion of the medical record should also include:(1)

   - identifying features, such as coat color or microchip number
   - client expectations for the patient: in this case, Samba is intended to be a companion, as opposed to a therapy dog or a working dog
   - lifestyle:

     - any plans for medical boarding or grooming?
     - any plans to frequent lakes/streams?

   - travel history:

     - Did Samba originate from this state/country? Or was he relinquished from another region?

   - travel, any plans to:

     - travel within the state?
     - travel out of state?
     - travel out of the country?

   - derological status
   - diet history
   - current medications, including over-the-counter vitamins and supplements
   - past pertinent health history, including familial, medical, surgical, and reproductive histories
   - vaccination status
   - current preventive care measures

- past pertinent diagnostic tests and tests results
- past pertinent therapeutic trials and outcomes.

6. By convention, sexual status is often abbreviated in the patient's signalment. Castrated male is typically abbreviated as MC in the United States or MN, which stands for male neutered.(1) Below are the common abbreviations for patients of other sexual statuses:(1)

- male intact (MI)
- female intact (FI)
- female spayed (FS) or female neutered (FN)

Outside of the United States, there is another term to denote that a patient is intact.(1) In England, for instance, a patient that is intact is said to be entire, as in an entire female or an entire male.

7. By convention, physical examination findings are listed in the "O" or objective section of the SOAP note.(1)

8. Based upon Samba's history and physical examination findings, I would prioritize CIRD as the most likely cause for the patient's chief complaint (cough). CIRD is often known as "kennel cough" among laypersons.(2) CIRD describes a common syndrome in clinical practice that causes outbreaks of respiratory disease in dogs.(3–7)
   CIRD may involve one or more of the following pathogens:(2, 6–11)

- bacterial

    - *Bordetella bronchiseptica*
    - *Mycoplasma* spp.
    - *Streptococcus equi* subsp. *zooepidemicus*

- viral

    - canine adenovirus-2 (CAV-2)
    - canine distemper virus (CDV)
    - canine herpesvirus
    - canine influenza (H3N8)
    - canine parainfluenza
    - canine respiratory coronavirus.

Co-infection with multiple infectious agents is common.(2) In addition, opportunistic invaders frequently invade the respiratory tract once it has been compromised by airway disease. These pathogens include:(2, 12, 13)

- *Escherichia coli*
- *Klebsiella pneumoniae*
- *Pasteurella* spp.
- *Pseudomonas* spp.
- *Staphylococcus* spp.

9. Young, stressed, and/or immunocompromized patients are most susceptible to CIRD.(4, 6, 13–15) Other risk factors include being in close contact with conspecifics or being housed in crowded conditions, such as pet shops, kennels, or shelters.

10. CIRD is associated with high morbidity.(4) It is highly infectious! Mortality is typically low when it comes to CIRD.(6) However, CIRD can potentially result in respiratory distress, pneumonia, and death.(16)

11. The incubation period depends upon the causative agent; however, it is typically on the order of 2 to 14 days, with active shedding for about the same amount of time post-infection.(4, 17, 18)

12. By convention, differential diagnoses are typically listed in the "A" section of the SOAP note. (1) The "A" stands for either assessment or analysis.(1) Each differential diagnosis that is listed in "A" is linked to one or more problems on the patient's problem list. Let's appreciate how that might work in Samba's case.

    Samba's primary problem is a cough. This presenting complaint would lead the "A" section of Samba's SOAP note. Following cough would be a list of differential diagnoses. CIRD would be at the top of that list. This might appear in the medical record like so:

    A:
       Cough
              DDx: CIRD

13. It may be tempting to zero in on this one differential diagnosis because CIRD is most likely given the patient's age, history, and physical exam findings. Pattern recognition helps seasoned clinicians work up clinical cases based upon prior experience and what is most likely. It is how I automatically jump to CIRD as the most probable cause for Samba's presenting complaint.

    Yet pattern recognition is imperfect. There are other causes of cough. These should be considered here, within the differentials list. Otherwise, I may miss something important in my quest to expedite case management and ultimately patient care.

14. New graduates do not have the same clinical acumen as seasoned practitioners. Novices often struggle with pattern recognition. They do not have an extensive case archive from which they can extrapolate the most likely cause of disease for the patient, based upon past experience and prior case outcomes.

    To facilitate keeping an open mind when it comes to compiling lists of differentials, several acronyms have been developed to guide novices through broad categories of disease to be considered. One such acronym is NITSCOMP DH.(1)

    - neoplasia
    - infectious
    - toxicities
    - structural
    - congenital
    - other
    - metabolic
    - parasitic
    - diet
    - husbandry.

This acronym encourages clinicians to think through other broad categories of disease that could, for instance, cause a cough. If we were to use this acronym to guide Samba's case management, we would find that we zeroed in on infectious causes of disease.

Could anything else cause Samba to cough?

Yes.

Lungworms are a differential diagnosis for parasitic causes of cough.(19) These include *Crenosoma vulpis* and *Eucoleus aerophilus* (syn. *Capillaria aerophila*), as well as the liver fluke, *Paragonimus kellicotti*.(19).

Another acronym that is taught as a tool for building lists of differentials is DAMNIT. There are several versions, depending upon how many of each letter (D, A, M, N, I, and T) are incorporated into the acronym. One example of the DAMNIT scheme has been outlined below:

    - degenerative
    - developmental
    - anomalous
    - autoimmune
    - metabolic
    - mental
    - nutritional
    - neoplastic
    - inflammatory
    - infectious
    - ischemic
    - iatrogenic
    - idiopathic
    - traumatic
    - toxicity.

15. By convention, next steps for diagnostic testing and/or therapeutic recommendations are listed in the "P" section of the SOAP note.(1) "P" stands for plan.

    Key aspects of client communication should also be documented in this section. For example, "client declined radiographs today, but will reconsider if . . ." is a critical aspect of the plan, moving forward, so that clinician and client are on the same page. Both have agreed to re-evaluate next steps if patient response to treatment is unsatisfactory as defined by the clinician. Remember that the medical chart constitutes a legal record. The general rule of thumb is that "if it isn't charted, it didn't happen."(20–25) Errors of omission weaken medical documentation and leave the practice open for litigation.(1)

Returning to Case 6: The Coughing Puppy

You discuss your clinical findings with Josh and Sabrina as well as the high index of suspicion that Samba has CIRD. They elect to proceed with a complete blood count (CBC), serum biochemistry panel, and two-view chest radiographs. Although auscultation of Samba's chest did not identify adventitious lung sounds, you had expressed concern that pneumonia may result from CIRD and that imaging the chest would be proactive as both a precaution and a baseline. (26)

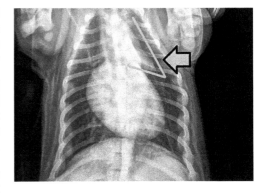

Figure 6.2 Ventrodorsal (V/D) thoracic radiograph.

The CBC is unremarkable. However, there is an elevation in alkaline phosphatase (ALP or ALK PHOS) on the serum biochemistry panel. The reference range for ALP in adults is 4–107 U/L; Samba's ALP measures 182 U/L.

Thoracic radiographs rule out an alveolar pulmonary pattern that is consistent with bacterial pneumonia.(26) Radiographs also rule out the interstitial pulmonary pattern that is sometimes seen early on in the disease process.(26)

When you review Samba's radiographs with the couple, Sabrina's eye catches an unusual structure of soft tissue opacity on the ventrodorsal (V/D) view (see Figure 6.2).

You will be asked to identify the structure in the question set below.

Round Two of Questions for Case 6: The Coughing Puppy

1. You did not hear adventitious lung sounds when you auscultated Samba's chest. What are adventitious lung sounds and what might their presence indicate?
2. What might you have expected to see on Samba's CBC that would have supported a diagnosis of bacterial pneumonia?
3. What is the most likely explanation for the elevation in Samba's ALP?
4. Samba does not appear to have bacterial pneumonia; however, in patients that do, which is the mostly likely pattern of distribution of lung lesions on thoracic radiographs: cranioventral or caudodorsal?
5. How might this pattern of distribution of lung lesions differ if Samba had aspiration pneumonia?
6. Which soft tissue structure on the V/D thoracic radiograph has caught Sabrina's attention? Is this structure something that we need to monitor and/or be concerned about?

Answers to Round Two of Questions for Case 6: The Coughing Puppy

1. When you auscultate the airway, you expect to hear certain sounds, which are considered normal, as opposed to adventitious sounds, which are not.(27) The most common adventitious lung sounds are crackles and wheezes.(27) The presence of one or both support a diagnosis of pneumonia.(28) Let's take a closer look at what these sounds refer to so that we understand how they arise.

    Crackles are "popping" sounds.(27) If you have ever eaten the Kellogg's brand of cereal, Rice Krispies, you will be familiar with its mascots, Snap, Crackle, and Pop. These gnome-like characters came into being to capture the sounds that result from pouring milk over crisped rice. In real life, crackles sound just like that when you auscultate airways that contain copious secretions. Crackles are the sounds that obstructed airways make when they finally open.(27)

    Wheezes are much more musical sounds than crackles.(27) Wheezes occur when previously collapsed airways open during inspiration or close during expiration.(27) Wheezes tell us that the airways have decreased diameter because they are reactive and thickened, or they have collapsed because of neighboring pulmonary disease.(27)

2. The presence of an inflammatory leukogram with pronounced neutrophilia would have been consistent with a diagnosis of bacterial pneumonia.(26) Sometimes, the bloodwork of a patient with pneumonia will also reflect a left shift.(26) This means that there is an increased number of immature leukocytes in circulation, primarily bands.(2, 26)

    Circulating neutrophils may also exhibit toxic changes.(26) This is a misnomer because the changes that you see are not necessarily associated with toxicity. Instead, toxic changes reflect abnormalities in the maturation process of a cell line, as might occur when the body's need for neutrophils expedites their production. This results in neutrophils prematurely entering into circulation before their nucleus and cytoplasm have fully matured.(29)

    Toxic changes include:(29)

    *   basophilic cytoplasm, due to the persistence of polyribosomes
    *   aggregates of rough endoplasmic reticulum within the cytoplasm – these are referred to as Döhle bodies
    *   an apparent frothiness to the cytoplasm, which results from lysosomal degradation
    *   lighter, coarsely clumped chromatin, which reflects nuclear immaturity.

3. Samba's elevation in ALP is most likely to be age-related and is in fact expected in a 12-week-old puppy.(30) The inducible enzyme, ALP, is synthesized by the following tissues:(29, 31)

    *   intestinal epithelium
    *   liver
    *   osteoblasts
    *   placenta
    *   renal epithelium.

    Of these tissues, the majority of serum activity comes from the liver.(29) Accordingly, ALP is one of several serum enzymes that is used to detect cholestasis in adults(29)

    ALP is elevated in both neonates and pediatric patients as compared to adults.(29–31) Colostrum is rich in ALP, so nursing pups are expected to have values that range from 1348–3715 U/L during the first three days of life.(30, 31)

    ALP decreases at 8 to 10 days of age so that it is no longer 30 times higher than adult values. However, ALP remains elevated for the first 16 weeks of life because the osseous isoenzyme is extremely active during periods of bone growth.(31)

4. A caudodorsal distribution of lung lesions is expected in cases of systemic infection and bronchopneumonia.(26)

5. A cranioventral distribution of lung lesions is expected in cases of aspiration pneumonia.(26) The right middle lung lobe is the primary target.(26)

6. The structure that caught Sabrina's eye on the V/D view is the thymus. The thymus is a normal structure in puppyhood.(32) It plays an important role in cell-mediated immunity.(33) T lymphocytes undergo a series of tests within the thymus, beginning with negative selection within the medulla.(33) Here, they are tested to see if they can distinguish self from non-self. If at any point they target self-antigens, they are destroyed.(33)

   Those that survive undergo a second round of testing within the cortex of the thymus.(33) Here, they undergo positive selection for those that exhibit moderate affinity to major histocompatibility class II (MHC II) molecules.(33) Survivors are swept into circulation to inhabit secondary lymphoid organs.(33)

   The thymus appears on radiographs as a triangular piece of soft tissue opacity within the cranial mediastinum.(32) Because of its geometric shape, it is often referred to as the "sail sign" when visualized on the V/D radiograph.(32) It widens at the mediastinum where it crosses near the cranial border of the heart to the left of midline. It involutes at or around 4 to 6 months of age.(32) Because Samba is only 12 weeks, this structure is expected to be present for another few months.

Returning to Case 6: The Coughing Puppy: Round Three of Questions

Josh and Sabrina are relieved to hear that Samba likely has an uncomplicated case of CIRD, but they need your help to identify next steps for the Marlowe family. When you ask what, if anything, concerns them, Sabrina shares that the following questions are weighing on their minds.

1. Because you said that CIRD can be caused by so many 'bugs', does it matter which 'bug' has made Samba sick? In other words, do we need to do any additional testing today?
2. Does Samba need antibiotics?
3. Does Samba need a cough suppressant?
4. If Samba does have kennel cough, is he infectious to Titan?
5. The shelter assured us that Samba had been given a shot for kennel cough. How can he have kennel cough if he's already been vaccinated against it? That doesn't make sense. Did the shelter lie to us about his vaccination record?

Answers to Round Three of Questions for Case 6: The Coughing Puppy

1. If we wanted to determine the etiologic diagnosis, then we would have to perform pathogen-specific diagnostic tests.(2) These may include, but are not limited to:(2)

   - bacterial cultures
   - virus isolation
   - respiratory panels to detect nucleic acid from pathogens, which typically requires an outside diagnostic lab to perform PCR.

   Samples for tests are typically acquired from:(2)

   - nasal swab
   - oropharyngeal swab
   - tracheal wash
   - bronchoalveolar lavage.

As with all test modalities, the diagnostic tools as listed above are imperfect.(2)

- A bacterial culture may report a false-negative result if the patient is in the early stages of CIRD and therefore bacterial load is low.
- Virus isolation may report a false-negative result if viral particles were damaged during transit
- PCR may report a false positive result if the patient was recently vaccinated with live-attenuated immunizations.(34)

When patients present with persistent clinical signs (i.e. lasting >7–10 days) or clinical signs are severe, then it is advised to obtain an etiologic diagnosis.(2) When patients present in the manner that Samba has, with mild clinical signs and without pyrexia or changes in appetite and activity level, it is reasonable to focus case management efforts on treatment.(2)

2. When disease is mild, treatment is supportive.(2) Treatment may include hydrating the patient by means of fluid therapy (as indicated) and nutritional support. Clients are often advised to switch out the leash and collar for a harness to minimize irritation to and tugging on the trachea.(2) Patients may require nebulization and coupage, both of which can be provided in the home environment.

   When disease is mild, antibiotic use is not indicated.(2, 35) Viruses are the primary infectious agent in the majority of cases, meaning that antibiotic use would be ineffectual.(35) Most of these viral cases are self-limiting and expected to spontaneously resolve within 10 days.(35)

   Antimicrobial agents are prescribed when patients present with fever and changes in activity and/or appetite. In the absence of a diagnosis of pneumonia, doxycycline may be prescribed as the first-line antibiotic.(35) Duration of therapy is typically on the order of 7–10 days; however, optimal duration is unknown.(35)

   Patient-specific factors may indicate the need for antibiotic use sooner. For instance, clinicians may be quicker to prescribe when case management involves the structural airway issues of brachycephalic dogs or the functional issues surrounding immune-compromised patients.(35)

   If patient response to the first line of antimicrobial therapy is poor, then a more extensive diagnostic work-up is indicated.(35)

3. Cough suppressants represent a gray zone. On one hand, it is thought that providing relief to dogs that are coughing through the night is beneficial to both the patient and the client.(2) After all, a dog with kennel cough that is not sleeping will likely keep the client awake at night as well. Clinicians may offer recommendations for over-the-counter anti-tussive agents to clients who are interested in pursuing this line of therapy. These products are mild and may take the edge off. However, prescription products such as hydrocodone are more efficacious.

   One concern about prescribing cough suppressants is that coughing serves an important purpose: clearing bacteria from the airway. If we turn off the body's protective function by suppressing the cough, then in theory the patient could be at greater risk for contracting secondary infections.(2, 12)

   Whether or not to use cough suppressants is in many cases a personal choice that should follow a discussion about risks versus benefits.

4. Yes, Titan is at risk of contracting kennel cough. It is highly infectious, dog to dog.(4) Titan has already been exposed so time will tell whether his body is able to fight it off or if he succumbs to CIRD.

5. It is unlikely that the shelter lied about administering the kennel cough vaccine to Samba. An important take-away message to share with Josh and Sabrina that kennel cough vaccines are not protective against all CIRD pathogens.(2) Most so-called kennel cough shots offer some degree of protection against *Bordetella bronchiseptica* and parainfluenza only. Separate vaccinations are required for canine influenza, canine adenovirus (CAV-2), and CDV.

It is also important that Josh and Sabrina understand that vaccines are imperfect, meaning that they do not come with a guarantee of immunity. Consider, for example, the human flu shot. Just because we may receive prophylaxis against the flu annually does not guarantee that we are immune to the flu. Instead, immunizations against the human flu or the canine kennel cough offer reduced duration of illness and severity of clinical signs.

If Samba does in fact have *Bordetella bronchiseptica* or parainfluenza, then it is likely that the kennel cough vaccine, which the shelter administered, contributed to him having mild signs. Other dogs have presented clinically much worse off than Samba. Although no one wants to see a sick pup, Samba is in good shape considering what the alternative could have been.

Once Samba has recovered, it is important that you revisit vaccination protocols with Josh and Sabrina when considering healthcare plans. Specifically, you can share how parenteral vaccines impact the immune system and contrast that with the immune response caused by intranasal or transoral vaccines. It is thought that mucosally administered vaccines speed protection against CIRD pathogens.(2) However, intranasal and transoral vaccines can also induce mild disease.(2) These are important considerations when selecting vaccines. As with every therapeutic recommendation, there are risks as well as benefits. Moving forward, it is critical to engage in open dialogue with Josh and Sabrina, elicit their perspective, and partner with them to develop a patient-specific plan that is mutually agreeable and beneficial to Samba.

CLINICAL PEARLS

- A common cause of cough in puppies is CIRD.

- CIRD is commonly referred to as "kennel cough."

- CIRD does not require kenneling to be contracted. Risk factors include contact with conspecifics as might occur within a household or between households, at dog parks, and at grooming facilities.

- CIRD includes several bacterial and viral pathogens that induce upper airway disease.

- The classic presentation for CIRD involves a harsh, dry, honking cough that is exacerbated by activity.

- CIRD is most often mild, self-limiting, and responsive to supportive care; however, it has the potential to progress to pneumonia.

- Clinical signs and/or physical exam findings that are suggestive of worsening disease include fever, anorexia, and lethargy.

- Thoracic auscultation and radiographs are important screening tools for bronchopneumonia.

- Antibiotic therapy is typically reserved for dogs with persistent and/or progressive clinical signs, fever, lethargy, and altered activity.

- Vaccinations are available to reduce severity of clinical disease, but they do not prevent CIRD.

- It is essential to communicate openly with clients about risk factors, clinical signs, disease progression, and vaccination strategies so that clients understand why we vaccinate.

References

1. Englar R. Writing skills for veterinarians. Sheffield: 5M Publishing; 2019.
2. Reagan KL, Sykes JE. Canine infectious respiratory disease. Vet Clin North Am Small Anim Pract 2020;50(2):405–18.
3. Hurley K. Canine infectious respiratory disease complex: Management and prevention in canine populations. DVM 2010;360.
4. Joffe DJ, Lelewski R, Weese JS, McGill-Worsley J, Shankel C, Mendonca S, et al. Factors associated with development of Canine Infectious Respiratory Disease Complex (CIRDC) in dogs in 5 Canadian small animal clinics. Can Vet J 2016;57(1):46–51.
5. Chalker VJ, Toomey C, Opperman S, Brooks HW, Ibuoye MA, Brownlie J, Rycroft AN. Respiratory disease in kennelled dogs: Serological responses to Bordetella bronchiseptica lipopolysaccharide do not correlate with bacterial isolation or clinical respiratory symptoms. Clin Diagn Lab Immunol 2003;10(3):352–6.
6. Nafe LA. Dogs infected with Bordetella bronchiseptica and Canine influenza virus (H3N8). Today's. Vet Pract 2014 (July/August):30–6.
7. Englar RE. Common clinical presentations in dogs and cats. Hoboken, NJ: Wiley/Blackwell; 2019.
8. Erles K, Brownlie J. Canine respiratory coronavirus: An emerging pathogen in the canine infectious respiratory disease complex. Vet Clin North Am Small Anim Pract 2008;38(4):815–25.
9. Dubovi EJ, Njaa BL. Canine influenza. Vet Clin North Am Small Anim Pract 2008;38(4):827–35.
10. Daniels J, Spencer E. Bacterial infections. In: Peterson ME, Kutzler MA, editors. Small animal pediatrics: The first 12 months of life. St. Louis, MO: Saunders; 2011. p. 113–8.
11. Evermann JF, Kennedy MA. Viral infections. In: Peterson ME, Kutzler MA, editors. Small animal pediatrics: The first 12 months of life. St. Louis, MO: Saunders; 2011. p. 119–30.
12. Thrusfield MV, Aitken CGG, Muirhead RH. A field investigation of kennel cough: Incubation period and clinical signs. J Small Anim Pract 1991;32(5):215–20.
13. Radhakrishnan A, Drobatz KJ, Culp WT, King LG. Community-acquired infectious pneumonia in puppies: 65 Cases (1993–2002). J Am Vet Med Assoc 2007;230(10):1493–7.
14. Priestnall SL, Mitchell JA, Walker CA, Erles K, Brownlie J. New and emerging pathogens in canine infectious respiratory disease. Vet Pathol 2014;51(2):492–504.
15. Holt DE, Mover MR, Brown DC. Serologic prevalence of antibodies against canine influenza virus (H3N8) in dogs in a metropolitan animal shelter. J Am Vet Med Assoc 2010;237(1):71–3.
16. Weese JS, Stull J. Respiratory disease outbreak in a veterinary hospital associated with canine parainfluenza virus infection. Can Vet J 2013;54(1):79–82.
17. Ellis JA, Krakowka GS. A review of canine parainfluenza virus infection in dogs. J Am Vet Med Assoc 2012;240(3):273–84.
18. Erles K, Toomey C, Brooks HW, Brownlie J. Detection of a group 2 coronavirus in dogs with canine infectious respiratory disease. Virology 2003;310(2):216–23.
19. Datz C. Parasitic and protozoal diseases. In: Peterson ME, Kutzler MA, editors. Small animal pediatrics: The first 12 months of life. St. Louis, MO: Saunders; 2011. p. 154–60.
20. Trossman S. The documentation dilemma: Nurses poised to address paperwork burden. Am Nurse 2001;33(5):1–18.
21. Page A, editor. Keeping patients safe: Transforming the work environment of nurses. Washington, DC; 2004.
22. Nguyen AVT, Nguyen DA. Learning from medical errors: Legal issues. Abingdon: Radcliffe; 2005.
23. Andrews A, St. Aubyn B. 'It it's not written down; it didn't happen.' J Commun Nurs 2015;29(5):20–2.
24. Catalano J. Nursing now! Today's issues, tomorrow's trends. 7th ed. Philadelphia, PA: F. A. Davis Company; 2015.
25. David G, Vinkhuyzen E. Medical records' dynamic nature. If it isn't written down, it didn't happen. And if it is written down, it might not be what it seems. J AHIMA 2013;84(11):32–5.
26. Dear JD. Bacterial pneumonia in dogs and cats. Vet Clin North Am Small Anim Pract 2014;44(1):143–59.
27. Englar RE. Performing the small animal physical examination. Hoboken, NJ: Wiley/Blackwell; 2017.
28. Herrtage M, Jones BR. Respiratory disorders: Diseases of the lower respiratory tract. In: Schaer M, editor. Clinical medicine of the dog and cat. Ames, IA: Iowa State Press; 2009. p. 197–211.

29. Thrall MA. Veterinary hematology and clinical chemistry. 2nd ed. Ames, IA: Wiley/Blackwell; 2012.

30. Center SA. The liver, biliary tract, and exocrine pancreas. In: Peterson ME, Kutzler MA, editors. Small animal pediatrics: The first 12 months of life. St. Louis, MO: Saunders; 2011. p. 368–90.

31. Gorman ME. Clinical chemistry of the puppy and kitten. In: Peterson ME, Kutzler MA, editors. Small animal pediatrics: The first 12 months of life. St. Louis, MO: Saunders; 2011. p. 259–75.

32. Mattoon JS. Radiographic considerations of the young patient. In: Peterson ME, Kutzler MA, editors. Small animal pediatrics: The first 12 months of life. St. Louis, MO: Saunders; 2011. p. 169–91.

33. Bird KE. The hematologic and lymphoid systems. In: Peterson ME, Kutzler MA, editors. Small animal pediatrics: The first 12 months of life. St. Louis, MO: Saunders; 2011. p. 305–27.

34. Ruch-Gallie R, Moroff S, Lappin MR. Adenovirus 2, Bordetella bronchiseptica, and parainfluenza molecular diagnostic assay results in puppies after vaccination with modified live vaccines. J Vet Intern Med 2016;30(1):164–6.

35. Lappin MR, Blondeau J, Boothe D, Breitschwerdt EB, Guardabassi L, Lloyd DH, et al. Antimicrobial use guidelines for treatment of respiratory tract disease in dogs and cats: Antimicrobial Guidelines Working Group of the International Society for Companion Animal Infectious Diseases. J Vet Intern Med 2017;31(2):279–94.

Case 7

The Diarrheic Puppy

It's a typical Monday morning at the clinic. Phones are ringing off the hook and you've already been asked to build two walk-in appointments into an overflowing schedule. At this rate, you're not sure how you're going to make it into the operating theatre by 10 A.M., and the surgical techs were counting on you to stay on track. Just when you think you're catching up, any and all progress that you've made towards the finish line is derailed. The third emergency of the morning walks into the waiting room. One of your customer service representatives triages the case and recognizes that the patient must be seen right away.

The patient is a puppy that is coated in fetid, liquified fecal matter. The client has carried him into the office, swaddled in a towel, but he struggles to get loose. As he squirms in the client's

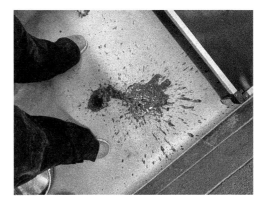

Figure 7.1 Diarrheic sample from your patient, a 10-week-old intact male mixed breed puppy. Courtesy of Rachel Sahrbeck.

arms to partially free himself of the towel, he lifts his tail and squirts diarrhea onto the waiting room floor. The unformed feces splatter on the tile. The smell is putrid. It fills the waiting room. It smells like decaying blood.

Your customer service representative recognizes the characteristic odor and expresses aloud her concern that this puppy could have an infectious disease. Without further delay, she whisks the patient and client duo into an exam room, then catches your attention between appointments to relay pertinent case details.

Your new client, Mrs. Kara Burch, adopted this puppy two days ago from a neighbor, who had taken in the pup's mother as a stray. Unbeknownst to the neighbor, the bitch was pregnant. She whelped six pups 10 weeks ago. Two of the six pups were weak at birth and reportedly "didn't make it." The remaining four appeared to be healthy, although neither the bitch nor the litter were evaluated by a veterinarian.

The neighbor assumed that the bitch was unowned and had not received prior medical attention. He had checked with local shelters for weeks now, and no one had ever called to claim her. He could not afford to keep all four pups plus mom, so he decided to rehome the litter. Kara agreed to take one off his hands. She has a 7-year-old son at home, Collin, who had been begging for a puppy for his eighth birthday. A free pup seemed like a sweet deal . . . until Jackson the pup took ill.

Jackson did not seem interested in dinner that first night in his new house. Kara chalked it up to being a difficult transition for him. After all, it was his first night away from his mother and brothers. But by morning, his appetite was still off, and he didn't have that spark that had attracted her to him in the first place. He seemed depressed and out of sorts.

Kara managed to coax him into ingesting a few pieces of kibble, which he promptly threw up. Shortly thereafter, he broke with yellow-grey diarrhea. He did not appear to be straining during this process. The diarrhea just poured out of him. One episode soon turned into two. By evening, she must have cleaned up four or five piles. She wasn't even sure how he could produce this much fecal matter when his intake had been next to nothing. What Jackson didn't pass out of one end, his rear, he brought up through the other. Vomiting continued overnight until there was nothing left to purge, but foamy froth.

By the time that Monday morning rolled around, it was clear that Kara had an emergency on her hands. She wrapped Jackson in a towel, propped him up in the passenger seat of her car, and drove him to the nearest clinic. Her husband, Steve, stayed behind with Collin. Collin's last words to Jackson were, "Feel better! I'll see you soon!"

Round One of Questions

1. Diarrhea is often defined by where it originates within the gut. Which are the characteristics that help you to distinguish between small bowel and large bowel diarrhea?
2. Based upon the information that you have been given in the clinical vignette, how would you characterize Jackson's diarrhea: is it most likely associated with the small bowel or large bowel?
3. Based upon your answer for Question #2 above, what is your list of differential diagnoses?
4. Of your list of differentials, which will you prioritize?

Answers to Round One of Questions for Case 7: The Diarrheic Puppy

1. Small bowel diarrhea is differentiated from large bowel diarrhea based upon the following characteristics:(1)

   - volume of fecal matter that is passed
   - frequency of defecation
   - whether or not the diarrhea is associated with weight loss
   - whether or not the diarrhea is associated with vomiting
   - whether or not the diarrhea is associated with copious amounts of mucous
   - whether or not blood is present

     - if blood is present, then is it frank blood?
     - or is it blood that has already been digested?

   In general, small bowel diarrhea involves the passage of large quantities of stool with only a mild increase (if any) in frequency of bowel movements.(1) A patient with small bowel diarrhea does not typically strain to defecate, and there is little to no fecal mucus.(1–4) If it persists, small bowel diarrhea is associated with weight loss.(2, 4, 5) If blood is present in the stool, then it will result in melena, black tarry feces.(1) The black tar appearance occurs because the blood has been digested before passage out of the digestive tract.(1)

   By contrast, large bowel diarrhea tends to involve copious fecal mucus, increased urgency and frequency of defecation, and tenesmus.(1) Fecal volume tends to be substantially less significant than is the case with small bowel diarrhea. Stool that is passed is often semi-formed or gelatinous. Blood may be present in large bowel diarrhea. However, it will pass out in the feces as fresh red streaks or drops of frank blood.(1) Large bowel diarrhea is not associated with weight loss.(1)

2. Jackson appears to be having small bowel diarrhea based upon the following details from the clinical vignette:

   - copious amounts of fecal matter
   - diarrhea is not associated with straining to defecate
   - diarrhea is associated with vomiting.

3. The list of differential diagnoses for small bowel diarrhea in a dog includes:(2–12)

- dietary indiscretion
- enteritis
    - bacterial
    - fungal:
        - histoplasmosis
        - phycomycosis
        - pythiosis
    - parasitic:
        - hookworms
        - protozoa
        - roundworms
        - tapeworms
    - viral:
        - canine parvovirus type 1 (CPV-1, minute virus)
        - canine parvovirus type 2 (CPV-2)
        - coronavirus
- exocrine pancreatic insufficiency (EPI)
- food allergy or intolerance
- hypoadrenocorticism
- hyperthyroidism
- pancreatitis
- portosystemic shunt
- protein-losing enteropathy (PLE)
    - inflammatory bowel disease (IBD)
    - intestinal lymphangiectasia
    - intestinal neoplasia, such as lymphoma
- small intestinal bacterial overgrowth (SIBO) as from malabsorptive small bowel disease
- toxicosis.

4. Of the differential diagnoses that are listed above, the following causes of small bowel diarrhea are most likely to occur in a puppy:(10)

- dietary indiscretion
- parasitic enteritis
- viral enteritis.

Of these three differentials, parvoviral enteritis is at the top of my list for any canine pediatric patient that presents with an acute onset of progressive vomiting and diarrhea, lethargy, and anorexia. The index of suspicion is heightened even further whenever I learn that the patient comes from an unknown background and that the vaccination statuses of the bitch and pup are both unknown.

Returning to Case 7: The Diarrheic Puppy

Kara agreed to have in-house point-of-care fecal tests run while waiting for you to evaluate Jackson. Both the in-house fecal analysis and the test for giardiasis are negative. However, the fecal enzyme-linked immunosorbent assay (ELISA) antigen test for parvovirus is positive (see Figure 7.2).

Round Two of Questions

1. What is the difference between canine parvovirus 1 (CPV-1; minute virus) and canine parvovirus 2 (CPV-2)?
2. Are there any apparent breed predispositions for CPV-2?
3. If this puppy had been vaccinated against CPV-2, what (if any) impact might that have had on diagnostic test results?
4. If the test results are accurate, and this patient is in fact infected with CPV-2, what might you expect to see on a CBC?
5. How does your understanding of the pathophysiology of CPV-2 support your anticipated findings with regards to this patient's hemogram and leukogram?

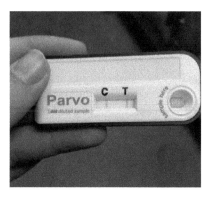

Figure 7.2 Point-of-care in-house test for parvovirus, demonstrating a (+) result.

Answers to Round Two of Questions for Case 7: The Diarrheic Puppy

1. Both CPV-1 (minute virus) and CPV-2 are nonenveloped, DNA viruses that preferentially replicate within rapidly dividing cells, such as the gut.(13)

    CPV-1 targets fetal and neonatal pups.(10, 13) Pups that are infected in utero often die before birth.(10) Those that are born alive are more likely to have birth defects and/or to succumb to so-called "fading puppy syndrome."(14) Neonates that are infected with CPV-1 often present with non-specific signs. They may exhibit generalized malaise. They often cry constantly and cannot be soothed. Some develop diarrhea and/or vomiting.(10) Others exhibit respiratory distress or sudden death.(10)

    Diagnostic tests are not available clinically for CPV-1.(10) There is no specific treatment other than supportive care, which is usually unsuccessful and disease progresses rapidly.(10) There is also not specific preventative measure to be taken against CPV-1 because there is currently no commercially available vaccination to address it.(10, 15)

    By contrast, CPV-2 targets unvaccinated pediatric patients and adults, and causes canine parvoviral enteritis.(10, 13) Historically, it only affected dogs.(13) However, newer strains 2a and 2b are capable of infecting felids.(13)

    Dogs that are infected with CPV-2 present with severe, progressive gastrointestinal signs. Bloody diarrhea and vomiting are commonly seen.(10, 13) Dehydration becomes a significant concern rapidly due to the amount of fluid that is lost through the digestive system over a very short period of time.(10, 13) CPV-2 can be fatal. When death occurs, it is typically due to sepsis, intestinal intussusception, and/or disseminated intravascular coagulation (DIC).(10, 13)

    As seen in this case, diagnosis of CPV-2 is made possible through in-house testing, which offers rapid turn-around time.(10, 13)

Treatment for CPV-2 is supportive and concentrates on correcting dehydration and any resultant electrolyte imbalance.(10, 13) Patients are typically prescribed prophylactic parenteral broad-spectrum antibiotic therapy to guard against sepsis.(10, 13)

Many patients that are afflicted with CPV-2 will survive if treatment is aggressive and instituted early on in the disease process.(10, 13)

Vaccinations are available to protect against CPV-2.(10, 13)

2. Rottweilers, Doberman Pinschers, Labrador retrievers, German shepherds, English springer spaniels, and Staffordshire terriers appear to be predisposed to infection with CPV-2.(10, 13, 16)

3. Administering a modified live virus (MLV) may cause the fecal ELISA antigen test to test false positive for parvovirus for 5 to 15 days post-vaccination.(10, 13, 17)

4. You might anticipate the following changes on Jackson's CBC:(10)

   • anemia
   • leukopenia

     • lymphopenia
     • neutropenia

   • hypoproteinemia.

5. CPV-2 causes the destruction of leukocyte precursors in circulation.(1) This causes a drop in the number of circulating white blood cells, including neutrophils and lymphocytes.(10)

   Anemia results from blood loss in small bowel diarrhea.(1)

   Small bowel diarrhea occurs because CPV-2 infects intestinal crypt cells.(1, 14) These cells are no longer able to keep up with normal cell turnover. The net result is that the intestinal villi shorten, collapse, and slough. Without this extensive population of fingerlike projections to increase surface area for absorption, patients cannot take in the nutrients that they need.(10) Temporarily, they experience PLE or so-called malabsorptive syndrome.(1)

Returning to Case 7: The Diarrheic Puppy

You examine Jackson and make the following notations in his medical record with regards to abnormal physical exam findings:

Body weight: 14 pounds (6.2 kilograms)

Mentation: Depressed

TEMPERATURE, PULSE, AND RESPIRATION (TPR)

T: 104.2°F (40.1°C)
P: 240 beats per minute
R: 22 breaths per minute

Mucous membrane color: pale pink

Capillary refill time (CRT): 3 seconds

General appearance:

   • BCS: 3/9

Integumentary system:

   • Fecal stained perineum and caudal thighs
   • Persistent skin tent

Eyes/ears/nose/throat (EENT):

   • Sunken eyes with prominent nictitans OU

Cardiovascular and respiratory systems:

- Grade 1/6 systolic murmur
- Tachycardia
- Weak, but synchronous femoral pulses

Gastrointestinal system:

- Dry and tacky mucous membranes
- Fetid smell to fecal matter
- Uncomfortable on abdominal palpation
- Diffusely thickened small bowel; bowel also feels fluid-filled

You share these findings with Kara as well as their significance. As you review Jackson's diagnosis and proposed case management, you express concern for Jackson's survival if he is not hospitalized straight away. You prepare an estimate and although Kara does a double take at the bottom line due to sticker shock, she agrees. Financially, it will be a stretch, but she knows how emotionally attached her son is to Jackson. To lose him now would devastate the family. She tells you to "do everything" and you admit him into the isolation ward immediately.

Round Three of Questions

1. How do you assess a dog's hydration status when performing a physical exam?
2. How might clinicopathologic data corroborate the veterinarian's findings that the patient appears to be dehydrated on physical exam?
3. How do you estimate the percentage by which the patient is dehydrated?
4. Based upon the physical exam findings that have been provided by way of clinical vignette, what is Jackson's estimated percent dehydration?
5. In anticipation of initiating fluid therapy, you need to place an intravenous (IV) catheter. What is/are an appropriate site(s) for IV catheter placement in a dog?
6. If IV access is not possible, what is an alternate route of fluid therapy administration that is appropriate for Jackson at this time, given the severity of his dehydration?
7. Which complication(s) of IV catheterization is/are Jackson at most risk of developing, given his current parvoviral infection?
8. Which type of IV fluid is the most appropriate choice to use to initiate fluid therapy: hypotonic, isotonic, or hypertonic?
9. When might you consider using a colloid in lieu of a crystalloid?
10. Which supplement(s) may be added to the fluid option that you selected in Question #8 (above)?
11. What is at least one important consideration with regards to rate of supplementation of electrolytes?
12. Calculate this patient's fluid deficit.
13. Over how long of a period will you replace the patient's fluid deficit?
14. Calculate this patient's maintenance IV fluid therapy rate in mL/day and mL/hour.
15. Because Jackson is significantly dehydrated, he will require far more than maintenance therapy. You decide that he could benefit from a shock bolus of crystalloids. What is the dosage for a shock bolus of crystalloids? Will you give this bolus all at once?
16. What could you measure to ensure that the patient is receiving adequate fluid replacement?
17. What are indicators on physical exam that the patient may be experiencing volume overload?
18. You need to cease Jackson's vomiting to reduce ongoing fluid losses through the digestive tract. There are many options to choose from. These have been outlined in the table opposite in terms of drug name and dose. Complete the table.
19. Using the dose provided in the table opposite, calculate the amount of maropitant citrate (in mg) that Jackson will require as an injectable once daily. If the concentration of maropitant citrate is 10 mg/mL, then how much volume will be administered to Jackson to achieve the calculated dose?

Table 10.1

Drug	Mechanism of action	Site of action	Dose
Maropitant citrate			1 mg/kg SQ q 24 h
Ondansetron			0.3–0.5 mg/kg SQ or IV q 8 h
Dolasetron			0.5–1.0 mg/kg SQ or IV q 24 h
Metoclopramide			CRI of 1–2 mg/kg/day

20. What is a valid concern about prescribing metoclopramide in a patient that has CPV-2?
21. You have elected to prescribe broad-spectrum bactericidal antibiotics because CPV-2 has disrupted the integrity of the digestive tract. This, in combination with Jackson's leukopenia, places him at great risk of contracting a secondary bacterial infection. There are many options of antibiotics to choose from. These have been outlined in the table below in terms of drug name and dose. Complete the table.

Table 10.2

Drug	Type of antibiotic	Dose	Adverse effects and/or contraindications to use
Ampicillin		10–20 mg/kg IV/IM/SQ q6-8 hours	
Ampicillin-sulbactam (Unasyn™)		50 mg/kg IV q8 hours	
Amoxicillin clavulanate		20 mg/kg IV q8 hours	
Amikacin		20 mg/kg IV/IM/SQ q24 hours	
Cefazolin		22 mg/kg IV/IM q8 hours	
Cefoxitin		22 mg/kg IV q6-8 hours	
Ceftriaxone		22 mg/kg IV q6-8 hours	
Enrofloxacin		5–10 mg/kg IV q24 hours	
Gentamicin		2 mg/kg IM/SQ q8 hours	

22. After weighing the pros and cons of each therapeutic agent, you elect to administer enrofloxacin. Using the low end of the dosing range that has been provided in the table above, calculate the amount of enrofloxacin (in mg) that Jackson will require as an injectable once every 24 hours. If the concentration of enrofloxacin is 22.7 mg/mL, then how much volume will be administered to Jackson to achieve the calculated dose?
23. Should Jackson be NPO (nil per os)? That is, should food and water be withheld?
24. While Jackson is in the hospital, what (if anything) should Kara do to clean up the home environment to reduce risk of re-exposure?
25. Kara's brother has a dog that sometimes visits the household. What can Kara do to assess that dog's risk of contracting CPV-2?
26. If Jackson recovers, Kara asks if it is possible for him to be re-infected with CPV-2?

Answers to Round Three of Questions for Case 7: The Diarrheic Puppy

1. Hydration status is assessed subjectively by evaluating the following physical exam parameters: (18, 19)

    - skin turgor
    - mucous membrane moistness
    - eye position within the orbits
    - heart rate
    - peripheral pulse quality
    - CRT
    - whether or not there is jugular distension.

    To recall how to assess skin turgor, review Case 5, The Snotty, Squinty Kitten.

2. Hydration status can also be assessed more objectively by evaluating clinicopathologic data. Patients that are clinically dehydrated tend to have the following changes on their lab work:(18)

    - hemoconcentration with increased total solids
    - azotemia
    - increased USG.

3. When dehydration is suspected based upon a patient's history, physical exam findings, and clinicopathologic data, an effort can be made to estimate the percentage by which the patient is dehydrated.(18)
    The smallest percentage at which dehydration is clinically detectable is 5%.(18) A patient that is 5% dehydrated has a subtle loss in skin elasticity. (18–20)
    Dehydration of 6–8% results in a delayed return of skin to normal positioning following an attempt to tent the skin.(20) The oral mucous membranes are beginning to get dry and CRT may be slightly prolonged.(19, 20) The eyes may be positioned slightly back in the orbits as if sunken; however, this is subtle.(20)
    A patient is said to be 10–12% dehydrated when there is persistent skin tenting and the oral mucous membranes are so dry that the veterinarian's fingers stick to them.(18) At this level of dehydration, the eyes appear sunken.(18) This makes the nictitans appear prominent bilaterally. (19) CRT is definitively prolonged.(20)
    A patient that is 10–12% dehydrated may experience signs of shock.(20) These include:(20)

    - tachycardia
    - weak pulses
    - cool extremities.

    Beyond 12% dehydration, survival is unlikely.(20)

4. Jackson's estimated percentage of dehydration is 10–12% based upon his sunken eyes, prominent nictitating membranes, tacky mucous membranes, weak pulses, tachycardia, and prolonged CRT.

5. Either the right or left cephalic vein is an appropriate choice for IV catheter placement in a canine patient. In a patient like Jackson, who is depressed and non-ambulatory, the right or left lateral saphenous vein would also be an appropriate choice were if not for the fact that he is diarrheic.
    Patients with diarrhea are more likely to soil the peripheral catheter site if the catheter has been inserted in the pelvic limb.(21) This is not ideal because it will increase the risk for an infection even if aseptic technique was used to place the catheter.(21)

6. The interosseous route of fluid administration is appropriate if IV access is not possible at this time.(22) Patients such as Jackson require rapid administration of fluids to correct severe dehydration and potentially severe derangements in electrolyte and acid-base status.(22) Because of this, subcutaneous therapy is not the best option for Jackson unless he is discharged home to the care of his owners against medical advice.

   Subcutaneous therapy is inappropriate when patients have significant volume deficits.(20) It is not possible for subcutaneous depots of fluid to be absorbed fast enough to improve the patient's clinical status. In addition, Jackson is in a state of shock. This means that he is experiencing peripheral vasoconstriction. This state further reduces the ability of his body to absorb subcutaneous fluid.(20)

   There is also concern that abscesses may result from subcutaneous fluid administration due to Jackson's immune-compromised state.(22, 23)

7. Puppies with parvovirus have significantly suppressed immune systems.(14, 22) This makes catheter-induced infections even more likely to occur if there is a breach in aseptic technique and/or catheter care.(14, 22) At minimum, these infections can result in phlebitis.(14) Severe cases may result in septic polyarthritis and/or discospondylitis.(22) Many of the bacteria that have been cultured from catheter tips are gram negative microbes with varying patterns of antimicrobial resistance.(14)

8. The most appropriate fluid choice at this time is an isotonic crystalloid solution.(22) Examples include:(22, 24)

   - 0.9% sodium chloride (NaCl)
   - lactated ringer solution
   - Plasma-Lyte-A®
   - Plasma-Lyte-148®

9. When a patient's TP drops below 35 g/L, particularly if albumin is less than 20 g/L, then it is time to consider the administration of hetastarch or dextran 70.(24) These are appropriate choices for colloidal therapy.

10. The following ingredients may need to be added to your isotonic crystalloid fluid of choice, based upon the patient's requirements:(22)

    - potassium chloride
    - dextrose.

11. Potassium must be diluted rather than administered directly as a concentrate. Concentrates of potassium induce cardiotoxicity by bringing atrial conduction to a standstill.(25) On ECG, this is evident as absent P waves.(25) Bradycardia will be pronounced.(25) Ultimately, the QRS complex merges with the T wave.(25) Soon after, the heart rhythm launches into ventricular fibrillation or ventricular asystole.(25) Death is imminent.(25)

    Because of this, the rate at which potassium chloride is administered to a patient must be monitored very carefully, even though it has been diluted out within a one-liter bag of isotonic crystalloid. If the rate of administration exceeds 0.5 mEq/kg/hour, then dysrhythmias and cardiac arrest may result.(22, 26)

12. Jackson's fluid deficit is 0.64 liters. The fluid deficit is determined by multiplying the patient's body weight (in kilograms) by the percentage dehydration.(20) The resultant answer carries the unit of measurement, liters.

13. Jackson is significantly dehydrated and would benefit from rapid replacement of his fluid deficit, particularly since his fluid losses are likely to be ongoing in the form of vomit and diarrhea until medical management can overcome the challenges caused by parvovirus. Ideally, Jackson's fluid

deficit should be replaced within the first 12–24 hours after admission to the isolation ward of the intensive care unit.

14. Jackson's maintenance IV fluid therapy rate is 384 mL/day or 15 mL/hour.

   Depending upon your reference, the maintenance rate of IV fluid administration is calculated using the following formula: 40–60 mL/kg/day.(20)

   I was trained to use the higher end (60 mL/kg/day), which is how I obtained the answer for this question. If you instead used the lower end of the formula (40 mL/kg/day), then Jackson's maintenance IV fluid therapy rate would be 255 mL/day or 10.6 mL/hour.

15. The dosage of a shock bolus for a dog is 90 mL/kg.(27)

   If we were to calculate that dosage for Jackson, then his full shock bolus would be 576 mL (roughly half of a liter).

   Every clinician has his/her own preference. I was trained to administer 1/4 of the shock bolus over 10–15 minutes and then reassess the patient for restoration of perfusion parameters.(27)

   If I were to follow this advice, then Jackson would receive a bolus of 144 mL over 10–15 minutes. This allows us to titrate the dose to effect.(27) If perfusion parameters have not normalized, then I would give another quarter of the shock bolus over 10–15 minutes and reassess.

   If the full shock bolus is administered and perfusion parameters remain subpar, then this likely reflects an ongoing intravascular volume deficit. Provided that the patient is not hypernatremic, you may need to administer hypertonic saline (7% NaCl) intravenously at 2–4 mL/kg over 10 minutes. To prevent interstitial dehydration, this must be given in combination with isotonic replacement crystalloids.(27)

   Alternatively, colloids may be given as an adjunctive fluid to assist with intravascular volume. (27)

16. You can and should also measure urine output to ensure that the patient is adequately receiving sufficient replacement fluids.(24) When a patient is euhydrated, it should produce on average a urine output of 1–2 mL/kg/hour.(24)

17. Clear nasal discharge and a sudden spike in respiratory rate may indicate that the patient is experiencing volume overload.(24)

18. The table has been completed below.(28, 29)

Table 10.3

Drug	Mechanism of action	Site of action	Dose
Maropitant citrate (Cerenia)	Neurokinin antagonist	CRTZ*** and emetic center	1 mg/kg SQ or IV q 24 h
Ondansetron	Serotonin antagonist	CRTZ	0.3–0.5 mg/kg SQ or IV q 8 h
Dolasetron	Serotonin antagonist	CRTZ	0.5–1.0 mg/kg SQ or IV q 24 h
Metoclopramide	Dopamine antagonist	CRTZ, GI smooth muscle	CRI of 1–2 mg/kg/day

Note: ***CRTZ = chemoreceptor trigger zone.

19. The dose of maropitant citrate is 1 mg/kg. Jackson weighs 6.4 kg, so his dose of maropitant citrate will be 6.4 kg × 1 mg/kg = 6.4 mg.

   If the concentration of maropitant citrate is 10 mg/mL, then Jackson will require 0.64 mL of maropitant citrate. In clinical practice, I would round this up to 0.65 mL for ease of administration.

20. A potential sequelae of CPV-2 is intussusception.(14, 22) Metoclopramide exerts its action by promoting gut motility within the upper intestinal tract.(22) The administration of metoclopramide may heighten the risk of intussusception.(22)

21. The table has been completed below.(14, 22, 28, 29)

Table 10.4

Drug	Type of antibiotic	Dose	Adverse effects and/or contraindications to use
Ampicillin	β-lactam antibiotic	10-20 mg/kg IV/IM/ SQ q6-8 hours	
Ampicillin-sulbactam (Unasyn™)	β-lactamase resistant	50 mg/kg IV q 8 hours	
Amoxicillin clavulanate	β-lactamase resistant	20 mg/kg IV q 8 hours	
Amikacin	Aminoglycoside	20 mg/kg IV/IM/SQ q 24 hours	Significant potential for nephrotoxicity; therefore, contraindicated until patient has been rehydrated.
Cefazolin	β-lactam antibiotic	22 mg/kg IV/IM q 8 hours	
Cefoxitin	β-lactam antibiotic	22 mg/kg IV q 6-8 hours	
Ceftriaxone	β-lactam antibiotic	22 mg/kg IV q 6-8 hours	
Enrofloxacin	Fluoroquinolone	5-10 mg/kg IV q 24 hours	May cause damage to the cartilage of juvenile animals
Gentamicin	Aminoglycoside	2 mg/kg IM/SQ q 8 hours	Significant potential for nephrotoxicity; therefore, contraindicated until patient has been rehydrated.

22. The dose of enrofloxacin is 5–10 mg/kg IV. We have been instructed to calculate for the low end of this dosing range. Jackson weighs 6.4 kg, so his dose of enrofloxacin will be 6.4 kg × (5 mg/kg) = 32 mg. If the concentration of enrofloxacin is 22.7 mg/mL, then Jackson will require 1.4 mL of enrofloxacin. This is calculated as follows: 32 mg × (1 mL/22.7 mg).

23. It is typical to withhold food and water when a patient is actively vomiting for 24–72 hours.(14, 22) However, there is relatively new evidence to support that dogs with parvovirus have speedier recoveries if we can get them eating sooner as opposed to later.(14, 22, 30) Enteral nutrition appears to play an important role in hastening repair of the gut and restoring its function.(14, 22) For this reason, it may be wise to consider placement of a nasoesophageal tube in Jackson on day one of treatment.(14, 30) This should help him to maintain his body weight, which will in turn facilitate recovery.(14)

24. CPV-2 is not easy to kill, so Kara should set to work straight away to decontaminate the home environment. Although viral shedding is short-lived, the virus is persistent in the environment for months to years if left untreated.(14) CPV-2 is susceptible to sodium hypochlorite (household bleach).(14) At-home surfaces, such as tile floors, can be sprayed with bleach that has been diluted 1:30.(14) Contact time is important. CPV-2 needs to be exposed to bleach for at least 10 minutes for bleach to be viricidal.(14)

Bleach may also be added to the washing machine when cleaning bedding and/or may be used to disinfect kitchenware – e.g. food and water bowels, kitchen utensils that may have come into contact with CPV-2.(14)

Boiling is also an effective method of killing CPV-2, so boiled water can be poured over tolerable dishware.(31)

25. I would strongly recommend that Kara ask her brother to review his dog's vaccination record with his veterinarian. If that dog has never been vaccinated against CPV-2, then he is at risk of contracting the disease. If on the other hand he had been vaccinated previously and is currently up to date on vaccinations against CPV-2, then his risk of contracting disease at this time is much reduced.

26. Assuming that Jackson makes a complete recovery, he should be immune from contracting CPV-2 for at least 20 months.(14) It is thought that immunity may even be life-long.(14) That being said, Jackson will still benefit from the combination vaccines, DHPP or DA2PP, where:

D = distemper
H = hepatitis
A2 = adenovirus Type 2
P = parvo
P = parainfluenza.

Recall that Jackson has no prior vaccine history and therefore he is immunologically naïve to every component of these combination vaccines except for parvovirus. Therefore, once Jackson is recovered from parvoviral enteritis, he will need to start his DA2PP series of vaccinations so that he receives adequate protection against the other components.

CLINICAL PEARLS

- History, signalment and the differentiation between small and large bowel diarrhea can significantly assist you in developing your list of differential diagnoses.

- Parvoviral enteritis is common among unvaccinated or improperly vaccinated puppies and young adult dogs.

- The hallmark clinical signs of parvoviral enteritis is acute onset of progressive bloody diarrhea and vomiting. Severe dehydration, lethargy, fever, and malaise ensue.

- The hallmark clinicopathologic abnormalities include anemia and leukopenia, particularly neutropenia and lymphopenia. Patients also develop hypoproteinemia (hypoalbuminemia) from the temporary damage that is done by the virus to intestinal crypt cells.

- Parvovirus is easily diagnosed via the in-house point-of-care fecal ELISA antigen test.

- Administering a modified live virus (MLV) may cause the fecal ELISA antigen test to test false positive for parvovirus for five to 15 days post-vaccination.

- Parvovirus is more easily prevented (through vaccination) than treated. Treatment requires supportive care and intensive fluid therapy.

- Fluid therapy must take into account fluid deficit at time of initial presentation, the patient's maintenance fluid therapy rate, whether or not the patient is in shock, and ongoing losses.

- Isotonic crystalloid therapy is the go-to fluid choice for intravenous administration. Colloidal therapy is indicated when hypoproteinemia is severe.

- Electrolyte imbalances (hypokalemia) and acid-base derangements are common, so intravenous fluid therapy must be customized to the patient. Potassium supplementation is common; however, rate of administration must be watched like a hawk.

- Antibiotics are administered prophylactically to protect against opportunistic invaders, given the degree of immunosuppression of parvovirus (+) patients.

References

1. Englar RE. Common clinical presentations in dogs and cats. Hoboken, NJ: Wiley/Blackwell; 2019.
2. Englar RE. Performing the small animal physical examination. Hoboken, NJ: Wiley; 2017.
3. Allenspach K. Diagnosis of small intestinal disorders in dogs and cats. Vet Clin North Am Small Anim Pract 2013;43(6):1227–40, v, v.
4. Gaschen F, editor. Small intestinal diarrhea – causes and treatment. WSAVA World Congress; 2006.
5. Greco DS. Diagnosis and dietary management of gastrointestinal disease: purina veterinary diets. Available from: https://www.purinaproplanvets.com/media/1202/gi_quick_reference_guide.pdf.
6. Marks SL, Kather EJ. Bacterial-associated diarrhea in the dog: a critical appraisal. Vet Clin North Am Small Anim Pract 2003;33(5):1029–60.
7. Greene CE. Enteric bacterial infections. In: Greene CE, editor. Infectious diseases of the dog and cat. St. Louis, MO: Saunders/Elsevier. p. 243–5; 1998.
8. Cave NJ, Marks SL, Kass PH, Melli AC, Brophy MA. Evaluation of a routine diagnostic fecal panel for dogs with diarrhea. J Am Vet Med Assoc 2002;221(1):52–9.
9. Guilford WG, Strombeck DR. Gastrointestinal tract infections, parasites, and toxicosis. In: Guilford WG, Center SA, editors. Stromback's small animal gastroenterology. 3rd ed. Philadelphia, PA: W. B. Saunders; 1996, p. 411–32.
10. Magne ML. Selected topics in pediatric gastroenterology. Vet Clin North Am Small Anim Pract 2006;36(3):533–48.
11. Matz ME. Chronic diarrhea in a dog. NAVC Clin's Brief 2006 (April):75–7.
12. Sokolow SH, Rand C, Marks SL, Drazenovich NL, Kather EJ, Foley JE. Epidemiologic evaluation of diarrhea in dogs in an animal shelter. Am J Vet Res 2005;66(6):1018–24.
13. McCaw DL, Hoskins JD. Canine viral enteritis. In: Greene CE, editor. Infectious diseases of the dog and cat. 3rd ed. St. Louis, MO: Saunders/Elsevier; 2006.
14. McCaw DL, Hoskins JD. Canine viral enteritis. In: Greene CE, editor. Infectious diseases of the dog and cat. 3rd ed. St. Louis, MO: Saunders/Elsevier; 2006. p. 63–72.
15. Hoskins JD, Dimski D. The digestive system. In: Hoskins JD, editor. Veterinary pediatrics. Philadelphia, PA: W.B Saunders; 1990. p. 133–87.
16. Glickman LT, Domanski LM, Patronek GJ, Visintainer F. Breed-related risk factors for canine parvovirus enteritis. J Am Vet Med Assoc 1985;187(6):589–94.
17. Rewerts JM, Cohn LA. CVT update: diagnosis and treatment of parvovirus. In: Bonagura JD, editor. Kirk's current veterinary therapy XIII. Philadelphia, PA: W.B. Saunders; 2000. p. 629–32.
18. Englar RE. Performing the small animal physical examination. Hoboken, NJ: Wiley/Blackwell; 2017.
19. DiBartola SP, Bateman S. Introduction to fluid therapy. In: DiBartola SP, editor. Fluid, electrolyte, and acid–base disorders in small animal practice. 3rd ed. St. Louis, MO: Saunders/Elsevier; 2006. p. 325–44.
20. DiBartola SP, Bateman S. Introduction to fluid therapy. In: DiBartola SP, editor. Fluid, electrolyte, and acid–base disorders in small animal practice. 3rd ed. St. Louis, MO: Saunders/Elsevier; 2006.
21. Hansen BD. Technical aspects of fluid therapy. In: DiBartola SP, editor. Fluid, electrolyte, and acid–base disorders in small animal practice. 3rd ed. St. Louis, MO: Saunders/Elsevier; 2006.
22. Goddard A, Leisewitz AL. Canine parvovirus. Vet Clin North Am Small Anim Pract 2010;40(6):1041–53.
23. Prittie J. Canine parvoviral enteritis: a review of diagnosis, management, and prevention. J Vet Emerg Crit Care 2004;14(3):167–76.

24. Mathews KA. Monitoring fluid therapy and complications of fluid therapy. In: DiBartola SP, editor. Fluid, electrolyte, and acid–base disorders in small animal practice. 3rd ed. St. Louis, MO: Saunders/Elsevier; 2006.

25. DiBartola SP, Autran de Morais H. Disorders of potassium: hypokalemia and hyperkalemia. In: DiBartola SP, editor. Fluid, electrolyte, and acid–base disorders in small animal practice. 3rd ed. St. Louis, MO: Saunders/Elsevier; 2006.

26. Brown AJ, Otto CM. Fluid therapy in vomiting and diarrhea. Vet Clin North Am Small Anim Pract 2008;38(3):653–75.

27. Day TK, Bateman S. Shock syndromes. In: DiBartola SP, editor. Fluid, electrolyte, and acid–base disorders in small animal practice. 3rd ed. St. Louis, MO: Saunders/Elsevier; 2006.

28. Plumb DC Stockholm WH, ed. Plumb's veterinary drug handbook. 9th ed. Hoboken, NJ: Pharma Vet, Inc; 2018.

29. Merck Vet Man. Whitehouse Station, NJ: Merck & Co., Inc. 2016.

30. Mohr AJ, Leisewitz AL, Jacobson LS, Steiner JM, Ruaux CG, Williams DA. Effect of early enteral nutrition on intestinal permeability, intestinal protein loss, and outcome in dogs with severe parvoviral enteritis. J Vet Intern Med 2003;17(6):791–8.

31. McGavin D. Inactivation of canine parvovirus by disinfectants and heat. J Small Anim Pract 1987;28(6):523–35.

Case 8

The Trembly Puppy

Carly Dickens had dreamed of owning a toy breed ever since she was a child. At 22 years old, she had finally moved out of her parents' home and into her own studio apartment. It seemed like the perfect time to add to her household of one. Never having owned a dog before, she wasn't sure where to look, so she pulled out her laptop computer and performed a google search for the query, "chihuahua puppies for sale near me."

Carly was blown away by the number of hits that were retrieved. It was overwhelming at first, and she didn't know where to begin. Then her eyes caught a post from a seller on Craigslist and she was sold. The breeder was located just a few blocks away and, as luck would have it, had two 8-week-old pups for sale. Carly telephoned and was encouraged to visit straight away.

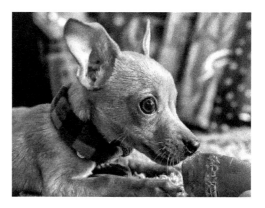

Figure 8.1 Your next patient, an 8-week-old intact male Chihuahua puppy.

When Carly arrived and the male pup was placed in her outstretched hands, she knew that she had found her match. He was the color of cinnamon and honey combined, and his eyes were so big that they melted her heart. When he licked the tip of her nose, she knew that he was coming home with her today! Carly had been warned by her parents to vet the breeder, but she wasn't sure what to ask and the pup seemed healthy enough, so she proceeded with the transaction. Eight hundred dollars (£640) seemed a bit steep, but she could swing it if she postponed purchasing furniture for the apartment. What she couldn't wait on was companionship.

Carly left the breeder's with Tiny Tim in hand and instructions to "feed him often." She was given several baggies of powdered milk replacer and told to sprinkle the contents over commercial canned food "generously." If he wouldn't eat puppy food, then she could try kitten chow. The breeder suggested that the higher protein content of cat food made it more palatable. If all else failed, it might tempt Tiny Tim to eat. Carly didn't think to ask what would happen if he refused the cat food. He had a nice rounded belly so, surely, he was getting enough?

Carly texted her friends once she got Tiny Tim settled into his new environment, and it wasn't long before they descended upon the household to introduce themselves to the new arrival. Tiny Tim played hard for several hours before he passed out from sheer exhaustion. Carly let him sleep through dinner.

By the time he woke, Carly was ready to call it a day. She cracked open a can of puppy food, stirred in some of the milk replacement powder, and offered it to him. She assumed that he'd eat. If anyone had worked up an appetite, he had! But Tiny Tim took one lick and refused. She dabbed a taste onto her index finger and offered her hand to him, hoping to coax him into dining. He took another lick, but ultimately that, too, backfired.

"Okay, fine, you win."

Carly retreated to the kitchen to collect a can of kitten food, then returned to the bedroom to empty its contents onto a nearby plate. Tiny Tim looked, but that was the extent of his interest.

"Then I guess you aren't that hungry after all! Goodnight, little man," she said, before turning out the light.

Morning came too soon to the Dickens household, particularly given that Tiny Tim whined all night. Carly tried everything. Initially, she had crated him. That was unpopular. So, she let him out, but he didn't like being alone in his doggie bed on the floor. He wanted up, in bed with her. She ultimately caved in and scooped him up into her arms. Then she spent half the night worrying about rolling over on him or him jumping off the bed. He also had several accidents throughout the night, which required her to strip her sheets – not once, but twice. No one had ever told Carly that having a puppy was this much work. She was starting to understand why her parents had always said "no."

Carly picked Tiny Tim down from the bed so that she could get ready for the day. She was surprised that he barely stirred beneath her touch. When Carly returned from the bathroom, dressed, he was still in his doggie bed on the floor. She called to him and he raised his head, but he seemed groggy.

"Wow, you're really not a morning person," She thought to herself. "Welcome to the club."

Carly became concerned only when Tiny Tim struggled to rise from his bed on the floor. He seemed weak and wobbly. At one point, he even toppled over. Panicked, she texted Jody, one of her closest friends, who suggested that Tiny Tim be evaluated by a veterinarian right away. Carly scooped him up and drove him to the nearest clinic. She is seated now, in your exam room, waiting to be seen on emergency.

Your technician initiates the intake appointment by taking Tiny Tim's vital signs:

Throughout data acquisition, the technician notices that Tiny Tim has intermittent muscle fasciculations associated with his muzzle and face. As soon as the TPR is obtained, these focal twitches progress into a whole-body convulsion that is best characterized as a generalized seizure.

Weight: 450 grams (0.45 kg)
Mentation: Depressed

TEMPERATURE, PULSE, AND RESPIRATION (TPR)

T: 101.2°F (38.4°C)
P: 168 beats per minute
R: 16 breaths per minute

Round One of Questions for Case 8: The Trembly Puppy

1. What is a seizure?
2. Describe the characteristics of a generalized seizure.
3. How does one distinguish syncope from a generalized seizure, given that both involve the patient collapsing?
4. How might you define protracted seizure activity?
5. What are the inherent dangers of protracted seizure activity?
6. Differentiate cluster seizures from status epilepticus.
7. Which is the first drug that you reach for in cases of status epilepticus?
8. Which is/are the route(s) of administration for this drug?
9. If this drug in and of itself is unsuccessful at ceasing seizure activity, which adjunctive therapies might you turn to?
10. Broadly speaking, what are intracranial causes of seizures?
11. Broadly speaking, what are extracranial causes of seizures?
12. Which are the most likely causes of seizures in pediatric patients?
13. Given Tiny Tim's signalment and history, which of these primary differential diagnoses is/are most likely?
14. What is your next step in terms of diagnostic plan to confirm your suspicion?

Answers to Round One of Questions for Case 8: The Trembly Puppy

1. A seizure is a clinical even that occurs when bursts of uncontrolled electrical activity cause involuntary motor activity.(1) This heightened motor activity is often described as being biphasic.(2) The tonic phase consists of prolonged muscular contraction by one or more muscle groups.(2, 3) This causes tightening of affected muscles. A clonic phase may follow, during which time affected muscles involuntarily jerk.(1–3)

2. Seizures may be focal or generalized. Generalized seizures are sometimes referred to as grand mal seizures.(2, 4) These involve both cerebral hemispheres.(2, 4) This impacts the entire body as opposed to focal involvement. A dog that presents in the midst of a generalized seizure will experience collapse and transient loss of consciousness.(5)

3. An episode of collapse is easy to recognize. The patient essentially falls to the ground due to loss of postural tone.(6–10)

   The cause of collapse is not always as easy to identify.(1) Collapse may be due to syncope or seizures.(6–8, 11, 12) These episodes may appear to be visually similar, particularly if witnessed by a novice or someone who is not in the medical field.(9, 12–14)

   Syncope ("fainting") occurs due to a lapse in perfusion of the brain.(11) This causes weakness and/or ataxia just before the patient passes out.(11) The episode is brief in duration.(11) Patients are most often flaccid when they collapse, only to promptly rise again as if everything is normal.(11)

   Generalized seizures, on the other hand, are characterized by stiffness rather than flaccidity.(1) The limbs tend to be toned.(1) Opisthotonus and extensor rigidity are common, and, if present, tonic-clonic actions cause the limbs to appear as if they are paddling.(4, 5)

   Autonomic activity during a generalized seizure is common.(1) Patients often lose bladder and bowel function.(4, 5)

   Many patients will also perform one or more of the following unconscious actions during a generalized seizure: (2)

   - chewing actions
   - grinding teeth
   - licking at the air
   - swallowing hard
   - vocalizing.

   Seizures often last longer than syncope, and seizing patients take more time to recover.(11) There is a so-called post-ictal period after a seizure, during which time the patient acts abnormally.(2, 4) This recovery phase is variable in duration, but typically is on the order of minutes to hours.(2, 4) During this time, patients may exhibit one or more of the following clinical signs:(2, 4, 15–18)

   - ataxia
   - blindness
   - circling
   - disorientation
   - lethargy
   - pacing.

4. Most seizures are self-limiting, meaning that patients recover on their own, without the need for medical intervention.(19) However, sometimes seizures are protracted. Protracted seizure activity means that either seizures are longer in duration than they ought to be, or the frequency with which they occur is on the rise.

113

5. Protracted seizure activity is concerning because it causes an excessive release of glutamate, which can irreversibly damage neurons.(19, 20) Once damaged, these neurons may form an abnormal cluster that is capable of initiating seizure activity in the future on its own.(19, 21)

    Patients that experience protracted seizure activity are also at risk of becoming dangerously hyperthermic.(4, 19, 21, 22) If a seizure persists long enough and core body temperature exceeds the high-end of its homeostatic setpoint for an extended period of time, then it is possible to essentially cook the brain. Thermal injury to the brain impacts the hippocampus, in particular, and has been linked to cognitive impairment in people.(23, 24)

    Protracted seizure activity may also cause arrhythmias and hypertension through mechanisms that have not yet been fully deduced.(4, 19, 21, 22)

6. When a patient has more than two seizures during a 24-hour period, the patient is said to be experiencing cluster seizures.(19) Cluster seizures may precipitate status epilepticus.(19) Status epilepticus refers to seizure activity that lasts for more than five minutes.(19) During status epilepticus, a patient may seize again and again without the opportunity to recover between episodes.(1)

7. Status epilepticus requires immediate medical intervention.(19, 25) The first drug that you reach for in this clinical situation is diazepam.(4, 19, 25–27)

8. Diazepam is typically administered intravenously; however, this can be challenging in a patient with generalized tonic-clonic activity. When intravenous access is not possible, rectal administration has been proposed.(19, 28)

    A single injection of diazepam may be insufficient. If patients are refractory to injectable diazepam, then continuous rate infusion (CRI) should be attempted.(1)

9. If patients are still refractory to treatment, then the following adjunctive therapies may be indicated:(19)

    - injectable phenobarbital
    - injectable levetiracetam
    - injectable propofol.

10. Intracranial causes of seizures include:(1, 4, 5, 25, 29–46)

    - anoxia
    - CNS trauma
    - idiopathic epilepsy
    - infectious disease:

        - bacterial:

            - *Escherichia coli*
            - *Staphylococcus* spp.
            - *Streptococcus* spp.

        - fungal:

            - blastomycosis
            - coccidioidomycosis
            - cryptococcosis

        - parasitic:

            - aberrant migration of cuterebra larvae
            - aberrant migration of adult *Dirofilaria immitis*

- protozoal:

    - neosporosis, caused by *Neospora caninum*
    - toxoplasmosis, caused by *Toxoplasma gondii*

- rickettsial:

    - ehrlichiosis
    - Rocky Mountain spotted fever (RMSF)

- viral:

    - canine distemper virus (CDV)
    - rabies virus

- neoplasia
- non-infectious inflammatory disease:

    - meningoencephalomyelitis
    - necrotizing encephalitis
    - necrotizing leukoencephalitis (NLE)
    - necrotizing meningoencephalomyelitis (NME)
    - pug dog encephalitis

- storage diseases
- structural diseases:

    - hydrocephalus
    - lissencephaly

- vascular accident.

11. Extracranial causes of seizures include:(1, 25, 29, 30, 37, 46)

- endocrinopathy:

    - hyperthyroidism
    - hypothyroidism

- hyperkalemia
- hypocalcemia
- hypoglycemia
- metabolic dysfunction:

    - portosystemic shunting and hepatic encephalopathy (HE)
    - uremia

- thiamine deficiency
- toxicosis:

    - chocolate
    - ethylene glycol
    - heavy metals
    - metaldehyde
    - tremorogenic mycotoxins

        - penitrem A
        - roquefortine

12. The following differential diagnoses are prioritized when seizures occur in pediatric patients:(1, 5)

- hydrocephalus
- hypoglycemia
- infectious disease
- lissencephaly
- portosystemic shunts.

13. Given that Tiny Tim is a toy breed and he has a history of decreased appetite progressing to inappetence over the past 24 hours or so, I am most concerned about hypoglycemia.

Given that he is a Chihuahua, I might also consider the differential diagnosis of hydrocephalus; however, it would have to be pretty severe because most patients with this condition are asymptomatic.(5) In order for hydrocephalus to cause seizure activity, I would expect to see a grossly abnormal contour of the skull on physical examination of Tiny Tim. A dome-shaped skull and/or prominent open fontanelle would raise my level of suspicion.(5)

Portosystemic shunts are possible, but more likely to occur in Yorkshire and Maltese terriers, and clinical signs related to the nervous system tend to occur after eating.(5) By contrast, Tiny Tim's history is that he has eaten very little in the last 24 hours.

14. To confirm my top differential diagnosis (hypoglycemia), I need to measure Tiny Tim's BG. I can perform this test easily using an in-house glucometer.

Returning to Case 8: The Trembly Puppy

Carly is petrified. She has never witnessed a seizure before, and she is beside herself with worry. She authorized the technician to whisk Tiny Tim into the back for stabilization and supportive care. While another team member is drawing up a dose of diazepam, the technician checks Tiny Tim's blood sugar using a glucometer (see Figure 8.2).

Round Two of Questions for Case 8: The Trembly Puppy

1. What type of blood do you need to run blood through a glucometer:

- whole blood?
- serum?
- plasma?

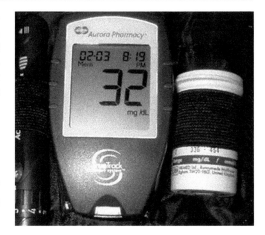

Figure 8.2 The in-house BG reading for Tiny Tim.

2. From which sites can you obtain a blood sample to assess BG in a dog? Cat? Consider how these sites may vary in the clinical setting (where technical staff are responsible for obtaining the sample) versus the home environment (where a client may be required to obtain a blood sample). Assume that the client has no training in venipuncture.
3. Based upon Tiny Tim's BG reading, would you classify him as being hyperglycemic, euglycemic, or hypoglycemic?
4. What is the normal reference range for BG in an 8-week-old puppy?
5. How does the normal reference range for BG change with age?
6. Which hormones regulate blood sugar?
7. What is the most likely explanation for Tiny Tim's BG level?
8. Is Tiny Tim's seizure activity likely to be related to his BG level? Why or why not?

9. What type of drug is diazepam?
10. What is the dose of diazepam?
11. Which side effects, if any, are associated with the administration of diazepam?
12. In addition to diazepam, which other drug(s) do you need to administer to Tiny Tim at this time? Provide a proposed dose and route of administration.
13. Once Tiny Tim is discharged to the care of his owner, what are your recommendations for Carly in terms of feeding instructions?
14. If Tiny Tim again goes off food at home and/or starts to act weak and lethargic, what could Carly do at home to intervene?

Answers to Round Two of Questions for Case 8: The Trembly Puppy

1. Glucometers require a sample of whole blood.

2. In a clinic setting, whole blood may be obtained through venipuncture, by drawing blood directly from a peripheral vessel, such as the cephalic vein or the lateral saphenous vein (canine)/medial saphenous vein (feline).

   In the home setting, the client may be trained to use a lancet to prick between the marginal ear veins and the edge of the ear, to obtain a sample of whole blood from a cat. Compare this approach with that of the canine patient. The inside of the dog's ear flap often yields a more consistent sample than using the outside of the ear flap as you would in a cat. In older dogs, elbow calluses are also a reasonable site to approach to collect a blood sample.

   Other helpful locations in dogs and cats, in the clinic and home environment, are the paw pads. However, patients typically resent this approach if the primary (weight-bearing) pads are used. Instead, make use of the pisiform pad, that is, the non-weight-bearing pad. This is better tolerated, even in those patients that dislike having their feet touched. Clients can be taught to use the "farrier technique": stand the pet up and flip the foot back towards you as you would to clean a horse's hoof. This facilitates blood collection.

3. Tiny Tim's BG is registering at 32 mg/dL. At this value, he is considered hypoglycemic.

4. Reference ranges vary somewhat depending upon which resource you refer to; however, in general, the BG of an 8-week-old pup tends to range from 122–159 mg/dL.(47)

5. As pups age, the lower end of the reference range drops. For example, between 4 and 6 months of age, the lower limit of BG averages 97 mg/dL.(47) By 7 to 12 months old, the lower limit is 76 mg/dL.(47) This stays relatively consistent through adult life.

6. The regulation of BG involves many players. Four hormones work in concert to increase BG levels as needed by the body:(48–52)

   - cortisol
   - epinephrine
   - glucagon
   - growth hormone.

   By contrast, only one hormone, insulin, is responsible for reducing circulating levels of BG.(48–51)

   Sometimes it helps to think of the major players, glucagon and insulin, as being on opposing teams: the former increases blood sugar, while the latter reduces it.

   Alternatively, think of the body's regulation of BG as a balancing act. When we check BG, we get a snapshot in time that reveals which "team" is winning in the moment.

7. The most likely explanation for Tiny Tim's BG level is transient juvenile hypoglycemia bought on by inappetence.(47, 50) This condition occurs primarily in miniature and toy breeds.(47, 52, 53)

   All pups have limited capacity to fast due to inadequate stores of glycogen. However, miniature and toy breeds are particularly deficient when it comes to energy reserves.(47) For starters, they are tiny. They have high surface area: volume ratios and very little fat. This means that they cannot generate their own fuel through the breakdown of adipose tissue when glucose is scarce.

   When miniature or toy breeds take in insufficient glucose in their diet because they are refusing to eat (or food has been taken away from them), they are also unable to efficiently generate their own glucose through gluconeogenesis.(47) In large part, this is because their liver is quite small by comparison to the adult dog, and their skeletal muscle mass is also minimal on account of age.(50) There is very little ability of the body to make its own sugar as a source of fuel. This is a concern because the brain requires glucose to function.(50) Without dietary glucose and without the ability to generate their own supply, these pups suffer from neuroglycopenia.(46, 51) Their brains essentially shut down. If the glucose deficit is not resolved promptly, neurons are unable to generate ATP and will die off due to increased vascular permeability, vascular dilation, and edema.(51) When a hypoglycemic episode such as this occurs in neonates, it is likely to result in permanent brain damage.(53, 54)

   Weakness, lethargy, dull mentation, muscle twitches, tremors, ataxia, collapse, and seizure activity are common clinical signs that are associated with transient juvenile hypoglycemia.(46, 50, 51) Patients are predisposed to this condition if they experience one or more of the following factors:(50, 51)

   - dehydration
   - diarrhea
   - hypothermia
   - inadequate quantity of food
   - infectious disease
   - poor quality food
   - prolonged fasting
   - stress
   - vaccinations
   - vomiting.

   Oftentimes, prolonged fasting is unintentional, meaning that the client is ill-informed. The client is unaware (or wasn't told!) that miniature and toy breed puppies cannot survive on just two meals a day. Twelve hours between breakfast and dinner is too great of a time to be without food. These pups require three to four feedings a day, at least through four to six months of age.(50)

8. Yes, it is likely that Tiny Tim is seizing because of hypoglycemia. When BG levels drop below 40 mg/dL in puppies that are less than six months of age, there is insufficient glucose to feed the brain.(50) This results in neuronal damage and brain injury as described in the answer to Question #7 above.

9. Diazepam (Valium) is a benzodiazepine.(5, 55, 56) Benzodiazepines tend to be effective anticonvulsant drugs because they potentiate the actions of gamma-aminobutyric acid (GABA), an inhibitory neurotransmitter.(5)

10. The dose of diazepam is 0.5 mg/kg when administered intravenously or 1–2mg/kg when administered rectally.(5, 55)

    If a CRI of diazepam is necessary because the patient is refractory to injectable therapy, then an infusion rate of 0.5 mg/kg/hour is appropriate.(5, 55)

11. The body develops tolerance to the use of benzodiazepines if they were used daily as part of maintenance therapy for epileptic individuals.(5) In addition, the effect of benzodiazepines in dogs is short-lived.(5) For both of these reasons, benzodiazepines are inappropriate for long-term use in outpatients to manage longstanding seizure disorders as part of a daily treatment regime.

12. Although the administration of diazepam should stop Tiny Tim's seizure activity, it does not address the underlying problem: transient juvenile hypoglycemia. Therefore, in addition to diazepam, Tiny Tim requires dextrose.

    Dextrose is available in high concentrations in the clinic setting. Most clinics carry solutions of 50% dextrose. If this concentration were administered directly into a vein, it would likely cause phlebitis and/or hemolysis.(51) To minimize this, 50% dextrose is diluted in sterile saline prior to injection.

    The dose of 50% dextrose is 0.5–1.0 mL/kg, diluted 1 : 2 with sterile saline and injected intravenously.(51)

    Patients are typically quick to respond and do so within five minutes of receiving the injection.(51) Patients such as Tiny Tim, with presumptive transient juvenile hypoglycemia, should perk up rather instantly. Appropriate mentation should be restored, and Tiny Tim may now show interest in eating.(51) Ideally, he should be offered a diet that contains complex carbohydrates so that it is broken down slowly and therefore blood levels of circulating glucose can be maintained for longer periods of time.(51) Even so, he needs frequent feedings.(51)

    If Tiny Tim does not want to eat on his own, then he will need to be admitted to the hospital until he proves that he is ready to take care of himself. To manage him as an inpatient, you will need to place an intravenous catheter so that he can receive a CRI of a balanced crystalloid solution that has been spiked with 2.5–5% dextrose.(51) The goal is to maintain BG between 60–150 mg/dL.(51) He can be weaned off gradually as he starts to show interest in eating on his own.

13. Once Tiny Tim is discharged to the care of his owner, Carly needs to offer him four meals per day. Feeding every six hours should prevent a recurrence of transient juvenile hypoglycemia.

14. If Tiny Tim again goes off food at home and/or starts to act weak and lethargic, Carly can apply corn syrup or honey to the lining of his cheek or directly to his gums.(51) Absorption through the oral mucosa is not ideal, so he will still require veterinary medical attention; however, this may buy time to get to the clinic.

CLINICAL PEARLS

- Miniature and toy breed puppies are predisposed to fasting hypoglycemia.

- If miniature and toy breed puppies do not receive frequent feedings, either because the client is misinformed and is only offering breakfast and dinner, or because the patients refuse to eat of their own accord, then they are at risk of developing neuropathy.

- The brain requires glucose as its sole fuel.

- Miniature and toy breed puppies are unable to produce adequate quantities of glucose on their own through gluconeogenesis and lipolysis because of their small size, small livers, small skeletal muscle mass, and inadequate fat depots.

- Without sufficient levels of circulating glucose, neurons cannot produce the ATP they need to sustain basic functions.

- Affected patients exhibit generalized signs of malaise, including weakness and lethargy.

- If BG drops below 40 mg/dL, then neurologic signs are imminent. These may include a dull or depressed mentation, ataxia, collapse, muscle fasciculations, convulsions, and/or seizure activity.

- BG levels can be measured in-house by testing whole blood samples using glucometers. This will confirm that the patient is experiencing a hypoglycemic state.

- Seizure activity should respond to intravenous or rectal administration of the benzodiazepine, diazepam; however, this does not address the underlying cause.
- Patients require intravenous dextrose diluted in saline to normalize BG.

References

1. Englar RE. Common clinical presentations in dogs and cats. Hoboken, NJ: Wiley/Blackwell; 2019.
2. Mariani CL. Terminology and classification of seizures and epilepsy in veterinary patients. Top Companion Anim Med 2013;28(2):34–41.
3. Chandler K. Canine epilepsy: what can we learn from human seizure disorders? Vet J 2006;172(2):207–17.
4. Thomas WB. Idiopathic epilepsy in dogs and cats. Vet Clin North Am Small Anim Pract 2010;40(1):161–79.
5. Lavely JA. Pediatric seizure disorders in dogs and cats. Vet Clin North Am Small Anim Pract 2014;44(2):275–301.
6. Kraus MS, editor. Syncope in small breed dogs. ACVIM; 2003. Available from: https://www.vin.com/Members/Proceedings/Proceedings.plx?CID=acvim2003&PID=pr03923&O=VIN.
7. Thawley V, Collapse SD. NAVC clinician's. Brief 2012 (November):14–5.
8. Estrada A. Differentiating syncope from seizure. NAVC Clin's Brief 2017 (July):50–5.
9. Barnett L, Martin MW, Todd J, Smith S, Cobb M. A retrospective study of 153 cases of undiagnosed collapse, syncope or exercise intolerance: the outcomes. J Small Anim Pract 2011;52(1):26–31.
10. Gurfinkel V, Cacciatore TW, Cordo P, Horak F, Nutt J, Skoss R. Postural muscle tone in the body axis of healthy humans. J Neurophysiol 2006;96(5):2678–87.
11. Schwartz DS, editor. The syncopal dog. World Small Animal Veterinary Association World Congress Proceedings, Sao Paulo, Brazil; 2009.
12. Dutton E, Dukes-McEwan J, Cripps PJ. Serum cardiac troponin I in canine syncope and seizures. J Vet Cardiol 2017;19(1):1–13.
13. Penning VA, Connolly DJ, Gajanayake I, McMahon LA, Luis Fuentes V, Chandler KE, Volk HA. Seizure-like episodes in 3 cats with intermittent high-grade atrioventricular dysfunction. J Vet Intern Med 2009;23(1):200–5.
14. Motta L, Dutton E. Suspected exercise-induced seizures in a young dog. J Small Anim Pract 2013;54(4):213–8.
15. De Risio L, Bhatti S, Muñana K, Penderis J, Stein V, Tipold A, et al. International veterinary epilepsy task force consensus proposal: diagnostic approach to epilepsy in dogs. BMC Vet Res 2015;11:148.
16. Berendt M, Gram L. Epilepsy and seizure classification in 63 dogs: a reappraisal of veterinary epilepsy terminology. J Vet Intern Med 1999;13(1):14–20.
17. Pákozdy A, Leschnik M, Tichy AG, Thalhammer JG. Retrospective clinical comparison of idiopathic versus symptomatic epilepsy in 240 dogs with seizures. Acta Vet Hung 2008;56(4):471–83.
18. Patterson EE, Armstrong PJ, O'Brien DP, Roberts MC, Johnson GS, Mickelson JR. Clinical description and mode of inheritance of idiopathic epilepsy in English springer spaniels. J Am Vet Med Assoc 2005;226(1):54–8.
19. Patterson EN. Status epilepticus and cluster seizures. Vet Clin North Am Small Anim Pract 2014;44(6):1103–12.
20. Huff JS, Fountain NB. Pathophysiology and definitions of seizures and status epilepticus. Emerg Med Clin North Am 2011;29(1):1–13.
21. Berg AT, Berkovic SF, Brodie MJ, Buchhalter J, Cross JH, van Emde Boas W, et al. Revised terminology and concepts for organization of seizures and epilepsies: report of the ILAE Commission on Classification and Terminology, 2005–2009. Epilepsia 2010;51(4):676–85.
22. Raith K, Steinberg T, Fischer A. Continuous electroencephalographic monitoring of status epilepticus in dogs and cats: 10 patients (2004–2005). J Vet Emerg Crit Care (San Antonio) 2010;20(4):446–55.
23. Scott RC. What are the effects of prolonged seizures in the brain? Epileptic Disord 2014;16;Spec No 1:S6–11.
24. Scott RC. Consequences of febrile seizures in childhood. Curr Opin Pediatr 2014;26(6):662–7.
25. Smith Bailey K, Dewey CW. The seizuring cat. Diagnostic work-up and therapy. J Feline Med Surg 2009;11(5):385–94.
26. Podell M. Antiepileptic drug therapy. Clin Tech Small Anim Pract 1998;13(3):185–92.
27. Platt S, Garosi L. Small animal neurological emergencies. London: Manson Publishing; 2012.

28. Podell M. The use of diazepam per rectum at home for the acute management of cluster seizures in dogs. J Vet Intern Med 1995;9(2):68–74.

29. Seizures CE. In: Côté E, editor. Clinical veterinary advisor Dogs and cats. 3rd ed. St. Louis. MO: Elsevier Mosby; 2013. p. 593–4.

30. Tilley LP, Smith FWK. The 5-minute veterinary consult: canine and feline. 3rd ed. Baltimore, MD: Lippincott Williams & Wilkins; 2004.

31. Thomas WB. Inflammatory diseases of the central nervous system in dogs. Clin Tech Small Anim Pract 1998;13(3):167–78.

32. Lowrie M. Infectious and non-infectious inflammatory causes of seizures in dogs and cats. Pract 2016;38(3):99–110.

33. Gaunt MC, Taylor SM, Kerr ME. Central nervous system blastomycosis in a dog. Can Vet J 2009;50(9):959–62.

34. Hecht S, Adams WH, Smith JR, Thomas WB. Clinical and imaging findings in five dogs with intracranial blastomycosis (Blastomyces dermatiditis). J Am Anim Hosp Assoc 2011;47(4):241–9.

35. Brömel C, Sykes JE. Epidemiology, diagnosis, and treatment of blastomycosis in dogs and cats. Clin Tech Small Anim Pract 2005;20(4):233–9.

36. Irwin PJ, Parry BW. Streptococcal meningoencephalitis in a dog. J Am Anim Hosp Assoc 1999;35(5):417–22.

37. Schriefl S, Steinberg TA, Matiasek K, Ossig A, Fenske N, Fischer A. Etiologic classification of seizures, signalment, clinical signs, and outcome in cats with seizure disorders: 91 cases (2000–2004). J Am Vet Med Assoc 2008;233(10):1591–7.

38. Barnes HL, Chrisman CL, Mariani CL, Sims M, Alleman AR. Clinical signs, underlying cause, and outcome in cats with seizures: 17 cases (1997–2002). J Am Vet Med Assoc 2004;225(11):1723–6.

39. Singh M, Foster DJ, Child G, Lamb WA. Inflammatory cerebrospinal fluid analysis in cats: clinical diagnosis and outcome. J Feline Med Surg 2005;7(2):77–93.

40. Quesnel AD, Parent JM, McDonell W, Percy D, Lumsden JH. Diagnostic evaluation of cats with seizure disorders: 30 cases (1991–1993). J Am Vet Med Assoc 1997;210(1):65–71.

41. Rand JS, Parent J, Percy D, Jacobs R. Clinical, cerebrospinal fluid, and histological data from twenty-seven cats with primary inflammatory disease of the central nervous system. Can Vet J 1994;35(2):103–10.

42. Troxel MT, Vite CH, Van Winkle TJ, Newton AL, Tiches D, Dayrell-Hart B, et al. Feline intracranial neoplasia: retrospective review of 160 cases (1985–2001). J Vet Intern Med 2003;17(6):850–9.

43. Barnes Heller H. Feline epilepsy. Vet Clin North Am Small Anim Pract 2018;48(1):31–43.

44. Schriefl S, Steinberg TA, Matiasek K, Ossig A, Fenske N, Fischer A. Etiologic classification of seizures, signalment, clinical signs, and outcome in cats with seizure disorders: 91 cases. Vet Med A 2008;233(10):1591–7.

45. Kline KL. Feline epilepsy. Clin Tech Small Anim Pract 1998;13(3):152–8.

46. Coates JR, Bergman RL. Seizures in young dogs and cats: pathophysiology and diagnosis. Compendium 2005:447–59.

47. Gorman ME. Clinical chemistry of the puppy and kitten. In: Peterson ME, Kutzler MA, editors. Small animal pediatrics: The first 12 months of life. St. Louis, MO: Saunders; 2011. p. 259–75.

48. Cunningham JG, Klein BG. Cunningham's textbook of veterinary physiology. 5th ed. St. Louis, MO: Elsevier/Saunders; 2013.

49. Singh B, Dyce KM. Dyce, Sack, and Wensing's textbook of veterinary anatomy, Missouri: Saunders. 854 Pages p. 5th ed.. ed. St. Louis 2018;xv.

50. Greco DS, Chastain CB. Endocrine and metabolic systems. In: Hoskins JD, editor. Veterinary pediatrics: Dogs and cats from birth to six months. 3rd ed. Philadelphia, PA: Saunders; 2001.

51. Idowu O, Heading K. Hypoglycemia in dogs: causes, management, and diagnosis. Can Vet J 2018;59(6):642–9.

52. van Toor AJ, van der Linde-Sipman JS, van den Ingh TS, Wensing T, Mol JA. Experimental induction of fasting hypoglycaemia and fatty liver syndrome in three Yorkshire Terrier pups. Vet Q 1991;13(1):16–23.

53. Vroom MW, Slappendel RJ. Transient juvenile hypoglycaemia in a Yorkshire Terrier and in a Chihuahua. Vet Q 1987;9(2):172–6.

54. Lopate C. The critical neonate: under 4 weeks of age. NAVC Clin's Brief 2009 (November):9–13.

55. Plumb DC. Plumb's veterinary drug handbook. 9th ed. Hoboken NJ: Pharma Vet Inc; 2018.

56. Shell L. Anticonvulsants or antiepileptic drugs. In Merck veterinary manual. Whitehouse Station, NJ: Merck & Co., Inc. 2016.

Case 9

The Ataxic Kitten

Until 4 months ago, Evelyn Carter was enjoying the quiet life as an empty nester and retiree. With her children grown and out of the house, Evelyn had looked forward to some alone time. She had a list of do-it-yourself projects that had fallen by the wayside years ago and that she was ready to breathe into being. She was quite handy, so nothing was out of the picture. She dreamed of building a terrace and planting a garden, but not just any backyard plot. She wanted a garden big enough that she could walk among the rows of lettuce and squash. Evelyn had the space to make it work; she'd just never had the time. Now was her opportunity to revive her passion for working with her hands.

Evelyn was just about to dust off her green thumb when Miss Priss, short for Priscilla, became a fixture at her back door. How she found the place was anyone's guess. Evelyn's home was tucked into a cul-de-sac that no one

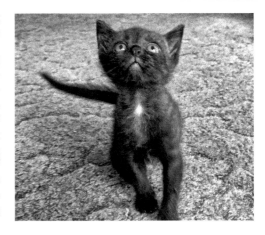

Figure 9.1 Your next patient, 8-week-old intact female domestic shorthaired (DSH) kitten. Courtesy of Sarah Greenway.

could seem to find, not even with GPS. Evelyn would later joke that Priss must have been drawn to an invisible sign in the yard that advertised a vacancy in the home. Priss had come from nowhere, so it seemed. Much like a weed, once her paws took hold of Carter soil, she was intent on staying.

Evelyn didn't feed her at first, hoping she'd go away. It wasn't that she didn't like cats. She just didn't want to be tied down to anything or anyone now that she finally had a breath of independence. But when Evelyn caught Priss breaking into the garbage can on day 3 to glean what little bit of meat there was on some old fish bones, her heart gave in. The mother in Evelyn took over, and she accepted Priss into her home.

Priss came and went as she pleased. She didn't look that bad for a stray. She wasn't skeletal, just unkempt. Evelyn assumed she'd gotten lost – and to that end, Evelyn put up fliers, but no one ever called upon her to claim Priss. Still, Priss was too socialized to be feral, and she certainly didn't have the hunting skills to support herself. Priss took after her name. She was snobby when it came to dining, but Evelyn indulged her. The way Evelyn saw it, this was her second chance in life. Might as well live it to the fullest.

After a few weeks, when it was clear that Priss was here to stay, Evelyn drove her to a vaccine clinic. Priss was tolerant and allowed a full exam. She tested negative for feline leukemia virus (FeLV) and feline immunodeficiency virus (FIV), and was vaccinated against rabies, feline viral rhinotracheitis-calicivirus-panleukopenia (FVRCP), and FeLV. Priss returned home to settle into a life of leisure. It wasn't long before she started to fill out nicely.

You can imagine Evelyn's surprise when one night, she heard muffled mews coming from the floor of the master bedroom closet. There, tucked in a makeshift nest of laundry, was Priss, surrounded by kittens! Evelyn had never seen ones so young, and she was glad that Priss seemed to know what to do. All seemed to be in order that first week or two. It was once the kittens started to move around that Evelyn grew concerned. Initially they all had sea legs, but two of the three kittens worked out the kinks rather quickly.

The third kitten seemed, well, different. She seemed shaky and unsure. When she stood, she hunkered low to the ground, and it was quite often that she would topple over. Her balance seemed to get worse when she was doing something. Eating, drinking, and scratching her post did not come easy to her. At times, she seemed like a drunken sailor. Evelyn worried about this little one – Pansy, she called her. She thought Pansy would grow out of it, but if anything, she seemed to be getting worse. Evelyn wondered if it was possible that Pansy had some kind of seizure disorder. At times, she did appear to go into fits or spasms. Her neighbor, a human nurse, didn't think so, and recommended that she seek veterinary care. Evelyn delayed the visit for as long as she could. She was deathly afraid that something was very wrong with Pansy. It was clear that she was not "normal" and that her "issue" wasn't going away.

By the time that Evelyn worked up the courage to schedule today's appointment, Pansy had turned 8 weeks old. The other two kittens had already been re-homed, but no one seemed to want Pansy. Evelyn is beside herself today, waiting for you to evaluate Pansy. She has already fallen in love with her, even though she promised herself that she wouldn't.

After taking a comprehensive patient history, you observe Pansy in the examination room. It is apparent that she has a form of dyskinesia.

Round One of Questions for Case 9: The Ataxic Kitten

1. Define dyskinesia.
2. In health, movement is a coordinated activity that requires different parts of the body to communicate with one another. What are the major players that are involved in this dynamic exchange of information?
3. Which types of neurons initiate and modulate movement?
4. Differentiate upper motor neurons (UMNs) from lower motor neurons (LMNs).
5. Does all movement require conscious thought?
6. How may dyskinesia resemble epilepsy?
7. How does dyskinesia differ from epilepsy?
8. Broadly differentiate primary from secondary dyskinesia.
9. Both primary and secondary dyskinesias often involve dystonia. Define dystonia and provide examples to illustrate how dystonia might present.

Answers to Round One of Questions for Case 9: The Ataxic Kitten

1. Dyskinesia is a broad term that is used to describe a number of involuntary movement disorders.(1)

2. The ability to initiate, sustain, and alter movement requires effective communication between the CNS, which constitutes the brain and spinal cord, and the peripheral nervous system (PNS).(1) These systems communicate with one another through an extensive network of neurons.(2–6)

3. In order for movement to occur, a specific type of neurons, motor neurons, must connect to and communicate with effector muscles.(2) When skeletal muscles receive signals from motor neurons, they must translate these signals into actions. The signals tell the muscle fibers to contract. This is the process by which the body can move.

    There are two types of motor neurons: UMNs and LMNs.(2, 5) Both play an important role in movement.(1)

4. UMNs originate from the CNS.(1) Specifically, UMNs arise from the brain. Their purpose is to connect different parts of the brain to different parts of the spinal cord in order to regulate posture, muscle tone, and gait.(2, 5)

    UMNs alone cannot reach the muscle fibers to tell them to contract to initiate movement. In order to send a signal to skeletal muscle, UMNs require intermediaries.(1) These messengers are LMNs. UMN axons may synapse directly onto LMNs or they may synapse onto one or more interneurons that pass the electrical signal to LMNs.(2, 4, 5) It is then the responsibility of LMNs to transmit the signal to muscle fibers.(2) LMNs make use of cranial or spinal nerves to reach their target effector.(2) When effectors are skeletal muscles, their response is to contract.(2)

5. No, all movement does not require conscious thought.(1) Consider reflexes. Reflexes occur when the body reacts to external or internal stimuli without cerebral input.(1) In that respect, reflexes are built-in responses.(5, 7, 8) We don't have to think about them for reflexes to happen. Somatic or spinal reflexes are a good example. These control muscle contraction, and are mediated by the brainstem and the spinal cord rather than the cerebrum.(9–11) They help to support the body against gravity at all times.(10) If we had to think about these reflexes for them to occur, then our body could not react as quickly or efficiently to external stimuli. Reflexes are a means of protecting our time so that we can focus our attention on what we need to, when we need to.

6. Certain types of dyskinesias may resemble epileptic episodes because both categories of medical conditions involve unusual, abnormal movements. Refer to Case #8 for a more complete discussion about seizures. However, to review, autonomic activity during a seizure is common. (1) Many patients with seizure disorders experience prolonged contraction of muscle groups, followed by a jerky muscular action.(1, 12, 13) When this occurs as part of a generalized seizure, many muscle groups are involved. The resultant limb paddling can be quite pronounced. Not all dyskinesias appear that dramatic. However, there are times when it may be difficult to distinguish dyskinesia from true epilepsy because clinical signs may overlap. An additional similarity is that both conditions are also episodic.

7. Although certain types of dyskinesias may resemble epileptic episodes, there are three important distinctions that can help to tell them apart:(1, 14, 15)

    A. Generalized seizure disorders involve a transient loss of consciousness because both cerebral hemispheres are involved.(12, 16, 17) Each episode is triggered by a burst of uncontrolled electrical activity.(1)

    By contrast, patients with dyskinesia do not lose consciousness.(1) They are aware of themselves and their surroundings. They simply experience involuntary muscle activity.(1)

    B. Patients with generalized seizure disorders often exhibit autonomic activity during and after an episode.(1, 18, 19) Most commonly, the sympathetic nervous system is activated, and the patient becomes tachycardic and hypertensive.(18) Human epileptic patients often report that their hearts seemed to be pounding from their chests.(19) Other autonomic signs that have been reported by and/or observed in people with epilepsy include:(19)

    - respiratory signs:

        - hyperventilation
        - post-seizure apnea

    - gastrointestinal signs:

        - nausea
        - retching
        - vomiting

- heartburn
- sensation of "butterflies" in the stomach (nervousness)
- sensation of abdominal distension or pressure

- cutaneous signs:

  - flushing of the skin
  - sweating
  - piloerection (development of "goosebumps" in people)

- urogenital signs:

  - urinary incontinence

- special senses:

  - bilateral mydriasis.

Many of these signs are observed in veterinary patients during an epileptic attack. In my clinical experience, mydriasis is quite common to witness in a patient that is actively seizing.

By contrast, patients with dyskinesia do not experience autonomic activity during involuntary muscle actions.(1)

C. Patients with generalized seizure disorders do not typically bounce back to normal after an episode. They need minutes to hours to recover.(12, 16, 20) This post-seizure recovery phase is referred to as the post-ictal period.(12, 16) During this phase, patients do not act clinically normal. They may experience one or more of the following signs:(12, 16, 21–24)

- ataxia
- blindness
- circling
- disorientation
- lethargy
- pacing.

By contrast, patients with dyskinesias do experience a post-ictal phase.(14, 15) Patients with dyskinesias are entirely normal between episodes.

8. Primary dyskinesias are inherited or idiopathic.(1) On the other hand, secondary dyskinesias result from structural lesions within the CNS, such as space-occupying masses.(25) Secondary dyskinesias may also be drug- or diet-induced.(25)

9. Dystonia refers to involuntary muscle contractions.(15, 26) These may be sustained or intermittent.(26)

Dystonia may present clinically in different ways:(15, 25–27)

- athetosis – twisting and writhing actions
- chorea – jerky movements involving the distal limbs and/or the face
- cramps – intense, painful muscular contractions that render a patient immobile during an episode
- fasciculations – subtle twitches of a fraction of muscle fibers just beneath the skin
- myokymia – constant rippling of the muscles just beneath the skin
- neuromyotonia – generalized stiffness due to delayed muscle relaxation
- tremor – involuntary quivering, caused by rhythmic muscle contractions.

Returning to Case 9: The Ataxic Kitten

You examine Pansy. Based upon her clinical presentation, you classify her dystonia as tremorgenic. More specifically, Pansy is experiencing so-called intention tremors.

In addition, you notice that Pansy is ataxic and hypermetric. Her default appears to be a broad-based stance that instantly takes you back to your introductory neurology course in vet school. You have seen her condition before, both in the lecture hall and in clinical practice.

Although you assure Evelyn that this condition is not terminal, Evelyn is understandably concerned about Pansy's future and whether she can still experience good quality of life. Help Evelyn to make sense of Pansy's condition and the most likely diagnosis.

Round Two of Questions for Case 9: The Ataxic Kitten

1. Define ataxia.
2. What are the three broad categories of ataxia?
3. What is meant by the clinical description, hypermetric gait?
4. What is an intention tremor?
5. An intention tremor is the result of dysfunction in which part of the brain?
6. Which medical condition is the most common cause of intention tremors in kittens?
7. Identify the infectious agent that is responsible for the medical condition that you named in Question #3 (above)
8. Describe the epidemiology of this infectious agent: how is the agent transmitted?
9. In brief, how does the agent impart disease?
10. How does the timing of infection (i.e. whether the patient is infected in utero versus as a neonate) impact the affected patient's clinical presentation?
11. How do you explain Pansy's clinical presentation? How did she most likely contract this condition?
12. Evelyn is not convinced that you are correct. She tells you that Pansy's two littermates are "fine" so how could your explanation possibly make sense? Wouldn't they all share the same experience?
13. If Pansy had instead contracted this condition as a young, unvaccinated kitten, how might her clinical presentation have been different from what you are seeing today? Consider clinical signs as well as physical exam findings that you would have anticipated.
14. If Pansy presented in the way that you described in Question #13 (above), what would you have expected her clinical laboratory findings to be?
15. Had Pansy presented like the kitten in Question #13 (above), how would you have tested her to confirm the diagnosis?
16. Evelyn appreciates the time that you have taken to share more with her about Pansy's condition. She asks you if it is likely that Pansy's condition will progress. How will you answer her?
17. Evelyn also asks if there is anything that she can do at home to help with Pansy's condition. What do you say?
18. Evelyn wants to know why the veterinarian did not know that Priss was pregnant at the time that she received her immunizations. She asks you if vaccinating Priss at that time constitutes malpractice. How do you respond?
19. Walk me through pregnancy detection by external palpation in a cat in terms of the timeline. When should you feel which structures, assuming that you have experience with pregnancy detection in cats?
20. Moving forward, are there any other vaccination-related concerns that you should keep in mind, if you end up working with clients with young (<4 weeks old) kittens in the future?

Answers to Round Two of Questions for Case 9: The Ataxic Kitten

1. Ataxia refers to an uncoordinated gait.(1, 28)

2. Three types of ataxia have been described in the veterinary medical literature:(29–31)

   - cerebellar ataxia
   - vestibular ataxia
   - proprioceptive (sensory) ataxia.

   Cerebellar ataxia involves the cerebellum.(1) The cerebellum is responsible for gait generation. (1) Therefore, a patient with cerebellar ataxia demonstrates an abnormal rate, range, or force of movement.(31) Sometimes these patients are described as having a classic "toy soldier" gait because they walk stiffly, with exaggerated flexion and over-reaching steps.(31, 32)

   Vestibular ataxia is caused by a dysfunctional vestibular system.(1) The vestibular system maintains the body's sense of balance as it moves through space, by coordinating body posture and eye position relative to where the head is positioned.(33–38) To be functional, the vestibular system requires communication between two components: the central and peripheral vestibular systems.(1) The central vestibular system is comprised of the brainstem, the cerebellum, and two caudal cerebellar peduncles.(39, 40) The peripheral vestibular system includes the middle and inner ear, as well as cranial nerve (CN) VIII, the vestibulocochlear nerve.(39–41) When either the central or peripheral vestibular system is compromised, then body posture, head posture, eye position, eye movement, and/or gait is altered.(33, 34, 37)

   A patient that exhibits vestibular ataxia has truly lost his or her balance.(31) In cases of unilateral disease, the patient will lean, if not fall, towards one side.(1) When vestibular disease is bilateral, the patient is reluctant to move, but may sway the head side to side.(29, 42)

   Proprioceptive (sensory) ataxia results from damage to the peripheral nerve, dorsal root, spinal cord, or brainstem. The affected patient no longer has a sense of where the affected limb is positioned relative to the rest of its body.(31) These patients will often "knuckle over," meaning that they scuff or stand upon the dorsal aspect of the affected foot or feet.

3. Hypermetria refers to a high-stepping gait.(1) Sometimes this is referred to as goose-stepping. It means that movement of the affected limbs is exaggerated. If you were to look at how a normal cat walks, for instance, you would see that the animal barely lifts it foot up off the ground. Movement is efficient and stride is succinct. When the gait becomes hypermetric, affected limbs are dramatically hiked up, much more so than is expected. The limbs are, in a sense, overreaching their goal.

4. There are many types of tremors. Some tremors occur at rest. Other tremors, such as intention tremors, are associated with certain actions.(25, 27) In other words, motion initiates the tremor.(1)

5. An intention tremor results from dysfunction within the cerebellum.(1)

6. Cerebellar hypoplasia is the most common cause of intention tremors in kittens.(1, 43–47)

7. When cerebellar hypoplasia occurs in kittens, they are most likely infected with feline panleukopenia virus.(1, 48) Because this is a type of parvovirus, the infectious agent is often referred to as feline parvovirus.(48)

8. Feline panleukopenia virus is ubiquitous in the environment.(48) It is stable in the environment and extremely infectious.(48–51) Most cats, including kittens, become exposed through the environment, by coming into contact with urine and/or feces from infected cats.(48) Feline panleukopenia virus is transmitted through the fecal-oral route.(48–50)

We can also play an accidental role in transmission if we handle infected kittens and cats and do not take care to decontaminate our hands and/or clothing.(48, 50) In this way, we can act as fomites for propagation of disease.(48, 50) Other sources of infection include contaminated food and water bowls, bedding, and even litter trays.(48)

Fetuses can also become infected in utero when queens become infected during pregnancy.(48)

9. All parvoviruses target rapidly dividing cells within their host's body.(48) In unvaccinated adult animals and kittens greater than six weeks of age, the following sites are often targeted because they have the greatest rate of mitotic activity:(48–50)

- bone marrow
- intestinal crypts
- lymph nodes and/or the thymus.

If the bone marrow is targeted, then the body's supply of stem cells will be under attack.(49) This will lead to neutropenia and, ultimately, both anemia and thrombocytopenia.(49)

Infection of the intestinal crypts will lead to shortening of the villi, the absorptive layer of the intestinal wall. This leads to poor absorption of nutrients and the clinical sign of diarrhea.(49)

If lymphoid tissue is targeted, then the thymus (in kittens) will atrophy prematurely, and patients will experience lymphopenia.(49) Adults that become infected can also experience lymphopenia if the virus causes apoptosis of circulating lymphocytes.(49)

10. The fetal cerebellum develops late in gestation.(48) If fetuses become infected during this time, then feline panleukopenia virus will preferentially attack this growing neural tissue.(48–50, 52) Specifically, the virus targets cortical cells within the cerebellum and hinders its development by replicating in Purkinje cells.(48, 49) The result is a poorly formed cerebellum that is hypoplastic.(48)

If the fetus becomes infected early in gestation, prior to cerebellar development, then the cerebellum will be spared at the expense of early developing neural tissues, including the spinal cord, optic nerve, and retina.(48) If neuropathy is severe, then fetuses may be aborted.(48, 50) In some cases, fetuses may grow to term, but have significant structural disease to overcome in neonatal life, including, but not limited to hydrocephalus and hydranencephaly.(48, 53) In cases of retinopathy, fetuses will grow to full-term, but they will be born with fundic lesions that represent discrete areas of retinal degeneration.(48)

11. In order for Pansy to demonstrate the neurologic signs that she is today, related to cerebellar dysfunction, Pansy's mom, Priss, would have had to have been infected with feline panleukopenia late in her pregnancy. This could have occurred through natural infection or infections could have been iatrogenic. We know from our comprehensive health history that Priss was vaccinated against FVRCP during pregnancy.

The FVRCP immunization is most often administered as a modified live vaccine (MLV).(48) Vaccinating a pregnant cat against FVRCP using a MLV may induce abortion or birth defects, including cerebellar dysfunction, depending upon when the vaccination was administered.(48, 54, 55)

12. I would agree with Evelyn that it is confusing why Pansy's littermates were unaffected. However, for reasons that we do not understand, not all littermates have to be affected by feline panleukopenia virus.(48, 52) Of those that are, it is not uncommon to see varying degrees of neurologic dysfunction.(48)

It has been hypothesized that littermates can be affected differently depending upon innate resistance.(50) Alternatively, it is possible that some kittens in utero may have acquired maternally derived antibodies while others did not.(50)

13. If Pansy had instead become infected with panleukopenia virus as a young, unvaccinated kitten, then she would have likely presented acutely for depression, lethargy, anorexia, and vomiting.(1, 48, 50, 56) The client may or may not have witnessed diarrhea. Not all kittens with panleukopenia are diarrheic.(48, 56) On presentation, I would have expected her to be febrile and dehydrated.(48) I would have expected to palpate diffusely thickened, ropy loops of small bowel.(48) Mortality rate is high in these cases and exceeds 90%.(49, 50)

14. If Pansy presented in the way that you described in Question #13 (above), I would have expected her to demonstrate one or more of the following changes in her leukogram (see figure 9.2):(48)

    • neutropenia
    • lymphopenia
    • leukopenia.

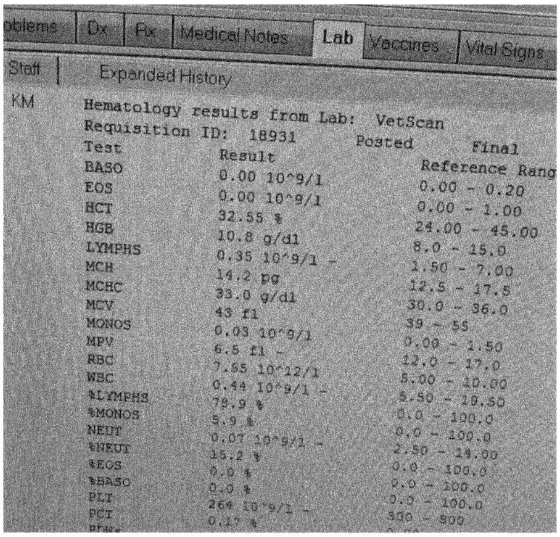

Figure 9.2 An example of an in-house complete blood count (CBC) for a kitten with panleukopenia. Courtesy of Allison Ward, DVM.

Anemia is not typically seen unless there is significant blood loss through the digestive tract.(48)
Thrombocytopenia may or may not be present.(48)
I would expect Pansy's serum biochemistry profile to demonstrate pre-renal azotemia, secondary to dehydration, and potentially mild to moderate elevations in aspartate aminotransferase (AST), alanine aminotransferase (ALT), or bilirubin.(48)

15. You can diagnose feline panleukopenia virus in kittens using the fecal enzyme-linked immunosorbent assay (ELISA) test for canine parvoviral antigen.(48, 49) However, it is important to understand that feline panleukopenia virus is typically shed for only 1 to 2 days in the feces of infected cats.(48, 56) Therefore, it is possible to obtain a false-negative result in a kitten that you suspect has feline panleukopenia virus.
    It is also important to know that MLV versions of the FVRCP vaccine can cause false positives up to 14 days post-immunization.(57, 58)

16. Although Pansy's condition will not get better, it almost certainly will not progress. The damage has already been done to her cerebellum, and those neurons will not regenerate. Therefore, whatever gait abnormalities she has will remain with her throughout life.

17. It is important to share with Evelyn that Pansy will not be in any pain from feline cerebellar hypoplasia.
    Like many other cats with cerebellar hypoplasia, Pansy will adapt to her condition and can lead a happy, healthy life.
    Evelyn can make the following adjustments in her management of Pansy's care to facilitate her adaptation to the Carter household.

    • Maintain Pansy's lifestyle as indoor-only.
    • Avoid trimming her nails super short because her claws will help her to gain traction as she moves around the house.
    • Consider investing in large litter boxes that are easy for her to get in and out.
    • Consider purchasing ramps to assist with getting on and off the furniture.

- Consider placing a baby gate at any stairwells to prevent Pansy from losing balance and accidentally falling down the steps.
- Consider the use of non-slip mats (including yoga mats) to provide traction on slippery floors.
- Avoid lots of vertical space because although cats love this design, there is too much opportunity for Pansy to injure herself.

18. It can be difficult to detect pregnancy in cats. Although the uterus is technically palpable during the pregnancy, it takes practice for a clinician to gain comfort, confidence, and accuracy with this skill.(59, 60).

    Many new graduates have never encountered an intact queen, let alone a pregnant one. Most of the cats that we see in general practice are in fact spayed. This reduces our opportunities to examine intact females and females that are definitively pregnant. So, it's not often that we get to practice our palpation skills for pregnancy detection unless we routinely work in the shelter environment.

19. If we were to confirm pregnancy through palpation, then technically we should be able to do so as early as day 14–17 of a 56–69 day gestation period.(28, 60, 61) During this time, each developing fetus is encased in its own spherical ball, which can be felt on abdominal palpation by an experienced practitioner.(60, 61) Sometimes these round structures are called "beads on a string" or "string of pearls." These become easier to appreciate on abdominal palpation between days 21–25 of pregnancy.(28, 59, 60)

    After day 35 to 45, it is difficult to appreciate the individual fetuses on abdominal palpation. (28) At this point, the placentas surrounding each fetal kitten are so large that the uterus palpates as one tubular structure rather than as individual sausage links.(60)

20. Cerebellar development begins in late gestation but continues through the first several weeks of neonatal life.(48) Therefore, it is possible to damage the cerebellum by vaccinating kittens that are younger than four weeks of age with a MLV vaccine.(48) If kittens are less than four weeks old and were deprived of colostrum, then historically it was common practice to administer an inactivated feline panleukopenia vaccine without ill effect.(48, 49) Inactivated vaccines produce less effective immunity; however, they will not cause cerebellar degeneration.(48, 49) Unfortunately, inactivated vaccines are rare finds in the present day. Most manufacturers have discontinued their production because vaccination with MLV provides more rapid protection.(49)

CLINICAL PEARLS

- Feline panleukopenia virus is a type of parvovirus that infects unvaccinated cats and kittens.

- Transmission of feline panleukopenia virus is via the fecal–oral route.

- Clinical signs of panleukopenia (+) cats or kittens vary significantly depending upon age at which they were infected.

  - Queens that become infected early in gestation may experience spontaneous abortion or kittens may be born with hydrocephalus or hydranencephaly.

  - Queens that become infected late in gestation will give birth to kittens that may exhibit signs of cerebellar hypoplasia. This is because the cerebellum is late to develop in fetal life and viral infection late in gestation will target that neural tissue specifically. Littermates are not necessarily all infected or infected to the same degree. Affected patients will present with varying degrees of cerebellar ataxia, hypermetria, intention tremors and a wide-based stance.

- Kittens under four weeks of age are still in the process of cerebellar development, so infection at this point can also lead to cerebellar hypoplasia.

- Kittens that are greater than or equal to six weeks of age and become infected more typically present with non-specific signs of malaise, depression, lethargy, vomiting, and anorexia, +/– diarrhea.

    - Mortality rate of this sector of the population is high.
    - Diagnosis of these kittens is made via the fecal enzyme-linked immunosorbent assay (ELISA) test for canine parvoviral antigen.

- Administration of the MLV during pregnancy can also cause fetal infection.

- Kittens that develop cerebellar hypoplasia secondary to feline panleukopenia virus can lead happy, healthy lives.

References

1. Englar RE. Common clinical presentations in dogs and cats. Hoboken, NJ: Wiley/Blackwell; 2019.
2. Molenaar GJ. The nervous system. In: Dyce KM, Sack WO, Wensing CJG, editors. Textbook of veterinary anatomy. 2nd ed. Philadelphia: W. B. Saunders Company; 1996. p. 259–324.
3. Behan M. Organization of the nervous system. In: Reece WO, editor. Dukes' physiology of domestic animals. 12th ed. Ithaca: Comstock Publishing Associates; 2004. p. 757–69.
4. Kitchell RL. Introduction to the nervous system. In: Evans HE, editor. Miller's anatomy of the dog. 3rd ed. Philadelphia: Saunders. p. 758–75.
5. Garosi L. Neurological examination of the cat. How to get started. J Feline Med Surg 2009;11(5):340–8.
6. Coates JR. The flaccid dog. DVM. 360 [Internet]; 2009. Available from: http://veterinarycalendar.dvm360.com/flaccid-dog-proceedings.
7. Jennings DP, Bailey JG. Spinal control of posture and movement. In: Reece WO, editor. Dukes' physiology of domestic animals. 12th ed. Ithaca, NY: Comstock Pub. Associates; 2004. p. 892–903.
8. Englar RE. Performing the small animal physical examination. Hoboken, NJ: Wiley; 2017.
9. Waldman SD. The spinal reflex arc. PAIN Review. Philaldephia, PA: Saunders; 2009.
10. Waterhouse J, Campbell I. Reflexes: principles and properties. Anaesth Intens Care Med 2017;18(5):270–5.
11. Millis DL, Mankin J. Orthopedic and neurologic evaluation. In: Millis DL, Levine D, editors. Canine rehabilitation and physical therapy. 2nd ed. Philadelphia, PA: Elsevier; 2014. p. 180–200.
12. Mariani CL. Terminology and classification of seizures and epilepsy in veterinary patients. Top Companion Anim Med 2013;28(2):34–41.
13. Chandler K. Canine epilepsy: what can we learn from human seizure disorders? Vet J 2006;172(2):207–17.
14. Akin E. Classifying paroxysmal dyskinesias. NAVC Clin's Brief 2017 (June):68–9.
15. Urkasemsin G, Olby NJ. Canine paroxysmal movement disorders. Vet Clin North Am Small Anim Pract 2014;44(6):1091–102.
16. Thomas WB. Idiopathic epilepsy in dogs and cats. Vet Clin North Am Small Anim Pract 2010;40(1):161–79.
17. Lavely JA. Pediatric seizure disorders in dogs and cats. Vet Clin North Am Small Anim Pract 2014;44(2):275–301.
18. Devinsky O. Effects of seizures on autonomic and cardiovascular function. Epilepsy Curr 2004;4(2):43–6.
19. Baumgartner C, Lurger S, Leutmezer F. Autonomic symptoms during epileptic seizures. Epileptic Disord 2001;3(3):103–16.
20. Schwartz DS, editor. The syncopal dog. Sao, Paulo: World Small Animal Veterinary Association World Congress Proceedings; 2009.
21. De Risio L, Bhatti S, Muñana K, Penderis J, Stein V, Tipold A, et al. International veterinary epilepsy task force consensus proposal: diagnostic approach to epilepsy in dogs. BMC Vet Res 2015;11:148.
22. Berendt M, Gram L. Epilepsy and seizure classification in 63 dogs: a reappraisal of veterinary epilepsy terminology. J Vet Intern Med 1999;13(1):14–20.

23. Pákozdy A, Leschnik M, Tichy AG, Thalhammer JG. Retrospective clinical comparison of idiopathic versus symptomatic epilepsy in 240 dogs with seizures. Acta Vet Hung 2008;56(4):471–83.

24. Patterson EE, Armstrong PJ, O'Brien DP, Roberts MC, Johnson GS, Mickelson JR. Clinical description and mode of inheritance of idiopathic epilepsy in English springer spaniels. J Am Vet Med Assoc 2005;226(1):54–8.

25. Lowrie M, Garosi L. Classification of involuntary movements in dogs: tremors and twitches. Vet J 2016;214:109–16.

26. Richter A, Hamann M, Wissel J, Volk HA. Dystonia and paroxysmal dyskinesias: under-recognized movement disorders in domestic animals? A comparison with human dystonia/paroxysmal dyskinesias. Front Vet Sci 2015;2:65.

27. Englar R. Evaluating the nervous system of the dog. In: Englar R, editor. Performing the small animal physical examination. Hoboken, NJ: John Wiley & Sons, Inc.; 2017. p. 412–31.

28. Englar RE. Performing the small animal physical examination. Hoboken, NJ: Wiley/Blackwell; 2017.

29. Thomas WB. Initial assessment of patients with neurologic dysfunction. Vet Clin North Am Small Anim Pract 2000;30(1):1–24, v, v.

30. Thomas WB, Dewey CW. Performing the neurologic examination. In: Dewey CW, editor. A practical guide to canine and feline neurology. 2nd ed. Ames, IA: Wiley/Blackwell; 2008. p. 53–74.

31. Casimiro da Costa R, editor. Ataxia – recognition and approach. World Small Animal Veterinary Association World Congress Proceedings; 2009.

32. Averill DR, Jr. The neurologic examination. Vet Clin North Am Small Anim Pract 1981;11(3):511–21.

33. Rossmeisl JH, Jr. Vestibular disease in dogs and cats. Vet Clin North Am Small Anim Pract 2010;40(1):81–100.

34. DeLahunta A, Glass E, Kent M. Veterinary neuroanatomy and clinical neurology. 4th ed.. ed. St. Louis. MO: Elsevier; 2015.

35. Angelaki DE, Cullen KE. Vestibular system: the many facets of a multimodal sense. Annu Rev Neurosci 2008;31:125–50.

36. Brandt T, Strupp M. General vestibular testing. Clin Neurophysiol 2005;116(2):406–26.

37. Thomas WB. Vestibular dysfunction. Vet Clin North Am Small Anim Pract 2000;30(1):227–49.

38. Troxel MT, Drobatz KJ, Vite CH. Signs of neurologic dysfunction in dogs with central versus peripheral vestibular disease. J Am Vet Med Assoc 2005;227(4):570–4.

39. Evans HE, DeLahunta A. Guide to the dissection of the dog. 6th ed. St. Louis, MO: Saunders; 2004.

40. Evans HE, Miller ME. Miller's anatomy of the dog. 4th ed. St. Louis, MO: Elsevier; 2013.

41. Rylander H. Vestibular syndrome: what's causing the head tilt and other neurologic signs? DVM360 [Internet]; 2012. Available from: http://veterinarymedicine.dvm360.com/vestibular-syndrome-whats-causing-head-tilt-and-other-neurologic-signs.

42. Parent JM. The cat with a head tilt, vestibular ataxia, or nystagmus. In: Rand J, editor. Problem-based feline medicine. Edinburgh. New York: Saunders; 2006. p. 835–51.

43. Lavely JA. Pediatric neurology of the dog and cat. Vet Clin North Am Small Anim Pract 2006;36(3):475–501, v, v.

44. Bagley RS. The cat with tremor or twitching. In: Rand J, editor. Problem-based feline medicine. St. Louis, MO: Saunders Elsevier; 2006. p. 852–69.

45. Hoskins JD, Shelton GD. The nervous and neuromuscular systems. In: Hoskins JD, editor. Veterinary pediatrics: dogs and cats from birth to six months. 3rd ed. Philadelphia, PA: Saunders; 2001. p. 425–62.

46. Blythe LL. The neurologic system. In: Peterson ME, Kutzler MA, editors. Small animal pediatrics: the first 12 months of life. St. Louis, MO: Saunders/Elsevier; 2011. p. 418–35.

47. Barone G. Neurology. In: Little SE, editor. The cat: clinical medicine and management. St. Louis. MO: Elsevier Saunders; 2012. p. 734–67.

48. Greene CE, Addie DD. Feline parvovirus infections. In: Greene CE, editor. Infectious diseases of the dog and cat. 3rd ed. St. Louis, MO: Saunders/Elsevier; 2006. p. 78–87.

49. Truyen U, Addie D, Belák S, Boucraut-Baralon C, Egberink H, Frymus T, et al. Feline panleukopenia. ABCD guidelines on prevention and management. J Feline Med Surg 2009;11(7):538–46.

50. Stuetzer B, Hartmann K. Feline parvovirus infection and associated diseases. Vet J 2014;201(2):150–5.

51. Kruse BD, Unterer S, Horlacher K, Sauter-Louis C, Hartmann K. Prognostic factors in cats with feline panleukopenia. J Vet Intern Med 2010;24(6):1271–6.

52. Greene CE, Addie DD. Feline parvovirus infections. In: Greene CE, editor. Infectious diseases of the dog and cat. 3rd ed. St. Louis, MO: Saunders/Elsevier; 2006. p. 78–88.

53. Sharp NJ, Davis BJ, Guy JS, Cullen JM, Steingold SF, Kornegay JN. Hydranencephaly and cerebellar hypoplasia in two kittens attributed to intrauterine parvovirus infection. J Comp Pathol 1999;121(1):39–53.

54. Scherk MA, Ford RB, Gaskell RM, Hartmann K, Hurley KF, Lappin MR, et al. 2013 AAFP Feline Vaccination Advisory Panel Report. J Feline Med Surg 2013;15(9):785–808.

55. Digangi BA, Gray LK, Levy JK, Dubovi EJ, Tucker SJ. Detection of protective antibody titers against feline panleukopenia virus, feline herpesvirus-1, and feline calicivirus in shelter cats using a point-of-care ELISA. J Feline Med Surg 2011;13(12):912–8.

56. Itenov TS, Jensen JU. Readmission after intensive care: frequent, hazardous, and possibly preventable. Crit Care Med 2015;43(2):504–5.

57. Neuerer FF, Horlacher K, Truyen U, Hartmann K. Comparison of different in-house test systems to detect parvovirus in faeces of cats. J Feline Med Surg 2008;10(3):247–51.

58. Patterson EV, Reese MJ, Tucker SJ, Dubovi EJ, Crawford PC, Levy JK. Effect of vaccination on parvovirus antigen testing in kittens. J Am Vet Med Assoc 2007;230(3):359–63.

59. Schaefers-Okkens AC, Kooistra HS. Female reproductive tract. In: Rijnberk A, van Sluijs FJ, editors. Medical history and physical examination in companion animals. St. Louis, MO: Saunders Elsevier; 2009.

60. Little SE. Female reproduction. In: Little SE, editor. The cat: clinical medicine and management. St. Louis, MO: Saunders Elsevier; 2012.

61. Feldman EC, Nelson RW. Canine and feline endocrinology and reproduction. 3rd ed. St. Louis, MO: Saunders; 2004.

Case 10

The Alopecic Kitten

Lyle Conway and his wife, Jodie, were surprised how quiet the house seemed when their third and last "child," Samantha, packed her bags and headed out of state to college for her freshman year. Samantha had always been the life of the party. As an all-season athlete and sports fanatic, her high school years had been a constant blur of meets, state championships, and end-of-season celebrations. Over the years, the Conway home had become a touchdown space for athletes and the cheer squad alike. Lyle and Jodie accepted everyone with open arms. They operated as one big happy family.

With Samantha away, the house was eerily still. Lyle and Jodie mentioned this to their next-door neighbor, who suggested that they foster through the local humane society. It was getting to be the peak of kitten season and the shelter was overrun with litters. There wasn't enough time or space to take them all in, so the shelter staff was looking for volunteers in the community

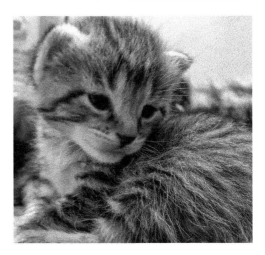

Figure 10.1 Your next patient. Image was taken when he was 3 weeks old. Domestic shorthaired (DSH) kitten. Courtesy of Sarah Greenway.

to share the load. Lyle and Jodie weren't quite ready to commit to adopting a pet, but they both agreed that fostering might be a good way to keep them busy. The idea of raising kittens underfoot appealed to them, and it was for a good cause. So, sure, why not!

Neither Lyle nor Jodie had experience rearing cats, but the shelter provided them with basic training and once they got their feet wet, they never looked back. Three litters later, they were sold on the process. Knock on wood, it had all been smooth sailing. Then Wilson came into their lives.

Wilson was one of a litter of three that came to stay with the Conways at 6 weeks of age. Mom had been a stray when she'd delivered him and his two brothers in the corner of a stranger's shed. When they were discovered, Animal Control was called and came to collect them. Mom and her kittens were given a safe place to sleep and a roof over their heads, but she never acclimated to mother-hood. She was a baby raising babies, and she had no patience for it. Wilson and his brothers were taken from mom, hand-reared, and bottle-fed. They'd made it to weaning but weren't old enough to be adopted. The Conway's home seemed like the perfect transition from the shelter. Besides, the shelter needed the space. Unexpectedly, it had taken in over 65 cats and 24 dogs from a hoarding case overnight, and it was more than they could handle. The new residents were riddled with illness and, not wanting them to jeopardize the health of the young and the old, Wilson and the others were fostered out.

The Conways picked up Wilson and his brothers just last weekend. All three kittens were settling in nicely and roughhousing like there was no tomorrow. When they played, they played hard – and then everyone passed out. Of the three, Wilson was the most outgoing when it came to people and he took a liking to Lyle. When his brothers would flop onto the rug for a midday nap, Wilson would seek Lyle out and request the pleasure of his lap. If Lyle weren't sitting, Wilson would climb up his pants leg until Lyle gave in. It became a daily ritual and Jodie was beginning to think that Wilson was there to stay.

About a week after the litter arrived at the Conways, Lyle noticed that Wilson was missing some fur along the back side of his right ear. He chalked it up to too much play. The way they tussled was at times merciless. And Wilson was the meeker one that usually found himself on the losing end of any brawl.

But then the spot got bigger. Overnight, it seemed to double. By the next day, it seemed to be somewhat red. There didn't appear to be any discharge, but the edges of skin at the perimeter of the hair loss seemed crusty. And, unless he was imaging things, Lyle thought that Wilson might be looking a little bit bald in terms of his face.

Lyle has brought Wilson in to see you today, and you have just completed your preliminary physical exam. You have documented your findings below, as Lyle waits patiently for you to interpret what you see:

Additional crusting is noted along the inner margin of the right pinnae, where the medial aspect of the ear attaches to the head. Areas of circular hypotrichosis appear dorsal to the right eye. There is a moth-eaten appearance to the rostral face. Examining his ears triggers pruritus.

Use the following questions to guide your diagnostic work-up of this case.

Weight: 1.3 lb
BCS: 3/9
Mentation: BAR

TPR

T: 101.2°F (38.9°C)
P: 180 beats per minute
R: 18 breaths per minute

Mucous membrane color: Light pink

Capillary refill time (CRT): < 2 seconds

Abnormal Findings: Large circular patch of focal alopecia along the external aspect of the right pinna. Centrally, the skin is hyperpigmented and scabbed over. Peripherally, the skin is erythematous. At the edges of the circle, there is crusting that extends up the lateral margin of the pinna (see **Plate 3**).

Round One of Questions for Case 10: The Alopecic Kitten

1. Define the following anatomical terms:

   - dorsal
   - focal
   - medial

   - lateral
   - peripheral
   - rostral.

2. Describe the following dermatologic terms:

   - alopecia
   - crust
   - erythema

   - hyperpigmentation
   - hypotrichosis
   - pruritus.

3. How can knowing the description or location of fur loss guide you in formulating your list of differential diagnoses?

4. What are major categories of differential diagnoses for thinning and/or loss of fur? Develop a comprehensive list.

5. Of the differential diagnoses that you outlined in Question #4, which broad categories are LEAST likely in this patient given the patient's signalment and health history? Explain your reasoning for each category that you are effectively ruling out.

6. Of the differential diagnoses that you outlined in Question #4, which broad category is most likely in this patient given the patient's signalment and health history?

7. Considering the category that you selected for Question #6, what is the most likely causative agent given the patient's signalment and health history?

8. You ask Lyle if either of Wilson's brothers have similar lesions. Why do you ask?

9. You ask Lyle if either he or his wife have developed skin lesions. Why is this important?

10. Lyle answers that, come to think of it, his wife has developed a rash on her forearm. She just attributed it to poisonous plants that she may have inadvertently encountered during gardening. He whips out his smart phone and shows you a photograph of the lesion. What is your advice to him?

11. Which screening tool can you perform in-house on Wilson that can potentially give you an immediate answer without requiring you to take samples of his skin, fur, or lesions?

12. If you perform this screening tool, what will a positive result look like?

13. How sensitive is the diagnostic test that you indicated you would like to perform in Question #11 (above)? Think in broad terms: is the test sensitivity high or low?

14. Define sensitivity. What does your answer in Question #13 (above) truly mean?

Answers to Round One of Questions for Case 10: The Alopecic Kitten

1. Define the following anatomical terms:
   - Dorsal means towards the patient's back as opposed to ventral, which means towards the belly of the patient.(2)
   - Focal is an adjective that is used to describe the distribution of a lesion that is circumscribed, as opposed to generalized, which means that lesions are dispersed all over the body.(3, 4)
   - Lateral means away from midline, whereas medial means towards midline.(2)
   - Peripheral refers to being located near the edge of something or away from its core, as opposed to something that is central, meaning near the center. If we refer to the periphery of a lesion, then we are describing something at the lesion's edge.
   - Rostral means towards the patient's nose.(2)

2. Describe the following dermatologic terms:
   - Thinning of the fur and complete fur loss are common clinical presentations in companion patients.(5–8) Hypotrichosis refers to the former condition. Alopecia refers to the latter.(6)
   - Crusts consist of dried exudate and keratin, as opposed to scabs, which are dried plugs of fibrin and platelets that cover the surface of a wound during the healing process, as a new layer of skin begins to form.(3)
   - Erythema refers to the reddening of the skin that results from acute injury, irritation, or inflammation.(3, 4) Capillaries dilate in response to inflammatory mediators. This increases

blood flow to the affected surface(s), causing the affected skin to pink up and appear red.

- Hyperpigmentation refers to the dark grey-black discoloration of the skin that develops as a response to chronic skin irritation and inflammation.(3)
- Pruritus is another way to describe itchiness.(2–4) Itchiness is an unpleasant sensation that makes Wilson want to scratch. Many skin conditions cause pruritus.

3. How can knowing the location of the fur loss guide you in formulating your list of differential diagnoses?

Hypotrichosis and alopecia are not pathognomonic for any one skin condition. In fact, both dermatologic presentations occur with many dermatopathies. However, when we apply descriptors to fur thinning or fur loss, we can more easily prioritize our list of differential diagnoses.

When we describe fur thinning or fur loss, we should consider the following:

- Is hypotrichosis/alopecia focal or generalized?
- What is the pattern of distribution of the hypotrichosis/alopecia?

  - Is it truncal?
  - Is it symmetrical?
  - Is it normal for the species?
  - Is it normal for the breed?

- Where specifically on the body is there hypotrichosis/alopecia?
- Did something specifically occur at the site(s) of hypotrichosis/alopecia?

  - Was a vaccine administered at that location?
  - Was a topical product applied to that location?

- Has the patient been observed to be grooming the site(s) of hypotrichosis/alopecia?

  - Does the patient appear to be overgrooming the location(s)?

- Is the hypotrichosis/alopecia paired with other primary or secondary dermatologic lesions?

  - Primary skin lesions include:(3, 4)

    - papules: small elevations of the skin
    - nodules: large papules
    - tumors: large nodules
    - pustules: pus-filled papules (so-called pimples)
    - vesicles: fluid-filled elevations that do not contain pus
    - bullae: large vesicles
    - wheals: pruritic, circumscribed areas of solid tissue that are raised in appearance due to dermal edema
    - plaques: thickened or raised circumscribed areas of solid tissue with flat tops that are not associated with dermal edema.

  - Secondary skin lesions include:(3, 4)

    - scales: loose flakes of skin; so-called dandruff
    - collarettes: circular lesions that are rimmed with scale; essentially what is left after pustules rupture
    - crusts: refer to definition in Question #2
    - scabs: refer to definition in Question #2
    - comedones: plugs of oil and dead skin cells; so-called blackheads
    - lichenification: thickened, leathery skin that develops as a response to chronic skin irritation or inflammation
    - hyperpigmentation: refer to definition in Question #2

- How long has the hypotrichosis/alopecia been present?
- Is the hypotrichosis/alopecia progressing?
- Is the hypotrichosis/alopecia seasonal?

These descriptors, along with pattern recognition, help seasoned clinicians narrow down their list of differentials (see Figures 10.2a–h).

For example, focal, symmetrical peri-aural (pre-auricular) alopecia is a normal physical exam finding in cats.(3, 4) Individual cats may vary in the degree to which this is exhibited, but all will have some degree of fur thinning in this region as compared to dogs. Clients that are new to owning cats and/or veterinary students who have never examined cats need to become familiar with this species-specific variation of normal anatomy so that they don't investigate something that is not a problem. (See Figure 10.2a)

Focal, symmetrical, seasonal, flank alopecia that is often paired with hyperpigmentation of the associated skin is another variation of normal that is seen in some, but not all, canine breeds, including English Bulldogs.(9–15) Fur loss occurs every season and does not require medical intervention. (See Figure 10.2b.)

Focal fur thinning or fur loss at a site where something was applied topically or administered as an injectable likely indicates an adverse reaction to therapy.(7) When fur loss occurs at the site of a vaccination, it is usually due to an immune-mediated aberrant response by the body. Vasculitis results in alopecia several weeks to months following immunization. In my experience, small-breed dogs are overrepresented, and the rabies vaccine seems more likely to trigger this response.

Adverse reactions can also occur when topical agents are applied.(16) The most commonly applied topical agent in cats in clinical practice is flea/tick/heartworm preventative. A study by Credille et al. reported that a formulation containing 39.6% spinetoram caused hypotrichosis/alopecia in 38% of cats within 72 hours of application. Biopsy results were consistent with alopecia due to barbering.(16) Discontinuation of the product led to fur regrowth.(16) Spinetoram is not the only product to cause hypotrichosis and/or alopecia in cats.(17) If fur loss occurs in a region of the body where topical agents are routinely applied, then the clinician should query the client to find out if and when a product was applied, and, if so, has this ever happened previously. (See Figure 10.2c.)

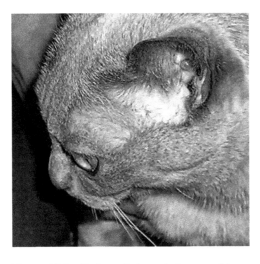

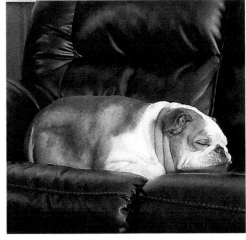

Figure 10.2a Peri-aural alopecia is normal in cats.

Figure 10.2b Seasonal flank alopecia is normal for certain breeds of dogs, such as English Bulldogs. Courtesy of Tara Beugel.

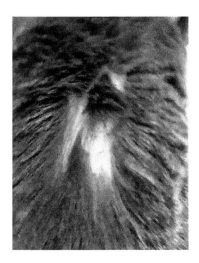

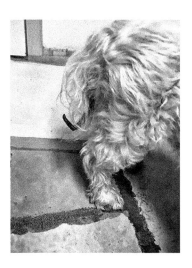

Figure 10.2c Alopecia at the site where topical over-the-counter flea preventative was applied to a cat. Courtesy of Andy and Kristina Burch.

Figure 10.2d Classic 'rat tail' alopecia consistent with endocrinopathy in a dog. Courtesy of Gail Nason.

Focal fur loss can also indicate other types of pathology, depending upon which region(s) of the body is/are affected. For example, when alopecia occurs at the tail base, concurrent with fleas or flea dirt, then flea allergy dermatitis is likely.(3, 4)

When alopecia is focal, truncal, and symmetrical, it is often associated with endocrinopathies.(3, 4, 18, 19) The classic example is bilaterally symmetrical flank alopecia in a dog with hypothyroidism.(20) Because the thyroid is a major player in the growth and replacement of fur, loss of thyroid hormone or function leads to several cutaneous manifestations of disease.(19, 21) In addition to flank alopecia, hypothyroid dogs often present with an alopecic patch outlining the neck ("ring around the collar"), and/or alopecic tails ("rat tail").(19) (See Figure 10.2d.)

Hypothyroidism is not the only condition that causes bilaterally symmetrical trunk alopecia. Estrogen-producing Sertoli cell testicular tumors induce a state of hyperestrogenism that also results in pattern alopecia.(22–29) So does hyperadrenocorticism, or Cushing's syndrome, albeit through a different mechanism. In the case of hyperadrenocorticism, excessive glucocorticoids, rather than sex steroids, leads to classic patterns of fur loss.(19, 30)

Focal alopecia is also present in infectious dermatological disease such as mange. For example, localized demodicosis preferentially targets the muzzle and feet as compared to sarcoptic mange, which tends to concentrate on the head, pinnae, elbows, and hock.(7, 31–34) Keep in mind that clinical presentations of mange can also be generalized. (See Figure 10.2e.)

Focal alopecia may also clue us in to internal pathology. In these clinical scenarios, the patient overgrooms the fur that overlies the region of the body that is uncomfortable in the same way we massage areas on our own body that hurt. For example, cats with chronic cystitis may present

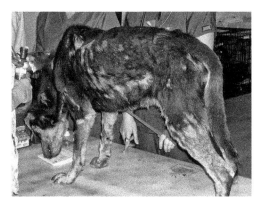

Figure 10.2e Classic distribution of patchy alopecia secondary to demodicosis in a dog. Courtesy of Laura Polerecky.

139

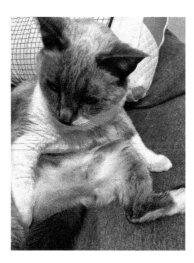

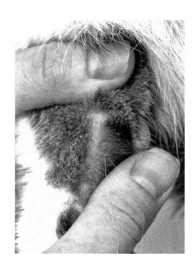

Figure 10.2f Caudoventral alopecia in the cat can be consistent with chronic cystitis. Courtesy of Jeri Altizer.

Figure 10.2g Alopecia over certain joints may indicate arthropathy. Overgrooming at these locations may indicate pain secondary to osteoarthritis. Courtesy of the Media Resources Department at Midwestern University.

for alopecia of the caudoventral abdomen (the groin) when in fact the fur loss is secondary to an underlying urinary condition.(3) (See Figure 10.2f.) Likewise, cats with arthralgia may overgroom in the region of painful joints. In my experience, many senior cats with tarsal arthritis present with hypotrichosis or alopecia of the affected hock(s). (See Figure 10.2g.)

Sometimes, fur loss is self-induced, but not because of an underlying medical condition. In this case, an owner may report overgrooming of a part of the body that, upon clinical examination, has no overt pathology. In this case, the hypotrichosis/alopecia is said to be psychogenic. This so-called fur mowing occurs more frequently in cats than dogs and may be precipitated by stress.(20, 35, 36). (See Figure 10.2h.)

There are too many examples to provide to cover the full range of dermatologic presentations and their classic appearance. However, the examples that have been provided above demonstrate why it is so important to describe a patient's fur loss in depth. The more details that we can gain from the patient profile and physical examination, the more likely we are to link what we find to a clinical diagnosis.

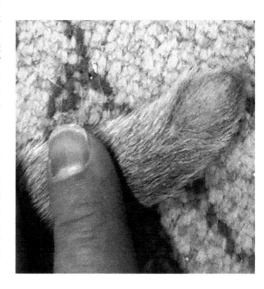

Figure 10.2h Alopecia at the tail tip in this instance represents a case of psychogenic alopecia in a cat.

4. The major categories of differential diagnoses for thinning of and/or loss of fur include:(3, 4)

- species-specific alopecia:
    - feline peri-aural (pre-auricular) alopecia
- tardive hypotrichosis or alopecia: patients are born with normal coats; however, the coats thin as they age:
    - pattern baldness:
        - pinnal alopecia: dogs (especially dachshunds) > cats
        - bald thigh syndrome: dogs (especially greyhounds)
    - black hair follicular dysplasia: abnormalities in hair shafts and follicles leads to loss of black fur only
    - color dilution alopecia: typically targets those with blue, red, and fawn coats
- non-color-linked, cyclical follicular dysplasias:
    - seasonal flank alopecia
- non-color-linked, non-cyclical follicular dysplasias:
    - alopecia X: typically targets Nordic breeds and others with plush coats
- non-endocrine, non-inflammatory hair loss:
    - congenital hypotrichosis and alopecia:
        - canine(37):
            - sub-Mexican hairless or xoloitzcuintli
            - Chinese crested
            - Inca hairless
            - Peruvian Inca orchid
        - feline:
            - Sphynx
            - Donskoy
            - the elf cat: a hybrid of the American Curl cat and the Sphynx
            - the Ukranian Levkoy: a hybrid of the Scottish Fold cat and the Sphynx
            - the bambino: a hybrid of the Munchkin and the Sphynx
- endocrine, non-inflammatory hair loss:
    - hyperadrenocorticism
    - hyperestrogenism
    - hypothyroidism
    - exposure to human topical hormone replacement therapy
- non-endocrine, inflammatory hair loss:
    - bacterial pyoderma
    - dermatophytosis
    - mange
- hepatocutaneous syndrome
- chemotherapy
- radiation therapy
- alopecia associated with topical medications
- non-medical causes of hair loss:
    - pressure alopecia

- nutritional causes of alopecia:

  - zinc deficiency
  - deficiency in linoleic acid

- environmental cause of alopecia
- compulsive and/or displacement disorders:

  - acral lick dermatitis
  - flank sucking
  - fur mowing.

5. Of the differential diagnoses that you outlined in Question #4 (above), the following categories are LEAST likely:

- species-specific alopecia – Wilson's fur loss does not have a peri-aural (pre-auricular distribution)
- tardive hypotrichosis or alopecia – Wilson's fur loss is associated with other lesions, whereas conditions like tardive hypotrichosis, such as pinnal alopecia, only involve loss of fur and/ or Wilson is also not experiencing fur loss that targets only one color of fur
- non-color-linked, cyclical follicular dysplasias – Wilson hasn't lived long enough for his hair loss to be seasonal
- non-color-linked, non-cyclical follicular dysplasias – Wilson is a cat; these conditions preferentially target Nordic breeds of dog
- non-endocrine, non-inflammatory hair loss – Wilson is not a hairless breed of cat
- endocrine, non-inflammatory hair loss – these conditions do not typically occur in pediatric patients, and Wilson has not been exposed to human topical hormone replacement therapy
- hepatocutaneous syndrome – this condition is rare and does not typically occur in pediatric patients. When it occurs, hepatocutaneous syndrome is often the result of hepatobiliary or pancreatic neoplasia
- chemotherapy – Wilson has not undergone chemotherapy
- radiation therapy – Wilson has not undergone radiation therapy
- alopecia associated with topical medications – Wilson has not been given any topical therapy, including flea/tick preventative
- non-medical causes of hair loss – Wilson does not wear clothing, collars, or harnesses, that can lead to pressure alopecia. Also, his alopecia is along his ear and face, rather than his body, where clothing could presumably play a role.
- nutritional causes of alopecia – Wilson is presumably receiving a nutritionally balanced diet that is appropriate for his life stage. He is also not a breed that is prone to zinc deficiency (i.e. Alaskan breeds of dog)
- environmental cause of alopecia – Wilson is not housed on hard surfaces that would cause pressure alopecia
- compulsive and/or displacement disorders – Although Wilson is pruritic, he does not appear to be obsessively scratching at his ears and he is unable to reach his ear with his tongue for fur mowing to be possible.

6. Of the differential diagnoses that you outlined in Question #4 (above), non-endocrine, inflammatory hair loss is most likely because it includes infectious diseases:

- bacterial pyoderma
- dermatophytosis
- mange.

Infectious diseases are the most likely cause of hypotrichosis and/or alopecia in a kitten of Wilson's age.

7. Considering the category that you selected for Question #6 (above), what is the most likely causative agent given the patient's signalment and health history?

Dermatophytosis ("ringworm") is the most likely cause of Wilson's fur loss. Whereas canine patients with ringworm tend to be infected with *Trichophyton mentagrophytes* or *Microsporum gypseum*, *Microsporum canis* is the primary source of ringworm in cats.(38–41)

Pyoderma is less likely. Pyoderma is a fancy way of describing a bacterial skin infection.(42) Papules and pustules are the classic textbook lesions for pyoderma in dogs.(4) Cats may also develop a papulopustular rash; however, in this species, pyoderma tends to present as superficial crusts, erosions, plaques, and/or ulcerations in a classic presentation that is referred to as military dermatitis.(4, 43, 44) These lesions arise secondary to allergic skin disease or mange mite infestations and classically appear as either "rodent ulcers" on the upper/lower lips or eosinophilic plaques along the ventrum and/or limbs.(43–48) This distribution of lesions does not fit Wilson's clinical picture.

Cats can develop mange; however, this condition occurs with less frequency than dermatophytosis. When I consider mange mites in the cat, the following four species come to mind:

- *Demodex* spp. – *Demodex felis*, *Demodex cati*, or *Demodex gatoi*(31, 49–53)
- *Sarcoptes scabiei*
- *Notoedres cati*
- *Cheyletiella* spp.

Demodicosis may result in localized or generalized disease. The face and forelimbs are often involved. Common lesions include erythema, hypotrichosis or alopecic patches with or without a papulopustular rash, folliculitis or furunculosis, scale, pododermatitis, and/or paronychia. (54–56) Some of these findings are consistent with Wilson's clinical picture, but not all.

Cats are rarely infested with *Sarcoptes scabiei*. When they are, lesions typically involve the bridge of the nose, feet, claws, and tail.(57–59) Neither of these locations fits with Wilson's clinical picture.

Notoedres cati is relatively rare, but can cause crusting and scaling of the face and pinnae as well as paronychia.(60, 61) Involvement of the pinnae fits with Wilson's clinical picture, but this condition is relatively rare, compared to dermatophytosis, which is quite common in catteries and shelters.(62)

Cheyletiella spp. do prefer the head and topline of cats, but they are surface dwellers only. (61) As they move up and down the trunk of the body, they create the appearance of "walking dandruff."(61) This is inconsistent with Wilson's clinical picture.

8. You ask Lyle if either of Wilson's brothers have similar lesions because dermatophytosis is highly contagious and can be spread cat-to-cat.(62)

9. You ask Lyle if either he or his wife have developed skin lesions because dermatophytosis is a zoonotic disease.(3, 4, 62, 63)

10. You explain to Lyle that if Wilson does in fact have ringworm, then, yes, it is possible for it to have spread to his wife. However, you need to emphasize that you are not a human medical professional and you have not received formal training in human medicine to accurately diagnose his wife. It is in fact illegal for you to do so. Although the lesions that are demonstrated in the photograph are consistent with what one might expect to see with ringworm in a person, strongly advise that Lyle's wife seek medical care as soon as possible. Instruct Lyle's wife to inform her physician that a kitten in the household is likely positive for ringworm.

11. An in-house screening tool that can potentially give you an immediate answer without requiring you to take samples of Wilson's skin, fur, or lesions is the Wood's lamp examination.(4, 62)

12. When you perform a Wood's lamp examination, lesions that are (+) for dermatophytosis will fluoresce an apple-green color.(4, 41, 62, 64)

13. The Wood's lamp examination has a relatively low sensitivity.(4, 41, 62)

14. The sensitivity of a diagnostic test explains how well the test can correctly identify those who have the condition. If the sensitivity for a given test is high, then few cases of disease are missed. Most of those with the disease are correctly identified as such, so few false negatives result.

    The Wood's lamp examination is said to have a low sensitivity because only 50% of *Microsporum canis* fluoresce.(4, 41, 62) Other dermatophyte species do not exhibit fluorescence.(4, 41, 62) This means that many patients will not test (+) on the Wood's lamp examination even though they have dermatophytosis. In other words, there will be a relatively high number of false negatives. Therefore, even if your patient tests (-) on the Wood's lamp examination, you cannot definitely rule out dermatophytosis.

Returning to Case 10: The Alopecic Kitten

You elect to use the Wood's lamp as an inexpensive, simple screening tool. Figure 10.3 is what you see.

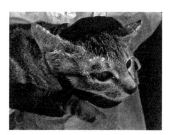 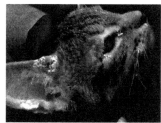 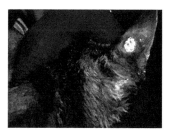

Figure 10.3a–c Using the Wood's lamp as a screening tool. Courtesy of Colleen Cook.

Round Two of Questions for Case 10: The Alopecic Kitten

1. Interpret the results of the Wood's lamp test.
2. Describe the Wood's lamp tool and how it works to produce fluorescence in patients with dermatophytosis.
3. What else on the patient's coat could potentially fluoresce, causing a false (+) test result?
4. User-error can play a role in any diagnostic test, particularly with the Wood's lamp. A patient may test (-) if we do not use the Wood's lamp properly. Provide at least one example of how using the lamp improperly may cause a false-negative test result.
5. If a Wood's lamp is not available to you, what is another simple, rapid, in-house test that can provide you with answers today?
6. Describe how to perform the diagnostic test that you identified in Question #5 (above).
7. What are you looking for when you evaluate your sample using the diagnostic test that you identified in Question #5?
8. Provide at least one reason why you might obtain a false-negative result when you perform the test that you identified in Question #5.
9. What is the sensitivity of the test that you identified in Question #5?

10. How could you increase the sensitivity of the test that you identified in Question #5?
11. Is the suggestion that you outlined in Question #9 practical in a clinic setting?

Answers to Round Two of Questions for Case 10: The Alopecic Kitten

1. Based upon the photographs that have been provided, Wilson tests (+) for the Wood's lamp examination.

2. The Wood's lamp is a hand-held device that emits ultraviolet (UV) radiation through a nickel or cobalt glass filter.(64, 65) It is not the same as a black light.(65) The filter that is associated with the Wood's lamp blocks out most wavelengths of light, with the exception of those that fall between 320 and 400 nm.(65) When light of these wavelengths comes across pteridine, a metabolic product of *M. canis*, the characteristic apple- or emerald-green color fluorescence is produced.(65) If the coat is long-haired and/or oily, then sometimes this color takes on the appearance of a bluer-green.(64)

3. A false (+) test may result from the presence of one or more of the following items on the patient's coat:(62, 64, 65)

   • scale
   • crusts
   • lint
   • soap residue
   • topical medications, such as tetracycline
   • some fabric fibers, especially those associated with synthetic carpets.

   In truth, these items fluoresce a different shade of green than pteridine.(65–68) They do not produce the characteristic apple-green or emerald-green that pteridine does.(65–68) However, a novice may find it difficult to tell the difference and may therefore diagnose a patient as being (+) for dermatophytosis by mistake.

4. The Wood's lamp needs to be turned on for 5 to 10 minutes before use.(64, 66, 67) This is because the wavelengths of light that are emitted depend upon temperature, so the Wood's lamp needs to warm up.(64) If you do not wait for it to warm up because you are in a rush to perform the test, then you may get a false (-).
   Other potential source of error include:(64)

   • not having the room dark enough
   • not taking enough time to perform a complete examination: you should expose the lesions to the Wood's lamp for a minimum of 3 to 5 minutes(64)
   • not allowing time for the examiner's eyes to adapt to darkness
   • not holding the lamp close enough: the Wood's lamp should be placed within a few inches of the lesions.(64)

5. If a Wood's lamp is unavailable to you today and you find yourself in need of another simple, rapid, in-house test that can provide you with answers today, then I would recommend a direct microscopic examination of hair or scales for dermatophytes.(41, 62, 64)

6. We can pluck hairs or scale from the edges of one or more of Wilson's lesions and evaluate these using light microscopy.(62, 64) A trichogram is a fancy name for microscopic examination of plucked hairs.(41)
   We can also perform a potassium hydroxide (KOH) prep in which several drops of 10–20% KOH are added to the slide, just enough to bathe the samples.(64) KOH destroys healthy skin

cells, leaving behind only fungal elements.(65, 69–71) Additional stains, such as lactophenol cotton blue or India Ink, may also improve visibility.(65, 71–73)

A glass cover-slip should be placed over the sample on the slide.(64)

Examine the slide first under low power, using the 4× or 10× objective.(64) This will help you to identify the abnormal hairs.(64) By contrast, higher power will facilitate identification of fungal spores, macro- and microconidia.(64)

7. When hair is infected with dermatophytes, the shafts themselves may appear wider, with coarse and irregular surfaces. Some people describe the affected shafts as appearing swollen or out of focus.(64) Some shafts may even appear to be frayed.(64)

   It is also possible via light microscopy to identify fungal elements, including hyphae and spores.(65) Hyphae are filamentous, branching structures of fungi. Spores are a means by which fungi asexually reproduce.

   Neither hyphae nor spores should be visible as structures within hair fragments in healthy, normal patients. Either may be present in patients with dermatophytosis.

   When KOH is added to hair shafts, only fungal elements remain. KOH makes these elements easier to visualize because the rest of the "background noise" has been removed.

8. You may get a false-negative result when you perform the direct microscopic examination for dermatophytes on hair and scale because of the following.

   • Of coat color. It may be harder to identify fungal elements on fur that is dark in color.(65)
   • Of inexperience. Many veterinary graduates do not feel comfortable performing or inter-preting this test. They do not always feel like they know what they are looking for, so it is possible for them to miss something of value.
   • Of insufficient prep time. It requires 20–30 minutes for KOH to thoroughly digest your sample and then the slide must be examined straight away.(64, 65) If this timeline isn't fol-lowed, then you may be prone to artifacts that make it difficult to decipher the results.(65)

9. The sensitivity of direct microscopic exam for dermatophytes on hair or scale is low.(62) One report by Sparkes et al. identified it as being 59%.(74)

10. Sensitivity of the direct microscopic exam for dermatophytes on hair or scale can be improved if you use fluorescence microscopy, which requires the stain, calcafluor white.(74) Calcafluor white binds to the fungal components chi-tin and cellulose, making fungal elements easier to detect.(74)

11. Fluorescence microscopy is not practical in a clinic setting. For that reason, its use is pri-marily restricted to academic use.

Returning to Case 10:
The Alopecic Kitten

You elect to perform direct microscopic exam-ination of hair and scale for dermatophytes as a second inexpensive, simple screening tool. This is what you see (see Figure 10.4).

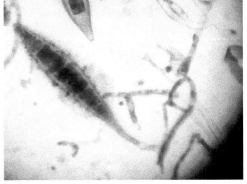

Figure 10.4 Findings from direct microscopic examination of hair and scale. Courtesy of Jennifer Lang.

Round Three of Questions for Case 10: The Alopecic Kitten

1. What is your diagnosis based upon your direct microscopic examination of hair and scale for dermatophytes?
2. What features did you notice that make you confident that your diagnosis is correct?
3. Despite the certainty with which you share your diagnosis with Lyle, he wants to be "sure." Historically, what has been considered the gold standard for the detection of dermatophytes?
4. Identify three ways to obtain a sample for the diagnostic test that you identified in Question #2?
5. Identify one potential downside to one of the methods of sample acquisition that you identified in Question #4.
6. What does dermatophyte test medium (DTM) contain to facilitate diagnosis of dermatophytosis?
7. How are fungal cultures stored?
8. How often should fungal cultures be examined?
9. How do you interpret the results of a fungal culture by visual inspection?
10. How can you cytologically examine the culture for pathogen identification?
11. You elect to proceed with this diagnostic test in order to give Lyle peace of mind; however, you have to inform him that he will not know the answer until when?

Answers to Round Three of Questions for Case 10: The Alopecic Kitten

1. Based upon the photograph that has been provided, my diagnosis is *Microsporum canis*.

2. I know this based upon the fungal structures that I see in the photograph. I see large spores – macroconidia – that are consistent with *Microsporum canis*. The macroconidia of *Microsporum canis* are spindle-shaped with thick walls.

3. Historically, the gold standard for the detection of dermatophytes is to culture hair and scale from suspect lesions onto a fungal culture plate.(65) As of the 2017 Clinical Consensus Guidelines of the World Association for Veterinary Dermatology by Moriello et al., there is no longer thought to be a "gold standard" test for dermatophytosis.(65) Diagnosis is best achieved by a combination of tests, including clinical response to therapy.(65)

   Despite these guidelines, fungal culture may still be prioritized by some practitioners today.
   The most commonly used media for fungal culture plates is DTM, which combines Sabouraud's dextrose agar with antimicrobials to inhibit growth of bacterial contaminants.(62, 64) Classically, these antimicrobials include cycloheximide, gentamicin, and chlortetracycline.(64)

   Other forms of media are commercially available, including a relatively recent product called Derm Duet.(64) This is a dual-compartment plate. DTM is seated on one side of the plate with rapid sporulating media (RSM) on the other side.(64) RSM expedites the development of spores.(64)

4. To perform a fungal culture, you may make use of one of three sampling techniques.(62, 64, 65)

   - You can pluck hairs and scale from the edges of presumptive lesions and apply these directly to the culture plate that contains DTM.
   - You can make use of an individually wrapped soft bristle toothbrush to brush the cat for approximately 2 to 3 minutes or until the bristles of the brush are full of fur. This method is particularly effective when you are presented with a subclinical patient but wish to screen for a carrier state.
   - You can take an approximate four-centimeter piece of acetate tape, press it over lesions, then press the same side onto the surface of the culture plate.

5. The toothbrush method tends to over-diagnose dermatophytosis because it is very effective at diagnosing spores on the hair coat; however, it does not differentiate true positive cats with clinical disease from those that are simply acting as mechanical carriers of spores.(1, 65)

6. DTM contains two ingredients that facilitate diagnosis of dermatophytosis:(64, 65)

    *   antibiotics, to suppress bacterial growth
    *   pH-color indicator that changes the medium from a visible yellow to red color that signifies fungal growth.

7. Cultures should be stored above room temperature in an incubator at 75°F (23°C).(62) This promotes fungal growth and sporulation.(62)

8. Cultures need to be examined every day for up to 21 days before they are reported as negative.(62) Certain dermatophyte species tend to be slow-growers/late-bloomers, including Trichophyton species.(62) You could miss these if you prematurely tossed out your culture.

9. Evaluate the culture plate every day for the presence of fungal colonies. Dermatophyte colonies are not pigmented and typically appear white-to-buff in color.(62) As these colonies grow, there should be a change in the media from yellow to red. Media color change should occur before or in concert with fungal colony growth.(62)

10. The presence of fungal colonies and the color change in DTM confirm the diagnosis of dermatophytosis. However, pathogens can only be identified cytologically via microscopy, meaning that you cannot diagnose *Microsporum canis* by gross inspection of the fungal culture alone. To examine the fungal culture cytologically, take acetate tape and brush the fungal colonies with the sticky side.(62) Take the sticky side of tape, which should now contain a sample from your fungal colony, and place it onto a microscope slide that contains a drop of lactophenol cotton blue.(62) An equally appropriate stain is new methylene blue.(62) Do not examine the slide immediately. Allow the slide to sit for about 5 to 10 minutes. This will allow the stain to seep into the fungal elements and improve visibility via light microscopy.(62) Each species of dermatophyte has its own characteristic shape for macro- and microconidia.

11. Technically, you need to wait a full 21 days before you can establish that the culture is truly negative. However, most cultures are (+) for *Microsporum canis* by day 14.(62) Given what you saw on Wilson's Wood's lamp examination and also on direct microscopic examination of hair and scale, you anticipate knowing results within the next 2 weeks.

    This concludes the case.

    For those who are interested in treatment options, please consult a dermatology or internal medicine text of your choice.

CLINICAL PEARLS

*   There are many causes of hypotrichosis and alopecia in kittens and cats. Of these, infectious causes are mostly likely in kittens.

*   Differential diagnoses for hypotrichosis and alopecia can be further narrowed down by considering the location(s) of hair loss as well as its distribution. For example, is it:

    *   focal or generalized
    *   symmetrical or asymmetrical.

- Feline dermatophytosis tends to target the following regions:(1)

  - muzzle
  - lips
  - periocular skin
  - pinnae
  - limbs
  - digits
  - tail.

- Dermatophytosis varies in terms of lesions that are present at the initial consultation; however, scale and crusts are commonly seen.

- Three dermatophytes are most commonly implicated in clinical cases:

  - *Microsporum canis*
  - *Trichophyton mentagrophytes*
  - *Microsporum gypseum.*

Of these, *Microsporum canis* is the primary source of ringworm in cats.

- The gold standard diagnostic test for dermatophytosis is fungal culture.

- Other in-house diagnostic tests, such as the Wood's lamp examination and the direct microscopic examination of hairs and scale, may provide more immediate (same day) results. However, these techniques are user-dependent, and both have relatively low sensitivity. Therefore, false negatives are common.

- Dermatophytes are zoonotic; clients need to be directed to seek medical attention from human healthcare providers.

References

1. Moriello K. Feline dermatophytosis: aspects pertinent to disease management in single and multiple cat situations. J Feline Med Surg 2014;16(5):419–31.
2. Englar R. Writing skills for veterinarians. Sheffield: 5M Publishing; 2019.
3. Englar RE. Performing the small animal physical examination. Hoboken, NJ: Wiley/Blackwell; 2017.
4. Englar RE. Common clinical presentations in dogs and cats. Hoboken, NJ: Wiley/Blackwell; 2019.
5. Moriello KA. Dermatology. In: Little SE, editor. The cat: clinical medicine and management. St. Louis: Elsevier Saunders; 2012. p. 371–424.
6. Breathnach RMS, Shipstone M. The cat with alopecia. In: Rand J, editor. Problem-based feline medicine. Toronto: Elsevier Saunders; 2006. p. 1052–66.
7. Kennis RA. Disorders causing focal alopecia. In: Morgan RV, editor. Handbook of small animal practice. 5th ed. St. Louis, MO: Saunders/Elsevier; 2008. p. 834–40.
8. Ghubash RM. Disorders causing symmetrical alopecia. In: Morgan RV, editor. Handbook of small animal practice. 4th ed. Philadelphia, PA: Saunders; 2003. p. 841–9.
9. Laffort-Dassot C, Beco L, Carlotti DN. Follicular dysplasia in five Weimaraners. Vet Dermatol 2002;13(5):253–60.
10. Curtis CF, Evans H, Lloyd DH. Investigation of the reproductive and growth hormone status of dogs affected by idiopathic recurrent flank alopecia. J Small Anim Pract 1996;37(9):417–22.
11. Müntener T, Schuepbach-Regula G, Frank L, Rüfenacht S, Welle MM. Canine noninflammatory alopecia: a comprehensive evaluation of common and distinguishing histological characteristics. Vet Dermatol 2012;23(3):206–e44.
12. Scott DW. Seasonal flank alopecia in ovariohysterectomized dogs. Cornell Vet 1990;80(2):187–95.
13. Miller MA, Dunstan RW. Seasonal flank alopecia in boxers and Airedale terriers: 24 cases (1985–1992). J Am Vet Med Assoc 1993;203(11):1567–72.
14. Waldman L. Seasonal flank alopecia in affenpinschers. J Small Anim Pract 1995;36(6):271–3.

15. Schmeitzel LP. Sex hormone-related and growth hormone-related alopecias. Vet Clin North Am Small Anim Pract 1990;20(6):1579–601.

16. Credille KM, Thompson LA, Young LM, Meyer JA, Winkle JR. Evaluation of hair loss in cats occurring after treatment with a topical flea control product. Vet Dermatol 2013;24(6):602–5.

17. Boy MG, Six RH, Thomas CA, Novotny MJ, Smothers CD, Rowan TG, Jernigan AD. Efficacy and safety of selamectin against fleas and heartworms in dogs and cats presented as veterinary patients in North America. Vet Parasitol 2000;91(3–4):233–50.

18. Zur G, White SD. Hyperadrenocorticism in 10 dogs with skin lesions as the only presenting clinical signs. J Am Anim Hosp Assoc 2011;47(6):419–27.

19. Frank LA. Comparative dermatology – canine endocrine dermatoses. Clin Dermatol 2006;24(4):317–25.

20. Medleau L, Hnilica KA. Small animal dermatology: A color atlas and therapeutic guide. 2nd ed. St. Louis, MO: Saunders Elsevier; 2006.

21. Baker K. Hormonal alopecia in dogs and cats. Pract 1986;8(2):71–8.

22. Hoskins JD. Testicular cancer remains easily preventable disease. DVM: 360 [Internet]; 2004. Available from: http://veterinarynews.dvm360.com/testicular-cancer-remains-easilypreventable-disease.

23. Lawrence JA, Saba CF. Tumors of the male reproductive system. In: Withrow SJ, Vail DM, Page RL, editors. Withrow and MacEwen's small animal clinical oncology. 5th ed. St. Louis, MO: Elsevier; 2013. p. 557–71.

24. Lipowitz AJ, Schwartz A, Wilson GP, Ebert JW. Testicular neoplasms and concomitant clinical changes in the dog. J Am Vet Med Assoc 1973;163(12):1364–8.

25. Huggins C, Moulder PV. Estrogen production by Sertoli cell tumors of the testis. Cancer Res 1945;5(9):510-and.

26. Zuckerman S, Groome JR. The ætiology of benign enlargement of the prostate in the dog. J Pathol 1937;44(1):113–24.

27. Zuckerman S, McKeown T. The canine prostate in relation to normal and abnormal testicular changes. J Pathol 1938;46(1):7–19.

28. Greulich WW, Burford TH. Testicular tumors associated with mammary, prostatic, and other changes in cryptorchid dogs. Am J Cancer 1936;28(3):496–511.

29. Paepe D, Hebbelinck L, Kitshoff A, Vandenabeele S. Feminization and severe pancytopenia caused by testicular neoplasia in a cryptorchid dog. VDT 2016;85(4):197–205.

30. Feldman EC, Nelson RW. Canine and feline endocrinology and reproduction. St. Louis, MO: W. B. Saunders; 2004.

31. Mueller RS. An update on the therapy of canine demodicosis. Compend Contin Educ Vet 2012;34(4):E1–4.

32. Scott DW, Miller WH, Griffin CE. Canine demodicosis. Muller and Kirk's small animal dermatology. Philadelphia, PA: W.B. Saunders; 2001. p. 457–74.

33. Pin D, Bensignor E, Carlotti DN, Cadiergues MC. Localised sarcoptic mange in dogs: a retrospective study of 10 cases. J Small Anim Pract 2006;47(10):611–4.

34. Scott DW, Miller WH, Griffin CE. Parasitic skin diseases. Muller and Kirk's Small Animal dermatology. Philadelphia, PA: W. B. Saunders; 2001.

35. Patterson AP. Psychocutaneous disorders. In: Small animal dermatology secrets. Philadelphia, PA: Hanley & Belfus; 2004. p. 324–32.

36. Schaer M. Clinical medicine of the dog and cat. 2nd ed. London: Manson Publishing, Ltd.; 2011.

37. Mecklenburg L. An overview on congenital alopecia in domestic animals. Vet Dermatol 2006;17(6):393–410.

38. Warren S. Claw disease in dogs: Part 2 – diagnosis and management of specific claw diseases. Companion Anim 2013;18(5):226–31.

39. Outerbridge CA. Mycologic disorders of the skin. Clin Tech Small Anim Pract 2006;21(3):128–34.

40. Colombo S, Nardoni S, Cornegliani L, Mancianti F. Prevalence of Malassezia spp. yeasts in feline nail folds: a cytological and mycological study. Vet Dermatol 2007;18(4):278–83.

41. DeBoer DJ, Moriello KA. Cutaneous fungal infections. In: Greene CE, editor. Infectious diseases of the dog and cat. 3rd ed. St. Louis, MO: Saunders/Elsevier; 2006. p. 551–69.

42. Summers JF, Hendricks A, Brodbelt DC. Prescribing practices of primary-care veterinary practitioners in dogs diagnosed with bacterial pyoderma. BMC Vet Res 2014;10:240.

43. Wildermuth BE, Griffin CE, Rosenkrantz WS. Feline pyoderma therapy. Clin Tech Small Anim Pract 2006;21(3):150–6.

44. Favrot C. Feline non-flea induced hypersensitivity dermatitis: clinical features, diagnosis and treatment. J Feline Med Surg 2013;15(9):778–84.

45. Ravens PA, Xu BJ, Vogelnest LJ. Feline atopic dermatitis: a retrospective study of 45 cases (2001–2012). Vet Dermatol 2014;25(2):95–102.

46. Vogelnest LJ, Cheng KY. Cutaneous adverse food reactions in cats: retrospective evaluation of 17 cases in a dermatology referral population (2001–2011). Aust Vet J 2013;91(11):443–51.

47. Yu HW, Vogelnest LJ. Feline superficial pyoderma: a retrospective study of 52 cases (2001–2011). Vet Dermatol 2012;23(5):448–e86.

48. Mueller RS. Bacterial dermatoses. In: Guagere E, Prelaud P, editors. A practical guide to feline dermatology. Paris: Merial; 1999. p. 6.1–6.11.

49. Taffin ER, Casaert S, Claerebout E, Vandekerkhof TJ, Vandenabeele S. Morphological variability of demodex cati in a feline immunodeficiency virus-positive cat. J Am Vet Med Assoc 2016;249(11):1308–12.

50. Neel JA, Tarigo J, Tater KC, Grindem CB. Deep and superficial skin scrapings from a feline immunodeficiency virus-positive cat. Vet Clin Pathol 2007;36(1):101–4.

51. Frank LA, Kania SA, Chung K, Brahmbhatt R. A molecular technique for the detection and differentiation of demodex mites on cats. Vet Dermatol 2013;24(3):367–9, e82, e82–3.

52. Cordero AM, Sheinberg-Waisburd G, Romero Núñez C, Heredia R. Early onset canine generalized demodicosis. Vet Dermatol 2018;29(2):173.

53. Bowden DG, Outerbridge CA, Kissel MB, Baron JN, White SD. Canine demodicosis: a retrospective study of a veterinary hospital population in California, USA (2000–2016). Vet Dermatol 2018;29(1):19–e10.

54. Mueller RS, Bensignor E, Ferrer L, Holm B, Lemarie S, Paradis M, et al. Treatment of demodicosis in dogs: 2011 clinical practice guidelines. Vet Dermatol 2012;23(2):86–96.

55. Rouben C. Claw and claw bed diseases. Clinician's. Brief 2016 (April):35–40.

56. Manning TO. Cutaneous diseases of the paw. Clin Dermatol 1983;1(1):131–42.

57. Huang HP, Lien YH. Feline sarcoptic mange in Taiwan: a case series of five cats. Vet Dermatol 2013;24(4):457–9.

58. Malik R, McKellar Stewart KM, Sousa CA, Krockenberger MB, Pope S, Ihrke P, et al. Crusted scabies (sarcoptic mange) in four cats due to Sarcoptes scabiei infestation. J Feline Med Surg 2006;8(5):327–39.

59. Hawkins JA, McDonald RK, Woody BJ. Sarcoptes scabiei infestation in a cat. J Am Vet Med Assoc 1987;190(12):1572–3.

60. Sivajothi S, Sudhakara Reddy B, Rayulu VC, Sreedevi C. Notoedres cati in cats and its management. J Parasit Dis 2015;39(2):303–5.

61. Arther RG. Mites and lice: biology and control. Vet Clin North Am Small Anim Pract 2009;39(6):1159–71.

62. Frymus T, Gruffydd-Jones T, Pennisi MG, Addie D, Belák S, Boucraut-Baralon C, et al. Dermatophytosis in cats: ABCD guidelines on prevention and management. J Feline Med Surg 2013;15(7):598–604.

63. Moriello KA, Kunkle G, DeBoer DJ. Isolation of Dermatophytes from the Haircoats of Stray Cats from Selected Animal Shelters in two Different Geographic Regions in the United States. Vet Dermatol 1994;5(2):57–62.

64. Moriello KA. Diagnostic techniques for dermatophytosis. Clin Tech Small Anim Pract 2001;16(4):219–24.

65. Moriello KA, Coyner K, Paterson S, Mignon B. Diagnosis and treatment of dermatophytosis in dogs and cats.: clinical Consensus Guidelines of the World Association for Veterinary Dermatology. Vet Dermatol 2017;28(3):266–68.

66. Asawananda P, Taylor CR. Wood's light in dermatology. Int J Dermatol 1999;38(11):801–7.

67. Caplan RM. Medical uses of the Wood's lamp. JAMA 1967;202(11):1035–8.

68. Keep J.M. The Epidemiology and control of Microsporum canis bodin in a CAT Community. Aust Vet J 1959;35:374–8.

69. Dasgupta T, Sahu J. Origins of the KOH technique. Clin Dermatol 2012;30(2):238–41; discussion 41–2.

70. Achten G. The use of detergents for direct mycologic examination. J Invest Dermatol 1956;26(5):389–97.

71. Robert R, Pihet M. Conventional methods for the diagnosis of dermatophytosis. Mycopathologia 2008;166(5–6):295–306.

72. Georg LK. The diagnosis of ringworm in animals. Vet Med 1954;49:157–66.

73. Taschdjian CL. Fountain pen ink as an aid in mycologic technic. J Invest Dermatol 1955;24(2):77–80.

74. Sparkes AH, Werrett G, Stokes CR, Gruffydd-Jones TJ. Improved sensitivity in the diagnosis of dermatophytosis by fluorescence microscopy with calcafluor white. Vet Rec 1994;134(12):307–8.

Case 11

Planning a Feline Castration

Stephanie Jackson and her boyfriend, Tom, had always dreamed of getting a dog. Not just any dog. A rough-and-tumble hiking buddy by day, and a couch potato at night. But the dream was misplaced from reality and would be for some time. Stephanie practically lived at law school, and as an emergency room nurse, Tom worked three 12-hour shifts that were anything but predictable. By the time Tom returned home at the end of a workday, he was headed to bed in preparation for the next one. On his days off, he found it difficult to motivate himself into action. He spent so many hours on his feet making life and death decisions that he treasured those quiet moments when the world did its own thing and all he had to do was watch from the sidelines. It was true that a dog would get him up out of bed because he would be responsible for it. But he and Steph both worried about the logistics of dog-ownership – who would take on which task and for how long before becoming resentful that the other was just skating by. Tom felt that Steph should take on more of a role in dog care because she could flex her schedule more easily than he could. Steph felt that her education was just like a job and could not be late to class if she had to walk the dog. At the end of the day, both felt it was unfair to adopt a dog that would be alone for most of his life, just so that they could have a weekend warrior to come home to.

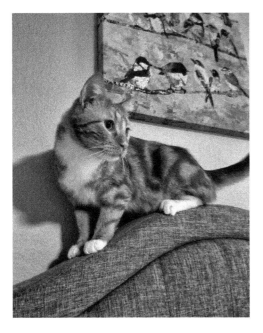

Figure 11.1 Meet your next patient, 16-week-old domestic medium-haired (DMH) kitten, Leonidas. Courtesy of Tim Gregory.

Just when they had made peace with their decision to hold off on being pet parents, Leonidas came into their lives. He appeared one day helping himself to the neighbor's trash across the street when Tom was pulling out of the driveway on his morning commute. By the next day, he was waiting on Tom's doorstep for someone to make an appearance. Tom tried to shoo him away – he wasn't really a cat person – but Leonidas seemed to think it was somewhat of a game and pounced on Tom's shoe before taking advantage of the open door to run inside the house. Tom was already late for work and wasn't in the mood for horsing around. It took some doing and a lot of cursing under his breath to extract the stranger from his home.

Ultimately, Leonidas was undeterred. He was waiting for Tom when Tom arrived home that night. Even though Tom shook his head in disbelief, something about Leo's boldness registered with Tom. For a kitten, he didn't seem at all afraid. That kind of gumption struck a chord within, and suddenly Tom found himself doing a 180 in both mind and heart. Crazier things could happen than adopting a kitten. Maybe, just maybe a cat could make a perfect addition to their home: just enough of a companion, yet independent enough to get by on his own for long stretches of time.

Tom talked it over with Steph, who was not hard to convince. She took one look at the little orange ball of fluff, scooped him up, and welcomed him home. Steph took him to the vaccine clinic in town that weekend to get him up to speed on his shots. The veterinarian on site estimated him to be about 12 weeks of age and deemed him healthy. He even remarked that Leonidas seemed like a perfect fit for a couple who wanted a dog but didn't have the schedule to support one now. Leonidas was more canine than feline. He was adventurous and inquisitive, interactive and dauntless. His favorite activity was playing fetch. He hadn't quite figured out how to mouth bouncy balls, but he loved retrieving cough drops. They had those little tabs at either end that he could hold onto.

Leonidas tested negative for feline leukemia (FeLV) and feline immunodeficiency virus (FIV) and was vaccinated against rabies and feline viral rhinotracheitis-calicivirus-panleukopenia (FVRCP) using recombinant and modified live virus (MLV) vaccines respectively. Steph was advised that he should return for a FVRCP booster in three to four weeks to complete the series and to discuss being neutered.

Before you can assist Steph and Tom with their decision making, it is important that you revisit feline male reproductive anatomy.

Round One of Questions for Case 11: Planning a Feline Castration

1. When is sexual maturity in the cat?
2. Which factors influence the onset of puberty in the cat?
3. What is a sexually mature, intact male cat called?
4. Describe the components of the male feline reproductive tract. Compare and contrast these with the male canine reproductive tract.
5. What is the os penis? Describe its function and location in the male cat.
6. Where are the testes located in an intact male cat? Compare and contrast this location with that in a male dog.
7. What is the male reproductive cell or gamete?
8. Where within the reproductive tract does the male gamete form?
9. Where within the reproductive tract does the male gamete undergo maturation?
10. How long does spermatogenesis take?
11. Track the path of the male reproductive cell through its exit point in the male reproductive tract.
12. What mixes with spermatozoa as they move through the male urogenital tract and why?
13. What happens to the sperm that have been produced if a patient is sexually inactive?
14. Compare and contrast the feline urethra with the same structure in the male dog.
15. Compare and contrast the feline penis with the same structure in the male dog.
16. What are penile spines?
17. If you were to extrude Leonidas' penis from the prepuce during this physical examination, would you expect to see penile spines? Why or why not?

Answers to Round One of Questions for Case 11: Planning a Feline Castration

1. Sexual maturity varies in onset between individuals, but is said to range between 4 and 12 months of age in the cat.(1) On average, onset of puberty occurs in the male cat at 6 months of age.(2)

2. The following factors may influence the onset of puberty in the cat:(1)

- season
- day length
- body weight
- breed.

On average, long-haired cats take longer to reach puberty than short-haired cats.(1)

3. A sexually mature, intact male cat is called a tomcat or, for short, a tom.(1)

4. The male feline reproductive tract includes:(2–5)

    *   external structures:

        *   scrotum
        *   paired testes
        *   prepuce, the sheath that contains the penis
        *   penis
        *   penile urethra

    *   internal structures:

        *   preprostatic urethra
        *   prostatic urethra
        *   postprostatic urethra
        *   accessory sex glands:

            *   prostate
            *   bulbourethral gland.

    As compared to the cat, the male canine reproductive tract only has one accessory sex gland, the prostate.(2–4)

5. The os penis, or baculum, is a bone that accompanies the penile urethra.(2, 6, 7) This mineralization is scant by comparison to the macroscopic os penis of the dog, and it does not appear to be present in all cats.(5, 6, 8, 9) When the os penis is present, it is seated dorsal to the canine urethra and ventral to the feline urethra within the glans, and it is not grooved, as it is in dogs, to accommodate the urethra.(2, 5, 9) It has been hypothesized that the os penis provides rigidity, which facilitates intromission.(2, 9) Others have proposed that the os penis maintains the patency of the urethra by preventing its collapse, so as to ensure delivery of semen to the female reproductive tract.(10)

6. The testes are located within the scrotum of an intact male cat, as is true of male dogs.(2–4, 7) The scrotum is a pouch of skin that hangs outside of the abdominal cavity.(2) This placement is essential for spermatogenesis, which is hindered when testicular temperatures exceed 104°F (40°C).(2)

    The location of the scrotum differs in cats and dogs. In the male dog, the scrotum is suspended between the thighs.(2–4) By contrast, the scrotum of the male cat is positioned within the perineum, ventral to the anus.(2–4) Therefore, the scrotum of a cat can only be seen when the cat is viewed from behind.(11) Note that the feline scrotum is heavily furred as opposed to the canine scrotum, which is not.(4) (See Figures 11.2a and 11.2b.)

7. The male reproductive cell or gamete is a spermatozoon.(2, 7, 12) The plural for this is spermatozoa. Sometimes we abbreviate this and simply refer to the male gamete as sperm.

8. Spermatozoa form within the seminiferous tubules of each testis.(2, 7)

9. Spermatozoa undergo maturation as they move through a coiled tube, the epididymis.(2–4) This firm structure runs along the dorsolateral surface of each canine testis, and the craniolateral surface of each feline testis.(3, 4, 11, 13)

    Each epididymis consists of a head, body, and tail.(3, 4) The tail is the most prominent portion of this structure and can be appreciated on physical exam.(3, 4) This is where the bulk of mature sperm are stored.(2) The tail of the epididymis is located at the caudalmost pole of the canine testis, and dorsally in the cat.(11, 13, 14)

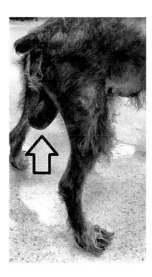

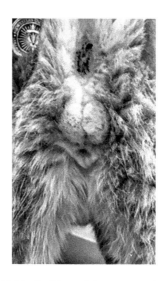

Figure 11.2a Position of the scrotum in an intact male dog. Courtesy of Beki Cohen Regan, DVM.

Figure 11.2b Position of the scrotum in an intact male cat.

10. Spermatogenesis takes approximately 47 days in the cat (15) as compared to 60 days in the dog.(2)

11. Spermatozoa originate within the seminiferous tubules and mature within the epididymis.(2) Spermatozoa then migrate out of the epididymis and into the vas deferens, a tubular one-way path to the urethra.(13) Spermatozoa arrive at the prostatic urethra. They then travel from the prostatic urethra to the postprostatic urethra, and ultimately to the penile urethra for exit from the body.(2)

12. As spermatozoa move through the urethra, they are mixed with seminal fluid from the accessory sex glands.(2) This seminal fluid has several purposes:(2, 7)

   • increase ejaculate volume
   • improve motility of spermatozoa
   • nourish spermatozoa
   • neutralize the acidity of urine within the urethra.

13. Sperm are voided in the urine if cats and dogs are sexually inactive.(2)

14. The canine urethra is much longer than feline urethra in the tom, but only one accessory sex gland contributes to urethral contents in the dog (the prostate) as opposed to two in the cat (the prostate and the bulbourethral glands).(2–4)

15. In both male dogs and cats, the penis is sheathed by the prepuce except during erection. This process requires the backwards-facing feline penis to curve downward and forward.(16)

    In the dog, the penis is slung between the thighs, whereas in the cat, the penis is said to point backwards.(2, 3) This means that the urogenital opening in cats arises from the perineum, from which the apex of the penis is directed caudoventrally.(3, 17) It is for this reason that sexual determination of kittens can be challenging.(3)

    A male dog has obvious external genitalia if one were to look between his legs. By contrast, male and female kittens tend to look alike, especially as neonates.(3) In the first few weeks of life, male kittens are differentiated from females primarily by eyeballing anogenital distance, which is greater in males than in females.(3) An increased anogenital distance in male cats allows their testes to sit dorsal to the urogenital opening.(3)

16. The glans penis of the tomcat is unique in that its surface contains 120–150 caudally directed keratinized papillae. (3, 4, 14, 18–22) These are sometimes called spikes or spines.(3, 4, 14, 18, 19, 22) These structures are visible with the naked eye after the penis has been extruded from its prepuce. (See Figure 11.3.)

    • The purpose of feline penile spines is to scrape the queen's reproductive tract during mating to induce ovulation.(14, 16–19, 21) Unlike many other species, female cats do not release oocytes without sexual stimulation.(16, 17, 21) Hence, queens are so-called induced ovulators.(3, 4)

17. Penile spines require testosterone in order to develop.(14, 20, 22) They are not apparent in a 12-week-old kitten, but are expected to be fully present by 6 or 7 months of age. (14, 20, 22) Leonidas is estimated to be four months old, so it is possible that his will be present. However, it would not be abnormal if they were absent.

    If they are present, they will regress as testosterone levels drop post-castration.(4) Note that regression is not instantaneous: it takes up to 6 weeks.(16, 17, 22)

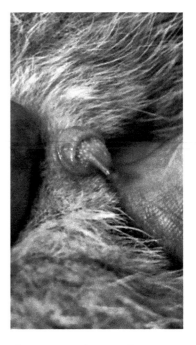

Figure 11.3 Feline penile spines. Courtesy of Joseph Onello, DVM.

Returning to Case 11: Planning a Feline Castration

You have examined Leonidas and he appears to be in good health. You make the following notations in his medical record concerning vital signs:

Leonidas does not have a heart murmur on thoracic auscultation and his lungs are clear. Based upon his physical exam today, he is a good candidate for castration. When you mention scheduling this procedure, Tom expresses several concerns. Help Tom to better understand the procedure by answering the questions below.

Weight: 3.8 pounds (1.7 kilograms)
BCS: 4/9
Mentation: BAR

TPR

T: 101.2°F (38.4°C)
P: 168 beats per minute
R: 16 breaths per minute

Round Two of Questions for Case 11: Planning a Feline Castration

1. What is the appropriate medical terminology for castration?
2. Tom has never owned a pet before, let alone a cat, so he is not sure what surgical castration involves. He asks if the procedure is essentially the same thing as having a vasectomy. How do you respond?

3. Tom isn't thrilled about having Leonidas undergo surgery at his young age. He asks if there is any other way to neuter him that does not require surgical intervention. What do you say?

4. Tom is still not convinced that Leonidas needs to be neutered. He understands now that removing the testicles will eliminate the chance of testicular cancer, but asks you, honestly, how common is that really?

5. What are the advantages of having Leonidas undergo this elective procedure?

6. What is/are potential health-related concern(s) about castration in general and how can the concern(s) be addressed?

7. What are the potential health-related concerns about castration specific to pediatric patients?

8. If Tom and Steph agree to proceed with castration, what is an essential component of your physical exam prior to Leonidas being anesthetized?

9. Tom is concerned about anesthetic risk. He wants a 100% guarantee that the anesthesia you will use on Leonidas is "safe." How do you respond?

10. What are the most common anesthetic risks in small animal practice?

11. How often does anesthetic death occur?

12. What are the most significant risk factors when it comes to anesthetic death in cats?

13. What steps can you take to improve the safety of the anesthetic event?

14. How will Leonidas be prepped for surgery?

15. Outline the surgical plan for orchiectomy. Include a comparison of open and closed castration techniques.

16. Will sutures be placed? If so, will they require removal?

17. What are potential complications of this procedure?

18. Are there any specific instructions for aftercare?

Answers to Round Two of Questions for Case 11: Planning a Feline Castration

1. Orchiectomy is the appropriate medical terminology for castration.(23–26)

2. I would explain that, no, a vasectomy is not the same procedure as orchiectomy. Orchiectomy refers to the surgical excision of both testes.(23–26) By contrast, vasectomy refers to the ligation of the vas deferens.(24) Both procedures are performed to inhibit fertility.(24) However, vasectomy does not eliminate the source of the patient's testosterone.(24) Therefore, testosterone levels remain within the normal reference range, and the patient is able to retain secondary sex characteristics and behavioral patterns.(24) By contrast, orchiectomy removes the source of testosterone through excision of both testicles. When performed on pediatric patients, orchiectomy prevents the development of secondary sex characteristics and behavioral patterns.

3. Non-surgical methods of reproduction control in cats have been described in the medical literature; however, although they avoid surgery, they are not all without risk.

Progestins can be administered as an alternative to orchiectomy.(27) These include megestrol acetate (MA), proligestone (PRG), and medroxyprogesterone acetate (MPA).(1) Such compounds inhibit the release of follicle-stimulating hormone (FSH) and luteinizing hormone (LH) from the anterior pituitary.(1)

In the tomcat, LH encourages the Leydig (interstitial) cells of the testes to produce testosterone.(7, 28) FSH promotes testicular growth and production of androgen-binding protein, an essential component for maturation of spermatozoa.(7, 28)

If the release of LH and FSH is inhibited, then the reproductive axis is effectively shut down for as long as inhibition persists. If sterilization is intended to be lifelong, then Leonidas would require lifelong medication.

Progestin administration will effectively reduce the following behaviors:(1)

- aggression
- marking with urine
- mating
- mounting.

However, adverse effects are not benign and include development of mammary tumors, and insulin resistant diabetes mellitus.(1)

Another non-surgical method of suppressing reproductive function is to subcutaneously implant a gonadotropin-releasing hormone (GnRH) agonist, such as deslorelin.(1) In health, GnRH is produced by the hypothalamus.(7, 28) It acts upon the anterior pituitary to release LH and FSH.(7, 28) If a patient is exposed to GnRH, then there will be an initial spike in LH and FSH.(1) This will lead to a transient increase in testosterone.(1) However, if exposure to GnRH persists, then pituitary GnRH receptors will eventually "tune out" the noise, that is they will be downregulated and testosterone concentrations will plummet over time.(1) In the tomcat, testosterone levels will mirror those achieved by surgical castration within four to eight weeks.(1) Testosterone levels will remain low for the lifetime of the implant, which averages 6 to 18 months.(1)

No adverse sequelae have been reported in toms that have received implants of GnRH agonists, and it is reversible – that is, the implant can be removed at any time in the event that it is not the right 'fit' for a given patient.(1) However, this does not offer the client a permanent solution.(1) The implant does not last for the lifetime of the cat.

Non-hormonal methods of contraception have also been explored. Male contraception by means of intratesticular or intraepididymal injections have been proposed for years in several species, not just cats, since the 1950s.(29–31) Many sclerosing agents have been investigated for their ability to achieve chemical castration. Proposed injectables have included:(31, 32)

- cadmium chloride
- calcium chloride dihydrate
- chlorhexidine digluconate
- clove oil
- dimethyl sulfoxide (DMSO)
- hypertonic saline
- zinc gluconate.

Of these agents, calcium chloride dihydrate and zinc gluconate have been tested as intratesticular injections in cats, and chlorhexidine digluconate has been tested as intraepididymal injections.(31)

The goal of these injectables is to replace functional testicular tissue with connective tissue to induce azoospermia.(31)

Primary advantages of chemical castration are that it is non-surgical and affordable as compared to surgical castration.(31) However, more research is necessary to perfect the technique. As of now, no standard guidelines have been published concerning volume, concentration, or formulation of the sclerosing agent(s).(31)

The need for analgesia and/or anesthesia remains unclear. Because afferent nerve endings for nociception are not located in testicular parenchyma, intratesticular injections do not typically induce immediate discomfort.(31, 33) However, pain receptors are present in the scrotal skin – meaning that the act of inserting the needle will be felt by the patient. Some degree of sedation, if not general anesthesia, may be of benefit, though not all protocols call for more than manual restraint.(30, 31, 34–36)

Pain receptors are also located within the testicular capsule, so patients are likely to experience pain when swelling causes both testicles to push against their capsules within 24 hours of the injection.(31) It does not appear that this pain precipitates self-trauma and mutilation. Biting and licking at the scrotum post-injection have not been reported.(36) However, iatrogenic scrotal injury is possible if the sclerosing agent leaks outside of the tunic during the injection process.(37)

Another concern about intratesticular and intraepididymal injections is that the testes continue to produce testosterone. This may not be ideal in a companion pet because sex steroid-induced behaviors, such as urine marking, mounting, and territorial aggression will persist.(31)

Finally, chemical castration is not immediate. On average, it takes four to six weeks to see a drop in sperm production.(30, 31, 36) Although this is unlikely to be of concern for Leonidas, given that he is four months old and has not yet reached sexual maturity, it isn't the instant fix that most people are hoping for.

Chemical castration is likely to evolve and may one day be considered superior to surgical castration; however, at this time, the methodology is not at a point where I would feel comfortable performing the procedure on Leonidas.

4. Tom is correct. Although veterinarians often claim that we neuter cats to reduce the rate of testicular cancer, the truth is that testicular tumors are rare in cats.(23, 38–45)

5. The advantages of having Leonidas undergo this elective procedure are primarily behavioral. By removing the source of testosterone, Leonidas will be less likely to:(25)

- act out aggressively
- become territorial
- roam
- urine-mark.

Castration in cats also contributes to their longevity. Neutered male cats have longer lifespans than their intact counterparts.(25)

In my experience, many clients also prefer neutered male cats because they lack the classic tomcat urine, which is particularly pungent.

6. Castrated cats are more likely to be obese.(25, 46) Obesity is a significant health concern because it predisposes cats to lameness, lower urinary tract disease, hepatic lipidosis, and diabetes mellitus.(47, 48) It has been estimated that over one-third of pet cats are overweight (>10% above ideal body weight) or obese (>20% above ideal body weight).(47, 49–51)

Obesity in castrated cats most likely results from over-eating. In my clinical experience, owners are not always advised (as they should be!) to reduce caloric intake after surgery. Neutered cats do not have the same requirement for caloric intake as intact cats. In fact, neutered cats require 28% less calories.(52) If we continue to feed them as if they are intact, then it is no surprise they will gain weight. We can easily right this wrong by providing owners with customized instructions for caloric reduction following spay/neuter. Reduced intake by calorie-restricting cats after they undergo elective sterilization should solve the problem of obesity in neutered cats by keeping them leaner post-operatively.

7. Concern has been expressed that pediatric spay/neuter may predispose patients to orthopedic disease. For example, we know that cats that are castrated before 7 months of age experience delays in physeal closure.(25) Theses delays may predispose them to growth plate fractures, of which the proximal femur is most often implicated. Of those cats that develop non-traumatic femoral capital physeal fractures – so-called slipped capital femoral epiphysis (SCFE) – young, neutered, obese male cats are overrepresented.(53–59)

SCFE may be unilateral or bilateral.(54, 56) Patients present with varying degrees of lameness associated with the affected pelvic limb(s).(4) On physical exam, patients react painfully to hip flexion and extension.(4, 60) It is common to palpate crepitus over the hip joint as the hip is carried through its normal range of motion.(4, 54) Palpation over the greater trochanter of the affected limb may also elicit pain.(4, 61)

Orthogonal radiographs of the pelvis and coxofemoral joints are performed under heavy sedation or general anesthesia.(4) Radiographic findings include loss of bone within the femoral neck, such that it begins to take on an "apple cored" appearance.(4)

Case management is most often surgical and involves femoral head ostectomy (FHO).(4)

Although orthopedic diagnoses such as SCFE are significant and serious when they arise, they are rare in occurrence. Benefits of sterilization appear to outweigh the risks in feline patients.

8. If Tom and Steph agree to proceed with castration, it is essential that you confirm Leonidas' sex and sexual status prior to him being anesthetized. Quite honestly, this should have been done during his initial physical examination. It's a bit late in the game to check now – but it is better now than never!

    I have witnessed clinic nightmares where sex of the patient was never confirmed, it was just assumed based upon the documentation that was provided at intake. Sometimes the clients themselves mistake the cat's sex. For instance, they might have listed male on the paperwork when in fact the cat is female. Or they might have listed female when in fact the cat is male. It works both ways.

    On other occasions, I've seen clients adopt or purchase a cat of a specified sex, only to find that the sex is wrong.

    Why does this matter? You don't want to trust the paperwork blindly and surgically open the abdomen of a cat to spay her, only to find that she is male. This will not sit well with the client, who expected you to be an expert. It pays to double-check or even triple-check. The opposite situation is nearly as bad. What if you were to trust the paperwork blindly and create an estimate for castration, if the cat is in fact female. Now you've anesthetized the supposedly male cat, looked under the tail to perform the castration, only to realize that he is female. Now you have to telephone the client to inform them about mistaken sexual identity, obtain permission to spay rather than castrate, and up the ante in terms of the procedural cost. Neither of these clinical scenarios sits well with a client. The client trusts you to be on top of these things. We all make mistakes, but don't let them happen when they are the easiest mistakes in veterinary practice to avoid!

    Sexing Leonidas requires only a brief, non-invasive examination of his perineum.

    If Leonidas is in fact male, then you need to go one step further on your examination: can you palpate two scrotal testes?

    Recall that canine and feline testes do not originate from the scrotum.(11, 13, 14) In the embryo, the testes develop near the caudal pole of each kidney.(13, 14, 62) They then must migrate to the scrotum through the inguinal canal before the canal closes between four and six months old.(11, 13, 14, 62–66) The inguinal canal is located in the groin as a passage through the abdominal wall.(13) This migration is facilitated by the gubernaculum, a fold of peritoneum that spans from the caudal pole of each testis to the scrotum.(13, 14, 62) During testicular migration, the gubernaculum enlarges. This dilates the inguinal canal, paving the way for testicular descent.(14, 62) The gubernaculum distal to the inguinal canal then pulls each testis towards the groin.(62) The gubernaculum shrinks down only after drawing the testes through the canal and into the scrotum.(62, 67–69)

    At birth, the gubernaculum is often palpable within the scrotum and may be mistaken for scrotal testes.(14, 62) In reality, most kittens lack scrotal testes at birth.(14, 62) Many testes drop into the scrotum between 3 and 10 days of age, but may move in and out of the scrotum until the inguinal canal closes at 4 to 6 months of age.(14, 62, 70, 71) At that point, feline testes should be scrotal.(14, 67, 70–74) If they are not, the patient is said to be cryptorchid.(14, 66, 67, 70–74)

    The incidence of cryptorchidism ranges from 3.3 and 6.8% in dogs as compared to 1.3 to 3.8% in cats.(64, 74–78) Patients may be unilaterally or bilaterally affected.(4) If one or both testes are not present within the scrotum, then they are "stuck" somewhere within the abdomen or inguinal canal.(62–64, 79–81) The "missing" testis/testes will require surgical extraction. This procedure is more complicated than a standard orchiectomy, which is why it is important that you know in advance whether this applies to your patient.

9. The most honest, direct answer is that, try as we might to select the safest selection of drugs and drug doses, no anesthetic protocol is ever 100% safe. That being said, there are ways that we can significantly improve the safety of our plan to optimize Leonidas' outcome. These will be

outlined in my response to Question #13 (below). However, in order to address Tom's concerns specifically, it would help to ask him to expand upon his fears. Open-ended statements that open the door to dialogue and elicit his perspective will be of benefit.

"Tell me more about what concerns you most," I might say, to encourage him to share. I want to know more about what's concerning him so that I can address it. Every client comes to me with different past experiences that have shaped his/her understanding of the present and the future.

If a client has experienced anesthetic death before – whether this involved a beloved pet or a friend/family member – then s/he may be concerned that this pet might share the same fate. Other clients may have no real life connection to anesthetic death but may fear based upon what they've heard from others, or what they've seen on television.

Sometimes when a client shares concern that anesthesia isn't "safe," we assume that s/he is talking about the risk of anesthetic death. That may or may not be the case. It behooves us to ask. I have had some clients not at all worried about death, but extremely concerned about post-operative pain or that the pet would wake up alone.

Everyone brings different concerns to the table. Even if two people share the same concern, they may not assign it the same level of importance. There are clients who are deathly afraid of anesthesia and will avoid it at all costs because they are afraid of death – even if the patient's condition will result in death if they do not undergo general anesthesia – and other clients who just want reassurance that appropriate measures are in place to minimize risk.

If we invite our clients to share, then we can:

* demonstrate that their concerns have been heard, through reflective (active) listening
* normalize their concerns: "It's normal to worry about . . ."
* validate their concerns: "No, you're not crazy to think that . . ."
* address their concerns: "Yes, it's true that . . ."
* take action on what can be done in the present and future to reduce risk.

Nowhere is client communication more important than prior to procedures that involve anesthesia.(82) The average veterinary client has minimal knowledge of what veterinary procedures involve, and may or may not understand that anesthetic agents could have adverse effects.(83) Of those clients that are concerned about their patient's treatment plan, not all choose to voice these concerns even when granted the opportunity. Others may instead rely upon alternate sources of information that may or may not be accurate. A recent study in the *Journal of the American Veterinary Medical Association* by Hofmeister et al. confirmed that 87% of veterinary clients rely upon the internet for veterinary medical information despite the fact that many sources are incomplete particularly when it comes to displaying information about general anesthesia in pets.(84) Eighteen percent of survey participants believed what they read online, that their pet was at increased risk of anesthesia because of breed – whether or not that information was backed up by scientific evidence.(84)

If we as professionals fail to address these misconceptions – or we inadvertently promote them by not entertaining client-initiated discussion about concerns – then we have failed to take advantage of the opportunity to educate and protect the patient. Our clients need to be informed of potential risks before they happen. They also need to be made aware of the preventative measures we take – and why we take them so that they understand how risks are managed.(83)

10. The primary anesthetic complications in veterinary medicine are intra-operative hypotension, (85–87) opioid-induced dysphoria,(88–90) cardiac dysrhythmias, (87) post-operative regurgitation and vomiting, (91) aspiration pneumonia,(92) cerebellar dysfunction,(93) blindness or deafness in cats,(94–96) and death.(97)

11. A recent study by Brodbelt et al. evaluated records from 98,036 dogs and 79,178 cats between June 2002 and 2004 in the UK and found that the overall risks of anesthetic death in dogs and

cats were 0.17% and 0.24%, respectively.(98) When patients were categorized by their health status, the risk of anesthetic death in healthy dogs and cats dropped to 0.05% and 0.11% compared to 1.33% and 1.40% in ill dogs and cats.(98) These percentages are much higher than those that have been reported for anesthetized people, 0.02–0.05%.(99–101)

12. In addition to health status,(97, 98, 102–105) the following are considered risk factors when considering anesthetic death in cats: body weight of less than 5 kg,(104) endotracheal intubation,(97, 103, 104) and concurrent intravenous fluid therapy.(102, 104) Certain breeds also increase anesthetic risk of death.(82, 97) So does age: those 12 years of age or older are considered to be at increased risk.(106)

13. There are several preoperative and intraoperative measures that we can take to improve the safety of Leonidas' anesthetic event.
     Pre-operative measures include the following.

     • Taking a comprehensive history.(107)

        • For example, we may find out that the patient has been short of breath or coughing – these could indicate airway disease that could decompensate under anesthesia. To improve safety of the anesthetic event, we would need to investigate and work-up the patient for these new findings before we can appropriately "clear" him/her for surgery.

     • Performing a thorough physical examination.(107)

        • For example, we may discover on thoracic auscultation that the patient has a grade 3/6 systolic heart murmur that requires imaging to evaluate the heart's structure and function before we can safely proceed.

     • Obtaining a minimum database.

        • As a veterinary student, I was taught that every minimum database included a complete blood count (CBC), chemistry panel, and urinalysis (UA) +/– imaging (thoracic radiographs +/– abdominal ultrasonography).(108)
        • Standardization of a minimum database encourages clinicians to share a similar approach to case management and provide equivalent care.(108, 109)
        • However, practices must also factor in client cost and what is deemed to be in the best interest of the patient.(109) Which diagnostic tests are essential to every patient? Which are essential for select patients? Should certain tests be prioritized? If so, do tests take priority always or only under certain circumstances? What, if any, are the exceptions to the rules?(108)
        • Evidence-based clear-cut guidelines for when to test which patient and for which diseases are hard to come by, but in general, organizations such as the American Animal Hospital Association (AAHA) are moving away from the one-size-fits-all patient database.(108, 110)
        • For young, healthy patients that are undergoing elective sterilization surgery, quick assessment tests (QATS) may be adequate:(107)

           • PCV
           • TP
           • blood glucose (BG)
           • Azostix® as a screening test for BUN (BUN and creatinine if Azostix® test is elevated)
           • USG.

     • Customize a multimodal approach to anesthesia, including pre-medications.(111)

- Pharmaceutical agents can be used synergistically to reduce the dose of each drug that is administered to the patient.
- Using more pharmaceutical agents in smaller amounts reduces adverse effects to the patient, which should improve patient outcomes.

- Calculate doses of emergency drugs just in case they are needed.
- Discuss risks with client.
- Establish the client's wishes for cardiopulmonary resuscitation (CPR) in the event of emergency. Each hospital has its own coding system for CPR designations. I was trained to use the stoplight method of green–yellow–red:

  - CODE RED = STOP = Do not resuscitate (DNR)
  - YELLOW = Closed-chest CPR
  - GREEN = Open-chest CPR.

- Acquire up to date day-of-procedure client contact information so that the client can be reached in the event of an emergency.

The importance of the pre-anesthetic evaluation cannot be understated even when the procedure is routine. Just because the procedure is routine does not mean that the anesthetic plan should not be tailored to the individual. Identifying patient risks before they become problems is half the battle. Anticipation paves the way for prevention. (82)

Intraoperative measures include:(112)

- anesthetic monitoring

  - heart rate (HR) and rhythm
  - respiratory rate (RR) and effort
  - pulse quality, rate, and strength
  - palpebral reflex
  - eye position
  - pupil size
  - mucous membrane color
  - capillary refill time (CRT)
  - electrocardiogram (ECG)
  - capnography
  - pulse oximetry
  - blood pressure (BP)
  - body temperature

    - esophageal thermometer is preferred because it will register the patient's core body temperature

- fluid therapy(107)
- patient warming devices, such as the Bair Hugger or the Hot Dog.

Finally, we can take measures to protect Leonidas during recovery from his procedure. Contrary to popular belief, most anesthetic deaths do not occur during induction or maintenance of anesthesia. The majority occur during recovery.(98) Stepping up patient monitoring in the post-operative period via pulse assessment and pulse oximetry can lessen risk.(104)

14. How tomcats are prepped for elective orchiectomy is extremely variable. The following components of the anesthetic and surgical prep may vary tremendously from practice to practice:

- whether an intravenous (IV) catheter is placed
- whether injectable anesthesia alone is used or in combination with inhalant anesthesia
- whether the patient receives inhalant anesthesia and flow-by oxygen via an oxygen mask or whether the patient is intubated

- whether the surgeon dons a surgical cap and mask
- whether surgical drapes are placed
- whether the patient is placed in dorsal or lateral recumbency with the hindlimbs pulled forward

    - right lateral recumbency tends to be preferred by right-handed surgeons.(23)

The feline scrotum is densely furred.(3) Scrotal fur should be removed before proceeding with orchiectomy.(23–26) Because clipping can irritate the thin skin of the scrotum, manual plucking of the fur is typically performed prior to prepping the perineum using aseptic technique.(23–26) In prepubertal patients, clipping may be required as opposed to plucking because there may be insufficient fur to grasp to make plucking a less traumatic technique.(24)

15. Feline orchiectomy can be performed using a closed or open castration technique. Let's start by defining what we mean.

    - In a closed castration, the vaginal tunic is not opened.(24) The vaginal tunic is serous membrane that encases each testis in a pouch within the scrotum. Because this membrane remains closed during the procedure, at no point does the surgeon enter the peritoneal cavity. This technique is expedient. However, there is the potential for hemorrhage because blood vessels that supply the testicles are indirectly ligated: the tunic is ligated rather than the vessels themselves.
    - In an open castration, the vaginal tunic is opened.(24) This allows for more complete visualization of and separation of the components of the spermatic cord for individual ligation. (24)

    Regardless of which technique is used, both versions of the feline orchiectomy start the same. One testicle is operated on at a time.(23–26)
    Start by applying pressure with your thumb and index finger over the base of the scrotum to push the testicle of interest to the surface.(23–26) Then incise the skin and subcutis from cranial to caudal over the center of the testicle.(23–26) The incision need not be large – 1 cm should be more than enough.(24) At this point, the procedural steps diverge depending upon which technique the surgeon prefers.(23–26)

    - Closed castration(23–26)

        - As you continue to apply pressure to the base of the scrotum, the testicle of interest should "pop" out of the incision. Sometimes you must incise a web of subcutaneous fascia to make this happen, but you must not cut through the tunic.
        - Use a square of sterile dry gauze to strip off the scrotal attachments of the testicle as you hold it in your hand. This should allow you to pull the testicle in one hand as you push against the cat's perineum with your other hand to break down the cremaster muscle. At this point, the testicle has been fully exteriorized and you have an appreciable length of spermatic cord to work with.
        - The overhand technique can then be applied using a closed curved hemostat to essentially tie the spermatic cord onto itself.

            - The curved closed hemostat is pointed downwards towards the cat.
            - The hemostat is then placed under, around, and over the cord. It is best to do this close to the hemostat's tips to facilitate the next step.
            - You then clamp the cord near the tips of the hemostat.
            - Transect the cord near the hemostat.
            - Using your fingers, push the cord off the hemostat to form a knot.
            - Tighten the knot by using your index finger and thumb on either side of the cord to push the knot towards the cat.

- Open the hemostat.
- Tuck the remnants of the cord back into the incision, taking care not to loosen the knot.

- Repeat the procedure for the second testicle.

- Open castration(23–26)

  - As you continue to apply pressure to the base of the scrotum, incise through the parietal aspect of the vaginal tunic to expose the testicle.
  - Pull the testicle out from the incision site for better exposure. You should now be able to visualize the spermatic cord.
  - Using your hands, separate the parietal aspect of the vaginal tunic from the testicle.
  - Using blunt dissection, separate the bundle of testicular vessels from the vas deferens. The vas deferens may be detached from the testicle at this time.
  - Tie the vas deferens to the vascular bundle. Form four throws for a total of two square knots.
  - Distal to your knots, transect.
  - Tuck the remnants back into the incision, taking care not to loosen the knot.
  - Repeat the procedure for the second testicle.

As a surgeon, I prefer to make use of the closed castration technique for kittens.

When cats are fully grown adults and/or especially if adult cats are well-endowed, then I prefer the open castration method because I find that my knots do not cinch down as tightly if I were to use the closed technique on these toms. The spermatic cords on these patients are so thick that I am not always convinced that I have indirectly ligated the bundle of testicular vessels through the cord if a closed technique is used.

16. Scrotal incisions in the cat are left open to heal. No sutures are placed, so no suture removal is required.(23–26)

17. Complications secondary to elective orchiectomy are rare.(23–26)

   - Perineal infection is rare if aseptic technique was used to prepare the site for surgery.
   - Hemorrhage is possible if the knot slipped. In the author's experience, this is more likely to happen with the closed castration technique. If this occurs, scrotal hemorrhage on the affected side will be apparent in the immediate post-operative period.

     - Sedate the patient.
     - Use a sterile hemostat to grasp blindly into the incision on the affected side. If you are lucky, you will find it.
     - However, the cord often retracts post-operatively, making it challenging to find.

       - If this occurs, place pressure on the inguinal and scrotal regions for 5–10 minutes to slow the bleeding.
       - Intraabdominal bleeding of significance is rare and would require abdominal surgery.
       - You can monitor serial hematocrits to be safe, watching for the development of anemia, which should not occur if the procedure had been routine.

18. Because the scrotal incisions are left open to the environment to heal on their own, paper litter is advised for several days – just until there is skin-to-skin apposition.(25) An Elizabethan collar may also be recommended to prevent excessive grooming, which could irritate the site and/or lead to perineal infection.

CLINICAL PEARLS

- The average age at which male cats reach sexual maturity is 6 months old. Sexually mature male cats are called toms.

- Testosterone is the hormone that is responsible for giving toms large jowls and barbed penises. It is also responsible for some of the behaviors that cat owners do not necessarily find appealing, including mounting, marking with urine, defending territories with aggression, and roaming.

- Surgical castration (orchiectomy) is a common elective procedure that permanently eliminates testosterone by removing both testes.

- Some clients think that castration is the same procedure as a vasectomy. It is important to clarify what is meant by "neutering" and to differentiate between the two procedures because vasectomies are performed in people and are reversible whereas orchiectomies are not.

- A primary advantage of orchiectomy is that by removing testosterone, the unwanted behaviors should cease, provided that they have not developed yet or have not become a part of the daily routine (that is, behaviors that have become "fixed").

- Removing testosterone will reduce resting and metabolic energy rate, which means that neutered cats require less calories to maintain body weight. If neutered cats are not calorie-restricted post-orchiectomy, then they are likely to gain weight. Obesity is a growing problem in pet populations globally.

- Although there is some concern that pre-pubertal surgical sterilization delays closure of growth plates, which could in turn result in physeal fractures, these orthopedic complications are rare in cats. For most feline patients, the benefits of surgical sterilization outweigh the risks.

- For those who are concerned about surgical sterilization, there are hormonal alternatives. In toms, these include progestins and GnRH agonists. The former has the potential for significant adverse effects; the latter is more typically used by breeders for studs for transient reduction in testosterone levels.

- Although chemical sterilization has been investigated for decades, the lack of standard protocols makes it a challenging sell for client-owned cats.

- Feline orchiectomy is performed via scrotal incision.

- Following scrotal incision, castration can be performed using a closed or open technique.

- Regardless of which technique (closed versus open) is used, synthetic ligatures are not typically placed. Instead, the spermatic cord is tied onto itself (in closed castration) and the vas deferens is tied to the bundle of testicular vessels (in open castration) so that the body's own tissues are used to form its own knots.

- Knot security is essential to prevent scrotal hemorrhage. For that reason, open techniques may be advised in larger toms because closed techniques only indirectly "ligate" the testicular vessels.

- Following castration, scrotal incisions are left open to heal on their own.

- Paper litter and Elizabethan collars in the immediate post-operative period may facilitate wound healing by decreasing risk of infection and/or self-mutilation.

- Clients are often concerned about anesthetic risk. Often, but not always, their concerns center around the risk of anesthetic death.

- It is important to be transparent about risk.

- It is also important to elicit clients' concerns using open-ended statements ("Tell me", "Share with me", and so forth) and to demonstrate that their concerns have been heard, through reflective (active) listening in order to normalize and validate their fears.

- Risk can never be 100% eliminated from any equation; however, it can be minimized by taking precautions in the pre-operative, peri-operative, intraoperative, and post-operative periods.

References

1. Goericke-Pesch S. Reproduction control in cats: new developments in non-surgical methods. J Feline Med Surg. 2010;12(7):539–46.
2. Aspinall V. Anatomy and physiology of the dog and cat II. The male reproductive system. Vet Nurs J. 2004;19(6):200–4.
3. Englar RE. Performing the small animal physical examination. Hoboken, NJ: Wiley/Blackwell; 2017.
4. Englar RE. Common clinical presentations in dogs and cats. Hoboken, NJ: Wiley/Blackwell; 2019.
5. Osborne CA, Caywood DD, Johnston GR, Polzin DJ, Lulich JP, Kruger JM, Ulrich LK. Feline perineal urethrostomy: a potential cause of feline lower urinary tract disease. Vet Clin North Am Small Anim Pract. 1996;26(3):535–49.
6. Evans HE, Miller ME. Miller's anatomy of the dog. 4th ed. St. Louis, MO: Elsevier; 2013.
7. Singh B, Dyce KM. Dyce, Sack, and Wensing's textbook of veterinary anatomy. 5th ed. St. Louis, MO: Saunders; 2018.
8. Piola V, Posch B, Aghte P, Caine A, Herrtage ME. Radiographic characterization of the os penis in the cat. Vet Radiol Ultrasound. 2011;52(3):270–2.
9. Tobon Restrepo M, Altuzarra R, Espada Y, Dominguez E, Mallol C. Novellas R. CT characterization of the feline os penis. J Feline Med Surg. 2019:X19873195:http://www.ncbi.nlm.nih.gov/pubmed/1098612.
10. Brassey CA, Gardiner JD, Kitchener AC. Testing hypotheses for the function of the carnivoran baculum using finite-element analysis. Proc Biol Sci. 2018;285(1887).
11. de Gier J, van Sluijs FJ. Male reproductive tract. In: Rijnberk A, Sluijs FJv, editors. Medical history and physical examination in companion animals. 2nd ed. New York: Saunders/Elsevier; 2009. p. 117–22.
12. Axnér E. Sperm maturation in the domestic cat. Theriogenology. 2006;66(1):14–24.
13. Evans HE, Christensen GC. The urogenital system. In: Evans HE, Miller ME, editors. Miller's anatomy of the dog. 3rd ed. Philadelphia, PA: W. B. Saunders; 1993, p. 494–558.
14. Englar RE. Performing the small animal physical examination. Hoboken, NJ: Wiley; 2017.
15. França LR, Godinho CL. Testis morphometry, seminiferous epithelium cycle length, and daily sperm production in domestic cats (Felis catus). Biol Reprod. 2003;68(5):1554–61.
16. Little SE. Male reproduction. In: Little SE, editor. The cat: clinical medicine and management. St. Louis, MO: Saunders Elsevier; 2012.
17. Dyce KM, Sack WO, Wensing CJG. Textbook of veterinary anatomy. 2nd ed. Philadelphia, PA: Saunders; 1996.
18. Hudson LC, Hamilton WP. Atlas of feline anatomy for veterinarians. Philadelphia, PA: Saunders; 1993.
19. Schatten H, Constantinescu GM. Comparative reproductive biology. 1st ed. Ames, IA: Blackwell; 2007.
20. August JR. Consultations in feline internal medicine. St. Louis, MO: Saunders; 2010.
21. Ettinger SJ, Feldman EC, Côté E. Textbook of veterinary internal medicine: diseases of the dog and the cat. 8th ed. 2 vols. St. Louis, MO: Elsevier; 2017.
22. Aronson LR, Cooper ML. Penile spines of the domestic cat: their endocrine-behavior relations. Anat Rec. 1967;157(1):71–8.

23. Friend EJ. Male genital tract. In: Langley-Hobbs SJ, Demetriou J, Ladlow JF, editors. Feline soft tissue and general surgery. Edinburgh. New York: Saunders/Elsevier; 2014.

24. Hedlund CS. Surgery of the reproductive and genital systems. In: Fossum TW, Duprey LP, O'Connor D, editors. Small animal surgery. 3rd ed. Boston, MA: Elsevier; 2007.

25. Tobias KM. Feline castration. In: Tobias KM, editor. Manual of small animal soft tissue surgery. Ames, IA: Wiley/Blackwell; 2010. p. 207–13.

26. Towle HA. Testes and scrotum. In: Tobias KM, Johnston SA, editors. Veterinary surgery: small animal. St. Louis, MO: Saunders; 2012. p. 1903–16.

27. Kutzler M, Wood A. Non-surgical methods of contraception and sterilization. Theriogenology. 2006;66(3):514–25.

28. Cunningham JG, Klein BG. Cunningham's textbook of veterinary physiology. 5th ed. St. Louis, MO: Elsevier/Saunders; 2013.

29. Freund J, Lipton MM, Thompson GE. Aspermatogenesis in the guinea pig induced by testicular tissue and adjuvants. J Exp Med. 1953;97(5):711–26.

30. Jana K, Samanta PK, Ghosh D. Evaluation of single intratesticular injection of calcium chloride for non-surgical sterilization of male Black Bengal goats (Capra hircus): a dose-dependent study. Anim Reprod Sci. 2005;86(1–2):89–108.

31. Kutzler MA. Intratesticular and intraepididymal injections to sterilize male cats: from calcium chloride to zinc gluconate and beyond. J Feline Med Surg. 2015;17(9):772–6.

32. Paranzini CS, Sousa AK, Cardoso GS, Perencin FM, Trautwein LGC, Bracarense APFRL, Martins MIM. Effects of chemical castration using 20% CaCl2 with 0.5% DMSO in tomcats: evaluation of inflammatory reaction by infrared thermography and effectiveness of treatment. Theriogenology. 2018;106:253–8.

33. Schummer A, Nickel R, Sak WO. The viscera of domestic animals. In: Schummer A, Nickel R, Sak WO, editors. Urogenital system: male genital organs of the carnivores. New York: Springer-Verlag; 1979. p. 324–8.

34. Pineda MH, Dooley MP. Surgical and chemical vasectomy in the cat. Am J Vet Res. 1984;45(2):291–300.

35. Fagundes AK, Oliveira EC, Tenorio BM, Melo CC, Nery LT, Santos FA, et al. Injection of a chemical castration agent, zinc gluconate, into the testes of cats results in the impairment of spermatogenesis: a potentially irreversible contraceptive approach for this species? Theriogenology. 2014;81(2):230–6.

36. Oliveira EC, Fagundes AK, Melo CC, Nery LT, Rêvoredo RG, Andrade TF, et al. Intratesticular injection of a zinc-based solution for contraception of domestic cats: a randomized clinical trial of efficacy and safety. Vet J. 2013;197(2):307–10.

37. Koger LM. Calcium chloride castration. Mod Vet Pract. 1978;59(2):119–21.

38. Lawrence JA, Saba CF. Tumors of the male reproductive system. In: Withrow SJ, Vail DM, Page RL, editors. Withrow and MacEwen's small animal clinical oncology. 5th ed. St. Louis, MO: Elsevier; 2013. p. 557–71.

39. Rosen DK, Carpenter JL. Functional ectopic interstitial cell tumor in a castrated male cat. J Am Vet Med Assoc. 1993;202(11):1865–6.

40. Cotchin E. Neoplasia. In: Wilkinson GT, editor. Diseases of the cat and their management. Oxford: Blackwell; 1984.

41. Miller MA, Hartnett SE, Ramos-Vara JA. Interstitial cell tumor and Sertoli cell tumor in the testis of a cat. Vet Pathol. 2007;44(3):394–7.

42. Miyoshi N, Yasuda N, Kamimura Y, Shinozaki M, Shimizu T. Teratoma in a feline unilateral cryptorchid testis. Vet Pathol. 2001;38(6):729–30.

43. Ferreira da Silva J. Tertoma in a feline unilateral cryptochid testis. Vet Pathol. 2002;39(4):516.

44. Benazzi C, Sarli G, Brunetti B. Sertoli cell tumour in a cat. J Vet Med A Physiol Pathol Clin Med. 2004;51(3):124–6.

45. Meier H. Sertoli-cell tumor in the cat: report of two cases. North Am Vet. 1956;37:979.

46. Nagakura AR, Clark TL. Positive effects of prepubertal neutering in dogs and cats. Iowa State Univ Vet. 1992;54(1).

47. Bjornvad CR, Nielsen DH, Armstrong PJ, McEvoy F, Hoelmkjaer KM, Jensen KS, et al. Evaluation of a nine-point body condition scoring system in physically inactive pet cats. Am J Vet Res. 2011;72(4):433–7.

48. Scarlett JM, Donoghue S. Associations between body condition and disease in cats. J Am Vet Med Assoc. 1998;212(11):1725–31.

49. Shoveller AK, DiGennaro J, Lanman C, Spangler D. Trained vs untrained evaluator assessment of body condition score as a predictor of percent body fat in adult cats. J Feline Med Surg. 2014;16(12):957–65.

50. Lund E, Armstrong PJ, Kirk C, et al. Prevalence and risk factors for obesity in adult cats from private US veterinary practices. Int J Appl Res Vet Med. 2005;3:88–96.

51. German AJ. The growing problem of obesity in dogs and cats. J Nutr. 2006;136(7);Suppl:1940S–6S SS-6 SS.

52. Romagnoli S. Early age neutering in dogs and cats: advantages and disadvantages. Rev Bras Reprod Anim. 2017;41(1):130–2.

53. Lafuente P. Young, male neutered, obese, lame? Non-traumatic fractures of the femoral head and neck. J Feline Med Surg. 2011;13(7):498–507.

54. McNicholas WT, Jr., Wilkens BE, Blevins WE, Snyder PW, McCabe GP, Applewhite AA, et al. Spontaneous femoral capital physeal fractures in adult cats: 26 cases (1996–2001). J Am Vet Med Assoc. 2002;221(12):1731–6.

55. Queen J, Bennett D, Carmichael S, Gibson N, Li A, Payne-Johnson CE, Kelly DF. Femoral neck metaphyseal osteopathy in the cat. Vet Rec. 1998;142(7):159–62.

56. Craig LE. Physeal dysplasia with slipped capital femoral epiphysis in 13 cats. Vet Pathol. 2001;38(1):92–7.

57. Beale BS, Cole G. Minimally invasive osteosynthesis technique for articular fractures. Vet Clin North Am Small Anim Pract. 2012;42(5):1051–68.

58. Fischer HR, Norton J, Kobluk CN, Reed AL, Rooks RL, Borostyankoi F. Surgical reduction and stabilization for repair of femoral capital physeal fractures in cats: 13 cases (1998–2002). J Am Vet Med Assoc. 2004;224(9):1478–82.

59. Forrest LJ, O'Brien RT, Manlet PA. Feline capital physeal dysplasia syndrome. Vet Radiol Ultrasound. 1999;40:672.

60. Chandler EA, Gaskell CJ, Gaskell RM RM. Feline medicine and therapeutics. Ames, IA: Iowa State Press; 2004.

61. Isola M, Baroni E, Zotti A. Radiographic features of two cases of feline proximal femoral dysplasia. J Small Anim Pract. 2005;46(12):597–9.

62. Romagnoli SE. Canine cryptorchidism. Vet Clin North Am Small Anim Pract. 1991;21(3):533–44.

63. Veronesi MC, Riccardi E, Rota A, Grieco V. Characteristics of cryptic/ectopic and contralateral scrotal testes in dogs between 1 and 2 years of age. Theriogenology. 2009;72(7):969–77.

64. Yates D, Hayes G, Heffernan M, Beynon R. Incidence of cryptorchidism in dogs and cats. Vet Rec. 2003;152(16):502–4.

65. Amann RP, Veeramachaneni DN. Cryptorchidism in common eutherian mammals. Reproduction. 2007;133(3):541–61.

66. Bushby PA. Cryptorchid surgery and simple ophthalmic procedures. DVM. 360 [Internet]; 2010. Available from: http://veterinarycalendar.dvm360.com/cryptorchid-surgery-and-simple-ophthalmic-procedures-proceedings.

67. Baumans V, Dijkstra G, Wensing CJ. Testicular descent in the dog. Anat Histol Embryol. 1981;10(2):97–110.

68. Baumans V, Dijkstra G, Wensing CJ. The effect of orchidectomy on gubernacular outgrowth and regression in the dog. Int J Androl. 1982;5(4):387–400.

69. Baumans V, Dijkstra G, Wensing CJ. The role of a non-androgenic testicular factor in the process of testicular descent in the dog. Int J Androl. 1983;6(6):541–52.

70. Kutzler MA. The reproductive tract. In: Peterson ME, Kutzler MA, editors. Small animal pediatrics: the first 12 months of life. St. Louis, MO: Elsevier Saunders; 2011.

71. Christensen BW. Disorders of sexual development in dogs and cats. Vet Clin North Am Small Anim Pract. 2012;42(3):515–26, vi, vi.

72. Peter AT. The reproductive system. In: Hoskins JD, editor. Veterinary pediatrics: dogs and cats from birth to six months. 3rd ed. Philadelphia, PA: Saunders; 2001. p. 463–75.

73. Rhoades JD, Foley CW. Cryptorchidism and intersexuality. Vet Clin North Am. 1977;7(4):789–94.

74. Meyers-Wallen VN. Gonadal and sex differentiation abnormalities of dogs and cats. Sex dev 2012;6(1–3):46–60.

75. Millis DL, Hauptman JG, Johnson CA. Cryptorchidism and monorchism in cats: 25 cases (1980–1989). J Am Vet Med Assoc. 1992;200(8):1128–30.

76. Richardson EF, Mullen H. Cryptorchidism in cats. Compend Contin Educ Pract Vet. 1993;15(10):1342–5.

77. Yates D, Hayes G, Heffernan M, Beynon R. Incidence of cryptorchidism in dogs and cats. Vet Rec. 2003;152(16):502–4.

78. Wallace JL, Levy JK. Population characteristics of feral cats admitted to seven trap-neuter-return programs in the United States. J Feline Med Surg. 2006;8(4):279–84.

79. D'Cruz AJ, Das K. Undescended testes. Indian J Pediatr. 2004;71(12):1111–5.

80. Docimo SG, Silver RI, Cromie W. The undescended testicle: diagnosis and management. Am Fam Phys. 2000;62(9):2037–44, 2047, 47–8.

81. Schindler AM, Diaz P, Cuendet A, Sizonenko PC. Cryptorchidism: a morphological study of 670 biopsies. Helv Paediatr Acta. 1987;42(2–3):145–58.

82. Bednarski R, Grimm K, Harvey R, Lukasik VM, Penn WS, Sargent B, et al. AAHA anesthesia guidelines for dogs and cats. J Am Anim Hosp Assoc. 2011;47(6):377–85.

83. 5 Common myths about veterinary anesthesia risks. DVM 360 [Internet]; 2011. Available from: http://veterinarybusiness.dvm360.com/5-common-myths-about-veterinary-anesthesia-risks.

84. Hofmeister EH, Watson V, Snyder LBC, Love EJ. Validity and client use of information from the World Wide Web regarding veterinary anesthesia in dogs. J Am Vet Med Assoc. 2008;233(12):1860–4.

85. Iizuka T, Kamata M, Yanagawa M, Nishimura R. Incidence of intraoperative hypotension during isoflurane-fentanyl and propofol-fentanyl anaesthesia in dogs. Vet J. 2013;198(1):289–91.

86. Anon. Hypotension during anesthesia in dogs and cats: recognition, causes, and treatment. Compend Contin Educ Pract Vet. 2001;23:728–37.

87. Gaynor JS, Dunlop CI, Wagner AE, Wertz EM, Golden AE, Demme WC. Complications and mortality associated with anesthesia in dogs and cats. J Am Anim Hosp Assoc. 1999;35(1):13–7.

88. Becker WM, Mama KR, Rao S, Palmer RH, Egger EL. Prevalence of dysphoria after fentanyl in dogs undergoing stifle surgery. Vet Surg 2013;42(3):302–7.

89. Väisänen M, Oksanen H, Vainio O. Postoperative signs in 96 dogs undergoing soft tissue surgery. Vet Rec. 2004;155(23):729–33.

90. Light GS, Hardie EM, Young MS, Hellyer PW, Brownie C, Hansen BD. Pain and anxiety behaviors of dogs during intravenous catheterization after premedication with placebo, acepromazine or oxymorphone. Applied Animal Behaviour Science. 1993;37(4):331–43.

91. Davies JA, Fransson BA, Davis AM, Gilbertsen AM, Gay JM. Incidence of and risk factors for postoperative regurgitation and vomiting in dogs: 244 cases (2000–2012). J Am Vet Med Assoc 2015;246(3):327–35.

92. Ovbey DH, Wilson DV, Bednarski RM, Hauptman JG, Stanley BJ, Radlinsky MG, et al. Prevalence and risk factors for canine post-anesthetic aspiration pneumonia (1999–2009): a multicenter study. Vet Anaesth Analg 2014;41(2):127–36.

93. Shamir M, Goelman G, Chai O. Postanesthetic cerebellar dysfunction in cats. J Vet Intern Med American College of Veterinary Internal Medicine. 2004;18(3):368–9.

94. Barton-Lamb AL, Martin-Flores M, Scrivani PV, Bezuidenhout AJ, Loew E, Erb HN, Ludders JW. Evaluation of maxillary arterial blood flow in anesthetized cats with the mouth closed and open. Vet J 2013;196(3):325–31.

95. Jurk IR, Thibodeau MS, Whitney K, Gilger BC, Davidson MG. Acute vision loss after general anesthesia in a cat. Vet Ophthalmol 2001;4(2):155–8.

96. Son WG, Jung BY, Kwon TE, Seo KM, Lee, I. Acute temporary visual loss after general anesthesia in a cat. J Vet Clin 2009;26:480–2.

97. Clark KW, Hall LW. A survey of anaesthesia in small animal practice: AVA/BSAVA report. J Vet Anaesth. 1990;17:4–10.

98. Brodbelt DC, Blissitt KJ, Hammond RA, Neath PJ, Young LE, Pfeiffer DU, Wood JL. The risk of death: the confidential enquiry into perioperative small animal fatalities. Vet Anaesth Analg. 2008;35(5):365–73.

99. Kawashima Y, Seo N, Morita K, Iwao Y, Irita K, Tsuzaki K, et al. Annual study of perioperative mortality and morbidity for the year of 1999 in Japan: the outlines – report of the Japan Society of Anesthesiologists Committee on Operating Room Safety. Masui 2001;50(11):1260–74.

100. Biboulet P, Aubas P, Dubourdieu J, Rubenovitch J, Capdevila X, d'Athis F. Fatal and non fatal cardiac arrests related to anesthesia. Can J Anaesth 2001;48(4):326–32.

101. Eagle CC, Davis NJ. Report of the Anaesthetic Mortality Committee of Western Australia 1990–1995. Anaesth Intensive Care 1997;25(1):51–9.

102. Brodbelt D. Feline anesthetic deaths in veterinary practice. Top Companion Anim Med 2010;25(4):189–94.

103. Dyson DH, Maxie MG, Schnurr D. Morbidity and mortality associated with anesthetic management in small animal veterinary practice in Ontario. J Am Anim Hosp Assoc 1998;34(4):325–35.

104. Brodbelt DC, Pfeiffer DU, Young LE, Wood JL. Risk factors for anaesthetic-related death in cats: results from the confidential enquiry into perioperative small animal fatalities (CEPSAF). Br J Anaesth 2007;99(5):617–23.

105. Hosgood G, Scholl DT. Evaluation of age and American Society of Anesthesiologists (ASA) physical status as risk factors for perianesthetic morbidity and mortality in the cat. Journal of Veterinary Emergency and Critical Care 2002;12(1):9–15.

106. Hosgood G, Scholl DT. Evaluation of age as a risk factor for perianesthetic morbidity and mortality in the dog. J Vet Emerg Crit Care. 1998;8(3):222–36.

107. Fossum TW. Preoperative and intraoperative care of the surgical patient. In: Fossum TW, Duprey LP, O'Connor D, editors. Small animal surgery. 3rd ed. Boston, MA: Elsevier; 2007.

108. Englar R. Writing skills for veterinarians. Sheffield. 5M Publishing; 2019.

109. Kipperman BS. The demise of the minimum database. J Am Vet Med Assoc. 2014;244(12):1368–70.

110. Bartges J, Boynton B, Vogt AH, Krauter E, Lambrecht K, Svec R, Thompson S. AAHA canine life stage guidelines. J Am Anim Hosp Assoc 2012;48(1):1–11.

111. Brown EN, Pavone KJ, Naranjo M. Multimodal general anesthesia: theory and practice. Anesth Analg 2018;127(5):1246–58.

112. Griffin B, Bushby PA, McCobb E et al. The Association of Shelter Veterinarians' 2016 Veterinary Medical Care Guidelines for Spay-Neuter Programs. *Journal of the American Veterinary Medical Association* 2016;249:165–88.

Case 12

Planning a Canine Castration

Primrose ("Prim") Malloy was more excited than her neighbor to find that an unplanned litter of pups was on its way. The neighbor, Judy, had intended on having her dog, Cricket, spayed, but as with many things in life, time got away from her. It wasn't until Judy saw a male dog from the next street over jump the fence that she realized her mistake. The scoundrel bred Cricket and she was now expecting.

Shortly after the dogs tied, Judy had contacted the veterinarian, who had assured her that they could proceed with spaying Cricket now to eliminate any pregnancy from developing. Cricket was healthy and young, with no additional risk factors that could complicate an anesthetic event. Judy had even considered it. It certainly would have been more convenient. She could barely handle one dog, let alone an entire pack. At the same time, she had mixed feelings about taking away Cricket's one and only chance at motherhood, and the neighbors had volunteered to take on the responsibility of adopting out the pups.

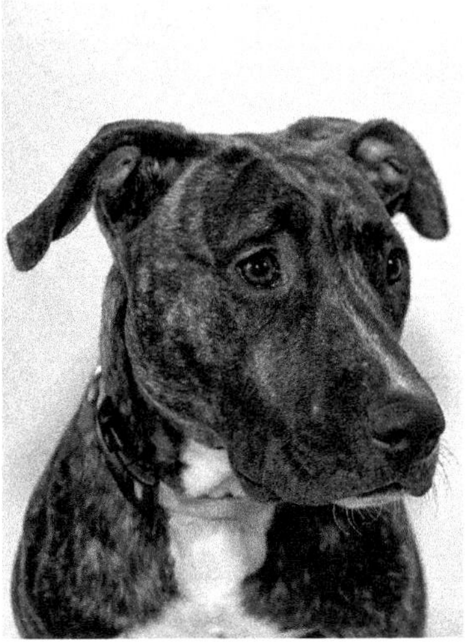

Prim was the first neighbor to reach out to offer assistance. As an obstetrics nurse, she was fascinated by labor and delivery and hoped to be present for the birth. She had helped to welcome several dozen humans into the world. Why not a litter of pups? More than ever, Judy appreciated the support. This was all very new to her and even though Prim's training was in

Figure 12.1 Meet your next patient, Tumbleweed, a 6-month-old intact male mixed breed dog. Courtesy of John Schwartz.

human medicine rather than veterinary, there was a certain comfort in knowing that medical assistance was just a house away. Prim also promised a good home for the firstborn in response for her help.

Two months later, octuplets entered the world. They were a motley crew for sure, given that neither parent was full-blooded anything. The best one could say is that most resembled Labrador-Boxer crosses, with a sprinkle of Staffordshire terrier. Their heads were blocky, and they were more muscle than anything else. They played hard, with spurts of energy that lasted late into the night. It wouldn't have been so bad except they were not the least bit gentle. The havoc that they caused was indescribable. Imagine a bull in a china shop. Now multiply that by eight.

Judy was used to Cricket's mild manners. The quiet life that they had built for themselves pretty much went out the window the day that the Heinz 57 collection arrived. The pups were dauntless, yet clunky. No object in the house was sacred. By the time the fourth lamp broke from a particularly rough bout of tussling, Judy was ready for them to be rehomed. She cried with joy the day the final pup packed its bags and headed off to new adventures.

True to her word, Prim adopted the eldest pup, whom she christened Tumbleweed. In the early days, Tumbleweed missed his littermates. It was a difficult transition to go from seven siblings to none. But Tumbleweed grew up with no shortage of love and, simply put, he grew. In just 6 months, he surpassed Cricket in height and weight, and it was time to think about neutering. Prim had no desire for him to follow in his father's footsteps.

Prim is here today to discuss surgical sterilization. She is familiar with this procedure in male cats, which she has owned before, but is unfamiliar how this procedure may differ in dogs.

You have examined Tumbleweed and he appears to be in good health. You make the following notations in his medical record concerning vital signs:

Tumbleweed does not have a heart murmur on thoracic auscultation and his lungs are clear. Based upon his physical exam today, he is a good candidate for castration. However, you identify two additional physical examination findings that you would like to discuss with Prim today relative to surgical planning:

- umbilical hernia (see Figure 12.2)
- cryptorchidism.

Weight: 55 lb (24.9 kg)
BCS: 4/9
Mentation: BAR

TPR

T: 100.6°F (38.1°C)
P: 86 beats per minute
R: panting

Round One of Questions for Case 12: Planning a Canine Castration

1. Define the abdominal cavity and its boundaries.
2. What is a synonym for the abdominal cavity?
3. Describe the normal anatomy of the abdominal wall.
4. Define hernia.
5. When we classify a hernia as being abdominal, what does that mean?
6. How do hernias develop?
7. How are hernias typically classified in clinical practice?
8. You identified an umbilical hernia in Tumbleweed. Where is this located?
9. What are other locations of hernias in the dog?
10. What are potential complications of hernias if they are not surgically repaired?
11. Can hernias spontaneously close on their own, without surgery?
12. What is the appropriate medical term for surgical repair of hernias?

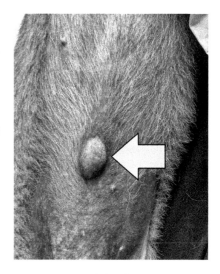

Figure 12.2 Umbilical hernia. Courtesy of Rachel Sahrbeck.

13. Case 11 (Planning for a Feline Castration) introduced the term, cryptorchidism. Review Round Two of Questions in Case 11 before proceeding.
14. What is the incidence of cryptorchidism in dogs?
15. Can a dog with cryptorchidism breed?
16. Should a dog with cryptorchidism be bred?
17. Is a dog with cryptorchidism fertile?
18. Are certain dog breeds overrepresented when it comes to cryptorchidism?
19. If one or both testes is/are not located within the scrotum, then where is/are it/they located?
20. How do you determine the location of the "missing" testis/testes?
21. Are cryptorchid patients at an increased risk of developing cancer if we choose not to surgically excise the missing testis/testes?
22. Has cryptorchidism been linked to medical conditions other than neoplasia?
23. Some clients have read online that cryptorchidism can be cured by administering hormone injections to the affected dog. Is this true?

Answers to Round One of Questions for Case 12: Planning a Canine Castration

1. The abdominal cavity is an organ-rich space that is bordered cranially by the muscular diaphragm, dorsally by the vertebral column, caudally by the pelvic floor, and ventrally by the abdominal wall.(1)

2. A synonym for the abdominal cavity is the peritoneal cavity. These spaces are one and the same.

3. The abdominal wall can be best thought of as layers of muscular sheets that form a collective barrier between the abdominal cavity and the outside world. These sheets are paired structures, with right and left halves that connect at ventral midline to a fibrous structure, the linea alba.(1–4)
    The linea alba is, as its name implies, a white band of tissue that begins at the xiphoid process of the sternum and runs in cranial to caudal fashion.(1–4) It is wider in cats than it is in dogs, but in both species it narrows appreciably as it approaches the brim of the pelvis. It is sandwiched on either side by the rectus abdominis,(3) and is of interest to surgeons because it is avascular. This makes it a preferred site for entering the abdominal cavity.
    The muscular sheets that contribute to the abdominal wall are:(1–4)

    - external abdominal oblique
    - internal abdominal oblique
    - transversus abdominis
    - rectus abdominis.

    The external abdominal oblique is the outermost layer of the abdominal wall. It originates from the lateral rib cage and thoracodorsal fascia. Its fibers are oriented caudoventrally towards midline in the same direction path that you would take to slide your fingers into the pockets of your pants.(1)
    The internal abdominal oblique is deep to the external abdominal oblique. The internal abdominal oblique originates primarily from the tuber coxa. Its fibers are oriented cranioventrally towards midline.(1)
    The transversus abdominis originates from the last ribs and the transverse processes of the lumbar vertebrae.(1) Its fibers are oriented in the same direction as one's waistline or how a belt loops around to the front of your pants.
    The rectus abdominis is a strap muscle that sits on either side of the linea alba and runs cranioventrally, much like suspenders, from the ventral rib cage to the pelvic brim. Its fibers are oriented parallel to the linea alba.(1)
    The rectus abdominis is surrounded by the so-called rectus sheath.(1–3) This is formed by aponeuroses of the aforementioned abdominal wall muscles and has two components:(1–3)

    - external rectus sheath
    - internal rectus sheath.

    The external rectus sheath is primarily formed by the external and internal abdominal obliques. (1–3) Near the pubis, there is a small contribution from the transversus abdominis.(1)
    Cranial to the umbilicus, the internal rectus sheath is formed by the internal abdominal oblique, the transversus abdominis, and transverse fascia. Caudal to the umbilicus, the internal abdominal oblique's contribution peters out. Near the pubis, only the transverse fascia remains. (1)
    This summary is intended to paint a clinical picture of what structures we are referring to when we are describing defects in the abdominal wall.
    This is not intended to be a comprehensive review of the origins and insertion points of the abdominal wall muscles. For that kind of depth, refer to an anatomy text of your choice.

4. A hernia is defined as an abnormal extension of tissue(s) and/or organ(s) outside of the borders of a cavity that normally contains it/them.(1–3)

5. An abdominal hernia means that tissue(s) and/or organ(s) that is/are normally housed in the abdominal cavity have abnormally breached that cavity's borders. An abdominal hernia may be:(4)

   • external
   • internal.

   External abdominal hernias occur when the abdominal wall is defective at one or more sites, causing abdominal cavity contents to spill outside of the cavity, between the abdominal wall and the skin.(4) Tumbleweed has this type of hernia, which is both visually apparent and palpable on physical examination.

   Internal abdominal hernias occur when tissues breach one or more borders of the abdominal cavity, without breaking through the abdominal wall.(4) For example, a diaphragmatic hernia occurs when abdominal contents encroach upon the thoracic cavity.(4) This is a type of internal abdominal hernia.

6. Hernias may be congenital or acquired. Acquired hernias may be traumatic or iatrogenic.(2)
   Congenital hernias are present at birth.(2, 4) Many result from problems that arise during the developmental stages of the embryo, some of which are inherited traits.(2, 4) Most umbilical hernias are both congenital and inherited.(4)

   In my experience, traumatic hernias occur more frequently in veterinary practice than iatrogenic. Hit-by-car clinical presentations are often associated with hernias. These may develop instantaneously, upon impact, or the hernia itself may be delayed in onset, occurring at a site of weakened tissue.

   An example of an iatrogenic hernia is one that arises at an incision site.(2) Consider, for example, an ovariohysterectomy. This procedure requires the abdominal wall to be sutured closed prior to recovery from general anesthesia. If for whatever reason there is premature breakdown of the suture at the linea alba, then the abdominal wall has essentially been reopened. This paves the way for tissue(s) and/or organ(s) to herniate through the opening in the abdominal wall and risk potential entrapment beneath the skin.

7. In broad terms, hernias can be classified by:(2, 3, 5–7)

   • size
   • location
   • consistency of the herniated contents
   • whether the herniated contents are reducible.

   Hernia size is subjective but can help clinicians to gauge how likely the patient is to experience serious complications.(7) For example, hernias that allow one human finger to slip through are at increased risk for bowel entrapment because the small intestine is roughly equal in size to the diameter of a loop of bowel in a small-to-medium-sized dog.(6, 7)

   In terms of location, external abdominal hernias can develop at any site within the abdominal wall.(7) However, the most common locations will be listed in the answer to Question #9 (below).

   Consistency of the hernia refers to whether the herniated contents are soft or firm.(7) Herniated contents should be soft and supple.(7) If at any point herniated contents become firm or tender, they may be becoming entrapped.(6, 7)

   Reducibility of a hernia refers to the ability of the tissue(s) or organ(s) to be replaced within the abdominal cavity using manual pressure.

- If a hernia is said to be reducible, then the herniated contents can be pushed back into the abdomen with ease.(2) For this to happen, the herniated contents must be freely moveable, meaning that they have not developed adhesions that keep them tethered to their new location outside of the abdominal cavity.(2)
- If a hernia is said to be non-reducible, then the herniated contents cannot be pushed back into the abdomen with ease.

8. Tumbleweed's umbilical hernia is located at his umbilicus, that is, his belly button. The umbilical aperture is a normal opening in the fetus.(4, 8) This provides a path for the umbilical blood supply, the vitelline duct, and the stalk of the allantois to reach the growing baby.(4, 8) At birth, these attachments are severed such that the neonate is no longer tethered to its dam.(4, 8) Delivery of the neonate should trigger the umbilical aperture to close.(4, 8) A hernia results when the aperture fails to contract down and scar over.(4, 8) A faulty aperture may also be too large to effectively close.(4, 8) In either situation, an umbilical hernia results.(4, 8) Umbilical hernias may also result from hypoplastic rectus muscles.(6)

9. Although external abdominal hernias may occur at any point along the abdominal wall, the most common sites are:(2–4, 7–10)

- anywhere along the ventral midline
- at the umbilicus (umbilical hernia)
- along the caudal rib margin (paracostal hernia)
- within the scrotum (scrotal hernia)
- within the groin (inguinal hernia).

At these locations, hernias tend to be congenital rather than traumatic.(6, 7, 11–13)
Other less common locations for external abdominal hernias include:(4)

- cranial public ligament hernias
- femoral hernias.

Internal abdominal hernias are relatively uncommon in companion animal practice, but include:(7)

- hiatal hernias
- traumatically induced diaphragmatic hernias(14–16)
- congenital peritoneopericardial hernias.(17)

10. What are potential complications of hernias if they are not surgically repaired?
The two most serious complications of hernias are:(3, 7)

- incarceration (or entrapment)
- strangulation.

Both complications are more likely to occur if hernias are non-reducible.(2, 3)
Herniated contents are said to be entrapped or incarcerated when they develop adhesions to surrounding tissues.(3, 7) Organs that are most likely to herniate through the abdominal wall include:(3)

- the urinary bladder
- small intestines
- the uterus.

Entrapment is potentially life-threatening because the affected organ(s) experience(s) altered function.(3) Consider, for example, a non-reducible hernia that contains portions of small bowel. If one or more portions of bowel becomes entrapped, then the lumen of the affected segment(s) narrow(s). This could lead to altered gut motility or even small bowel obstruction.

Strangulation often occurs secondary to entrapment.(3) When herniated contents are strangulated, their blood flow is compromised.(3) Arterial or venous supply may be impacted, or both.(3) Typically venous obstruction occurs first, then back pressure on the capillary beds leads to stagnation of blood within the arteries.(3) If this vascular occlusion persists and/or if collateral circulation is not adequate, then the organ(s) will become necrotic and may even rupture.(3) Necrotic tissue takes on the color of black or dark brown.

It is important to note that traumatic hernias may not show signs of incarceration or strangulation immediately; however as adhesions form during wound healing, one or both of these complications may arise.(3) It is therefore prudent to be cautious about prognosis following events such as automobile trauma because the patient may look stable at initial presentation only to decompensate over the first few days. Aggressive monitoring is indicated so that if either complication arises, surgical intervention can be expedient.

11. It is possible for small umbilical hernias (<2–3 mm) to spontaneously seal at or before six months of age.(3)

12. Herniorrhaphy is the appropriate medical term for surgical repair of hernias.

13. Cryptorchidism is more likely to occur in dogs than cats.(7, 9) The incidence of cryptorchidism varies based upon the study that is referenced, but it typically ranges between 3.3% and 6.8% in dogs as compared to 1.3–3.8% in cats.(18–23)

    Canine presentations of cryptorchidism are more often unilateral than bilateral.(7, 9) For reasons that have yet to be determined, the right testis is less likely to descend into the scrotum than the left.(23–26)

14. Yes, it is physically possible for a dog with cryptorchidism to breed. Dogs that are cryptorchid still produce testosterone and may still have the drive to breed although libido may be reduced as compared to a dog without this condition.(27)

15. Dogs that are cryptorchid should not be bred because the condition is believed to be heritable.(4) The trait is thought to be sex-linked and autosomal recessive.(4)

16. Whether cryptorchid dogs are sterile depends largely upon whether the condition is unilateral or bilateral.(27)

    If a dog is bilaterally affected and both testicles are located within the abdomen, then spermatogenesis will be significantly compromised.(27) Spermatozoa do not develop and mature properly if they are subjected to core body temperature.(27) This is why canine and feline spermatogenesis occur in the testicles outside of the abdominal cavity, within the thermally distinct scrotum. A dog with bilateral cryptorchidism is therefore sterile.(9, 25, 27–30)

    If a dog is unilaterally affected, meaning that one testicle is scrotal and one is not, then fertile sperm will be produced by the scrotal testicle.(27) This will mix with sterile sperm from the non-scrotal testicle, reducing fertility. Additional obstacles that unilateral cryptorchid dogs have to overcome concerning fertility include:(27)

- decreased testosterone, which results in decreased libido
- decreased semen volume
- decreased numbers of viable sperm
- decreased motility of sperm
- increased numbers of misshapen, dysfunctional, or otherwise abnormal sperm.

Although most cryptorchid patients can achieve erection, they may not ejaculate.(25, 30, 31) Of those that do, ejaculates may or may not contain live sperm.(25, 30) When they do, progressive motility of sperm is often impaired.(25, 30)

Pregnancy is possible, but perhaps more challenging to achieve.(25, 28)

17. Pedigreed pets are overrepresented among cryptorchid patients.(25, 32) Roughly three out of every four dogs with cryptorchidism are purebred.(9) The following canine breeds may be more likely to develop this condition:(23, 29, 33–37)

- Boxer
- Chihuahua
- Cocker Spaniel
- English Bulldog
- German shepherd
- Maltese
- Miniature Dachshund

- Old English Sheepdog
- Pekingese
- Pomeranian
- Poodle
- Shetland sheepdog
- Yorkshire terrier.

Small-breed dogs are also overrepresented.(23, 29, 35, 36, 38, 39)

18. Cryptorchid testes may be found along the path by which they are supposed to descend from the abdomen into the scrotum. Recall from embryology that the testes develop within the abdomen, near the caudal pole of each kidney.(25, 28, 40) This means that a wayward testis may be found anywhere from the ipsilateral kidney all to the way to the ipsilateral inguinal canal.

    The most common presentation of cryptorchidism in the dog finds the "missing" testis in the right inguinal canal.(23–26) The second most common location is right-sided abdominal.(23–26)

19. If you are fortunate, the cryptorchid testicle will be palpable within the ipsilateral groin. In my experience, this may or may not be possible with the patient in a standing position. Positioning the patient in dorsal recumbency may facilitate palpation of the "missing" testis. To be most successful, the patient should be relaxed. Kicking of the back feet and/or tensing the legs may hinder palpation of the groin. Sometimes for this reason, it is not possible to exclude an inguinal location until the patient has been placed under general anesthesia. Without muscular tension, palpation of the groin is often much more revealing.

    If you do not palpate an inguinal testis, then you will need to enter the abdomen to locate it. Although this may seem like an insurmountable task, it is not too difficult to locate an abdominal testis if you recall basic anatomy. Recall that the vas deferens enters the urethra at the prostate, and that the vas deferens can be found dorsal to the urinary bladder. To find the vas deferens, retroflex the urinary bladder.(41) Now trace the vas deferens from the prostatic urethra to the "missing" testicle.(41)

    If when you follow the vas deferens you reach a dead end and the "missing" testis disappears from sight, then it has tucked into the inguinal canal.(41) In this case, the "missing" testis cannot be accessed through the abdominal cavity and will require an inguinal incision.(41)

20. Cryptorchid patients are more likely to develop testicular cancer.(23, 25, 26, 29, 35, 36, 38, 42–44) The rate of testicular cancer in cryptorchid dogs is 13.6 times greater than in dogs without this condition.(43) The chance that a cryptorchid will develop a Sertoli cell tumor is five times greater than the general population; the chance that a cryptorchid will develop a seminoma is three times greater (33). In addition, the retained testis is more likely to experience torsion.(24, 25, 29, 45–47)

21. Cryptorchidism has been associated with the following congenital defects:(25)

- hernias:

    - inguinal

    - umbilical

- hypospadias:

    - the urethral opening should be located at the tip of the penis
    - in a patient with hypospadias, the urethral opening is in an abnormal location

- patellar subluxation.

22. Hormonal attempts to correct testicular descent are ineffective in the dog and should be discouraged by the veterinary team because the patient carries a heritable trait.(25, 33, 48)

Returning to Case 12: Planning a Canine Castration

After discussing Tumbleweed's physical exam findings with Prim, Prim agrees that it is best for his health to proceed with bilateral castration and herniorrhaphy. Tumbleweed returns the following morning to be prepped for surgery. When he is placed in lateral recumbency under general anesthesia, you find that his right testis is both visible and palpable in the subcutaneous tissues associated with the right groin (see Figure 12.3.)

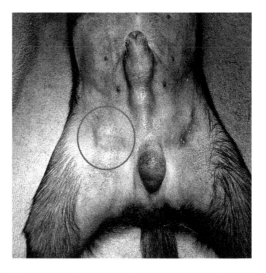

Figure 12.3 Cryptorchid patient prepped for surgery. Note that the right testis is grossly apparent. Courtesy of Shannon Carey, DVM.

Round Two of Questions for Case 12: Planning a Canine Castration

1. How common is testicular cancer in dogs?
2. Other than preventing testicular cancer, what behavioral and health-related benefits have been ascribed to canine castration?
3. The risk of which medical conditions in dogs may be increased by castration?
4. Why is it so challenging to identify with certainty how castration impacts canine health?
5. How does this uncertainty about the risks and benefits of canine castration challenge clinical communication? What is our role in presenting this information to our clients and which communication skill will facilitate these kinds of conversations?
6. What is your surgical approach for excising Tumbleweed's scrotal testis?
7. What is an alternate approach for excising Tumbleweed's scrotal testis?
8. When is it appropriate to perform a concurrent scrotal ablation?
9. What are potential postoperative complications of scrotal orchiectomy?
10. Are there any specific instructions for Tumbleweed's aftercare?

Answers to Round Two of Questions for Case 12: Planning a Canine Castration

1. It is true that the testes are the most common site of primary reproductive neoplasia in the male dog.(43, 44, 49–52) However, testicular tumors rarely cause terminal disease in dogs.(53–55) Less than one percent of dogs with testicular tumors will die from their primary cancer.(53–55) Testicular cancer is relatively easy to cure in dogs with castration.(53) So it is a hard sell to suggest that your client must castrate her dog to save her dog from testicular disease.

2. Other than preventing testicular cancer, the benefits that have been attributed to canine castration include:(53, 56)

   • improved behavior:***

      • reduced inter-dog aggression(57)

- decreased roaming(57)
- decreased mounting(57)

- improved longevity(58)
- reduction in clinical signs for benign prostatic hyperplasia (bph):

  - an estimated three out of every four intact male dogs by age 6 will have some degree of bph and associated clinical signs:(59, 60)

    - tenesmus
    - dysuria
    - hematuria
    - urethral discharge

  - an estimated 95% of intact male dogs by age nine will have some degree of bph (59)
  - bph predisposes intact males to other prostatic disease:(53, 61–64)

    - prostatic abscesses
    - prostatitis
    - prostatic cysts
    - paraprostatic cysts

  - within 3 weeks of castration, prostate size is reduced by 50%(56)
  - within 2 to 3 months of castration, clinical signs resolve(56)

- resolution of perianal adenomas.

Note: ***Several question marks may be raised when we suggest that castration improves behavior because in truth there are mixed reviews concerning behavioral outcomes. Although castration does appear to reduce objectional behaviors such as mounting, roaming, and inter-dog aggression, there is some concern that prepubertal castration in dogs may in fact increase aggression towards people (family members and strangers).(65, 66)

3. Canine castration may increase the risk of developing the following medical conditions:(53, 56)

    - cranial cruciate ligament injuries(67–70)
    - elbow dysplasia(70)
    - hip dysplasia(67, 70, 71)
    - lymphoma:

      - one study reports that intact male dogs are at increased risk as compared to those that are neutered(72)
      - a conflicting study reports that neutered vizlas are at greater risk(73)
      - yet another study suggests that the risk to male golden retrievers can be reduced if they are castrated just after one year of age(67)

    - osteosarcoma(53, 56, 74, 75)
    - prostatic carcinoma(53, 56)
    - transitional cell carcinoma.(53, 56)

4. One of the major challenges when reviewing the current veterinary medical literature is that breed-specific studies abound, yet cannot always be extrapolated to the entire species, dogs, because breeds are likely to have their own unique risk factors and predispositions to disease.(53) We must therefore take breed-specific research with a grain of salt. It may be that as a general rule, it is considered safe to castrate male dogs at or over 6 weeks of age, but that we might do well to exert caution and potentially postpone castration in specific (often larger) breeds.(53)

Another major challenge is that many of the conditions listed above are multifactorial.(53) In other words, it is difficult to examine the risk of one factor in isolation when multiple factors play a role in many of the diseases that are listed above. For example, how much of a role does BCS and obesity play in the development of orthopedic diseases? How might these variables have impacted the outcomes of the studies that were trying to isolate sexual status and evaluate it as a standalone risk factor?

The studies that I have cited here are a mere fraction of what has been reported in the veterinary medical literature. These studies do what they can to provide unbiased answers, yet, if anything, these studies raise more questions.

5. This inherent uncertainty can make our task as clinicians that much more difficult because at the end of the day, medicine is rarely black or white. We all operate to some degree in shades of grey. So, what then is our role? How do we best serve our clients and our patients?

    We serve clients best by being transparent. We need to help them understand what we know and, more commonly, what we don't know so that we are both on the same page. It may well be that castration reduces the risk of one type of cancer while increasing the risk of another. In that case, all we can do is present the options that are available to us and partner with our clients to determine which is considered to be the greatest risk to the individual patient.

6. My surgical approach to excising Tumbleweed's scrotal testis is to make a pre-scrotal midline incision with the patient in dorsal recumbency after the patient has been prepped and draped using aseptic technique.(27, 41, 56) For this approach to castration, the scrotum is not clipped to prevent scrotal irritation that might encourage self-mutilation in the post-operative period.(56)

    Prior to making my initial incision, I would push the scrotal testicle cranially towards the pre-scrotal incision site. At this point, I can choose to perform either a closed or open castration.

    In a closed castration, the vaginal tunic is not opened.(41) The vaginal tunic is serous membrane that encases each testis in a pouch within the scrotum. Because this membrane remains closed during the procedure, at no point does the surgeon enter the peritoneal cavity. This technique is expedient. However, there is the potential for hemorrhage because blood vessels that supply the testicles are indirectly ligated: the tunic is ligated rather than the vessels themselves.

    In an open castration, the vaginal tunic is opened.(41) This allows for more complete visualization of and separation of the components of the spermatic cord for individual ligation.(41)

    If we were to proceed with a CLOSED castration, then I would adopt the following procedure.(27, 41, 56)

- Incise the subcutaneous tissues over the testicle, taking care not to incise the parietal vaginal tunic.
- Use both hands to "pop" the scrotal testicle out from the incision site.
- Use a square of sterile dry gauze to strip off the scrotal attachments of the testicle as you hold it in your hand. This should allow you to pull the testicle in one hand as you push against the dog's perineum with your other hand to break down the cremaster muscle. At this point, the testicle has been fully exteriorized, and you have an appreciable length of spermatic cord to work with.
- Make use of a three-clamp technique in preparation for ligature placement.
- Place one circumferential ligature around the spermatic cord and tunic proximal to the bottom clamp, that is, the clamp nearest to the patient's body. Use absorbable suture for your ligature.
- Remove the most proximal clamp.
- Place a second circumferential ligature around the spermatic cord and tunic in the crush line where the bottom clamp had been. This second ligature will be seated distal to the first ligature. Use absorbable suture for your ligature.
- Consider the placement of transfixation ligatures, taking care to pass the needle through the

cremaster muscle, if there is bulk to the cord and concern that mass ligatures will not be sufficient to indirectly ligate the vascular bundle. Use absorbable suture for your ligature.

- Transect between the two clamps, distal to your ligatures.
- Use thumb forceps to grasp the "stump" of the transected spermatic cord that will be returned to the scrotum through the pre-scrotal incision site.
- Remove the clamp.
- Inspect the "stump" for bleeding.
- Release the "stump" back into the incision. You may need to "tuck" it out of site gently.
- If Tumbleweed were not cryptorchid, then you would repeat this procedure on the second scrotal testicle.
- Close the incision. Skin sutures are not typically placed. A subcuticular pattern that buries the final knot offers a pleasing aesthetic look that does not require suture removal.

If we were to proceed with an OPEN castration, then the steps I would take are as follows.(27, 41, 56)

- Incise the subcutaneous tissues over the testicle.
- Incise the parietal vaginal tunic.
- Use both hands to "pop" the scrotal testicle out of the tunic. You may need to extend the tunic incision with scissors in order to achieve better visualization of the vascular bundle.
- Using blunt dissection, separate the vascular bundle from the cremaster muscle.
- Circumferentially ligate the parietal tunic and cremaster muscle together.
- Place two circumferential ligatures on the vascular bundle using the 3-clamp technique described for closed castration.
- Consider the placement of transfixation ligature as needed.
- Transect between the two clamps, distal to your ligatures.
- Use thumb forceps to grasp the "stump" of the transected tissues that will be returned to the scrotum through the pre-scrotal incision site.
- Remove the clamp.
- Inspect the "stump" for bleeding.
- Release the "stump" back into the incision. You may need to "tuck" it out of site gently.
- If Tumbleweed were not cryptorchid, then you would repeat this procedure on the second scrotal testicle.
- Close the incision. Skin sutures are not typically placed. A subcuticular pattern that buries the final knot offers a pleasing aesthetic look that does not require suture removal.

7. An alternate approach for excising Tumbleweed's scrotal testis is to perform a scrotal castration. This technique is commonly used in high-quality, high-volume spay/neuter programs with success.(76) The details of this technique will not be described here because I personally have yet to perform it myself. However, my colleagues share that the procedure is well-tolerated. Incisions are either left to heal via second intention, as is considered standard practice for feline orchiectomies or the skin may be closed by means of a surgical grade adhesive.(76)

   When performed by experienced surgeons, scrotal castrations take less time than pre-scrotal castrations.(76) Swelling and/or bruising at the incision site and peri-incisional dermatitis are rare occurrences in the post-operative period.(76) Patients that undergo scrotal castrations are also less likely to self-mutilate.(76) This is contrary to popular thought. For decades, veterinary students have been taught to never incise the scrotum because of its thin skin and inherent sensitivity. In actuality, scrotal incisions are handled well by the patient.

   Accordingly, scrotal castrations are now considered to be an acceptable practice in accordance with the Association of Shelter Veterinarians' Veterinary Medical Care Guidelines for Spay-Neuter Programs.(77)

8. Scrotal ablation in dogs is not typically performed as standard practice for orchiectomy.(27, 41) Scrotal ablation is typically reserved for dogs that have sustained significant trauma to the scrotum

and/or have cancer that involves the scrotal sac.(27, 41) Scrotal ablation is also sometimes performed in older adult dogs that are well-endowed at the time of sterilization surgery to avoid potential postoperative complications, such as scrotal hemorrhage.(27) In my experience, clients of older adult large-breed dogs may also request this procedure because it is thought to result in a more cosmetic outcome than a large, floppy, empty scrotal sac.

9. Postoperative complications of scrotal orchiectomy include:(27, 56)

    • dehiscence at the surgical site
    • infection at the surgical site
    • scrotal swelling:

        • scrotal swelling may be more likely to occur after open castrations(56)

    • scrotal bruizing
    • scrotal irritation
    • scrotal hematoma (see Figure 12.4).

Intra-abdominal hemorrhage is rare, but occurs when a vascular pedicle that has been improperly ligated retracts into the abdomen.(56)

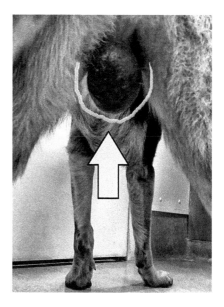

Figure 12.4 Scrotal hematoma, post-orchiectomy. Courtesy of Jackie Kukscar.

10. Aftercare for Tumbleweed's herniorrhaphy is minimal. The client should be instructed to monitor the surgical site daily for signs of infection.(3) Likewise, the client can be taught to monitor the inguinal as well as the pre-scrotal (or scrotal) incision sites for increased redness, swelling, discomfort, and/or the development of incisional site discharge.

Restricting exercise in the immediate postoperative period is likely to reduce the degree to which the scrotum swells.(27, 56) In the event of scrotal swelling that causes discomfort, cold packs may be used to reduce edema, but their efficacy depends largely upon the patient's tolerance.(56)

Elizabethan collars are often prescribed for 10–14 days, during wound healing, to reduce the chance of self-mutilation at the surgical site, specifically the pre-scrotal or scrotal sites.(56) Constant licking at any surgical site may precipitate dermatitis and/or secondary skin infection, which could ultimately contribute to dehiscence.

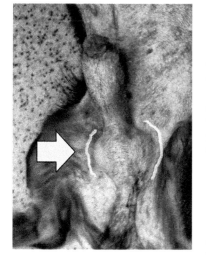

Figure 12.5 Post-operative swelling at the base of the prepuce. Note that this patient is not actually Tumbleweed.

Returning to Case 12: Planning a Canine Castration

Tumbleweed re-presents to your clinic three days post-operatively. Although Tumbleweed's attitude has been stellar and he does not appear to be in any discomfort, Prim has noticed an intermittent swelling near the surgical site. This concerns her. She doesn't want to doubt you yet cannot help but question whether you did in fact neuter Tumbleweed. She points out the swelling that she has noticed at the base of his prepuce (see Figure 12.5).

Round Three of Questions for Case 12: Planning a Canine Castration

1. What is the swelling that Prim has identified?
    Prim is still doubtful. Thankfully, you can prove that you neutered Tumbleweed because, as luck would have it, you preserved his testicles in formalin for teaching purchases (see Figure 12.6).

2. Which testicle, the one on the left or the one on the right, represents the cryptorchid one?

Answers to Round Three of Questions for Case 12: Planning a Canine Castration

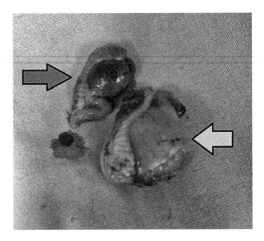

Figure 12.6 Surgically excised testicles. Courtesy of Shannon Carey, DVM.

1. The structure that Prim is referring to sits at the base of the penis and is called the bulbus glandis. The bulbus glandis is a vascular structure. Its purpose is to fill with blood during erection to form a prominent ring-like structure at the penile base.(78) Sometimes this swelling is called a knot.(9) This swelling allows dogs to "tie" during mating, meaning that the male is transiently locked inside of the female to facilitate transfer of semen from one reproductive tract to another.(79–81) Dogs may remain in this "tie" for minutes to an hour or so, until detumescence causes the bulbus glandis to become dislodged from the female reproductive tract.(9)

    Although the bulbus glandis is a predominantly sexual structure, it is important to note that in the male dog, the bulbus glandis may also swell in response to generalized excitement.(9) This explains why we may see swelling of the bulbus glandis in non-sexual situations as well as in neutered males.(9)

    It is not unusual to see intermittent swelling of the bulbus glandis in the immediate post-operative period following castration.(9) It is thought that manipulation of this region of the body during surgery and the associated post-operative swelling may put pressure on this structure, causing it to enlarge.(9)

    Note that when the bulbus glandis swells in a non-erect dog, the glans penis remains hidden within the preputial sheath.(9) This causes two discrete swellings to form under the skin at the base of the penis.(9) To an untrained eye, these two swellings might appear to be testicles.(9) You need to convince Prim that they are not, and that they are part of Tumbleweed's normal anatomy.(9)

2. The testicle on the left is the cryptorchid one because it is smaller in size. This is typical of cryptorchid testicles, which may also appear misshapen and softer in texture than scrotal testicles.(41)

CLINICAL PEARLS

- Canine castration has been associated with behavioral and health-related benefits.

- Most canine castrations are performed in prepubertal patients. However, there is some growing concern in the veterinary medical literature that there may be breed-specific disadvantages to pediatric orchiectomy.

- Certain breeds of dog, particularly large-breed dogs, may be at greater risk for development of certain cancers and orthopedic development disease. So, it is critical to keep an eye out for additional studies to guide decision making.

- As with any other procedure, it is critical to discuss patient-specific risks and benefits.

- Transparency is an important skill to facilitate clinical conversations in which there is no one "right" answer.

- When you and the client do agree to proceed with castration, it is imperative that you perform a comprehensive pre-operative physical exam on the patient and confirm the presence of two scrotal testicles.

- Testicles arise within the abdomen near the kidneys in embryonic life and must migrate to the scrotum.

- Testicles are not typically present in the scrotum at birth; however, they ought to be present by six months of age.

- If one or both testicles is/are not present in the scrotum by this age, then the patient is said to be cryptorchid.

- Cryptorchidism is thought to be inherited and has been associated with other defects, including umbilical hernias.

- Cryptorchid dogs should not be bred. They exhibit reduced fertility and libido.

- Cryptorchid dogs are at a significantly increased risk of developing testicular cancer and testicular torsion.

- Cryptorchid dogs may be unilaterally or bilaterally affected. The former is more common; the right testicle is more often the one that is "missing."

- "Missing" testicles can be found anywhere from their site of origin in the abdomen near the kidney to the inguinal canal.

- Even if a patient is unilaterally cryptorchid, he should undergo bilateral castration.

- Historically, orchiectomy in dogs has been performed via a pre-scrotal approach and incision site. However, scrotal incisions in dogs have been studied extensively, particularly in the growing area of shelter medicine.

- Scrotal incisions are not associated with higher post-operative complication rates. In fact, scrotal castrations appear to take less time when performed by an experienced surgeon, and cause minimal post-operative discomfort as compared to the traditional approach.

- Hernia repair can be performed at the same time as orchiectomy.

- Hernias can be described by their location, size, and reducibility.

- If left unrepaired, external abdominal hernias risk the herniation of abdominal contents into the space between the skin and the body wall.

- Herniated contents may become entrapped and/or strangulated. Both represent medical emergencies.

References

1. Evans HE, Miller ME. Miller's anatomy of the dog. 4th ed. St. Louis, MO: Elsevier; 2013.

2. Pratschke KM. Abdominal wall hernias and ruptures. In: Langley-Hobbs SJ, Demetriou J, Ladlow JF, editors. Feline soft tissue and general surgery. New York: Saunders/Elsevier; 2014.

3. Smeak DD. Abdominal wall reconstruction and hernias. In: Tobias KM, Johnston SA, editors. Veterinary surgery: small animal. Two. St. Louis, MO: Saunders; 2012. p. 1353–79.

4. Fossum TW. Surgery of the abdominal cavity. In: Fossum TW, Duprey LP, O'Connor D, editors. Small animal surgery. 3rd ed. Boston, MA: Elsevier; 2007.

5. Hoskins JD, Partington BP. Physical examination and diagnostic imaging procedures. In: Hoskins JD, editor. Veterinary pediatrics: dogs and cats from birth to six months. 3rd ed. Philadelphia, PA: Saunders Elsevier; 2001. p. 6–7.

6. Smeak DD. Abdominal wall reconstruction and hernias. In: Tobias KM, Johnston SA, editors. Veterinary surgery: small animal. 2. St. Louis, MO: Saunders Elsevier; 2012. p. 1353–79.

7. Englar RE. Performing the small animal physical examination. Hoboken, NJ: Wiley/Blackwell; 2017.

8. Tobias KM. Umbilical hernias. In: Tobias KM, editor. Manual of small animal soft tissue surgery. Ames, IA: Wiley/Blackwell; 2010.

9. Englar RE. Common clinical presentations in dogs and cats. Hoboken, NJ: Wiley/Blackwell; 2019.

10. Tobias KM. Inguinal hernias. In: Tobias KM, editor. Manual of small animal soft tissue surgery. Ames, IA: Wiley/Blackwell; 2010.

11. Hermanson JW, Evans HE. The muscular system. In: Evans HE, editor. Miller's anatomy of the dog. 3rd ed. Philadelphia, PA: Saunders Elsevier; 1993. p. 258–384.

12. Dyce KM, Sack WO, Wensing CJG. Textbook of veterinary anatomy. 2nd ed. Philadelphia, PA: Saunders; 1996.

13. Pratschke KM. Abdominal wall hernias and ruptures. In: Langley-Hobbs SJ, Demetriou JL, Ladlow JF, editors. Feline soft tissue and general surgery. St. Louis, MO: Saunders Elsevier; 2014. p. 269–80.

14. Voges AK, Bertrand S, Hill RC, Neuwirth L, Schaer M. True diaphragmatic hernia in a cat. Vet Radiol Ultrasound 1997;38(2):116–9.

15. Worth AJ, Machon RG. Traumatic diaphragmatic herniation: pathophysiology and management. Comp Cont Educ Pract 2005;27(3):178.

16. Schmiedt CW, Tobias KM, Stevenson MA. Traumatic diaphragmatic hernia in cats: 34 cases (1991–2001). J Am Vet Med Assoc 2003;222(9):1237–40.

17. Fossum TW. Pleural and extrapleural diseases. In: Ettinger SJ, Feldman EC, editors. Textbook of veterinary internal medicine. Philadelphia, PA: Saunders; 2000. p. 1098.

18. Millis DL, Hauptman JG, Johnson CA. Cryptorchidism and monorchism in cats: 25 cases (1980–1989). J Am Vet Med Assoc 1992;200(8):1128–30.

19. Meyers-Wallen VN. Gonadal and sex differentiation abnormalities of dogs and cats. Sex Dev 2012;6(1–3):46–60.

20. Richardson EF, Mullen H. Cryptorchidism in cats. Compend Contin Educ Pract Vet 1993;15(10):1342–5.

21. Yates D, Hayes G, Heffernan M, Beynon R. Incidence of cryptorchidism in dogs and cats. Vet Rec 2003;152(16):502–4.

22. Wallace JL, Levy JK. Population characteristics of feral cats admitted to seven trap-neuter-return programs in the United States. J Feline Med Surg 2006;8(4):279–84.

23. Yates D, Hayes G, Heffernan M, Beynon R. Incidence of cryptorchidism in dogs and cats. Vet Rec 2003;152(16):502–4.

24. Foster RA. Common lesions in the male reproductive tract of cats and dogs. Vet Clin North Am Small Anim Pract 2012;42(3):527–45.

25. Romagnoli SE. Canine cryptorchidism. Vet Clin North Am Small Anim Pract 1991;21(3):533–44.

26. Reif JS, Brodey RS. The relationship between cryptorchidism and canine testicular neoplasia. J Am Vet Med Assoc 1969;155(12):2005–10.

27. Towle HA. Testes and scrotum. In: Tobias KM, Johnston SA, editors. Veterinary surgery: small animal. Two. St. Louis, MO: Saunders; 2012. p. 1903–16.

28. Evans HE, Christensen GC. The urogenital system. In: Evans HE, Miller ME, editors. Miller's anatomy of the dog. 3rd ed. Philadelphia, PA: W. B. Saunders; 1993. p. 494–558.

29. Birchard SJ, Nappier M. Cryptorchidism. Compend Contin Educ Vet 2008;30(6):325–36; quiz 36–7.
30. Kawakami E, Tsutsui T, Yamada Y, Yamauchi M. Cryptorchidism in the dog: occurrence of cryptorchidism and semen quality in the cryptorchid dog. Nihon Juigaku Zasshi 1984;46(3):303–8.
31. Davidson AP. Canine cryptorchidism. NAVC Clin's Brief 2014 (January):102–4.
32. Cox VS, Wallace LJ, Jessen CR. An anatomic and genetic study of canine cryptorchidism. Teratology 1978;18(2):233–40.
33. Kutzler MA. The reproductive tract. In: Peterson ME, Kutzler MA, editors. Small animal pediatrics: the first 12 months of life. St. Louis, MO: Saunders/Elsevier; 2011. p. 405–17.
34. Pullig T. Cryptorchidism in cocker spaniels. J Hered 1953;44(6):250–.
35. Hayes HM, Wilson GP, Pendergrass TW, Cox VS. Canine cryptorchism and subsequent testicular neoplasia: case-control study with epidemiologic update. Teratology 1985;32(1):51–6.
36. Pendergrass TW, Hayes HM. Cryptorchidism and related defects in dogs: epidemiologic comparison with man. Teratology 1975;12(1):51–5.
37. Graves TK. Diseases of the testes and scrotum. In: Birchard SJ, Sherding RG, editors. Saunders manual of small animal practice. St. Louis, MO: Elsevier; 2006. p. 963.
38. Veronesi MC, Riccardi E, Rota A, Grieco V. Characteristics of cryptic/ectopic and contralateral scrotal testes in dogs between 1 and 2 years of age. Theriogenology 2009;72(7):969–77.
39. Johnston SD, Root Kustritz MV, Olson PNS. Disorders of canine testes and epididymes. Canine and feline theriogenology: W.B. Saunders; 2001. p. 312–32.
40. Englar RE. Performing the small animal physical examination. Hoboken, NJ: Wiley; 2017.
41. Hedlund CS. Surgery of the reproductive and Ge nital systems. In: Fossum TW, Duprey LP, O'Connor D, editors. Small animal surgery. 3rd ed. Boston, MA: Elsevier; 2007.
42. Wolff A. Castration, cryptorchidism, and cryptorchidectomy in dogs and cats. Vet Med Small Anim Clin 1981;76(12):1739–41.
43. Hayes HM, Jr., Pendergrass TW. Canine testicular tumors: epidemiologic features of 410 dogs. Int J Cancer 1976;18(4):482–7.
44. Hohšteter M, Artuković B, Severin K, Kurilj AG, Beck A, Šoštarić-Zuckermann IC, Grabarević Ž. Canine testicular tumors: two types of seminomas can be differentiated by immunohistochemistry. BMC Vet Res 2014;10:169.
45. Pearson H, Kelly DF. Testicular torsion in the dog: a review of 13 cases. Vet Rec 1975;97(11):200–4.
46. Hayes HM, Wilson GP, Pendergrass TW, Cox VS. Canine cryptorchism and subsequent testicular neoplasia: case-control study with epidemiologic update. Teratology 1985;32(1):51–6.
47. Pendergrass TW, Hayes HM. Cryptorchism and related defects in dogs: epidemiologic comparisons with man. Teratology 1975;12(1):51–5.
48. Little SE. Male reproduction. In: Little SE, editor. The cat: clinical medicine and management. St. Louis: Saunders Elsevier; 2012.
49. Lawrence JA, Saba CF. Tumors of the male reproductive system. In: Withrow SJ, Vail DM, Page RL, editors. Withrow and MacEwen's small animal clinical oncology. 5th ed. St. Louis, MO: Elsevier; 2013. p. 557–71.
50. Cotchin E. Testicular neoplasms in dogs. J Comp Pathol 1960;70:232–48.
51. von Bomhard D, Pukkavesa C, Haenichen T. The ultrastructure of testicular tumours in the dog: I. Germinal cells and seminomas. J Comp Pathol 1978;88(1):49–57.
52. Liao AT, Chu PY, Yeh LS, Lin CT, Liu CH. A 12-year retrospective study of canine testicular tumors. J Vet Med Sci 2009;71(7):919–23.
53. Howe LM. Current perspectives on the optimal age to spay/castrate` dogs and cats. Vetmed (Auckl) 2015;6:171–80.
54. DC, JS R, RS B, H.K. Epidemiological analysis of the most prevalent sites and types of canine neoplasia observed in a veterinary hospital. Cancer Res 1997;34:2859–68.
55. Johnston SD, RKM, Olson PN. Disorders of the canine testes and epididymes. In: Johnston SD, RKM, Olson PN, editors. Canine and feline theriogenology. Philadelphia; 2001. p. 312–32.
56. Tobias KM. Canine castration. In: Tobias KM, editor. Manual of small animal soft tissue surgery. Ames, IA: Wiley/Blackwell; 2010.
57. Hart BL. Problems with objectionable sociosexual behavior of dogs and cats: therapeutic use of castration and progestins. Compend Contin Educ Pract 1979;1:461–5.

58. Hoffman JM, Creevy KE, Promislow DE. PLOS ONE 2013;8(4):e61082.

59. Barsanti JA, Finco DR. Canine prostatic diseases. Vet Clin North Am Small Anim Pract 1986;16(3):587–99.

60. Johnston SD, Kamolpatana K, Root-Kustritz MV, Johnston GR. Prostatic disorders in the dog. Anim Reprod Sci 2000;60–61:405–15.

61. Berry SJ, Coffey DS, Strandberg JD, Ewing LL. Effect of age, castration, and testosterone replacement on the development and restoration of canine benign prostatic hyperplasia. Prostate 1986;9(3):295–302.

62. Berry SJ, Strandberg JD, Saunders WJ, Coffey DS. Development of canine benign prostatic hyperplasia with age. Prostate 1986;9(4):363–73.

63. Black GM, Ling GV, Nyland TG, Baker T. Prevalence of prostatic cysts in adult, large-breed dogs. J Am Anim Hosp Assoc 1998;34(2):177–80.

64. Bray JP, White RA, Williams JM. Partial resection and omentalization: a new technique for management of prostatic retention cysts in dogs. Vet Surg 1997;26(3):202–9.

65. Roll A, Unshelm J. Aggressive conflicts amongst dogs and factors affecting them. Appl Anim Behav Sci 1997;52(3–4):229–42.

66. Spain CV, Scarlett JM, Houpt KA. Long-term risks and benefits of early-age gonadectomy in dogs. J Am Vet Med Assoc 2004;224(3):380–7.

67. Torres de la Riva G, Hart BL, Farver TB, Oberbauer AM, Messam LL, Willits N, Hart LA. Neutering dogs: effects on joint disorders and cancers in golden retrievers. PLOS ONE 2013;8(2):e55937.

68. Whitehair JG, Vasseur PB, Willits NH. Epidemiology of cranial cruciate ligament rupture in dogs. J Am Vet Med Assoc 1993;203(7):1016–9.

69. Slauterbeck JR, Pankratz K, Xu KT, Bozeman SC, Hardy DM. Canine ovariohysterectomy and orchiectomy increases the prevalence of ACL injury. Clin Orthop Relat Res 2004;429(429):301–5.

70. Hart BL, Hart LA, Thigpen AP, Willits NH. Long-term health effects of neutering dogs: comparison of Labrador Retrievers with Golden Retrievers. PLOS ONE 2014;9(7):e102241.

71. van Hagen MA, Ducro BJ, van den Broek J, Knol BW. Incidence, risk factors, and heritability estimates of hind limb lameness caused by hip dysplasia in a birth cohort of boxers. Am J Vet Res 2005;66(2):307–12.

72. Villamil JA, Henry CJ, Hahn AW, Bryan JN, Tyler JW, Caldwell CW. Hormonal and sex impact on the epidemiology of canine lymphoma. J Cancer Epidemiol 2009;2009:591753.

73. Zink MC, Farhoody P, Elser SE, Ruffini LD, Gibbons TA, Rieger RH. Evaluation of the risk and age of onset of cancer and behavioral disorders in gonadectomized Vizslas. J Am Vet Med Assoc 2014;244(3):309–19.

74. Cooley DM, Beranek BC, Schlittler DL, Glickman NW, Glickman LT, Waters DJ. Endogenous gonadal hormone exposure and bone sarcoma risk. Cancer Epidemiol Biomarkers Prev 2002;11(11):1434–40.

75. Ru G, Terracini B, Glickman LT. hosts. Vet J 1998;156(1):31–9.

76. Miller KP, Rekers WL, DeTar LG, Blanchette JM, Milovancev M. Evaluation of sutureless scrotal castration for pediatric and juvenile dogs. J Am Vet Med Assoc 2018;253(12):1589–93.

77. Association of Shelter, Griffin B, Bushby PA, McCobb E, White SC, Rigdon-Brestle YK et al. The Association of Shelter Veterinarians' 2016 Veterinary Medical Care Guidelines for Spay-Neuter Programs. J Am Vet Med Assoc 2016;249(2):165–88.

78. Kutzler MA. Semen collection in the dog. Theriogenology 2005;64(3):747–54.

79. The urogenital apparatus. In: Dyce KM, Sack WO, Wensing CJG, editors. Textbook of veterinary anatomy. 4th ed. Philadelphia, PA: Saunders; 2009.

80. Evans HE, Christensen GC. The urogenital system. In: Evans HE, Miller ME, editors. Miller's anatomy of the dog. 3rd ed. Philadelphia, PA: W. B. Saunders; 1993. p. 494–554.

81. Hart BL. The action of extrinsic penile muscles during copulation in the male dog. Anat Rec 1972;173(1):1–5.

Case 13

Planning a Feline Spay

Keleigh Downey was a rising star within her firm as a promising young attorney. Although she had a gentle exterior and a reserved approach to personal conflict, she could be ruthless in the courtroom as a prosecutor and already had quite a few wins to show for it. If she continued her performance at this pace and with this track record, she would be promoted in record time. She aspired to make partner by age 35 and her vision of "retirement" was being a Supreme Court justice.

Keleigh was by far the most ambitious of her peer group. Friends would remark that she was an old soul trapped in a young body. While everyone else was out on the town, the bar scene wasn't her style. What most people didn't understand about her was that she chose this lifestyle – and happily so. It was more empowering than a margarita and a one-night stand. Life in the court-

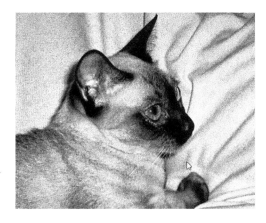

Figure 13.1 Meet your next patient, Bailey's Crème Brûlée, a 4-month-old intact female Siamese kitten.

room was the adrenaline ride that she needed. She worked hard to play hard. And although from time to time she missed out on human companionship, she decided that she didn't need a relationship with a man; she needed a kitten.

Keleigh had always planned on adopting. In fact, rescues were all that she'd known as a child. But now that Keleigh was all grown up, she was looking for more than an aloof furry "sibling" to share her day bed. Keleigh wanted a feline friend that was unlike any other cat that she had ever owned. She wanted a dog in a cat's body. So it was that she found herself stumbling across an advertisement online for a Siamese cattery.

Keleigh had long been a fan of the color-point coat. She preferred the seal point over the flame point but was not particularly picky about coat color provided that the kitten of her choice was female. She'd just purchased her first home and had heard that male cats were more likely to spray. So, she settled on the idea of purchasing a female kitten that could perhaps be more easily persuaded to abide by house rules.

Keleigh contacted the cattery and was excited to hear that a litter of kittens was available for purchase. Only one of the four kittens was female. If she wanted the female to be hers, she had to visit straight away. Keleigh didn't need much convincing to hop in the car. A little over an hour later, she arrived at the cattery and held Bailey's Crème Brûlée for the very first time. Bailey was shy, but sweet. It wasn't long before she warmed up to Keleigh's lap.

Keleigh spent the next 2 hours talking with the breeder to get a sense of the cattery's history and Bailey's pedigree. She didn't care about Bailey's ancestry from the perspective of maintaining her line. Bailey would be strictly a companion. Keleigh had no intentions of showing or breeding her. Yet Keleigh had heard horror stories about inbreeding and wanted to do her homework. Before she signed her life away on the dotted line of any contract, Keleigh wanted to be sure that Bailey's genetics were sound and that she came from a good home, raised underfoot rather than in a cage or behind closed doors. When Keleigh was certain that she had asked all the right questions, she agreed to take on Bailey's care.

One week later, after Keleigh had purchased all the new kitten essentials, Bailey came home with her. She was initially soft-spoken, but it wasn't long before she learned how to make her demands heard. She soon trained Keleigh to meet her every need, as soon as she required it, and if Keleigh didn't comply, immediately, then she would hear all about it!

Bailey was certainly agitated now, in the clinic setting, pitching a fit from her cat carrier as she waited for today's exam. Keleigh had brought Bailey in to finalize her last round of kitten shots and to discuss having her spayed. Your technician remarks that her vocal cords are certainly in good working order as he documents her vital signs in the medical record:

Weight: 4.6 lb (2.1 kg)
BCS: 4/9
Mentation: BAR

TPR

T: 100.4°F (38.0°C)
P: 202 beats per minute
R: 18 breaths per minute

Work through the following questions as you review Bailey's chart to prepare you for this consultation.

Note that the first half of the questions pertain to Bailey's breed. It is important that you familiarize with any breed that will be presenting to you so that you are aware of any breed-specific traits and/or medical conditions that may impact the health and well-being of the patient.

Round One of Questions for Case 13: Planning a Feline Spay

1. What are so-called points in Siamese cats?
2. What causes point coloration in Siamese cats?
3. What are the major point colors in Siamese cats?
4. Are points present at birth?
5. Do points change color as Siamese cats age?
6. How does geography play a role in point coloration?
7. How might clipping Bailey's coat affect her point coloration?
8. Do any other cat breeds develop point coloration?
9. Why is it important to familiarize yourself with breed-specific characteristics, such as points?
10. Breed-specific predispositions to disease have been established in both cats and dogs. Which medical and/or behavioral conditions are more likely to occur in Siamese?
11. What is the relationship between a cat's intact sexual status and its likelihood of developing mammary neoplasia?
12. How common is mammary neoplasia in cats relative to dogs?
13. How common is malignancy when it comes to mammary neoplasia in cats?
14. Bailey is female, but can and do male cats also get mammary cancer?
15. What is the typical presentation for mammary neoplasia in cats?
16. Which behavioral and health-related benefits have been ascribed to spaying cats?
17. How does this compare to reported behavioral and health-related benefits in spayed dogs?
18. The risk of which medical conditions may be increased by spaying cats?
19. How does this compare to reported behavioral and health-related risks in spayed dogs?
20. Explain the link between sterilization and obesity.
21. How common is obesity in companion cats?
22. Differentiate ovariohysterectomy from ovariectomy. What are the advantages and disadvantages of each procedure?
23. Describe a ventral midline surgical approach to ovariohysterectomy.
24. How might your ventral midline surgical approach differ if Bailey were a dog instead of a cat?

25. What are potential surgical and/or postoperative complications of ovariohysterectomy?
26. In the unlikely event that you need to perform a blood transfusion, which blood type is Bailey most likely to be?
27. Are there any specific instructions for Bailey's aftercare?

Answers to Round One of Questions for Case 13: Planning a Feline Spay

1. Points refer to certain regions of the body that are darker than others. In the Siamese cat, points include the face and extremities – the ears, paws, and tails.(1, 2)

2. Points arise from acromelanism, a condition in which temperature plays a role in the development of pigment on the coat.(2–7) Cats with points have inherited a mutation of the albino gene. (1, 2) This mutation results in temperature-dependent tyrosinase.(2, 5) Tyrosinase is an enzyme that catalyzes the production of one specific type of pigment, melanin, within the hair bulb.(2, 5, 7–11) Melanin is dark brown to black in color.(2) In color-point cats, tyrosinase activates at cool temperatures only, causing the extremities to darken.(2, 8–11)

3. Siamese cats are typically characterized into four groups based upon their point coloration:(1, 2)

    - seal points (brown)
    - flame points (red-orange)
    - blue points (grey)
    - lilac (lavender) points.

4. No, points are not present at birth.(1, 2) Siamese kittens are white when they are born because during fetal life, their bodies are bathed in a uniformly warm environment, the queen's uterus. (1, 2) This warm body temperature inactivates tyrosinase such that pigment production does not occur until after birth.(1, 2)

5. As neonates, kittens are exposed to a much different environment than their mom's womb. This environment is not uniformly warm. In fact, different regions of the body are exposed to slightly different temperatures. The face, muzzle, and extremities, including the tail, are slightly cooler than core body temperature.(1, 2) This change in temperature is significant enough to activate tyrosinase.(1, 2) When tyrosinase is activated, it causes pigment formation within these cooler regions of the body, causing them to darken relative to the torso, which remains light.(1, 2) Color points are overt by the time Siamese kittens reach 4 weeks of age.(1, 2) As Siamese cats age, their points darken.(1, 2)

6. Color-point cats that live in cooler climates (particularly those who spend a significant time outdoors) tend to develop darker points more quickly than those that live in warmer climates. (1, 2) Exposure to chronically cold temperatures may inspire the development of dark pigmentation along the trunk and flanks.(1–4, 6) Exclusively outdoor color-point cats may even lose their points altogether as their entire coat darkens.(1, 2, 6)

7. Coat clipping is likely to influence coat color.(2) Even something as transient as shaving the ventral abdomen to spay a color-point cat chills the skin at the surgical site.(2) This is enough to activate thermally dependent tyrosinase.(2) Once activated, tyrosinase will enhance pigment production within the hair bulbs at the site of the spay.(2) As fur regrows, it is likely to grow back darker than it had been before. This change in coat color will persist until the next hair cycle.(1–4)

8. In addition to Siamese cats, the following breeds are known for point coloration:(1, 2, 4, 8, 12)

   - Balinese
   - Birman
   - Burmese
   - Himalayan
   - Singapura
   - Tonkinese.

9. Clients expect you to be familiar with their breed and breed-associated characteristics. If you do not see many exotic breeds of cats at your clinic, then chances are you are going to be unfamiliar with several of their features and quirks. In those circumstances, the client and/or the breeder may be more of an expert in the exam room than you are, at least concerning the breed standard. As you start to see more cats in your exam room, you will learn that "cat people" are often very excited to share their love for and knowledge of the breed. It is important to take the time to listen because these types of conversations build partnership and establish confidence in your client that you are indeed willing to listen. Not all cats are cut from the same cloth. Not all breeds share the same traits or characteristics. The names for points are often breed-specific, and cat fanciers will care how you refer to them. There are no "seal point" Tonkinese cats, for instance.(1, 2) Although they may resemble seal point Siamese cats, their coats are referred to as champagne.(1, 2) This may seem like a small distinction to you, and one of clinical insignificance. But most clients do care and are more than willing to share if you simply take the time to ask.

10. Breed-specific predispositions to disease have been established in both cats and dogs. Siamese cats are said to be predisposed to the following conditions:(13)

    - dermatopathies:
      - periocular leukotrichia: the development of white fur around the eyes(14, 15)
      - pinnal alopecia: thinning of the fur along the dorsal aspects of both ears(16)
      - vitiligo: a condition in which whole patches of skin lose their pigment(17, 18)
    - gastrointestinal conditions:
      - amyloidosis(19)
      - cleft palate(20)
      - congenital megaesophagus(21)
      - congenital portosystemic shunts(22, 23)
      - pyloric dysfunction(21, 24–26)
      - small intestinal adenocarcinoma(27–29)
    - neoplasia:
      - basal cell tumor(30)
      - mammary tumors(31–36)
      - mast cell tumors(37, 38)
    - neurological conditions:
      - hyperesthesia syndrome(39–41)
      - myasthenia gravis(42)
    - obsessive-compulsive behaviors:
      - psychogenic alopecia(43)
      - wool sucking(44)

- ocular conditions:

  - convergent strabismus(2, 45)
  - corneal sequestrum(46, 47)
  - nystagmus(2, 45)

- orthopedic conditions:

  - hip dysplasia(48)
  - mucopolysaccharidosis VI(49)

- respiratory conditions:

  - feline asthma.(50, 51)

11. Intact cats are seven times more likely to develop mammary cancer than neutered cats.(31, 32, 35, 52–54) Cats that are spayed before 6 months of age have a 91% risk reduction.(31)

    The degree of protection is reduced as the patient ages.(2, 31, 35, 54–56) Cats that are spayed between 7 and 12 months old have a risk reduction of 86%, whereas cats that are spayed between 13 months old and 2 years of age have a risk reduction of only 11%.(31) There does not appear to be any protective benefit from spay relative to mammary neoplasia after a cat exceeds two years old.(31)

12. Mammary cancer occurs less frequently in cats than dogs.(2, 31, 55)

13. Mammary neoplasia is more likely to be malignant in cats than in dogs.(2, 31, 35, 55, 57, 58) Between 85% and 93% of mammary masses are malignant in cats.(35, 59)

14. Yes, male cats can and do develop mammary cancer, although this occurrence is more commonly seen in females.(2)

    Recall from basic anatomy that females are not the only sex to have mammary glands. All cats, regardless of sex, have mammary glands.(1, 2) Most cats have four sets for a total of eight glands and their associated nipples.(1, 2, 35, 60–62) The nipples are often difficult to see because they are hidden within the fur that lines the ventral abdomen.(1, 2, 61)

    Male cats have the same number of mammary glands as females.(1, 2) The primary difference is that these glands do not develop secretory tissue in males with healthy, functional endocrine systems.(2, 61, 63)

15. Most mammary masses in cats are firm and discrete, and easily palpated.(2, 31) At time of diagnosis, most cats present with more than one.(2, 31, 64) If the tumor(s) has/have developed a secondary bacterial infection, then the affected surface(s) may be ulcerated.(31, 35)

    Ipsilateral lymph node involvement is likely.(31) Always palpate for axillary and inguinal lymph nodes in these patients.(2) Even though neither set should be palpable in health (1), many cats with mammary malignancies will develop enlargements of the lymph nodes that drain the affected gland(s).

    Venous return from the pelvic limbs may be compromised by inguinal mammary masses as they enlarge.(35) Affected cats develop edema at one or both hind limbs.(35)

16. Other than significantly reducing the risk of mammary neoplasia, the following behavioral and health-related benefits have been ascribed to spaying cats:

- spaying increases life expectancy(65)
- spaying eliminates the risk of pyometra (if an ovariohysterectomy is pursued):(55)

  - Siamese cats, Korats, Ocicats, and Bengals are predisposed(66)

- when they present with pyometra, these overrepresented breeds tend to be younger in age than is true of the general population(66)

- spaying prevents unplanned and/or unwanted pregnancies.(55, 65, 67, 68)

17. The same behavioral and health-related benefits have been ascribed to spaying dogs. However, dogs are much more likely than cats to develop pyometra.(2, 55, 61, 69, 70) Pyometra occurs in 2.2% of intact queens by the time they reach 13 years of age (2, 61), compared to 25–66% of dogs over 9–10 years old.(55, 70, 71) Therefore, the protective benefits of ovariohysterectomy relative to this risk is much greater in dogs.

18. Spayed cats may be at increased risk of:
    - delayed physeal closure(72–74)
    - diabetes mellitus(65, 75–77)
    - obesity.(65, 72, 78, 79)

19. The following health-related risks may be associated with spaying dogs:
    - cranial cruciate ligament injury(80, 81)
    - hip dysplasia(82)
    - increased aggression(83–87)
    - osteosarcoma(55, 88, 89)
    - peri-vulvar dermatitis(65)
    - recessed vulva(65)
    - transitional cell carcinoma (TCC)(65, 90)
    - urethral sphincter-associated urinary incontinence.(55, 91–97)

20. Neutered cats are more likely to be overweight or obese.(72, 79) Cats that are sterilized between the ages of 7 weeks and 7 months weigh more than intact cats of the same age and also have greater accumulation of falciform fat.(72, 73, 98, 99) This predisposition for obesity has been attributed to the loss of sex hormones from gonadectomy. In health, estrogen contributes to appetite regulation and satiety through interactions with the hormone, leptin.(78, 100)

    Although clients are not always informed about this at discharge from surgery, the maintenance energy requirement (MER) in neutered cats is significantly less than what they required preoperatively.(79) MER is in fact one-quarter less than what has previously been recommended by the National Research Council.(79)

    If clients are not instructed to restrict intake in the immediate postoperative period, then their neutered pets are likely to experience weight gain and obesity.(79) More specifically, caloric intake should be reduced by 30% to prevent weight gain post-spay.(78)

21. Obesity is a significant problem in companion cats.(1, 72, 78) Within the US alone, 30–40% of cats are overweight or obese.(78, 101, 102) Many cats present to veterinary clinics with an estimated 50% body fat, if not higher.(103, 104)

22. An ovariohysterectomy refers to the traditional spay procedure, which involves surgical excision of both ovaries and the uterus.(105) This procedure is still recommended by the majority of veterinary colleges within the US and Canada,(106) and many practitioners consider it to be the gold standard for surgical sterilization of female cats and dogs.

    An ovariectomy is an acceptable surgical alternative to ovariohysterectomy, and has been adopted throughout many parts of Europe as the new standard of care.(106–108) This procedure involves excision of both ovaries and is uterine-sparing.(105)

    Historically, ovariohysterectomy has been preferred over ovariectomy due to fear that patients who undergo the latter procedure risk the development of uterine disease because the uterus remains intact.(109) Some practitioners have expressed concern that leaving the uterus behind could predispose the patient to:(106)

- cystic endometrial hyperplasia-pyometra complex:

    - however, removal of both ovaries eliminates the endogenous source of progesterone that is required for this condition to materialize.(105)

- uterine neoplasia:

    - however, most tumors of the uterus occur in dogs, not cats
    - of these, most are benign leiomyomas(65, 110–113)
    - of those that are malignant, metastasis is rare, such that surgical excision of the uterus at the time of diagnosis is considered curative.

Both ovariohysterectomy and ovariectomy take approximately the same amount of surgical time to perform.(106, 114)

Skin and fascial incisions are smaller for ovariectomy than ovariohysterectomy.(106, 114) Ovariectomy would therefore be considered minimally invasive by comparison to the traditional approach, particularly if ovariectomy is combined with laparoscopic technique.(108, 115)

23. If you were to proceed with ovariohysterectomy, then your ventral midline surgical approach to spaying Bailey is as follows.(105, 115–117)

- Anesthetize the patient.
- Place the patient in dorsal recumbency.
- Prep and drape the patient using aseptic technique.

    - Fur is routinely clipped, beginning cranial to the xiphoid and extending caudal to the pubis.

- Using your "imaginoscope," divide the distance between the umbilicus and the pubis into thirds.
- Make a ventral midline incision through the skin and subcutaneous tissues in the middle third.

    - As a point of reference, some surgeons propose that you make your incision two fingers' width caudal to the umbilicus.
    - In kittens less than 3 months old, the incision is a bit more caudal. It is estimated to begin two-thirds of the distance between the umbilicus and the pelvis.

- Tent the linea alba with Adson rat-toothed forceps.
- Invert the scalpel so that the blade is pointing up and pierce through the linea alba to enter the abdomen.
- Use Mayo scissors to extend the incision through the linea alba to improve exposure and visualization.
- Find the uterus through gentle digital exploration of the abdomen.

    - Reflect the urinary bladder to find the uterine body sandwiched between the urinary bladder and the colon.
    - The uterine horns are dorsal to the uterine body.
    - Exteriorize the uterus.

- Alternatively, you may find the uterus using a spay-hook, a so-called Snook hook.

    - Run this tool down the abdominal wall, with the hook facing the lateral (outermost) aspect of the abdominal cavity.
    - Near the floor of the abdominal cavity, turn the hook medially.

- Lift the hook gently to see if you successfully snared the uterus. This may take several attempts.
- Never yank on the Snook hook. Use caution because it is possible to inadvertently hook and tear the ureter.

- Follow one uterine horn cranially to the ipsilateral ovary.
- Stretch the suspensory ligament and/or break it down if necessary, to improve exposure of the ovary.
- Make a nick in the mesovarium to assist with clamp placement.
- Use a three-clamp technique (or an acceptable alternative) to place hemostats across the ovarian pedicle dorsal to the ovary, taking care not to inadvertently include a portion of the ovary in the clamped tissue.
- Place your first circumferential ligature proximal to the hemostats or in the crush of the most proximal hemostat.

  - Use caution because feline tissue is thin and easy to tear inadvertently with suture if you do not use gentle tissue handling.

- Place a second circumferential ligature distal to the first.
- Use your scalpel to transect between the distal-most and middle clamp.
- Use thumb forceps to grasp the "stump" of the transected pedicle that will be returned to the abdominal cavity.
- Remove the clamp.
- Inspect the "stump" for bleeding.
- Release the "stump" back into the abdomen. You may need to "tuck" it out of site gently.
- Leave the distal clamp on the part of the female reproductive tract that will be eventually leaving the body so that this tissue does not hemorrhage while you repeat the procedure for the opposite ovary.
- Now exteriorize the uterus so that you can see the uterine bifurcation. Doing so may require you to use blunt dissection to break down the broad and round ligaments.
- Use a three-clamp technique (or an acceptable alternative) to place hemostats across the uterine horns, proximal to the cervix.

  - Use caution if the uterus is friable.
  - If it is, then you may inadvertently cut through it with your clamps rather than crushing it.
  - If you are concerned about the integrity of the uterus, then proceed with ligation without using clamps.

- Place two circumferential ligatures around the uterine body or place one of this type and one transfixation ligature. Consult a surgical text of your choice to revisit this technique.

  - Transfixation is recommended if the uterus is very vascular because it more directly achieves ligation of the vascular bundle.
  - Transfixation is also recommended if the uterus is very large.

- Use your scalpel to transect between the second and the most distal hemostat.
- Use thumb forceps to grasp the "stump" of the transected uterine body that will be returned to the abdominal cavity.
- Remove the clamp.
- Inspect the "stump" for bleeding.
- Release the "stump" back into the abdomen. You may need to "tuck" it out of site gently.
- Remove the excised ovaries and uterus from the abdominal cavity for disposal.
- Examine the abdomen for evidence of active bleeding.
- Use a two-layer closure for the abdominal wall:

- linea alba and rectus fascia
- skin.

- In lieu of skin sutures, you may choose to place a subcuticular stitch, which allows for skin-to-skin apposition without necessitating skin sutures and their subsequent removal.

24. In general, a female cat's reproductive tract is a lot "stretchier" and more mobile than a dog's reproductive tract. As compared to a cat, it is often difficult to visualize and exteriorize canine ovaries.(115) To facilitate surgery, you often need to begin your incision at the umbilicus.(115) Therefore, your incision will be more cranial in a dog than in a cat.(105, 115, 117)

    Another potential challenge in the dog as compared to the cat is entering the abdominal cavity through the linea alba.(115) Recall from basic anatomy that the linea alba is a white band of tissue that begins at the xiphoid process of the sternum and runs in cranial to caudal fashion. (118–121) Because it is wider in cats than it is in dogs, it may be more difficult to find. It is often hidden by subcutaneous fat that has attached to midline.(115) Such attachments will need to be transected before you can enter the abdomen through midline. On occasion, the abdomen is entered accidentally by incising muscle layers rather than the linea alba. In these cases, the surgeon thinks that s/he is cutting through the linea when in fact s/he is on a muscle plane. It is not as easy as it sounds to tell the two apart when working through subcutaneous fat and tissue bleeding, particularly in large-breed, deep-chested dogs.

    Another challenge in dogs is that one or both ovaries often cannot be exteriorized without breaking down the suspensory ligament. This can be a scary step in the surgical process, particularly for novices. It is an uncomfortable feeling to exert controlled pressure on something to break it down without being able to see it in the process.(115) Vessels may be torn prematurely if caution is not exercised during this step.(115) This is a concern because the vascular bundles have not been ligated at this point.

    Transfixation ligatures are used more commonly in dogs to tie off ovarian pedicles and the uterine body because these tissues tend to be thicker and more friable. There is a concern that circumferential ligatures may not adequately occlude vascular supply if tissues are appreciably thick, which could cause the ligatures to slip off, resulting in hemorrhage.

    The canine abdomen is typically closed in three layers:(117)

- linea alba
- subcutaneous tissue
- skin.

In lieu of skin sutures, you may choose to place a subcuticular stitch, which allows for skin-to-skin apposition without necessitating suture removal.

25. Potential intra-operative and post-operative complications of ovariohysterectomy include:(105, 115–117)

- abdominal hemorrhage
- abdominal wall dehiscence:

    - incisional hernia
    - evisceration

- granuloma formation:

    - pedicle site(s)
    - uterine stump

- inadvertent ureteral ligation
- seroma formation
- skin dehiscence

- skin infection
- suture reaction
- urinary incontinence
- vaginal bleeding.

26. In the current veterinary medical literature, 100% of Siamese cats are reported to be blood type A.(122, 123) Ideally, all transfusions would be performed after blood typing. However, in the event of an emergency, I would feel comfortable with administering type A blood to Bailey and monitoring her closely for signs of transfusion reactions.

27. Aftercare is minimal. The client should be instructed to monitor the surgical site daily for signs of increased redness, swelling, discomfort, and/or the development of incisional site discharge, which could indicate a brewing surgical site infection.

    Elizabethan collars are often prescribed for 10–14 days, during wound healing, to reduce the chance of self-mutilation at the surgical site. Constant licking at any surgical site may precipitate dermatitis and/or secondary skin infection, which could ultimately contribute to dehiscence.

Returning to Case 13: Planning a Feline Spay

Keleigh presents Bailey 4 weeks later for unusual behavior. Although Bailey has been in good spirits, she seems to be exhibiting an unusual behavior that she wasn't exhibiting before surgery. On occasion, she rolls side to side. Keleigh describes that she sometimes lowers her front end and "sticks her butt up in the air" while she treads with her pelvic legs. Keleigh is not sure if Bailey is playing and is seeking your input.

Round Two of Questions for Case 13: Planning a Feline Spay

1. It sounds as though Keleigh may be describing mating behavior. Lordosis is a common posture in female cats that are receptive to mating. Define lordosis.
2. If Bailey is in fact displaying mating behavior, what is the most likely explanation in a spayed cat?
3. What are your recommendations for confirming your presumptive diagnosis?

Answers to Round Two of Questions for Case 13: Planning a Feline Spay

1. Lordosis in cats refers to females lowering their front end, elevating their hindquarters, and depressing the lumbar spine, like a horse with swayback.(2)

2. Bailey most likely has ovarian remnant syndrome (ORS). ORS is an uncommon surgical complication that occurs when a fraction of one or both ovaries is left inside of the abdomen.(2, 116, 124, 125) Even though the patient has been spayed, meaning that she cannot become pregnant or sustain a pregnancy, she is still producing estrogen from her residual ovarian tissue.(2) The presence of estrogen triggers behavioral signs of estrus.(2, 124)

    Errors in surgical technique increase the likelihood of ORS.(2, 124) For example, an incision that is too small may prevent the surgeon from adequately visualizing and exteriorizing one or both ovaries.(2, 124) When poor visualization occurs intraoperatively, a sliver of one or both ovaries may accidentally become incorporated into a ligature.(2, 124) This remnant of tissue remains vascularized by the omentum.(124) Vascularized, vital tissue is hormonally active and will produce estrogen.(2)

Cats with ORS are likely to demonstrate sexual receptivity in one or more of the following ways.(2, 61, 124–128)

- They may develop vulvar discharge.
- They may attract tomcats.
- They may exhibit lordosis.
- They may roll side to side.
- They may tread with the hind limbs.
- They may tuck their tail to the side in preparation for mating.
- They may tolerate mounting by the male.
- They may even tolerate intromission.

3. What are your recommendations for confirming your presumptive diagnosis?
    ORS can be confirmed by:(124, 127, 129)

- hormone assays
- ultrasonography
- vaginal cytology.

Note that many practitioners do not feel comfortable evaluating vaginal cytology in a cat because this procedure is not commonly performed in clinical practice unless you work very closely with cat breeders or are yourself a theriogenologist.

Because Bailey was recently spayed and her behavior is consistent with estrus, there is a high index of suspicion that she has ORS. This suspicion warrants an exploratory laparotomy to find and remove the remnant(s).(2) Unless the remnant(s) is/are removed, Bailey will continue to exhibit estrous behavior.(2)

CLINICAL PEARLS

- Clients that present purebred patients to the clinic appreciate when you take the time to familiarize yourself with breed characteristics and/or breed predispositions to disease.

- It's not possible to know everything about every breed and there have been instances when I actually knew nothing about the breed that was standing before me. In those cases, it helps to be transparent about your knowledge gap. ("I would like to know more about this breed, but I've never met a cat like this before . . .").

- Communication skills that will help include (1) eliciting the client's perspective ("May I ask what made you decide upon this breed?") and (2) assessing the client's knowledge ("Can you tell me more about this breed?").

- Clients will appreciate that you (1) make the effort when possible to do your homework and (2) include them in the conversation as an expert in their own right. Cat fanciers may well know more about their breed than you do, and it is important that we take the time to listen.

- Breed characteristics are not just about aesthetics, such as points and coat color, although knowledge of these basics helps to establish trust and create a connection between you and the client.

- There are often breed-specific predispositions to disease. Siamese cats, for instance, are predisposed to mammary neoplasia, among other potentially life-limiting conditions.

- Intact female cats are at an increased risk for development of mammary neoplasia.

- When cats develop mammary cancer, the condition is almost always malignant.

- Spaying cats is protective against mammary cancer. This protective benefit decreases as cats age, which is why many practitioners recommend prepubertal sterilization.

- Spaying cats traditionally has been defined as ovariohysterectomy. However, an acceptable alternate approach that is growing in popularity and is considered to be the standard of care in much of Europe is the ovariectomy.

- Although historically ovariectomies have raised concern that the patients are at risk of developing uterine pathology, the risk is in fact quite low. Pyometras are relatively uncommon in cats and can be surgically or medically managed. Uterine cancer is uncommon and when it occurs, hysterectomy is often curative.

- Ovariectomies are minimally invasive as compared to ovariohysterectomies, especially when performed using laparoscopy.

- Abdominal hemorrhage is a potential surgical complication. When it occurs due to sterilization surgery in female cats, it may be due to slipped ligatures. Transfixation ligatures may provide greater security when it comes to fully occluding the vascular ovarian pedicle and/or uterine body.

- Abdominal hemorrhage can also result from accidentally cutting through the ovarian pedicle or uterine body with clamps. These tissues are more fragile and thinner in the cat than in the dog and may more easily tear. If you are concerned about the potential for shearing through rather than crushing these tissues with clamps, then ligate without them.

- ORS is a relatively uncommon condition in which a sliver of ovarian tissue is left behind in the patient. This tissue can remain vital due to omental blood supply, allowing for continued production of estrogen. This will result in the continuation of estrous behaviors post-spay that will persist until the remnant(s) is/are removed.

- Exploratory laparotomy allows for diagnostic confirmation and resolution by finding and excising the remnant(s).

References

1. Englar RE. Performing the small animal physical examination. Hoboken, NJ: Wiley/Blackwell; 2017.
2. Englar RE. Common clinical presentations in dogs and cats. Hoboken, NJ: Wiley/Blackwell; 2019.
3. Maxie MG. Jubb, Kennedy, and Palmer's pathology of domestic animals. 6th ed. 3 vols. St. Louis, MO: Elsevier; 2016.
4. Miller WH, Griffin CE, Campbell KL, Muller GH, Scott DW. Muller and Kirk's small animal dermatology. 7th ed. St. Louis, MO: Elsevier; 2013.
5. van Grouw H. What colour is that sparrow? A case study: colour aberrations in the house sparrow Passer domesticus. Intern Stud Sparrows 2012;36(1):30–55.
6. McCannon-Collier M, Davis KL. Siamese cats: everything about Acquisition, care, nutrition, behavior, health care, and breeding. Hauppauge, NY: Barron's Educational Series, Inc.; 1992.
7. Kaas JH. Serendipity and the Siamese cat: the discovery that genes for coat and eye pigment affect the brain. ILAR J 2005;46(4):357–63.
8. Stokking LB, Campbell KC. Disorders of pigmentation. In: Campbell KC, editor. Small animal dermatology secrets. Philadelphia, PA: Hanley & Belfus; 2004. p. 352–5.
9. Association CF, Cat Colors FAQ. Cat color genetics. n.d. Available from: http://www.fanciers.com/other-faqs/color-genetics.html.

10. Lyons LA, Imes DL, Rah HC, Grahn RA. Tyrosinase mutations associated with Siamese and Burmese patterns in the domestic cat (Felis catus). Anim Genet 2005;36(2):119–26.

11. Ye XC, Pegado V, Patel MS, Wasserman WW. Strabismus genetics across a spectrum of eye misalignment disorders. Clin Genet 2014;86(2):103–11.

12. Gebhardt RH, Pond G, Raleigh I. A Standard guide to cat breeds. New York: McGraw-Hill; 1979.

13. Gough A, Thomas A, O'Neill D. ed., Breed predispositions to disease in dogs and cats. 3rd ed. Hoboken, NJ: Wiley; 2018.

14. Friberg C. Feline facial dermatoses. Vet Clin North Am Small Anim Pract 2006;36(1):115–40.

15. Foil CS. Facial, pedal, and other regional dermatoses. Vet Clin North Am Small Anim Pract 1995;25(4):923–44.

16. Ashley P. Non-endocrine alopecia. In: Coyner KS, editor. Clinical atlas of canine and feline dermatology. Hoboken, NJ: John Wiley & Sons, Inc.; 2020.

17. Bystryn JC. Immune mechanisms in vitiligo. Clin Dermatol 1997;15(6):853–61.

18. Naughton GK, Mahaffey M, Bystryn JC. Antibodies to surface antigens of pigmented cells in animals with vitiligo. Proc Soc Exp Biol Med 1986;181(3):423–6.

19. van der Linde-Sipman JS, Niewold TA, Tooten PC, de Neijs-Backer M, Gruys E. Generalized AA-amyloidosis in Siamese and Oriental cats. Vet Immunol Immunopathol 1997;56(1–2):1–10.

20. Loevy HT. Cytogenetic analysis of Siamese cats with cleft palate. J Dent Res 1974;53(2):453–6.

21. Forbes DC, Leishman DE. Megaesophagus in a cat. Can Vet J 1985;26(11):354–6.

22. Lamb CR, Forster-van Hijfte MA, White RN, McEvoy FJ, Rutgers HC. Ultrasonographic diagnosis of congenital portosystemic shunt in 14 cats. J Small Anim Pract 1996;37(5):205–9.

23. Kyles AE, Hardie EM, Mehl M, Gregory CR. Evaluation of ameroid ring constrictors for the management of single extrahepatic portosystemic shunts in cats: 23 cases (1996–2001). J Am Vet Med Assoc 2002;220(9):1341–7.

24. Moses L, Harpster NK, Beck KA, Hartzband L. Esophageal motility dysfunction in cats: a study of 44 cases. J Am Anim Hosp Assoc 2000;36(4):309–12.

25. Pearson H, Gaskell CJ, Gibbs C, Waterman A. Pyloric and oesophageal dysfunction in the cat. J Small Anim Pract 1974;15(8):487–501.

26. Syrcle JA, Gambino JM, Kimberlin WW. Treatment of pyloric stenosis in a cat via pylorectomy and gastroduodenostomy (Billroth I procedure). J Am Vet Med Assoc 2013;242(6):792–7.

27. Turk MA, Gallina AM, Russell TS. Nonhematopoietic gastrointestinal neoplasia in cats: a retrospective study of 44 cases. Vet Pathol 1981;18(5):614–20.

28. Cribb AE. Feline gastrointestinal adenocarcinoma: a review and retrospective study. Can Vet J 1988;29(9):709–12.

29. Patnaik AK, Liu SK, Johnson GF. Feline intestinal adenocarcinoma. A clinicopathologic study of 22 cases. Vet Pathol 1976;13(1):1–10.

30. Diters RW, Walsh KM. Feline basal cell tumors: a review of 124 cases. Vet Pathol 1984;21(1):51–6.

31. Sorenmo KU, Worley. Dr, Goldschmidt MH. Tumors of the mammary gland. Withrow and MacEwen's small animal clinical oncology. 5th ed. St. Louis, MO: Elsevier Saunders; 2013. p. 538–56.

32. Hayes HM, Jr., Milne KL, Mandell CP. Epidemiological features of feline mammary carcinoma. Vet Rec 1981;108(22):476–9.

33. Ito T, Kadosawa T, Mochizuki M, Matsunaga S, Nishimura R, Sasaki N. Prognosis of malignant mammary tumor in 53 cats. J Vet Med Sci 1996;58(8):723–6.

34. Patnaik AK, Liu SK, Hurvitz AI, McClelland AJ. Nonhematopoietic neoplasms in cats. J Natl Cancer Inst 1975;54(4):855–60.

35. Giménez F, Hecht S, Craig LE, Legendre AM. Early detection, aggressive therapy: optimizing the management of feline mammary masses. J Feline Med Surg 2010;12(3):214–24.

36. Silva MN, Leite JS, Mello MF, Silva KV, Corgozinho KB, de Souza HJ, et al. Histologic evaluation of Ki-67 and cleaved caspase-3 expression in feline mammary carcinoma. J Feline Med Surg 2017;19(4):440–5.

37. Miller MA, Nelson SL, Turk JR, Pace LW, Brown TP, Shaw DP, et al. Cutaneous neoplasia in 340 cats. Vet Pathol 1991;28(5):389–95.

38. Schmidt JM, North SM, Freeman KP, Ramiro-Ibañez F. Feline paediatric oncology: retrospective assessment of 233 tumours from cats up to one year (1993 to 2008). J Small Anim Pract 2010;51(6):306–11.

39. Ciribassi J. Understanding behavior: feline hyperesthesia syndrome. Compend Contin Educ Vet 2009;31(3):E10.

40. de Lorimier LP. Feline hyperesthesia syndrome. Compend Contin Educ Vet 2009;31(6):E4.

41. Tuttle J. Feline hyperesthesia syndrome. J Am Vet Med Assoc 1980;176(1):47.

42. Hague DW, Humphries HD, Mitchell MA, Shelton GD. Risk factors and outcomes in cats with acquired myasthenia gravis (2001–2012). J Vet Intern Med 2015;29(5):1307–12.

43. Sawyer LS, Moon-Fanelli AA, Dodman NH. Psychogenic alopecia in cats: 11 cases (1993–1996). J Am Vet Med Assoc 1999;214(1):71–4.

44. Borns-Weil S, Emmanuel C, Longo J, Kini N, Barton B, Smith A, Dodman NH. A case-control study of compulsive wool-sucking in Siamese and Birman cats (n = 204). J Vet Behav 2015;10(6):543–8.

45. Glaze MB. Congenital and hereditary ocular abnormalities in cats. Clin Tech Small Anim Pract 2005;20(2):74–82.

46. Laguna F, Leiva M, Costa D, Lacerda R, Peña Gimenez T. Corneal grafting for the treatment of feline corneal sequestrum: a retrospective study of 18 eyes (13 cats). Vet Ophthalmol 2015;18(4):291–6.

47. Laguna F, Leiva M, Costa D, Lacerda R, Peña Gimenez T. Corneal necrosis and sequestration in the cat: a review and record of 100 cases. Veterinary Ophthalmol 1988;29(7):476–86.

48. Keller GG, Reed AL, Lattimer JC, Corley EA. Hip dysplasia: a feline population study. Vet Radiol Ultrasound 1999;40(5):460–4.

49. Crawley AC, Muntz FH, Haskins ME, Jones BR, Hopwood JJ. Prevalence of mucopolysaccharidosis type VI mutations in Siamese cats. J Vet Intern Med 2003;17(4):495–8.

50. Dye JA, McKiernan BC, Rozanski EA, Hoffmann WE, Losonsky JM, Homco LD, et al. Bronchopulmonary disease in the cat: historical, physical, radiographic, clinicopathologic, and pulmonary functional evaluation of 24 affected and 15 healthy cats. J Vet Intern Med 1996;10(6):385–400.

51. Moise NS, Wiedenkeller D, Yeager AE, Blue JT, Scarlett J. Clinical, radiographic, and bronchial cytologic features of cats with bronchial disease: 65 cases (1980–1986). J Am Vet Med Assoc 1989;194(10):1467–73.

52. Dorn CR, Taylor DO, Schneider R, Hibbard HH, Klauber MR. Survey of animal neoplasms in Alameda and Contra Costa Counties, California. II. Cancer morbidity in dogs and cats from Alameda County. J Natl Cancer Inst 1968;40(2):307–18.

53. Misdorp W, Romijn A, Hart AA. Feline mammary tumors: a case-control study of hormonal factors. Anticancer Res 1991;11(5):1793–7.

54. Overley B, Shofer FS, Goldschmidt MH, Sherer D, Sorenmo KU. Association between ovarihysterectomy and feline mammary carcinoma. J Vet Intern Med 2005;19(4):560–3.

55. Howe LM. Current perspectives on the optimal age to spay/castrate dogs and cats. Vetmed (Auckl) 2015;6:171–80.

56. Overley B, Shofer FS, Goldschmidt MH, Sherer D, Sorenmo KU. Association between ovarihysterectomy and feline mammary carcinoma. J Vet Intern Med 2005;19(4):560–3.

57. Straw RC. The cat with skin lumps and bumps. In: Rand J, editor. Problem-based feline medicine. Edinburgh. New York: Saunders; 2006. p. 1067–80.

58. Tilley LP, Smith FWK. Mammary gland tumors – cats. In: Tilley LP, Smith FWK, editors. The 5-minute veterinary consult: canine and feline. 3rd ed. Baltimore, MD: Lippincott Williams & Wilkins; 2004. p. 804–5.

59. Lana SE, Rutteman GR, Withrow SJ. Tumors of the mammary gland. In: Withrow SJ, Vail DM, editors. Withrow and MacEwen's small animal clinical oncology. 4th ed. ed. St. Louis, MO: Saunders; 2007. p. 629.

60. Rijnberk A, Sluijs FJ. Medical history and physical examination in companion animals. 2nd ed. New York: Saunders/Elsevier; 2009.

61. Englar RE. Performing the small animal physical examination. Hoboken, NJ: Wiley; 2017.

62. Rutteman GR, Teske E. Mammary glands. In: Rijnberk A, van Sluijs FJ, editors. Medical history and physical examination in companion animals. Philadelphia: Elsevier; 2009. p. 132–4.

63. Evans HE, Christensen GC. The urogenital system. In: Evans HE, Miller ME, editors. Miller's anatomy of the dog. 3rd ed. Philadelphia: W. B. Saunders; 1993. p. 494–558.

64. Hayes AA, Mooney S. Feline mammary tumors. Vet Clin North Am Small Anim Pract 1985;15(3):513–20.

65. Reichler IM. Gonadectomy in cats and dogs: a review of risks and benefits. Reprod Domest Anim 2009;44;Suppl 2:29–35.

66. Hagman R, Ström Holst B, Möller L, Egenvall A. Incidence of pyometra in Swedish insured cats. Theriogenology 2014;82(1):114–20.

67. Root Kustritz MV. Population control in small animals. Vet Clin North Am Small Anim Pract 2018;48(4): 721–32.

68. McKenzie B. Evaluating the benefits and risks of neutering dogs and cats. CAB Rev 2010;5(45).

69. Biddle D, Macintire DK. Obstetrical emergencies. Clin Tech Small Anim Pract 2000;15(2):88–93.

70. Dow C. The cystic hyperplasia-pyometra complex in the bitch. J Comp Pathol 1959;69:237–50.

71. Johnson SD, Root Kustritz MV, Olsen PN. Disorders of the canine uterus and uterine tubes (oviducts). In: Johnston SD, Root Kustritz KM, Olson PN, editors. Canine and feline theriogenology. Philadelphia, PA: W.B. Saunders; 2001. p. 206–20.

72. Kustritz MV. Early spay-neuter: clinical considerations. Clin Tech Small Anim Pract 2002;17(3):124–8.

73. Stubbs WP, Bloomberg MS, Scruggs SL, Shille VM, Lane TJ. Effects of prepubertal gonadectomy on physical and behavioral development in cats. J Am Vet Med Assoc 1996;209(11):1864–71.

74. Root MV, Johnston SD, Olson PN. The effect of prepuberal and postpuberal gonadectomy on radial physeal closure in male and female domestic cats. Vet Radiol Ultrasound 1997;38(1):42–7.

75. McCann TM, Simpson KE, Shaw DJ, Butt JA, Gunn-Moore DA. Feline diabetes mellitus in the UK: the prevalence within an insured cat population and a questionnaire-based putative risk factor analysis. J Feline Med Surg 2007;9(4):289–99.

76. Panciera DL, Thomas CB, Eicker SW, Atkins CE. Epizootiologic patterns of diabetes mellitus in cats: 333 cases (1980–1986). J Am Vet Med Assoc 1990;197(11):1504–8.

77. Prahl A, Guptill L, Glickman NW, Tetrick M, Glickman LT. Time trends and risk factors for diabetes mellitus in cats presented to veterinary teaching hospitals. J Feline Med Surg 2007;9(5):351–8.

78. Belsito KR, Vester BM, Keel T, Graves TK, Swanson KS. Impact of ovariohysterectomy and food intake on body composition, physical activity, and adipose gene expression in cats. J Anim Sci 2009;87(2):594–602.

79. Mitsuhashi Y, Chamberlin AJ, Bigley KE, Bauer JE. Maintenance energy requirement determination of cats after spaying. Br J Nutr 2011;106;Suppl 1:S135–8.

80. Torres de la Riva G, Hart BL, Farver TB, Oberbauer AM, Messam LL, Willits N, Hart LA. Neutering dogs: effects on joint disorders and cancers in golden retrievers. PLOS ONE 2013;8(2):e55937.

81. Slauterbeck JR, Pankratz K, Xu KT, Bozeman SC, Hardy DM. Canine ovariohysterectomy and orchiectomy increases the prevalence of ACL injury. Clin Orthop Relat Res 2004;429(429):301–5.

82. Hart BL, Hart LA, Thigpen AP, Willits NH. Long-term health effects of neutering dogs: comparison of Labrador Retrievers with Golden Retrievers. PLOS ONE 2014;9(7):e102241.

83. Luescher A. Behavioral disorders. In: Ettinger SJ, Feldman EC, editors. Textbook of veterinary internal medicine. One. St. Louis, MO: Elsevier; 2005. p. 183–9.

84. O'Farrell V, Peachey E. Behavioural effects of ovariohysterectomy on hitches. J Small Anim Pract 1990;31(12):595–8.

85. Podberscek AL, Serpell JA. The English Cocker Spaniel: preliminary findings on aggressive behaviour. Appl Anim Behav Sci 1996;47(1–2):75–89.

86. Wright JC, Nesselrote MS. Classification of behavior problems in dogs: distributions of age, breed, sex and reproductive status. Appl Anim Behav Sci 1987;19(1–2):169–78.

87. Kim HH, Yeon SC, Houpt KA, Lee HC, Chang HH, Lee HJ. Effects of ovariohysterectomy on reactivity in German Shepherd dogs. Vet J 2006;172(1):154–9.

88. Cooley DM, Beranek BC, Schlittler DL, Glickman NW, Glickman LT, Waters DJ. Endogenous gonadal hormone exposure and bone sarcoma risk. Cancer Epidemiol Biomarkers Prev 2002;11(11):1434–40.

89. Ru G, Terracini B, Glickman LT. Host related risk factors for canine osteosarcoma. Vet J 1998;156(1):31–9.

90. Knapp DW, Glickman NW, Denicola DB, Bonney PL, Lin TL, Glickman LT. Naturally-occurring canine transitional cell carcinoma of the urinary bladder A relevant model of human invasive bladder cancer. Urol Oncol 2000;5(2):47–59.

91. Beauvais W, Cardwell JM, Brodbelt DC. The effect of neutering on the risk of urinary incontinence in bitches – a systematic review. J Small Anim Pract 2012;53(4):198–204.

92. Stöcklin-Gautschi NM, Hässig M, Reichler IM, Hubler M, Arnold S. The relationship of urinary incontinence to early spaying in bitches. J Reprod Fertil Suppl 2001;57:233–6.

93. Thrusfield MV, Holt PE, Muirhead RH. Acquired urinary incontinence in bitches: its incidence and relationship to neutering practices. J Small Anim Pract 1998;39(12):559–66.

94. Arnold S, Arnold P, Hubler M, Casal M, Rüsch P. [Urinary incontinence in spayed female dogs: frequency and breed disposition]. Schweiz Arch Tierheilkd 1989;131(5):259–63.

95. Coates JR, Kerl ME. Micturition disorders. In: Morgan RV, editor. Handbook of small animal practice. St. Louis, MO: Saunders Elsevier; 2008. p. 540–50.

96. Gregory SP. Developments in the understanding of the pathophysiology of urethral sphincter mechanism incompetence in the bitch. Br Vet J 1994;150(2):135–50.

97. de Bleser B, Brodbelt DC, Gregory NG, Martinez TA. The association between acquired urinary sphincter mechanism incompetence in bitches and early spaying: a case-control study. Vet J 2011;187(1):42–7.

98. Howe LM, Slater MR, Boothe HW, Hobson HP, Fossum TW, Spann AC, Wilkie WS. Long-term outcome of gonadectomy performed at an early age or traditional age in cats. J Am Vet Med Assoc 2000;217(11):1661–5.

99. Root Kustritz MV. Early spay-neuter in the cat: effect on development of obesity and metabolic rate. Vet Clin Nutr 1995;2:132.

100. Cooke PS, Naaz A. Role of estrogens in adipocyte development and function. Exp Biol Med (Maywood) 2004;229(11):1127–35.

101. Lund EM, Armstrong PJ, Kirk CA, Klausner JS. Prevalence and risk factors for obesity in adult cats from private US veterinary practices. Int J Appl Res Vet Med 2005;3:88–96.

102. Scarlett JM, Donoghue S, Saidla J, Wills J. Overweight cats: prevalence and risk factors. Int J Obes Relat Metab Disord 1994;18;Suppl 1:S22–8.

103. German AJ, Holden SL, Moxham GL, Holmes KL, Hackett RM, Rawlings JM. A simple, reliable tool for owners to assess the body condition of their dog or cat. J Nutr 2006;136(7);Suppl:2031S–3S SS.

104. Bjornvad CR, Nielsen DH, Armstrong PJ, McEvoy F, Hoelmkjaer KM, Jensen KS, et al. Evaluation of a nine-point body condition scoring system in physically inactive pet cats. Am J Vet Res 2011;72(4):433–7.

105. Fransson BA. Ovaries and uterus. In: Tobias KM, Johnston SA, editors. Veterinary surgery: small animal. St. Louis, MO: Saunders; 2012.

106. DeTora M, McCarthy RJ. Ovariohysterectomy versus ovariectomy for elective sterilization of female dogs and cats: is removal of the uterus necessary? J Am Vet Med Assoc 2011;239(11):1409–12.

107. Van Goethem B, Schaefers-Okkens A, Kirpensteijn J. Making a rational choice between ovariectomy and ovariohysterectomy in the dog: a discussion of the benefits of either technique. Vet Surg 2006;35(2):136–43.

108. van Nimwegen SA, Kirpensteijn J. Laparoscopic ovariectomy in cats: comparison of laser and bipolar electrocoagulation. J Feline Med Surg 2007;9(5):397–403.

109. Furneaux RW. Ovariectomy or ovariohysterectomy? J Feline Med Surg 2011;13(3):162.

110. Klein MK. Tumors of the female reproductive system. In: Withrow S, Vail D, editors. Small animal clinical oncology. 4th ed. St. Louis, MO: Elsevier Science; 2007. p. 613–4.

111. Ortega-Pacheco A, Segura-Correa JC, Jimenez-Coello M, Linde Forsberg C. Reproductive patterns and reproductive pathologies of stray bitches in the tropics. Theriogenology 2007;67(2):382–90.

112. Brodey RS, Roszel JF. Neoplasms of the canine uterus, vagina, and vulva: a clinicopathologic survey of 90 cases. J Am Vet Med Assoc 1967;151(10):1294–307.

113. Cotchin E. Neoplasia in the dog. Vet Rec 1954;66:382–90.

114. Peeters ME, Kirpensteijn J. Comparison of surgical variables and short-term postoperative complications in healthy dogs undergoing ovariohysterectomy or ovariectomy. J Am Vet Med Assoc 2011;238(2):189–94.

115. Tobias KM. Ovariohysterectomy. In: Tobias KM, editor. Manual of small animal soft tissue surgery. Ames, IA: Wiley/Blackwell; 2010.

116. Langley-Hobbs SJ. Female Ge nital Tract. In. In: Langley-Hobbs SJ, Demetriou J, Ladlow JF, editors. Feline soft tissue and general surgery. New York: Saunders/Elsevier; 2014.

117. Hedlund CS. Surgery of the reproductive and Ge nital systems. In: Fossum TW, Duprey LP, O'Connor D, editors. Small animal surgery. 3rd ed. Boston, MA: Elsevier; 2007.

118. Evans HE, Miller ME. Miller's anatomy of the dog. 4th ed. St. Louis, MO: Elsevier; 2013.

119. Pratschke KM. Abdominal wall hernias and ruptures. In: Langley-Hobbs SJ, Demetriou J, Ladlow JF, editors. Feline soft tissue and general surgery. New York: Saunders/Elsevier; 2014.

120. Smeak DD. Abdominal wall reconstruction and hernias. In: Tobias KM, Johnston SA, editors. Veterinary surgery: small animal. Two. St. Louis, MO: Saunders; 2012. p. 1353–79.

121. Fossum TW. Surgery of the abdominal cavity. In: Fossum TW, Duprey LP, O'Connor D, editors. Small animal surgery. 3rd ed. Boston, MA: Elsevier; 2007.
122. Giger U, Bucheler J, Patterson DF. Frequency and inheritance of A and B blood types in feline breeds of the United States. J Hered 1991;82(1):15–20.
123. Silvestre-Ferreira AC, Pastor J. Feline neonatal isoerythrolysis and the importance of feline blood types. Vet Med Int 2010;2010:753726.
124. Demirel MA, Acar DB. Ovarian remnant syndrome and uterine stump pyometra in three queens. J Feline Med Surg 2012;14(12):913–8.
125. Heffelfinger DJ. Ovarian remnant in a 2-year-old queen. Can Vet J 2006;47(2):165–7.
126. Miller DM. Ovarian remnant syndrome in dogs and cats: 46 cases (1988–1992). J Vet Diagn Invest 1995;7(4):572–4.
127. Wallace MS. The ovarian remnant syndrome in the bitch and queen. Vet Clin North Am Small Anim Pract 1991;21(3):501–7.
128. Rota A, Pregel P, Cannizzo FT, Sereno A, Appino S. Unusual case of uterine stump pyometra in a cat. J Feline Med Surg 2011;13(6):448–50.
129. DeNardo GA, Becker K, Brown NO, Dobbins S. Ovarian remnant syndrome: revascularization of free-floating ovarian tissue in the feline abdominal cavity. J Am Anim Hosp Assoc 2001;37(3):290–6.

Part 3

Common Cases in Adult and Geriatric Canine and Feline Medicine

Case 14

Adult Feline Wellness and Behavior

Like many cats, Ragu was an unexpected addition to the family. At the time of his arrival, his owner, Brad Greyson, had just finalized his divorce from Scarlett, his wife of 10 years. Brad was just getting his feet back under him and was not looking for any additional commitments. He lived alone, and neither he nor Scarlett shared children. He appreciated that his life as a bachelor was quiet and predictable. Brad's work as a financial analyst for a Fortune 500 company kept him tethered to his computer. If he was not busy crunching numbers, then he was advising the portfolio manager or meeting with investors. Brad travelled on business unpredictably, so a dog didn't quite fit into his fly by-the-seat-of-his-pants lifestyle, but a cat had not been entirely ruled out of the picture.

As if on cue, Ragu appeared. At 2 or 3 months of age, he appeared on Brad's doorstep. He was a persistent orange ball of fluff, and Brad had never been good at saying "no." It wasn't long before Ragu pushed his way past the foyer and made himself at home.

For the most part, Ragu has been the prototypical cat – independent and aloof. He does as he pleases, when he feels like it, and seeks attention when it is in his best interest.

Brad lives at the end of a cul-de-sac, adjacent to a natural preserve. Environmental enrichment is aplenty. Ragu spends most days roaming free, returning home every night. Ragu doesn't ask for much. Then again, he has everything he needs.

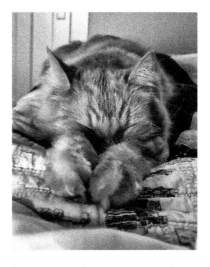

Figure 14.1 Meet your next patient, Ragu Greyson, a 4.5-year-old indoor-outdoor castrated male domestic medium-haired (DMH) cat. Courtesy of Tim Gregory.

Brad tended to Ragu's veterinary needs as a kitten. Ragu tested negative for feline leukemia (FeLV) and feline immunodeficiency virus (FIV). At 6 months old, he was neutered, and Brad has made a point to keep him up to date on his vaccinations. Ragu has been vaccinated against rabies, feline rhinotracheitis – calicivirus – panleukopenia (FVRCP), and FeLV. He is maintained on "seasonal" monthly topical flea and tick preventative – and Brad has been known to skip a dose or two. Ragu has been remarkably healthy.

Brad has no complaints other than Ragu's poor attitude at the veterinary clinic. Every time he is taken in to be examined, Ragu has an increasingly short fuse. Brad is starting to dread the annual visit because everyone at the clinic has heard about Ragu. Even though he's only been there a handful of times, those visits were more than enough for him to be labeled as "difficult" and "fractious" on his chart. It's to the point that everyone assumes Ragu will act out and be "bad." One of the veterinary assistants even called him the "devil's cat." This year, Brad scheduled Ragu's visit elsewhere. He hopes that a change in scenery might improve the experience for all involved.

Brad has arrived at your clinic on-time for Ragu's appointment today. At check-in, he makes no mention of the cat's history or "cattitude." He notes only that Ragu is unusually quiet and he is hoping that "it stays that way." Your technician is the first to evaluate Ragu. She reports back to you that Ragu appears to be "scared," but that she was able to obtain the following vital signs.

When you enter the consultation room, you find Ragu outside of his carrier, which is seated on the exam room floor, and the door to its entrance has been closed. Ragu has flattened himself at the edge of the examination table. Brad remarks that "he's never been this calm before!" You explain to Brad that Ragu is far from calm. He is visibly "stressed," and his body language exudes fear.

Weight: 12.6 lb (5.7 kg)
BCS: 5/9
Mentation: QAR

TPR

T: 100.4°F (38.0°C)
P: 240 beats per minute
R: 56 breaths per minute

Round One of Questions for Case 14: Feline Adult Wellness and Behavior

1. The clinic is often a stressor for veterinary patients.(1) Define stressor.
2. What are three main categories of stressors? Provide examples of each category. Which category(ies) include(s) the clinic?
3. Stressors elicit the so-called stress response. At its most basic level, what does this response involve?
4. True or false: The stress response can be triggered in response to a perceived threat, even if that perception proves to be incorrect.
5. What hormone mediates the stress response when stress is acute? Where in the body is this hormone produced?
6. In response to release of the hormone that you identified in Question #5 (above), which physiologic responses occur immediately in response to perceived stress?
7. What is the normal TPR for an adult cat?
8. Based upon your knowledge of reference ranges for TPR in an adult cat, how likely are the physiologic responses that you identified in Question #6 (above) to be occurring in Ragu?
9. How does stress impact your ability to deliver high-quality care today?
10. How does the stress that Ragu is experiencing today impact your ability to deliver high-quality care at his next visit?
11. Chronic stress may occur with hospitalization or with frequent veterinary visits.(2) Which hormone(s) mediate(s) chronic stress?
12. What are the long-term effects of chronic stress?
13. Differentiate fear from anxiety.
14. How can we tell the difference between fear and anxiety in our patients?
15. Provide five examples of body language that you would like to see in Ragu, which, if present, would indicate that he is relaxed.
16. Consider signs of relaxation in a different species, the dog. How might a dog's body language convey that he is relaxed?
17. Your technician picks up on the fact that Ragu the cat is "scared." Provide five examples of feline body language that your technician might have witnessed that indicate fear, anxiety, or stress (FAS).
18. Consider signs of FAS in a different species, the dog. How might a dog's body language convey that he is experiencing fear, stress, or anxiety?
19. Identify four broad categories of behaviors that dogs and cats exhibit in response to FAS. Identify which categories are most commonly observed in cats.
20. The veterinary experience can contribute to FAS by triggering various sensory pathways: sight,

sound, scent, taste, and touch. Explain how each sensory system may be adversely impacted in a clinical setting.

21. Strategize how to improve the hospital experience in each category outlined in Question #20 (above).

Answers to Round One of Questions for Case 14: Feline Adult Wellness and Behavior

1. A stressor is something that is disruptive to homeostasis, the body's steady state at which physiologic processes are able to function normally.(2–4)

2. Stressors can be categorized as follows:(1, 2, 5–7)

   - environmental – examples include confinement, noise (such as barking), and odors (such as anal glands)
   - physiologic stressors – examples include painful stimuli, thirst, and hunger
   - psychosocial stressors – examples include forced isolation or forced interactions with strangers, including physical touch (handling).(8)

   The clinic includes all three categories of stressors.

3. The stress response involves an awareness of the stimulus followed by one or more reactions to address that which has caused alarm.(9) In this way, the stress response can be thought of as being adaptive.(6) The patient's physiologic and/or behavioral reactions attempt to reset the body to its normal state of functioning.(2, 9) The ultimate goal is to return the body to baseline.(2) If this does not occur and stress persists or in fact escalates, then the patient is said to be in distress. (2) The fight, flight, or freeze response occurs in patients that are distressed.(2, 6)

4. True. Perceived threats as well as actual threats can elicit the stress response.

5. Epinephrine, sometimes referred to as adrenaline, is released by the adrenal medulla in response to stimulation from the sympathetic nervous system.(2–4, 6)

6. Epinephrine causes the following physiologic responses to occur in response to acute stress:(2–4, 6, 10–12)

   - increased energy substrates through

     - increased glycolysis
     - increased gluconeogenesis
     - increased lipolysis

   - hyperglycemia
   - tachycardia (increased heart rate [HR])
   - increased cardiac output
   - tachypnea (increased respiratory rate [RR])
   - peripheral vasoconstriction.

7. The normal reference range for feline rectal temperature is 100.5–102.5°F (38.1–39.2°C), although this range varies somewhat depending upon your choice of reference text.(13, 14)

   HR for a cat is largely dependent upon sympathetic tone. The resting HR of an adult cat in its home environment is 120–140 beats per minutes.(15) The HR of an adult cat in a clinic setting typically averages 180–220 beats per minute.(14) Stress activates the sympathetic nervous system, causing the heart to beat faster and with greater force. This pathway is particularly accentuated in cats. Stress elicits tachycardia and hypertension.(14) Collectively, this is referred to as "white coat syndrome."(14)

The normal reference range for RR of an adult cat is 20–40 breaths per minute.(16, 17)

8. Ragu is both tachycardic and tachypneic. Given his past experiences at the veterinary clinic, it is likely that both physiologic responses are secondary to stress.

9. It is difficult to deliver high-quality care to patients that are experiencing stress or are distressed. (2) These patients are likely to resist handling and/or may be intolerant of physical examination. (2) This may result in abbreviated consultations that could potentially miss out on identifying key abnormalities that require attention. For example, a significant heart murmur may be missed in a cat that is growling and/or hissing.

Patients that refuse to be examined may also prevent the veterinary team from pursuing diagnostics, even if these are rapid in-house tests that are relatively non-invasive. Again, this may lead to missed diagnoses and missed opportunities at early detection.

Certain patients may require specific testing to monitor conditions. For instance, pets with hypertension benefit from routine assessment of blood pressure (BP). If these patients are stressed, then any attempt to measure BP will be pointless because the stress response will result in epinephrine, which will create physiologic hypertension. At that point, it is difficult to assess whether BP is high chronically, due to disease, despite ongoing medical management, or whether medical management at home is effective, but momentarily lapsed due to being faced with a stressful situation.

10. Veterinary patients recall fearful situations because fear is ingrained in memories.(2) Patients remember people, objects, and places that inspire fear, such that they may be quicker to respond fearfully at the next visit. These pets may appear to have a "shorter fuse" at each subsequent visit. Indeed they do, because fear overrides learned behavior.(2) Pets like Ragu are more reactive and startle more easily because they have easy-to-retrieve memories of what happened to them at the last visit, whether those threats were real or perceived.(2) Members of the veterinary team are at increased risk of injury to themselves when they find themselves in the position of having to handle and restrain reactive patients.(1) Cats, in particular, are notorious for redirecting aggression towards their handlers.(18)

Clients also perceive when veterinary visits are stressful to their cats and may elect to spare their cats the stress by opting not to pursue follow-up, including essential check-ups and routine preventative care.(1, 11, 19, 20) This occurs more often in cats than dogs because cat-owning clients recognize that most veterinary visits take a significant toll on their pets' wellbeing.(14) As a testament to that, the Bayer Veterinary Care Usage Study asked nearly 2,000 cat-owning clients to create a collage representing their perception of their cats' experience at the veterinary clinic. The majority of cat owners used pictures from horror films.(20) Fifty-eight percent of cat owners described their cats as hating veterinary visits.(21) This perception influences how likely the pet owner is to return to the clinic for continued care. If Ragu's distress persists, then Ragu is at risk of being lost to follow-up because Brad may no longer be motivated to take him in unless he becomes significantly unwell.

11. Chronic stress causes the hypothalamus to release corticotropin-releasing factor (CRF).(3, 4) CRF stimulates the pituitary gland to release adrenocorticotropic hormone (ACTH).(3, 4) ACTH acts upon the adrenal glands to release cortisol.(3, 4)

12. Chronic stress may contribute to or exacerbate:(2–4, 6, 22)

- behavioral problems
- delayed wound healing

- feline interstitial cystitis (FIC), sometimes referred to as feline lower urinary tract disease (FLUTD) or feline urologic syndrome (FUS)
- gastric ulceration
- immunosuppression
- inappropriate behavior
- inflammatory bowel disease (IBD).

13. Fear is an emotional response to an actual threat.(2, 23) For example, Ragu may be afraid of needles because he remembers that being poked by them hurts. Anxiety is the state of anticipation of something unpleasant that is expected to occur.(2, 23) Ragu may become anxious when he is placed in the carrier for transport because he anticipates that his arrival at the clinic will be unpleasant. Both fear and anxiety trigger the stress response.

14. Our patients cannot tell us in words whether they are fearful or anxious. They can only demonstrate states that are consistent with stress through body language. These cues are recognizable to observant veterinary team members as signs of so-called FAS.

15. If Ragu were relaxed, then we would expect to observe the following:(2, 14)

- lack of tension in his face
- his mouth is closed
- his ears are forward
- his paws, legs, and tail are away from his body
- his tail is up
- the tip of the tail is shaped like the curled edge of a question mark or an inverted-u
- his pupils are shaped like vertically placed almonds as opposed to dilated saucers
- he might solicit petting, i.e. bunting.

16. If Ragu were instead a dog and that dog were relaxed, then we would expect to observe the following:(2, 14)

- lack of tension in his face
- lack of tension in his mouth, with an open mouth and loose lips
- his pupils are round, but not dilated
- his gaze is soft, rather than a fixed stare with hard eyes
- his ears are forward or midway on the head – note that this will depend somewhat upon ear carriage as defined by the breed
- his tail is level with his topline and it may wag – note that this will depend somewhat upon tail carriage as defined by the breed.

17. Your technician picks upon the fact that Ragu the cat is "scared." Signs of FAS in the cat include:(2, 14, 23, 24)

- arching of the back
- tense face
- tense jaw
- lowering of the head
- mydriatic (dilated) pupils
- "airplane ears," i.e. ears that swivel such that the inner pinna face sideways, in opposite directions, or are completely back and flattened against the skull
- open mouth, associated with growling, hissing, or spitting
- the body is tucked up to appear smaller and feet are hidden underneath of the body
- the cat may be exhibiting piloerection of fur along the topline

- the tail is curled around the body; the tail may or may not be piloerect
- the tail may be thwacking rhythmically against the exam room table.

18. Sigs of FAS in the dog include:(2, 14)

- tension in the face
- wrinkled brow
- tension in the mouth
- the mouth is usually closed (initially)
- the dog may be growling and/or barking
- the dog may exhibit lip-licking, panting, yawning, and/or paw lifting
- the lips are pulled back and may be lifted
- mydriasis
- fixed stare with hard eyes
- "whale eye" or "crescent moon eye" – that is, the sclera of both eyes is much more prominent, causing the "whites" of the eyes to visible
- rigid posture
- lowered body
- variable ear position: ears may be forward, backwards, or sideways
- variable tail position: tail may be tucked or tail may be positioned above topline.

19. Dogs and cats exhibit four main responses to FAS:(2, 6, 23)

- fight*
- flight*
- freeze*
- fidget

The starred items (*) are most likely to be observed in cats. Cats like Ragu, that are frozen on the examination room table, are often mistaken for compliant. Brad has made that mistake here.

20. The veterinary experience can contribute to FAS by triggering various sensory pathways:(2, 14)

- sight:
    - bright fluorescent overhead lights and continuous light exposure (the tapetum lucidum in companion animals intensifies their perception of light and they may be averse to lighting that is comfortable to humans) (14, 25, 26)
    - other animals in the parking lot and waiting areas
    - light reflection against stainless steel cages creates glare
    - white coat
    - strangers
    - hands of strangers coming towards them, strangers leaning over them and/or generalized lack of personal space
    - rapid motions of strangers coming towards them
- sound:
    - constant barrage of noise (i.e. several telephones ringing off the hook, the sound of the dental machine and/or drill, the sound of struggling with other patients in the treatment area)
    - other animals in the parking lot and waiting areas
    - unfamiliar voices
    - strangers shushing them ("shhhhhhhhhhhhhhhhhh" sounds remarkably like hissing!)

- scent***:
  - smells of urine, feces, and/or anal glands are aversive
  - smells of disinfectants, cleaners, and air fresheners that contain citrus, aloe, pine, or eucalyptus are aversive(23)
  - cats that have not been around or experienced dogs may experience FAS if they smell dogs in the clinic
  - cats hate the smell of rubbing alcohol(14, 30)
- taste – if medication is hidden in food and the pet tastes the medication, then the pet may associate this food with medication and discontinue eating it
- touch:
  - cold and slippery stainless steel exam room tables do not provide comfort or traction
  - being handled by strangers may be scary.

Note: ***Compared to humans, who have 2–4 cm² of olfactory epithelium, cats are estimated to have 20 cm².(14) Cats rely heavily on olfaction to communicate.(14) Unlike visual cues, which are fleeting, olfactory messages persist in the environment.(14) Veterinary professionals often forget that these olfactory cues can overwhelm feline patients because the scents are much less intense to the human nose.(14, 27–29)

21. We can improve the hospital experience in each sensory category as follows.(1, 2, 11, 14, 23)

- Sight:
  - We can adapt cats to carriers by leaving them out in the home environment.
  - We can segregate waiting areas (dedicated cat space versus dedicated dog space).
  - We can usher cats directly into examination rooms so that they do not have to wait in a shared space with other pets.
  - We can provide additional chairs or some form of customized shelf to allow clients in waiting areas to position the cat carrier high, thus making effective use of vertical space.
  - We can use towels over cat carriers to block views of hospital shared spaces that contain other pets.
  - We can use towels in the examination room to allow our patients to hide under, thus blocking them from view.
  - We can use towels over cage doors to block visual stimuli from inpatients.
  - We can provide hide spaces, such as disposable cardboard boxes, within cages so that inpatients have a place to escape to.
  - We can arrange our inpatient hospital cages in such a way that they do not face one another.
  - We can invest in cages that have been built with laminate materials instead of stainless steel because light does not bounce off of the former to create glare.
  - We can dim the lights to improve patient comfort.
  - We can take off our white coat.
  - Avoid rapid motions.
  - Make use a "slow blink" to suggest that you are not a threat.
  - Avoid direct stares.
- Sound:
  - We can use our "indoor voice" – that is, we can talk softly.
  - Use low pitch rather than high squeals when talking to the cat.
  - We can avoid shushing at cats.
  - We can make use of calm and relaxing background music:

- in both shelter and kennel environments, hard rock and heavy metal music induces stress whereas classical music induces calm(31, 32)
- consider the species that you are working with and, in the case of cats, avoid background music that emphasizes the sound of water (rain, streams, and oceans).

- Scent:

  - Recommend that clients bring objects that carry a familiar scent (i.e. a scent from home or an article of clothing that carries the scent of a favorite person).
  - Avoid placing cats in unclean exam rooms.
  - Avoid cleaning agents and disinfectants that contain citrus, aloe, pine, or eucalyptus. (23)
  - Avoid the use of rubbing alcohol when possible.
  - Avoid exposing feline patients to canine scent.
  - Prepare feline-dedicated ("cat-only") examination rooms.
  - Wipe down any and all exposed surfaces between patients: not just the floor, but also walls and cabinets.(30)
  - Use synthetic feline facial pheromone.

    - Cats possess five functional pheromones in their facial secretions: F1-F5.(33)
    - Cats preferentially deposit the F3 fraction on familiar objects, so it is thought that the F3 fraction induces a sense of security.(14)
    - The F3 fraction has been commercially produced for use in veterinary medicine (Feliway; Ceva Santé Animale) as a diffuser, carrier wipe, and/or spray.(14, 23, 34)

- Taste:

  - We can offer our patients tasty treats.(35)
  - Clients can be instructed to withhold food before a visit so that the patient comes to the clinic hungry and therefore may be more tempted to sample treats.

- Touch:

  - Avoid dumping cats out of carriers onto cold examination room tables. Instead, suggest that clients purchase carriers with removable tops. The carrier can be deconstructed around the cat such that the cat can be examined in the bottom of the carrier.
  - Some cats prefer to be examined on the clinician's lap rather than on the table. If so, allow the cat to face the client.
  - Cats typically only exhibit allorubbing and allogrooming towards those within their social group.(14) When cats exhibit these behaviors towards members of the same species, they typically limit themselves to the head and neck.(14, 23) Likewise, cats prefer the same locations when they accept physical touch from humans.(23, 28) Therefore, if you are trying to introduce yourself to a cat, start out by attempting contact in these agreeable zones rather than trying to stroke the belly.(36)
  - Use low-stress handling techniques.(23, 24)

    - Use only as much pressure as is necessary.
    - Use a touch gradient.

  - Avoid poking when you are palpating – apply gentle, even pressure.
  - Touch least sensitive areas of the body first.
  - Touch most sensitive areas of the body last (ventrum, base of tail, paws, claws, ears, peri-anal and genital regions).(1, 2, 8)
  - Use non-slip mats on exam room tables.

Returning to Case 14: Feline Adult Wellness and Behavior

You find that Ragu prefers to tuck himself out of view by hiding beneath a towel. He tolerates your cursory examination so long as he remains largely hidden, and if you approach him from behind rather than facing him head-on. You continuously assess your needs versus wants when examining Ragu and decide that you don't need to create trouble by trying to examine his face. Physical examination is unremarkable except for the endoparasites that you find adhered to Ragu's perineal fur (see Figure 14.2).

When you discuss your findings with Brad, he balks at the idea that Ragu could have worms. "How could this have happened?"

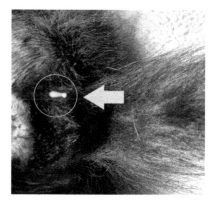

Figure 14.2 Example of the endoparasites that you find adhered to Ragu's perineal fur. For the purpose of orientation, this feline model is in dorsal recumbency and its tail is to the right.

Round Two of Questions for Case 14: Feline Adult Wellness and Behavior

1. In broad terms, which type of endoparasite have you diagnosed in Ragu?
2. What is the appropriate medical term for the segment of endoparasite that you have identified?
3. In addition to visible segments adhered to perineal fur, what other clinical signs may be suggestive of endoparasitism?
4. What are the two most common types of this parasite when it is found in cats?
5. Describe the life cycle for each parasite that you identified in Question #4 (above). Be sure to include intermediate hosts.
6. What is the pre-patent period for each parasite that you identified in Question #4 (above)?
7. How can you presumptively differentiate between the two parasites that you identified in Question #4?
8. How can you definitively differentiate between the two parasites that you identified in Question #4?
9. Is this parasite zoonotic?
10. How can you prevent this kind of parasite in Ragu?

Answers to Round Two of Questions for Case 14: Feline Adult Wellness and Behavior

1. Figure 14.2 demonstrates that Ragu has tapeworms.(14, 37, 38)

2. The tapeworm segment that you have identified is called a proglottid.(14, 37, 38) This is a terminal segment in which tapeworm eggs are stored.(14, 37, 38) Once a proglottid is full of eggs, it detaches and is shed in the host's feces. Proglottids are visible to the naked eye and may resemble grains of white rice or cucumber seeds.(38, 39)

3. Tapeworms in adult cats and dogs are usually more of an aesthetic issue and an inconvenience for the owner than it is pathological to the patient.(38) However, proglottids are mobile and may wander across the perineum. This may cause patients to experience mild itch at the rear end. (37) Affected patients may scoot.(37)

Occasionally, tapeworms become unattached from the intestines and migrate retrograde to the stomach. This may cause gastric irritation, which elicits vomiting.(37) It is possible for cat to vomit tapeworms that are several centimeters long!

Severe endoparasitism is usually more problematic in pediatric patients, whose tapeworm burden may overwhelm to the degree that they experience weight loss. (37) These patients may appear unthrifty and potbellied.(37) Their coats may be dull. They may present with diarrhea or constipation. Tapeworms may be abundant in the feces (see Figure 14.3).

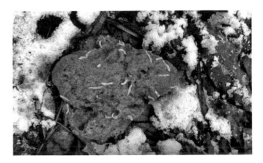

Figure 14.3 Soft stool of cow paddy consistency from a dog with significant cestodiasis. Courtesy of Michelle Lugones, DVM.

4. The most common (and therefore clinically relevant) tapeworms in dogs and cats are:(37, 40)

   • *Dipylidium caninum*
   • *Taenia taeniaeformis*.

5. The life cycles for both *D. caninum* and *T. taeniaeformis* will be discussed in brief here.

   D. caninum eggs are released into the environment when proglottids break open.(37, 38) The larval stages of the cat flea, *Ctenocephalides felis*, become infected when they consume these eggs.(37, 38) Inside of the larval cat flea, the *D. caninum* egg matures into a larval stage, the cysticercoid.(37, 38) Each flea may contain dozens of cysticercoids, each of which is capable of infecting a cat when a cat ingests the flea during grooming.(37, 38)

   Note that the flea is an important intermediate host for *D. caninum*.(37, 38) Cats cannot become infected by eating tapeworm segments or eggs.(37, 38) Cats only become infected with *D. caninum* when they ingest an infected flea.(37, 38)

   By contrast, the intermediate hosts for *Taenia* spp. are mice, birds, or rabbits.(37, 38) When these intermediate hosts ingest Taenia eggs, the eggs hatch within their digestive tract. The hatchlings then enter the intestinal wall of the intermediate host and migrate to the liver, among other tissues.(38) Within these preferential tissues, the embryos differentiate into second-stage larva, which are capable of infecting others.(38) Cats become infected with Taenia when they hunt and consume infected prey.(37, 38) Cats that are avid hunters are predisposed to reinfection.(37, 38)

6. *D. caninum* has a pre-patent period of 2 to 4 weeks.(38, 41, 42)

   By contrast, the pre-patent period for *T. taeniaeformis* in cats is 6 to 9 weeks.(38, 43) Without medical intervention, infections with Taenia may be patent for 7 to 34 months.(38)

7. Both *D. caninum* and *Taenia* spp. produce proglottids. In general, the proglottids of *D. caninum* tend to be longer than they are wide, such that they look like grains of white rice. By contrast, the proglottids of *Taenia* spp. tend to be wider than they are long. However, this is a subjective evaluation that can be challenging to discern, particularly as tapeworm segments dry out in the environment and shrivel up.

   Cats with known hunting histories are at risk of developing endoparasitism with *T. taeniaeformis*. The presence of fleas or flea dirt on physical examination are supportive of endoparasitism with *D. caninum*.(37) It is possible for cats to be infected with both.(37)

8. Definitive diagnosis is achieved by identifying eggs on fecal exam. Eggs of *D. caninum* and *Taenia* spp. are visibly distinct when they are examined via light microscopy.

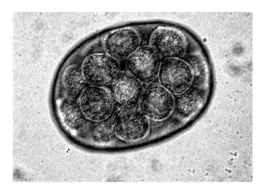

Figure 14.4 *Dipylidium caninum* egg packet. Courtesy of Dr. Araceli Lucio-Forster, Cornell University College of Veterinary Medicine.

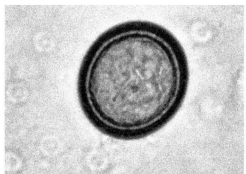

Figure 14.5 Egg of *Taenia taeniaeformis*.

Each proglottid of *D. caninum* contains egg packets, each of which houses 5–30 hexacanth ova.(38) (see Figure 14.4).

Compare Figure 14.4 with Figure 14.5, which depicts a typical *Taenia* egg.(38)

9. Yes, tapeworms are zoonotic.(37, 38) People primarily become infected when they unknowingly ingest whole fleas that contain *D. caninum*.(37, 44–46) This more commonly occurs in children, in whom hand hygiene may not be ideal.(37) Affected children may develop peri-anal pruritus and diarrhea.(37, 47)

   T. taeniaeformis is also zoonotic and isolated reports of infection in people have been published in the medical literature. These infections are rare, but can cause cysts to form within the central nervous system, eye, muscle, or subcutaneous tissues.(37, 47)

   Infection of people with other *Taenia* spp., such as *T. saginata* and *T. solium,* through the ingestion of beef or pork, tends to be more of a concern to public health.

   Infection of people with another type of tapeworm, *Echinococcus granulosus*, is of even greater concern because it causes the development of cysts in the liver and other viscera.(47) This is referred to as hydatid disease, which occurs primarily in the northern US, Canada, and Alaska.(47) Dogs (rather than cats) become infected when they are fed viscera of moose and caribou.(47) These dogs then become a source of exposure for the people with whom they interact.(47)

10. Administration of a cestodicidal drug, such as praziquantel, will eliminate immature and adult *D. caninum* and *T. taeniaeformis*.(37, 38) This drug may be given alone. However, praziquantel is frequently administered in combination with pyrantel pamoate and febantel to broaden coverage against additional endoparasites. Note that unless the source of tapeworms is removed, tapeworm reinfection will occur.(37, 38) If cats are avid hunters, for example, then they are likely to re-infect themselves with *T. taeniaeformis* unless they are prophylactically dewormed on a schedule that has been established by the veterinary team in accordance with best practices. Client communication plays an essential role in maintaining effective preventative care. Reinfection can be frustrating if clients are led to believe that a one-time treatment will be sufficient.

Returning to Case 14: Feline Adult Wellness and Behavior

After you explain tapeworm transmission to Brad, he acknowledges that he has been inconsistent with administering topical flea/tick preventative. This represents a gap in preventative care that may have led to infection with Dipylidium caninum. In addition, Ragu is a successful hunter and frequently brings home (and ingests!) his kills. Brad agrees to treat tapeworms at today's visit and that, moving forward, he needs to administer prophylactic dewormer to prevent reinfection. He elects to purchase Profender® (emodepside and praziquantel) and administer this drug topically once a month. In addition, he will recommit himself to administering once a month Frontline Plus (fipronil and (S)-methoprene) to prevent fleas and, by association, *D. caninum*.

In addition to Ragu's medical needs, you want to address his fear and anxiety to make future visits less stressful. Brad is amenable to partnering with you to improve Ragu's experience so that healthcare delivery is not hindered in the future. You discuss preparing Ragu for his next veterinary visit by acclimating him to the carrier. (Refer to Case #4 for additional information).

You also open the door to dialogue concerning recommendations to prescribe an anxiolytic agent to manage Ragu's fear prior to his next veterinary visit.

RoundThree of Questions for Case 14: Feline AdultWellness and Behavior

1. In broad terms, how do anxiolytic agents work?
2. What are broad categories of anxiolytic agents that are typically prescribed to veterinary patients? Give an example of a medication from each category.
3. What medication(s) might you prescribe for Brad to administer at home to reduce Ragu's anxiety the next time that he must be transported to the clinic?
4. What is pre-visit test dosing and why is it important for Brad to perform?
5. Brad recalls that a long time ago, he owned a dog that was exceptionally "stressed" in the veterinary clinic. The veterinarian prescribed "ace" (i.e. acepromazine). He asks if that is something that you could prescribe today. He says that it seemed to work well. How do you respond?
6. Diazepam is a type of benzodiazepine. True or false: Diazepam is safe to be given orally to cats.
7. Brad asks if there are any nutraceuticals that could work instead of these medications or to supplement them. He prefers an "all natural" approach. What do you tell him?

Answers to RoundThree of Questions for Case 14: Feline Adult Wellness and Behavior

1. Anxiolytic agents target key chemical messengers in the brain to tone down overstimulation.

2. Broad categories of anxiolytic agents include:(6, 23, 48, 49)

    - antidepressants (e.g. fluoxetine) – typically increase neurotransmitters, such as serotonin, norepinephrine, and dopamine

      - denzodiazepines (e.g. alprazolam) – typically increase gamma-aminobutyric acid (GABA), an inhibitory neurotransmitter, which reduces brain activity
      - anticonvulsants, such as gabapentin, also have anxiolytic properties.

3. In cats, I typically prescribe combination therapy that includes either:(48, 49)

    - a benzodiazepine and trazodone:

      - alprazolam: 0.125–025 mg/CAT given 30–60 minutes before needed
      - trazodone: 50mg/CAT given 1–2 hours before needed.

    - a benzodiazepine and gabapentin:

- • alprazolam: 0.125–025 mg/CAT given 30–60 minutes before needed
  - • gabapentin: 50–100 mg/CAT given 1–2 hours before needed.
- • trazodone and gabapentin:
  - • trazodone: 50mg/CAT given 1–2 hours before needed
  - • gabapentin: 50–100 mg/CAT given 1–2 hours before needed.

I have provided those drug doses that I have found to be successful to my work in clinical practice. However, to select a starting dose, I would encourage you to seek out your preferred drug handbook.

4. Keep in mind that there is individual variability in terms of response to each drug in isolation or in combination.(48) For this reason, it is important to instruct Brad to do a "test run" or trial prior to the next visit.

    Pre-visit test dosing will help you and Brad to finetune drug choice and dose before the day of the visit.(48) Pre-visit test dosing will also help Brad to know what to expect when his Ragu is medicated. If a side effect, such as paradoxical excitation, is possible, then it is important that you make him aware of what to look for and to communicate that to you so that you can work with him to adjust the dose or change the medication(s) altogether.

5. "Ace" (i.e. acepromazine) used to be prescribed in clinical practice as a sole agent because it appeared to reduce anxiety. However, it has since been discovered that acepromazine, in and of itself, is not anxiolytic. It immobilizes patients but does not reduce their fear or anxiety. It is therefore no longer advisable to prescribe ace in isolation.(48) Ace also can cause sensitivity to sound and may increase aggression.(48)

    That being said, ace can be effectively combined with other pre-visit pharmaceutical drugs to achieve both sedation and reduced anxiety.(48)

6. False. Diazepam is not recommended to be given orally to cats. Although reports in the veterinary medical literature are sporadic, diazepam has been linked to idiosyncratic liver failure in cats that have been administered it orally.(49)

7. Natural products may successfully reduce FAS, particularly if FAS is mild. However, not all natural products have been proven to be efficacious. The following products may be of benefit:(48)

- • alpha-casozephine
- • L-theanine
- • L-tryptophan.

Advise Brad that individuals respond to these products differently, and that pre-visit pharmaceuticals may still be necessary.(48) Given that Ragu's FAS is moderate to severe, you suspect that he will still require pre-visit pharmaceuticals to reduce FAS to the levels that are needed to improve his clinical experience.

CLINICAL PEARLS REGARDING BEHAVIOR

- Fear is an emotional response to a threat. Anxiety is anticipation that something unpleasant will occur.

- Stress is the body's natural response to fear and anxiety.

- The stress response attempts to restore the body to its steady state.

- In response to acute stress, epinephrine triggers the following changes in the body:

    - tachycardia
    - tachypnea
    - hypertension.

- These changes in physiologic parameters facilitate the fight-or-flight response, the purpose of which is survival.

- In addition to fight or flight, dogs and cats can freeze or fidget. Cats that freeze are often mistaken as compliant when in fact they are petrified.

- It is important that practitioners learn how to recognize body language cues that are suggestive of FAS.

- Fear-free and feline-friendly practice emphasize low-stress handling techniques in which the veterinary team adapts to the patient. This may require team members to reassess needs versus wants.

- The veterinary team should partner with the client to determine how to make the veterinary visit less stressful for the patient. This begins at home. Cats should be acclimated to carriers long before they travel.

- Patients may also benefit from the administration of pre-visit pharmaceuticals (PVPs). These exert primarily anxiolytic actions and may facilitate the delivery of care.

CLINICAL PEARLS REGARDING GASTROINTESTINAL ENDOPARASITISM

- The two most common tapeworms in cats are *D. caninum* and *T. taeniaeformis*.

- Fleas are the intermediate host for *D. caninum*. Cats (and people!) become infected when they ingest an infected flea.

- Prevention of *D. caninum* requires eradication of fleas to prevent re-infection.

- There are many intermediate hosts for *T. taeniaeformis*. Birds, mice, and rabbits are the most common among these when cats become infected with *T. taeniaeformis*. Infected cats have consumed infected prey.

- Prevention of *T. taeniaeformis* requires routine deworming among avid hunters; otherwise, cats will simply be re-infected.

- Diagnosis is straightforward: proglottid segments of either may be observed adhered to the patient's perineal fur. These segments are mobile and may cause peri-anal pruritus and/or scooting.

- Proglottid segments of *D. caninum* are longer than they are wide and resemble grains of white rice.

- Proglottid segments of *T. taeniaeformis* are wider than they are long.

- Definitive diagnosis of the species of tapeworm is obtained through fecal analysis. Ova of each have a distinct appearance.

- Both *D. caninum* and *T. taeniaeformis* are zoonotic.

References

1. Mariti C, Bowen JE, Campa S, Grebe G, Sighieri C, Gazzano A. Guardians' perceptions of cats' welfare and behavior regarding visiting veterinary clinics. J Appl Anim Welf Sci 2016;19(4):375–84.
2. Fear Free, LLC. Module 1: Fear free efforts to prevent and alleviate fear, anxiety, and stress. Available from: https://fearfreepets.com/.
3. Cunningham JG, Klein BG. Cunningham's textbook of veterinary physiology. 5th ed. St. Louis, MO: Elsevier/Saunders; 2013.
4. Reece WO, Erickson HH, Goff JP, Uemura EE. Dukes' physiology of domestic animals. Ames, IA: John Wiley & Sons, Inc.; 2015.
5. Kogler L, Müller VI, Chang A, Eickhoff SB, Fox PT, Gur RC, Derntl B. Psychosocial versus physiological stress – Meta-analyses on deactivations and activations of the neural correlates of stress reactions. Neuroimage 2015;119:235–51.
6. Levine ED. Feline fear and anxiety. Vet Clin North Am Small Anim Pract 2008;38(5):1065–79, vii, vii.
7. Clark JD, Rager DR, Calpin JP. Animal well-being. II. Stress and distress. Lab Anim Sci 1997;47(6):571–9.
8. Ellis SLH, Thompson H, Guijarro C, Zulch HE. The influence of body region, handler familiarity and order of region handled on the domestic cat's response to being stroked. Appl Anim Behav Sci 2015;173:60–7.
9. Ursin H, Eriksen HR. The cognitive activation theory of stress. Psychoneuroendocrinology 2004;29(5):567–92.
10. Currie WB. Structure and function of domestic animals. Boston, MA: Butterworths; 1988.
11. Nibblett BM, Ketzis JK, Grigg EK. Comparison of stress exhibited by cats examined in a clinic versus a home setting. Appl Anim Behav Sci 2015;173:68–75.
12. Quimby JM, Smith ML, Lunn KF. Evaluation of the effects of hospital visit stress on physiologic parameters in the cat. J Feline Med Surg 2011;13(10):733–7.
13. Rijnberk A, Stokhof AA. General examination. In: Rijnberk A, van Sluijs FJ, editors. Medical history and physical examination in companion animals. New York: Elsevier Limited; 2009.
14. Englar RE. Performing the small animal physical examination. Hoboken, NJ: Wiley/Blackwell; 2017.
15. The Merck veterinary manual. Whitehouse Station, NJ: Merck & Co.; 2016.
16. Rijnberk A, van Sluijs FS. Medical history and physical examination in companion animals. Amsterdam: Elsevier; 2009.
17. Cote E, MacDonald KA, Meurs KM, Sleeper MM. Feline cardiology. Ames, IA: Wiley/Blackwell; 2011.
18. Moffat K. Addressing canine and feline aggression in the veterinary clinic. Vet Clin North Am Small Anim Pract 2008;38(5):983–1003.
19. Volk JO, Felsted KE, Thomas JG, Siren CW. Executive summary of the Bayer veterinary care usage study. J Am Vet Med Assoc 2011;238(10):1275–82.
20. Volk JO, Thomas JG, Colleran EJ, Siren CW. Executive summary of phase 3 of the Bayer veterinary care usage study. J Am Vet Med Assoc 2014;244(7):799–802.
21. Volk JO, Felsted KE, Thomas JG, Siren CW. Executive summary of phase 2 of the Bayer veterinary care usage study. J Am Vet Med Assoc 2011;239(10):1311–6.
22. Stella J, Croney C, Buffington T. Effects of stressors on the behavior and physiology of domestic cats. Appl Anim Behav Sci 2013;143(2–4):157–63.

23. Rodan I, Sundahl E, Carney H, Gagnon AC, Heath S, Landsberg G, et al. AAFP and ISFM feline-friendly handling guidelines. J Feline Med Surg 2011;13(5):364–75.

24. Moody CM, Picketts VA, Mason GJ, Dewey CE, Niel L, Dewey CE, Niel L. Validating negative responses to restraint in cats. Appl Anim Behav Sci 2018;204:94–100.

25. Gunter R. The absolute threshold for vision in the cat. J Physiol Lond 1951;114(1–2):8–15.

26. Miller PE, Murphy CJ. Vision in dogs. J Am Vet Med Assoc 1995;207(12):1623–34.

27. Scherk M. The cat-friendly practice. In: Harvey A, Tasker S, editors. BSAVA manual of feline practice: A foundation manual. Gloucester: British Small Animal Veterinary Association; 2013.

28. Rodan I. Understanding feline behavior and application for appropriate handling and management. Top Companion Anim Med 2010;25(4):178–88.

29. Overall KL. Clinical behavioral medicine for small animals. St. Louis, MO: Mosby; 1997.

30. Herron ME, Shreyer T. The Pet-friendly veterinary practice: A guide for practitioners. Vet Clin N am. Small 2014;44(3):451.

31. Wells DL, Graham L, Hepper PG. The influence of auditory stimulation on the behaviour of dogs housed in a rescue shelter. Anim Welf 2002;11(4):385–93.

32. Kogan LR, Schoenfeld-Tacher R, Simon AA. Behavioral effects of auditory stimulation on kenneled dogs. J Vet Behav 2012;7(5):268–75.

33. Pereira JS, Fragoso S, Beck A, Lavigne S, Varejão AS, da Graça Pereira G. Improving the feline veterinary consultation: The usefulness of Feliway spray in reducing cats' stress. J Feline Med Surg 2016;18(12):959–64.

34. Da Graça Pereira G, Fragoso S, Morais D, Villa de Brito MT, de Sousa L. Comparison of interpretation of cat's behavioral needs between veterinarians, veterinary nurses, and cat owners. J Vet Behav 2014;9(6):324–8.

35. Westlund K. To feed or not to feed: Counterconditioning in the veterinary clinic. J Vet Behav 2015;10(5):433–7.

36. Heath S.. Aggression in cats. In: DH, D M, editors. BSAVA manual of canine and feline behavioural medicine. 2nd ed. Gloucester: British Small Animal Veterinary Association; 2009.

37. Englar RE. Common clinical presentations in dogs and cats. Hoboken, NJ: Wiley/Blackwell; 2019.

38. Bowman DD, Georgi JR. Georgis' parasitology for veterinarians. 9th ed. St. Louis, MO: Saunders/Elsevier; 2009.

39. Griffiths HJ. Handbook of veterinary parasitology. Minneapolis, MN: University of Minnesota; 1978.

40. Magne ML. Selected topics in pediatric gastroenterology. Vet Clin North Am Small Anim Pract 2006;36(3):533–48.

41. Boreham RE, Boreham PFL. Dipylidium-caninum – Life-cycle, epizootiology, and Control. Comp cont. Educ Pract 1990;12(5):667.

42. Fourie JJ, Crafford D, Horak IG, Stanneck D. Prophylactic treatment of flea-infested cats with an Imidacloprid/flumethrin collar to forestall infection with Dipylidium caninum. Parasit Vectors 2012;5:151.

43. Williams JF, Shearer AM. Longevity and productivity of Taenia taeniaeformis in cats. Am J Vet Res 1981;42(12):2182–3.

44. Traversa D. Fleas infesting pets in the era of emerging extra-intestinal nematodes. Parasit Vectors 2013;6:59.

45. Dobler G, Pfeffer M. Fleas as parasites of the family Canidae. Parasit Vectors 2011;4:139.

46. Kramer F, Mencke N. Flea biology and control. Berlin, Germany. Berlin: Springer-Verlag; 2001.

47. Schantz PM. Zoonotic parasitic infections contracted from dogs and cats: How frequent are they? DVM.360 [Internet]; 2007. Available from: http://veterinarymedicine.dvm360.com/zoonotic-parasitic-infections-contracted-dogs-and-cats-how-frequent-are-they.

48. Fear Free, LLC. Module 7a: Pre-visit protocols: complementary therapeutics, products, and pharmaceuticals. Available from: https://fearfreepets.com/.

49. Plumb DC. Plumb's veterinary drug handbook. 9 ed. Hoboken, NJ,: Pharma Vet Inc; 2018.

Case 15

Adult Canine Wellness and Weight Management

You have known Baguette since she was 3 months old. Her owner, Nora Parsons, has been a fan of Boxers for as long as she can remember. Her earliest memories center around the family's two Boxers, Harriet and Greta, but she had never owned her own. It was a dream of hers that had always seemed so out of reach. As a middle-school teacher just beginning her career in the field of education, Nora didn't have a lot of disposable income. Her friends had all either fostered from the local shelter or taken in rescues. They were of the mantra, "Don't shop, adopt," so part of her felt guilty even thinking about spending that kind of money on a dog when there were so many in need of a good home. Then she met Baguette, and everything changed. Baguette needed a home just like any other dog. More than that, she had been brought into this world by a responsible breeder, who had worked hard to find not just any home for her, but the right

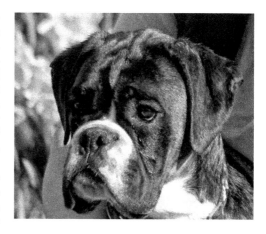

Figure 15.1 Meet your next patient, Baguette, a 4.5-year-old spayed female Boxer dog. Courtesy of Jayne Regan.

home. Nora had put in her application as soon as she saw Baguette's photo online, and she was ecstatic when the breeder chose her.

Nora made good on her promise to raise Baguette in a loving home. For the past 4 years, Baguette has never known a shortage of love. She has been reared underfoot as the only "child" and has access to everything that a dog (or even a human!) could possibly want.

Baguette has visited you over the years for routine health visits as needed, but she has never been ill. She is vaccinated against rabies, distemper-adenovirus-parvovirus-parainfluenza (DA2PP), Bordetella bronchiseptica, leptospirosis, and Lyme disease. She receives year-round monthly topical flea/tick/heartworm preventative (when Nora remembers to administer it). Sometimes Nora skips a dose here or there, but the doses that are skipped are never back to back.

Baguette presents today for wellness examination and to update her immunizations. Your technician greets Nora and Baguette in the waiting area and accompanies them to the consultation room to take Baguette's vital signs.

Baguette is her usual happy, bouncy self and it is a challenge to get her to settle for the technician to take an accurate reading on the scale. Nora jokes that "no one likes scales – and for good

Weight: 72.4 lb (32.9 kg)
BCS: 7/9
Mentation: BAR

TPR

T: 102.8°F (39.3°C)
P: 126 beats per minute
R: Panting

reason!" The technician agrees that Baguette will not be too happy with her weight because it has gone up "significantly" since last year. He asks if Baguette is "eating more than usual" because she has gained 10 lb(!) since she visited the clinic a year ago.

"That's nearly one pound of weight gain each month!" The technician remarks. "If she wants her beach body back by the time that summer rolls around, then she needs to go on a diet!"

The technician intended this to be a playful joke, but Nora bristles. She asks if last year's number could have been documented incorrectly. Baguette only looks "one or two pounds heavier" to her and "that's probably because it's been unseasonably rainy this week, so she's been pent up inside."

The technician asks, "What do you feed Baguette?" Nora is quick to respond with, "Brubaker's Adult Large Breed dry, 2 cups, breakfast and dinner. Same as always."

When the technician asks Nora if anything has changed at mealtime, she says, "no," and that "if anything, Baguette gets more exercise than she ever did before!"

Your technician updates you before you enter the room. He tells you to go easy on discussing Bageutte's weight because Nora seems "defensive."

Round One of Questions for Case 15: Adult Canine Wellness and Weight Management

1. BCS was introduced in Case 3. Review this case to refresh your understanding of how visual and palpable landmarks play a role in determining this patient-specific score. For each BCS that falls above a 5/9, the patient is an additional _____% overweight.
2. Your technician has assigned Baguette a BCS of 7/9. This means that Baguette is _____% overweight.
3. Based upon your answer for Question #2 (above), what should Baguette's ideal body weight be? Include your estimate in terms of pounds and kilograms to gain practice with conversions.
4. Differentiate overweight from obese.
5. Based upon the definition that you provided for Question #4 (above), how would you classify Baguette?
6. How common is obesity among the general pet population?
7. Which risk factors predispose patients to obesity?
8. Which disease states has obesity been associated with in companion animal patients?
9. What additional risks does obesity present for dogs like Baguette, that are brachycephalic?
10. In general, how does the client's perception of obesity compare to that of the veterinary team's?
11. It is critical that you obtain a complete diet history from Nora. Nora has already shared what Baguette eats in terms of brand name, amount, and meals. What additional information do we need to be certain that our history is comprehensive?
12. In addition to caloric consumption, what other broad category of historical information is essential to gain a clinical picture of this patient's lifestyle in its home environment?
13. Question design has a significant impact on the dietary information that you can solicit during veterinary consultations. Explain how to phrase your inquiry about the patient's diet history in order to gain the most amount of information. Be specific. Tell me exactly what words you will use.
14. Dialogues surrounding weight can be challenging.

    a. How might you seek permission to broach this topic with Nora? Give an example of the words you will choose.
    b. How might you elicit Nora's perspective about Baguette's weight gain. Give an example of the words you will choose.
    c. How might you express empathy concerning how difficult it is to manage Baguette's weight?
    d. How might you express partnership to help Nora to understand that she is not alone?

15. Define RER.
16. How do you calculate RER?
17. What is Baguette's RER?
18. Define MER.
19. How do you calculate MER?
20. What is Baguette's MER?
21. Nora claims to feed two cups of Brubaker's Adult Large Breed dry, twice daily. If each cup of this brand of food contains 340 kcal, then how many kilocalories is Baguette eating per day, assuming Nora measures out the food?
22. Assuming that Baguette is not ingesting any other source of calories, how does Baguette's intake compare to her MER?
23. Is your answer in Question #22 (above) in agreement with her weight gain? In other words, based upon what the client is reporting as her caloric intake, should Baguette be gaining?
24. How might you account for the discrepancy in Question #23 (above)?
25. Why is it important that Nora measure out Baguette's food using a digital scale?
26. What, if any, underlying medical condition(s) could be contributing to Baguette's weight gain?

Answers to Round One of Questions for Case 15: Adult Canine Wellness and Weight Management

1. For every BCS value that is above a 5/9, the patient is considered to be an additional 10% over-weight.(1) A dog that has a BCS of 6/9 is 10% overweight; a dog that has a BCS of 7/9 is 20% overweight; a dog that has a BCS of 8/9 is 30% overweight; and a dog that has a BCS of 9/9 is 40% overweight. Scoring systems for BCS have been validated for use in patients with <45% body fat.(2, 3) When the percentage of body fat in veterinary patients exceeds 45%, the 9-point scale falls short of accurately predicting body composition. At that point, body composition could only be accurately determined in the laboratory by means of DEXA.(2)

2. Baguette is 20% overweight.

3. Baguette's ideal body weight is 80% of her current weight.

   72.4 lb × 0.8 = 57.92 lb

   For convenience, let's round that to 58 lb even. Recall that 1 kg is equivalent to 2.2 lb. Therefore, 58 lb = 26.4 kg

4. Companion animal patients are considered overweight if they weigh in at over 10% but less than 20% of their ideal body weight.(4, 5) Patients that are at or exceed 20% of their ideal body weight are considered obese.(4, 5)

5. Baguette is obese.

6. Canine obesity is a common medical disease throughout the globe.(6–23) A 2010 study of dogs in the UK revealed that 59% of those surveyed were overweight or obese (21), and it has been estimated that as many as one-half of the pets in the US are obese.(24)

7. The following risk factors have been associated with obesity.(4)
   - Age – dogs that are overweight or obese are more likely to be older.(21)
   - Age of owner – dogs that are overweight or obese tend to be owned by older clients.(21)

- Income of owner – risk of obesity increases as owner income increases.(21)
- Sex and sexual status:(21)

  - female spayed (FS) dogs are more likely to be overweight or obese than castrated male dogs
  - spayed and castrated dogs are more likely to be overweight or obese than intact dogs.

- Having an overweight or obese owner.
- Having a sedentary lifestyle.

8. Obesity has been associated with the following medical conditions:(4, 25)

- cranial cruciate ligament rupture
- decreased immune function
- dermatitis
- diabetes mellitus(18, 26)
- heatstroke
- hypercholesterolemia(27)
- hyperinsulinemia(27)
- hypertension(28–30)
- hypertriglyceridemia(27)
- hypothyroidism
- increased anesthetic risk
- increased resting heart rate(28–30)
- insulin resistance(26)
- intervertebral disc disease(31, 32)
- lameness
- laryngeal paralysis
- neoplasia:

  - mammary
  - urinary

- osteoarthritis(18, 31, 33)
- pancreatitis
- reduced lifespan(34)
- reduce quality of life(35)
- tracheal collapse.

9. Baguette is a Boxer, and this breed of dog is brachycephalic. Brachycephalic dogs are known for their foreshortened faces and shallow orbits, which gives them a "bug-eyed" appearance.(1, 36–39) This "pushed in" facial appearance has underlying structural consequences. Although the length of the skull is short, the associated soft tissue structures have not been proportionally reduced.(40–42) This excessive tissue bulges into the airway lumen, increasing the chance of airway obstruction.(40) Other potential structural defects that collectively comprise so-called brachycephalic airway syndrome include:(36, 40, 41, 43–46)

- abnormal conchae
- elongated soft palate
- everted laryngeal saccules
- laryngeal collapse
- laryngeal edema
- stenotic nares.

Being overweight or obese is likely to exacerbate pre-existing structural airway disease, particularly since obesity has in and of itself been associated with tracheal collapse and laryngeal paralysis.

10. Clients are more likely to underestimate body weight than members of the veterinary team.(12, 13, 47–49)

11. In addition to brand name and amount fed, we need to know the following information to make our dietary history complete.(15, 50)

    - Whether the pet tends to be a grazer or a gorger?
    - How is the pet fed?

        - "Free-fed" (ad libitum) or meal-fed? In this vignette, Baguette is reportedly meal-fed (twice daily).
        - If there are multiple pets in the household, are they fed in separate rooms or in separate crates, or can they steal each other's food? In this vignette, Baguette is the only "child."

    - Does the pet have access to food preparation areas (i.e. the kitchen) in the home?
    - Does the pet have access to food consumption areas (i.e. the dining room) in the home?
    - Who is responsible for feeding the pet and is this the same person who has presented the patient for consultation? In this vignette, only Nora is responsible for Baguette's care.
    - What is the consistency of the food: kibble, canned, or a mixture of both?
    - Is the amount fed measured?

        - Is it "eyeballed"?
        - Is it weighed using a digital scale?

    - Is the dog food a commercially sold brand or is it homemade?
    - Is the current dog food a prescription diet that is required to maintain the patient's health or could it be changed if needed?
    - Whether anything else other than "dog food" is fed to the patient, for example:

        - dog treats
        - chew toys
        - human treats
        - table scraps
        - flavored medications
        - flavored oral preventatives (i.e. heartworm prophylaxis)
        - nutraceuticals, including vitamins and supplements.

    - Whether the patient gets into any other sources of "food":

        - garbage
        - hunting
        - scavenging
        - neighbor's pet food.

12. In addition to caloric consumption, it is important to know the patient's activity level.(15) Patients that are sedentary are at greater risk of becoming obese.(6, 15, 21, 22, 51)

13. Question design has a significant impact on the dietary information that you can solicit during veterinary consultations. In order to gain the most amount of information, you should phrase your line of questioning as follows: "Tell me everything he/she eats throughout a day, starting first thing in the morning right through to the end of the day."(52, 53)

    Veterinarians are more likely to ask a "what?" question, such as "What kind of food is he/she on?"(52, 53) When the patient's diet history is solicited in this manner, using a closed-ended question, it is rare that clients offer up more than one or two food items as answers.(52, 53) Human snacks and table scraps were only measured in 8% of consultations in which diet history was phrased this way.(52, 53)

The use of an open-ended statement, "Tell me," more effectively encourages the client to share.(52, 53) Clients are more likely to identify the patient's main diet as well as add-ons, including treats, human food, medications, and supplements.(52–54)

14. Dialogues surrounding weight can be challenging.

    a. To seek permission to broach this topic with Nora, you might ask one of the following questions.

        i. Would you be open to discussing Baguette's weight today?
        ii. Are you up to chatting about Baguette's weight?
        iii. Do you have time to talk about Baguette's weight?

    b. To elicit Nora's perspective about Baguette's weight gain, you might ask one or more of the following questions.

        i. What do you think about Baguette's weight?
        ii. What are your concerns about Baguette's weight?
        iii. I am concerned that Baguette's weight is causing some of her other health conditions. What are your thoughts about that?
        iv. Moving forward, what is going to be the biggest challenge for you?
        v. How can we make changes that set you up for success?

    c. To express empathy concerning how difficult it is to manage Baguette's weight, you might offer one or more of the following statements.

        i. I can see how difficult this is for you.
        ii. I can see how frustrated you are with this situation.
        iii. I know that this feels like a lot of work and it's not easy.
        iv. I understand that this can feel overwhelming.
        v. I know that it's hard to work on this when you have so much else going on.

    d. To express partnership so that Nora understands that she is not alone, you may offer one or more of the following statements.

        i. Let's come up with a plan that we can work on together to set Baguette up for success.
        ii. I am going to be with you each step of the way so that we move forward together, in the direction that you want for Baguette.
        iii. We're in this together. What can I do for you to help you through this?
        iv. How can I be of help so that we get through this together?

15. RER stands for resting energy requirement. This refers to the caloric intake that a patient needs to perform vital functions such as respiration and digestion.(55–57)

16. RER is calculated using the following equation: $70 \times$ (patient's body weight in kilograms)$^{3/4}$.

    For example, the RER for a 10 kg dog is equal to 70(10)3/4. The answer is approximately 400 kcal.

    This isn't the easiest formula to remember. If your patient is medium-sized, that is if s/he weighs between 2–45 kg, you can make use of the following equation, which is much more user-friendly:(58)

$$30 \times \text{(body weight in kg)} + 70$$

If we make use of that same patient in our example, then using this formula that 10 kg patient would consume 30(10) + 70 = 300 + 70 = 370 kcal.

17. Baguette's RER is:

   30 × (body weight in kg) + 70

   30(32.9) + 70 = 1057 kcal

18. MER is short for maintenance energy requirement. RER implies that the patient is exclusively at rest. However, any form of activity requires supplemental energy to sustain. Certain life stages and physiologic states (i.e. lactation) are also associated with greater metabolic demands and energy requirements. Patients that are very active (i.e. working dogs) will also require greater caloric intake. Even sedentary patients require slightly more calories than RER allows for to maintain their body weight.

19. To determine MER, you calculate RER by a specified factor. These factors vary based upon the following:(58)

   - species
   - life stage
   - sexual status
   - activity level.

   Multiplication factors can be outlined for ease as follows.(58, 59)

   - For critical care/hospitalized/recumbent patients, the multiplication factor is 1.
   - For dogs that are attempting to achieve weight loss, the multiplication factor is 1.
   - For relatively inactive dogs, the multiplication factor is 1.2.
   - For neutered adult dogs, the multiplication factor is 1.6.
   - For intact adult dogs, the multiplication factor is 1.8.
   - Pregnant dogs require a multiplication factor that ranges between 1.6 and 2.0.
   - For dogs that perform light work, the multiplication factor is 2.0.
   - Puppies and kittens require a multiplication factor that ranges between 2.0 and 3.0 because they are in a stage of active growth.
   - Lactating dogs require a multiplication factor that ranges 2–6.
   - For dogs that perform heavy work, the multiplication factor is 4–8.

   Note that these factors should not be memorized. They can be retrieved easily from any veterinary nutritional text.

20. Using the multiplication factor of 1.6 to signify that Baguette is a neutered adult dog, her MER is equal to RER × 1.6 = 1057 × 6 = 1691.2 kcal, which we can round to 1691 kcal.

21. Nora claims to feed two cups of Brubaker's Adult Large Breed dry, twice daily. If each cup of this brand of food contains 340 kcal, then Baguette is eating 1360 kcal per day, assuming Nora measures out the food.

22. Baguette is consuming LESS calories than what we calculated as her MER.

23. This is not consistent with Baguette's history of weight gain.

24. There could be several reasons for the inconsistency that was noted in Question #23.

   - The client may be underestimating how much food she is feeding Baguette. Nora claims to be feeding two cups twice/day, but is she actually measuring them or does she guestimate two "scoops" at each meal?
   - The client may not have shared a complete diet history. Nora may have shared only what Baguette consumes as meals, but left out all other edible items, including snacks.

- MER is imperfect. It provides a starting point, but by no means is it definitive. It gets the pet in the right "zip code", per se, in terms of how many calories that pet should aim to consume. However, the margin for error is significant. Patients may vary in their caloric needs by as much as 50% of the calculated value.(59) In Baguette's case, MER may have overestimated caloric intake.
- The client may have overestimated Baguette's activity, in which case a lower multiplication factor should have been applied to the equation for calculating MER.

25. It is important that Nora measure out Baguette's food using a digital scale because substantial inaccuracies abound when veterinary clients try to eyeball the correct amount. A 2019 study by Coe et al. asked clients to use three measuring tools (a 2-cup scoop to measure dry goods; a 2-cup liquid measuring cup; and a 1-cup plastic dry measuring cup) to measure three different amounts of food (1/4 cup, 1/2 cup, and 1 cup).(60) Each amount was then assessed with an electronic gram scale to determine each participant's accuracy.(60) Accuracy ranged from 48% to 152%.(60) The implications for clinical practice are alarming. A dog that is only supposed to get one cup of food could in theory be measured out the equivalent of 1.52 cups. It is easy to see how this amount, when fed long-term, contributes to weight gain. Instructing clients to measure out food on a digital scale should guard against unintentional excessive caloric intake.(60)

26. Baguette could in theory have an underlying medical condition that causes and/or exacerbates weight gain. Acquired hypothyroidism is a relatively common endocrinopathy that is associated with weight gain in predominantly middle-aged to older canine patients.(1, 61) These patients have a sluggish metabolism, such that they gain weight even when their caloric intake is appropriate.

    Hyperadrenocorticism is a second endocrinopathy that can cause weight gain because the excessive cortisol triggers polyphagia.(5) However, these patients tend to have a classic weight distribution pattern in that they often accumulate fat at and around the belly. Baguette has not taken on that Cushingoid appearance.

Returning to Case 15: Adult Canine Wellness and Weight Management

You greet Nora and Baguette in the consultation room and explain that you need to expand upon some of questions that the technician had asked. Your plan is to solicit a diet history using a different approach. You convert "What do you feed Baguette?" into an open-ended question that begins with "Tell me . . ."

Nora confirms that Baguette eats four cups of kibble per day, but she also adds that Baguette is a "beggar" and it is hard to turn her away. In addition to meals, Baguette consumes the following every day:

- a few tablespoons of cooked oatmeal at breakfast, with brown sugar topping
- one hotdog at lunch (plus the bun)
- peanut butter to coat her daily multivitamin
- three Milk-Bone® treats after her morning walk
- two sausages after her evening walk
- a "few" potato chips as snacks
- a quarter-cup of vanilla ice cream at night for dessert.

After Nora outlines the above, she pauses for moment, then acknowledges that "perhaps I'm overdoing it a bit." Although you cannot rule out endocrinopathy or other causes of weight gain without a diagnostic work-up, you agree that the most likely cause of Baguette's weight loss is overeating, particularly when many of the extras are energy dense. You offer baseline bloodwork to assess Baguette's overall health and a thyroid panel to rule out hypothyroidism. Nora agrees with your assessment that caloric intake is the most likely culprit and elects to enroll Baguette in a customized weight loss plan. If Baguette's weight barely budges after implementing this plan, then she will reconsider diagnostic testing.

Nora says she feels guilty that she "let it get this bad," but "it is just so hard to say 'no'." You validate the challenges that she has faced up to this point and commend her for being willing to set new goals for the future. "After all, you're here now," you share with her. "That's what matters."

You reassure Nora that you'll come up with the best plan for everyone involved. "Remember: dieting is not fun, but it's not about cutting out everything, it's about moderation." Nora seems agreeable. She says that she is willing to try.

Round Two of Questions for Case 15: Adult Canine Wellness and Weight Management

1. You tell Nora that weight loss is a marathon, not a sprint. What is the ideal rate of weight loss per week for dogs and cats?
2. If your patient exceeds the rate of weight loss that you outlined in Question #1 (above) as your target, then what are the potential consequences?
3. How might we propose to restrict caloric intake using RER or MER?
4. What is an alternate approach to restricting caloric intake without calculating MER?
5. Does Baguette have to switch to a prescription weight loss diet to achieve weight loss?
6. What are the advantages of switching to a prescription weight loss diet?
7. What are potential disadvantages of switching to a prescription weight loss diet?
8. Does Baguette have to switch to a canned diet to achieve weight loss?
9. What are the advantages of switching to a canned diet?
10. What are the disadvantages of switching to a canned diet?
11. What are some examples of low-calorie snacks that Nora could test out as substitutes for energy-dense treats?
12. What about snacks can you take advantage of as a strategy for increased diet adherence?
13. In addition to caloric restriction, what else is an important part of a successful weight loss plan?

Answers to Round Two of Questions for Case 15: Adult Canine Wellness and Weight Management

1. Ideally, dogs and cats should aim to lose no more than 0.5–2% of their body weight each week. (4, 62–64) This means that if Baguette were to max out on the high end of this range, then she should expect to lose only 1.4 lb during her first week of her weight loss plan. Note that each plan must still be customized to the patient. For instance, patients with comorbidities may require even more gradual weight reduction, that is, at a rate slower than 0.5% body weight per week.(64)

2. If your patient exceeds the ideal rate of weight loss that was outlined in Question #1 (above) as its target, potential consequences include weight loss at the expense of lean body mass and nutrient deficiencies as well as the potential for rebound weight gain (in cats).(4, 65)

3. In many clinical cases, including Baguette's, it may be difficult to quantify the exact caloric intake because there are so many treats and snacks to factor into the equation. Although it is possible to track down the ingredient label for every item, it can be tiresome, and clients may be tempted to take shortcuts to obtain an answer faster. Rather than counting each item on the pre-diet menu, we may elect to approach the situation using MER. Recall that MER = RER ×

[specified factor]. Recall also that the specified factor for the MER equation for weight loss is 1. Therefore, for the purposes of weight loss, MER = RER. As calculated previously, Baguette's RER for her present weight is:

30 x (body weight in kg) + 70

30(32.9) + 70 = 1057 kcal/day

However, we would like to calculate RER for her ideal body weight. Recall that Baguette's ideal body weight is 80% of her current weight:

72.4 lb × 0.8 = 57.92 lb

Therefore, Baguette's RER for her ideal body weight is:

30 × (body weight in kg) + 70

30(26.3) + 70 = 859 kcal/day

For Baguette to lose weight, she should consume somewhere between RER for her current weight and RER for her ideal weight.(4, 66) This range suggests that Baguette should eat between 859–1057 kcal/day.

The high-end may not be sufficient to allow for weight loss.(67) Therefore, in clinical practice I tended to calculate caloric intake so that it more closely matched RER for the patient's ideal body weight.

Using the selected value (i.e. 859 kcal/day), you can then develop a daily meal planner with individual items that add up to this amount. For patients like Baguette, who are used to being fed snacks quite frequently, it is important that you remember to build these snacks into the planner so that they are accounted for. Remember, it's not about cutting everything. It's about reducing. So instead of eating a whole hot dog for lunch, maybe she gets a 1 cm cube of hotdog. Or instead of eating a quarter-cup of vanilla ice cream, maybe she gets to lick the spoon.

No one is perfect. There will be cheat days. But as long as the overall plan is maintained and the client feels supported throughout the process, then the patient will be moving in the right direction.

4. For pets that have measured out meals and truly do not do a lot of snacking, it is a lot easier to quantify their current intake. If this were the case, then it is appropriate to restrict caloric intake by 20%.(4) This numerical value provides a starting point, from which adjustments can be made.

5. No, Baguette does not have to switch to a prescription weight loss diet to achieve weight loss.

6. Advantages of switching to a prescription weight loss diet are these foods tend to be high in fiber, which enhances satiety. Diets that are high in insoluble fiber with ingredients like cellulose are significantly less energy dense.(64) This means that pets can eat more of it, yet take in fewer calories.(64) Additionally, fiber takes a longer time to digest, such that patients feel fuller for longer stretches of time.(64) This feeling of fullness is enhanced because fiber digestion increases the concentration of satiety-inducing hormones, including peripheral peptide tyrosine-tyrosine and glucagonlike peptide 1.(64) When patients feel less hungry, then they beg less, which makes it easier for the client to adhere to the plan.

7. One potential downside to feeding a prescription weight loss diet is that much of what is ingested is not digested fully, causing a significant increase in fecal bulk.(64) Patients often defecate more

frequently and in larger volumes. This may be displeasing to the client, who has to dispose of this additional waste.

8. No, Baguette does not have to switch to a canned diet to achieve weight loss.

9. The advantages of switching to a canned diet is that canned food contains a high percentage of water.(64) Water is filling and therefore contributes to satiety.(64)

10. The downside to feeding a canned diet for a dog of Baguette's size is cost.(64) You're paying for mostly water and Baguette is going to require a large number of cans per day because canned food is less energy dense than dry.

11. The following are low-calorie snacks that Nora could test out as substitutes for energy-dense treats:

- baby carrots or carrot sticks
- cucumber or zucchini slices
- celery
- green beans
- peas
- broccoli
- asparagus
- rice cakes
- unbuttered, unsalted popcorn.

Fruit, such as apple slices, blueberries, cranberries, cantaloupe, and watermelon, can also be given; however, these tend to be high in sugars and calories can also add up quickly if clients are not aware of portion sizes.

12. Remind clients that dieting is about giving their dogs a taste of something amazing without going overboard. For example, if I myself were dieting, a spoonful of chocolate chip cookie dough ice cream would taste the same to me as the whole pint. If I can learn to savor the taste and slow down eating my ration of a tasty treat, then I will still feel like I got something, rather than feeling deprived.

    The same is true in terms of what we want our pets to experience. Nora doesn't want Baguette to feel cheated. Being able to offer her this list of snacks still provides her with a means of using food to reward Baguette, while cutting back on calories.

    It is important to partner with the client to create a so-called food allowance when formulating a weight loss plan for Baguette.(64) A food allowance provides for flexibility. Consider, for example, a situation in which daily treat allowance is a total of 100 kcal. What if Baguette's favorite chew is 300 kcal? Does that mean that Baguette can never again have this chew treat? No. What it means is that the client will have to prioritize the chew treat. How valuable is it to Baguette? Is it essential? If so, then Baguette can have it – but having it comes at a cost. If she gets the chew treat today, then that means for the next three days, she gets no additional treats because the chew treat essentially "cost" her 3 days' worth of snacks.

    A food allowance is a win–win. It allows clients to make room in the meal planner for special items that are facilitating the human–animal bond. And it helps our patients to continue enjoying what they love – but in moderation.

13. Frequent check-ins are part of a successful weight loss plan. Check-ins help the clients to feel accountable – and they allow for you, the clinician, to make adjustments when indicated. Check-ins also provide clients with support. Weight loss is rarely easy, and clients need to feel that they are a part of a team approach. Clients need to feel understood and respected for trying to take steps in the right direction, even if for every two steps forward, there is a step backwards. Clients need to be rewarded for their intentions, and assisted through the obstacles.

CLINICAL PEARLS

- Increased body weight is a common clinical presentation in companion animal practice.

- A patient is said to be overweight when s/he weighs between 10 and 20% more than what his/her ideal body weight should be.

- A patient is said to be obese when s/he weighs at or over 20% above what his/her ideal body weight should be.

- Patients may be overweight or obese because of underlying disease processes, such as endocrinopathy.

- Although a diagnostic work-up is always advised to provide a baseline for the patient, it is essential that you take a comprehensive diet history.

- The way you phrase your questions when taking a diet history significantly impacts the responses that you will get from the client.

- Using an open-ended statement is much more effective than "What do you feed?"

- Tell me everything he/she eats throughout a day, starting first thing in the morning right through to the end of the day.

- Clients are much more likely to provide an extended answer that includes the main food source as well as extras (i.e. treats, snacks, table scraps, and human food).

- Ideal body weight is a subjective guestimate at best. However, it provides a target weight when customizing a weight loss plan for any given patient.

- When there is no underlying medical reason for the patient to be overweight or obese, obesity most often stems from excessive caloric intake.

- Caloric restriction can be achieved by reducing intake by 20% or through calculations of MER using a multiplication factor of 1 and the patient's ideal body weight.

- Calculations are imperfect because every patient is an individual. Be prepared to adjust frequently. Schedule follow-up visits often.

References

1. Englar RE. Common clinical presentations in dogs and cats. Hoboken, NJ: Wiley/Blackwell; 2019.
2. Witzel AL, Kirk CA, Henry GA, Toll PW, Brejda JJ, Paetau-Robinson I. Use of a novel morphometric method and body fat index system for estimation of body composition in overweight and obese dogs. J Am Vet Med Assoc 2014;244(11):1279–84.
3. Toll PW, Yamka RM, Schoenherr WD, et al. Obesity. In: Hand MS, Thatcher CD, Remillard RL, et al., editors. Small animal clinical nutrition. Topeka, KS: Mark Morris Institute; 2010. p. 501–42.
4. Linder D, Mueller M. Pet obesity management: beyond nutrition. Vet Clin North Am Small Anim Pract 2014;44(4):789–806, vii, vii.
5. German AJ. Obesity prevention and weight maintenance after loss. Vet Clin North Am Small Anim Pract 2016;46(5):913–29.
6. Robertson ID. The association of exercise, diet and other factors with owner-perceived obesity in privately owned dogs from metropolitan Perth, WA. Prev Vet Med 2003;58(1–2):75–83.
7. Anderson RS. Obesity in the dog and cat. Vet Ann 1973;1441:82–186.

8. Crane SW. Occurrence and management of obesity in companion animals. J Small Anim Pract 1991;32(6):275–82.

9. Sloth C. Practical management of obesity in dogs and cats. J Small Anim Pract 1992;33(4):178–82.

10. Wolfsheimer KJ. Obesity in dogs. Compend Contin Educ Pract Vet 1994;16(8):981-and.

11. Colliard L, Ancel J, Benet JJ, Paragon BM, Blanchard G. Risk factors for obesity in dogs in France. J Nutr 2006;136(7);Suppl:1951S–1954S.

12. McGreevy PD, Thomson PC, Pride C, Fawcett A, Grassi T, Jones B. Prevalence of obesity in dogs examined by Australian veterinary practices and the risk factors involved. Vet Rec 2005;156(22):695–702.

13. Robertson ID. The association of exercise, diet and other factors with owner-perceived obesity in privately owned dogs from metropolitan Perth, WA. Prev Vet Med 2003;58(1–2):75–83.

14. Holmes KL, Morris PJ, Abdulla Z, Hackett RM, Rawlings JM. Risk factors associated with excess body weight in dogs in the UK. J Anim Physiol Anim Nutr 2007;91(3–4):166–7.

15. Murphy M. Obesity treatment: environment and behavior modification. Vet Clin North Am Small Anim Pract 2016;46(5):883–98.

16. Krook L, Larsson S, Rooney JR. The interrelationship of diabetes mellitus, obesity, and pyometra in the dog. Am J Vet Res 1960;21:120–7.

17. McGreevy PD, Thomson PC, Pride C, Fawcett A, Grassi T, Jones B. Prevalence of obesity in dogs examined by Australian veterinary practices and the risk factors involved. Vet Rec 2005;156(22):695–702.

18. Lund EM, Armsstrong PJ, Kirk CA. Prevalence and risk factors for obesity in adult dogs from private US veterinary practices. Int J Appl Res Vet Med 2006;4(2):177–86.

19. Colliard L, Ancel J, Benet JJ, Paragon BM, Blanchard G. Risk factors for obesity in dogs in France. J Nutr 2006;136(7);Suppl:1951S–1954S.

20. Corbee RJ. Obesity in show dogs. J Anim Physiol Anim Nutr (Berl) 2013;97(5):904–10.

21. Courcier EA, Thomson RM, Mellor DJ, Yam PS. An epidemiological study of environmental factors associated with canine obesity. J Small Anim Pract 2010;51(7):362–7.

22. Mao J, Xia Z, Chen J, Yu J. Prevalence and risk factors for canine obesity surveyed in veterinary practices in Beijing, China. Prev Vet Med 2013;112(3–4):438–42.

23. Heuberger R, Wakshlag J. The relationship of feeding patterns and obesity in dogs. J Anim Physiol Anim Nutr (Berl) 2011;95(1):98–105.

24. Churchill J, Ward E. Communicating with pet owners about obesity: roles of the Veterinary Health Care Team. Vet Clin North Am Small Anim Pract 2016;46(5):899–911.

25. German AJ, Woods GRT, Holden SL, Brennan L, Burke C. Dangerous trends in pet obesity. Vet Rec 2018;182(1):25.

26. Clark M, Hoenig M. Metabolic effects of obesity and its interaction with endocrine diseases. Vet Clin North Am Small Anim Pract 2016;46(5):797–815.

27. Jeusette IC, Lhoest ET, Istasse LP, Diez MO. Influence of obesity on plasma lipid and lipoprotein concentrations in dogs. Am J Vet Res 2005;66(1):81–6.

28. Chandler ML. Impact of obesity on cardiopulmonary disease. Vet Clin North Am Small Anim Pract 2016;46(5):817–30.

29. Truett AA, Borne AT, Poincot MA, West DB. Autonomic control of blood pressure and heart rate in obese hypertensive dogs. Am J Physiol 1996;270(3 Pt 2):R541–9.

30. Van Vliet BN, Hall JE, Mizelle HL, Montani JP, Smith MJ, Jr. Reduced parasympathetic control of heart rate in obese dogs. Am J Physiol 1995;269(2 Pt 2):H629–37.

31. Frye CW, Shmalberg JW, Wakshlag JJ. Obesity, exercise and orthopedic disease. Vet Clin North Am Small Anim Pract 2016;46(5):831–41.

32. Packer RM, Hendricks A, Volk HA, Shihab NK, Burn CC. How long and low can you go? Effect of conformation on the risk of thoracolumbar intervertebral disc extrusion in domestic dogs. PLOS ONE 2013;8(7):e69650.

33. Marshall WG, Hazewinkel HA, Mullen D, De Meyer G, Baert K, Carmichael S. The effect of weight loss on lameness in obese dogs with osteoarthritis. Vet Res Commun 2010;34(3):241–53.

34. Kealy RD, Lawler DF, Ballam JM, Mantz SL, Biery DN, Greeley EH, et al. Effects of diet restriction on life span and age-related changes in dogs. J Am Vet Med Assoc 2002;220(9):1315–20.

35. German AJ, Holden SL, Wiseman-Orr ML, Reid J, Nolan AM, Biourge V, et al. Quality of life is reduced in obese dogs but improves after successful weight loss. Vet J 2012;192(3):428–34.
36. Englar RE. Performing the small animal physical examination. Hoboken, NJ: Wiley; 2017.
37. Phillips H. Brachycephalic syndrome. NAVC Clin's Brief 2016 (September).
38. Schuenemann R, Oechtering GU. Inside the brachycephalic nose: intranasal mucosal contact points. J Am Anim Hosp Assoc 2014;50(3):149–58.
39. Evans HE, Miller ME. Miller's anatomy of the dog. 4th ed. St. Louis, MO: Elsevier; 2013.
40. Tilley LP, Smith FWK. The 5-minute veterinary consult: canine and feline. 3rd ed. Baltimore, MD: Lippincott Williams & Wilkins; 2004.
41. Fasanella FJ, Shivley JM, Wardlaw JL, Givaruangsawat S. Brachycephalic airway obstructive syndrome in dogs: 90 cases (1991–2008). J Am Vet Med Assoc 2010;237(9):1048–51.
42. Wykes PM. Brachycephalic airway obstructive syndrome. Probl Vet Med 1991;3(2):188–97.
43. Miller J, Gannon K. Perioperative management of brachycephalic dogs. NAVC Clin's Brief 2015 (April): 54–9.
44. Ginn JA, Kumar MSA, McKiernan BC, Powers BE. Nasopharyngeal turbinates in brachycephalic dogs and cats. J Am Anim Hosp Assoc 2008;44(5):243–9.
45. Koch DA, Arnold S, Hubler M, Montavon PM. Brachycephalic syndrome in dogs. Comp Cont Educ Pract 2003;25(1):48.
46. Findji L, Dupre G. Brachycephalic syndrome: innovative surgical techniques. NAVC Clin's Brief 2013 (June):79–85.
47. Scarlett JM, Donoghue S, Saidla J, Wills J. Overweight cats: prevalence and risk factors. Int J Obes Relat Metab Disord 1994;18;Suppl 1:S22–8.
48. Courcier EA, Mellor DJ, Thomson RM, Yam PS. A cross sectional study of the prevalence and risk factors for owner misperception of canine body shape in first opinion practice in Glasgow. Prev Vet Med 2011;102(1):66–74.
49. White GA, Hobson-West P, Cobb K, Craigon J, Hammond R, Millar KM. Canine obesity: is there a difference between veterinarian and owner perception? J Small Anim Pract 2011;52(12):622–6.
50. Eirmann L. Nutritional assessment. Vet Clin North Am Small Anim Pract 2016;46(5):855–67.
51. Bland IM, Guthrie-Jones A, Taylor RD, Hill J. Dog obesity: owner attitudes and behaviour. Prev Vet Med 2009;92(4):333–40.
52. MacMartin C, Wheat HC, Coe JB, Adams CL. Effect of question design on dietary information solicited during veterinarian-client interactions in companion animal practice in Ontario, Canada. J Am Vet Med Assoc 2015;246(11):1203–14.
53. Coe JB, editor. Practical communication tips for partnering with clients in framing their nutrition truths. Hill's global symposium: harnessing the power of the microbiome; July 14–15, 2019, Toronto, Canada.
54. Coe JB, O'Connor RE, MacMartin C, Verbrugghe A, Janke KA. Effects of three diet history questions on the amount of information gained from a sample of pet owners in Ontario, Canada. J Am Vet Med Assoc 2020;256(4):469–78.
55. Cunningham JG, Klein BG. Cunningham's textbook of veterinary physiology. 5th ed. St. Louis, MO: Elsevier/Saunders; 2013.
56. Currie WB. Structure and function of domestic animals. xiii. Boston: Butterworths, 443 p. p.; 1988.
57. Reece WO, Erickson HH, Goff JP, Uemura EE. Dukes' physiology of domestic animals. Ames, IA: John Wiley & Sons Inc; 2015.
58. Carlson E. Calculate the perfect portions for pets. DVM. 360 [Internet]; 2017. Available from: https://www.dvm360.com/view/calculate-perfect-portions-pets.
59. Center TOSUVM. Basic calorie calculator. Available from: https://vet.osu.edu/vmc/companion/our-services/nutrition-support-service/basic-calorie-calculator.
60. Coe JB, Rankovic A, Edwards TR, Parr JM. Dog owner's accuracy measuring different volumes of dry dog food using three different measuring devices. Vet Rec 2019;185(19):599.
61. Frank LA. Comparative dermatology--canine endocrine dermatoses. Clin Dermatol 2006;24(4):317–25.
62. Butterwick RF, Hawthorne AJ. Advances in dietary management of obesity in dogs and cats. J Nutr 1998;128(12);Suppl:2771S–5S.

63. Laflamme DP, Kuhlman G, Lawler DF. Evaluation of weight loss protocols for dogs. J Am Anim Hosp Assoc 1997;33(3):253–9.

64. Linder DE, Parker VJ. Dietary aspects of weight management in cats and dogs. Vet Clin North Am Small Anim Pract 2016;46(5):869–82.

65. Laflamme DP, Hannah SS. Increased dietary protein promotes fat loss and reduces loss of lean body mass during weight loss in cats. Int J Appl Res Vet Med 2005;3(2):62–8.

66. Burkholder WJ, Bauer JE. Foods and techniques for managing obesity in companion animals. J Am Vet Med Assoc 1998;212(5):658–62.

67. Blanchard G, Nguyen P, Gayet C, Leriche I, Siliart B, Paragon BM. Rapid weight loss with a high-protein low-energy diet allows the recovery of ideal body composition and insulin sensitivity in obese dogs. J Nutr 2004;134(8):2148S–50S.

Case 16

Feline Weight Loss

You have known Figaro and his owner, Kat Stevens, for the past 9 years. He'd been purchased as a kitten as a wedding gift from Kat's late husband, Jay. They had intended to grow the family together, beginning with Figaro. Kat never imagined that one day it would just be her and the cat.

These days, Figaro is a welcome distraction from the past 6 months of bereavement. Kat thinks of Figaro as her child. Since Jay's untimely passing, Kat's love for Figaro has only grown. Figaro now represents a tie to the past and in that way bridges the pain of the present to the hope of the future. Kat would do anything within her power for Figaro. He is her motivation for living.

As the fog of grief begins to lift, Kat has noticed that Figaro is exhibiting unusual behavior. He has always been a foodie, but his appetite

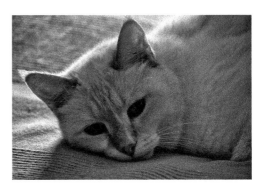

Figure 16.1 Meet your next patient, Figaro Stevens, an indoor-only, 9-year-old castrated male flame point Siamese cat. Courtesy of Kathy Knowles and Fletcher.

has recently taken an upswing. For the past month, he acts like he is starving "all the time." Every time Kat turns around, the shiny metal bottom of the food bowl is peering back at her. He's chowing down the food like there's no tomorrow, yet he doesn't appear to be putting on any weight. Kat is a stress eater, so she can relate to his binging. At the same time, it seems to have gotten out of hand. Figaro is now waking her up in the middle of the night, demanding to be fed. Kat tells the technician that "this has got to stop. I barely get any sleep as it is."

Kat also reports that Figaro is more active than usual. It's as if he's gotten a second wind. Kat shares her surprise that "he's acting like a kitten all over again!" Still, he seems "thinner" than before, almost "lankier." For a cat that used to preen meticulously, he's also looking a bit rough in the grooming department. As the technician takes Figaro's vital signs, he agrees that the cat is a bit unkempt.

BCS: 3/9
Muscle condition score: Moderate muscle loss
Mentation: BAR
Systolic BP: 220 mmHg

TPR

T: 100.6°F (38.1°C)
P: 212 beats per minute
R: 30 breaths per minute

The technician reviews the chart to consider how Figaro's body weight has changed over the past five years.

Today's Body Weight: 9.8 lb (4.5 kg)

Last Year (5/20/2019): 12.5 lb (5.7 kg)

Two Years Ago (5/22/2018): 12.7 lb (5.8 kg)

Three Years Ago (5/18/2017): 13 lb (5.9 kg)

Four Years Ago (5/12/2016): 12.8 lb (5.8 kg)

Five Years Ago (5/01/2015): 12.6 lb (5.7 kg)

The technician confirms Kat's suspicions: Figaro has in fact lost 2.7 lb (1.2 kg) of weight since his last visit. This is significant. He reassures Kat that you will "get to the bottom of this." Consider the following list of questions to help you work through this clinical case.

Round One of Questions for Case 16: Feline Weight Loss

1. Identify broad mechanisms by which weight loss occurs.
2. Of the broad mechanisms that you listed in Question #1 (above), which is LEAST likely in this patient? Explain why.
3. What are additional questions that you would like to ask Kat to investigate if one or more of the other mechanisms that you listed in Question #1 could be at play?
4. Kat reports that Figaro is "always hungry." What is the medical term for increased appetite?
5. What, if any, medications may cause increased appetite?
6. Do we know if Figaro is taking any medications that cause polyphagia? What do we need to ask the owner and why?
7. Which differential diagnoses are consistent with a feline history of weight loss despite the cat having a normal-to-increased appetite?
8. For each differential diagnosis that you listed in Question #7 (above), what are the primary historical and/or physical examination features that you would expect to hear and/or see (in addition to weight loss and polyphagia)?
9. Other than the differential diagnoses that you listed in Question #7, what is another possible explanation for Figaro's unkempt appearance?
10. After history-taking, what is your next step in the diagnostic plan?

Answers to Round One of Questions for Case 16: Feline Weight Loss

1. Broad mechanisms by which weight loss occurs include:

   - decreased consumption of food:

     - reduced appetite (and therefore, reduced caloric intake):

       - change in brand, protein source, carbohydrate source, texture or consistency; new food is less palatable
       - Illness: fever; gastrointestinal (GI) distress (nausea, vomiting, diarrhea); space-occupying mass within GI tract such that the patient feels full

     - reduced access to food
     - reduced quality of food with substandard nutritional plane

   - increased metabolic requirements:

     - increased metabolic activity
     - increased metabolic rate

   - decreased absorption of nutrients and/or increased loss of nutrients:

     - through GI tract (i.e. protein-losing enteropathy (PLE); inflammatory bowel disease (IBD), exocrine pancreatic insufficiency (EPI); endoparasitism)
     - through the urinary tract (i.e. protein-losing nephropathy).

2. Of the mechanisms outlined above, decreased consumption of food is LEAST likely in this patient. The patient history reveals that Figaro is eating MORE than usual.

3. I would like to investigate the possibility that Figaro is not absorbing nutrients and/or is losing nutrients. The history does not report any indication of GI upset. However, to be thorough, we need to ask the following questions.

    *   Have you noticed Figaro vomiting? If so:

        *   Is he truly vomiting (as opposed to regurgitating)?
        *   What is the frequency of vomiting?
        *   Has the frequency of vomiting changed?
        *   What does he vomit? (i.e. food, hairball, fluid) / What does the vomitus look like?
        *   Is there any obvious blood in the vomit?
        *   Are there any parasites in the vomit (i.e. roundworms, tapeworms)?

    *   Tell me about Figaro's bowel movements.

        *   What is the frequency of his bowel movements?
        *   Has the frequency of bowel movements changed?
        *   What is the consistency of his bowel movements?
        *   Has the consistency of bowel movements changed?
        *   Is there any frank (red) blood in the stool?
        *   Does the stool look like melena (black tar)?

Nutrients can also be lost through the urinary tract, so it is important that we invite dialogue about Figaro's urinary habits as well.

*   Tell me about Figaro's urinary habits.
*   How often do you scoop his litter?
*   Has your frequency of scooping the litter changed? If so, why has it changed?
*   Does Figaro appear to be urinating more? / Are there MORE clumps than normal in the litter box? / Are the clumps in the litter box LARGER than normal?

Thirst is also tied to urination, so we need to ask questions about how much Figaro drinks. This is not always easy to quantify in a cat. Clients may or may not notice changes in thirst. However, some changes are pronounced, so it is important to ask the following.

*   Tell me about Figaro's thirst?
*   Have you seen Figaro drink water?
*   How often are you refilling his water bowl(s)?
*   Does Figaro appear to be drinking more than normal?

I would also want to circle back to ask the following questions about his eating habits.

*   How is Figaro fed? Ad libitum or meal-fed?

    *   If meal-fed, how much food does he get at each meal?
    *   Does Kat measure the amount of food that is fed at each feeding?
    *   How is the food measured? Is it eye-balled or is there a digital scale?

*   What does Figaro eat?

As we learned in Case 15, question design has a significant impact on the diet history that you can solicit during veterinary consultations. To gain the most amount of information, you should phrase your line of questioning as follows: "Tell me everything he/she eats throughout a day, starting first thing in the morning right through to the end of the day."(1, 2)

*   Has Kat recently changed brand(s) of foods?
*   Is Figaro eating his cat food? Is he holding out for table scraps? Is he doing both?

4. The appropriate medical term for increased appetite is polyphagia.(3)

5. Glucocorticoids, such as prednisolone, cause polyphagia.(4, 5)

6. It is unlikely that Figaro is taking glucocorticoids. For one thing, because they cause polyphagia, their use is often associated with weight gain. Figaro's history of weight loss does not fit the typical clinical picture. Furthermore, you have known Figaro for nine years and based upon the details that have been provided in this clinical vignette, you have not prescribed any new medications recently.

    However, it is imperative that you ask the client if Figaro has been seen elsewhere. If so, what was his presenting complaint? Were any medications administered? Which medication were prescribed, at what dosing, at what frequency of administration, and over how long of a period? Is Figaro still taking the medication(s)?

7. Feline weight loss despite a normal-to-increased appetite can be due to:(4, 6–8)

    - endocrinopathy

        - diabetes mellitus
        - hyperadrenocorticism
        - hyperthyroidism

    - EPI
    - IBD
    - intestinal parasites
    - protein-losing nephropathy

        - glomerulonephritis.

8. Considering each differential diagnosis, I would expect to see the following historical and/or physical exam features, in addition to weight loss and polyphagia:(4, 6, 9–11)

    - diabetes mellitus:

        - expected historical features:

            - usually (but not always) older, obese, neutered male cats
            - breed predisposition: Burmese
            - PU/PD (polyuric/polydipsic)
            - history may be suggestive of urinary tract infection (UTI), which is a common sequela of this endocrinopathy. Clients may report urinary accidents (house-soiling), pollakiuria, straining to urinate, etc.

        - anticipated physical exam findings:

            - dull coat
            - muscle atrophy
            - dehydration (if systemically unwell)
            - pot-bellied appearance (if hepatomegaly)
            - pelvic limb weakness and plantigrade stance secondary to diabetic neuropathy

    - hyperadrenocorticism:(12)

        - expected historical features:

            - sex predisposition: female cats are more likely to develop this condition
            - PU/PD
            - history may be suggestive of UTI, which is a common sequela of this endocrinopathy.

Clients may report urinary accidents (house-soiling), pollakiuria, straining to urinate, etc.

- anticipated physical exam findings:
  - alopecic patches
  - delayed wound healing
  - dull coat
  - muscle atrophy
  - thin, shiny, fragile skin that tears easily (do not scruff these cats!)
  - increased tendency to bruise
  - pot-bellied appearance
  - palpable hepatomegaly

- hyperthyroidism:(8, 13)
  - expected historical features:
    - older (usually >8-year-old) cat
    - weight loss is progressive
    - appetite is ravenous – clients may report that the cat acts like s/he's on a diet – always scrounging around, looking for food
    - activity level is increased
    - clients may report that the cat acts like a kitten
    - clients may share that the cat appears restless
    - clients may report less grooming activity
    - PU/PD
    - +/– vomiting
    - +/– diarrhea
  - anticipated physical exam findings:
    - unkempt coat
    - +/– dehydration
    - muscle atrophy
    - tachycardia
    - systolic heart murmur
    - +/– gallop rhythm
    - +/– palpable thyroid nodule on one or both sides along the ventral neck
    - +/– retinal hemorrhages and other ocular changes (if persistent systemic hypertension)

- EPI:(14)
  - expected historical features:
    - stool may be normal or it may be unformed
    - +/– steatorrhea
    - +/– watery diarrhea
    - lethargy
    - vomiting
  - anticipated physical exam findings:
    - poor hair coat

- IBD:
  - expected historical features:

- - most commonly occurs in middle-aged to older cats
  - +/– vomiting
  - +/– diarrhea
  - clinical signs may wax and wane
- anticipated physical exam findings:
  - relatively unremarkable
  - patients may resent abdominal palpation if there is GI discomfort
  - small bowel may be palpably thickened
- intestinal parasites:
  - expected historical features:
    - usually kittens or young adults
    - usually cats with exposure to outdoors
    - +/– vomiting
    - +/– diarrhea
    - client may report seeing what looks like "white rice" at or around the rear end
    - client may report seeing worms in the vomitus
    - patient may have a history of fleas
    - patient may have a history of being an avid hunter and/or ingesting prey
  - anticipated physical exam findings:
    - dull coat
    - +/– potbellied appearance (common with ascarids)
    - +/– fleas or flea dirt (if tapeworms)
    - +/– pale mucous membranes (if hookworms)
    - +/– melena (if hookworms)
    - +/– peri-anal pruritus (if tapeworms)
    - proglottids may be visible adhered to perineum or perineal fur
- protein-losing nephropathy:
  - expected historical features:
    - rare – mostly occurs in young male cats
    - PU/PD
    - +/– vomiting
    - +/– diarrhea
    - anorexia as disease progresses
    - depression as disease progresses
  - anticipated physical exam findings:
    - ascites
    - subcutaneous edema
    - abnormal kidney size (usually small)
    - abnormal kidney contour (usually irregular)
    - +/– retinopathy (secondary to systemic hypertension due to renal dysfunction).

9. Osteoarthritis can result in decreased grooming in older cats.(15) Osteoarthritis is associated with the stiffening of affected joints, which in turn reduces flexibility. It may be difficult for cats to access certain areas of their body and/or it may physically be painful to do so. When the spine and/or hips are involved, affected cats may find it challenging to reach the lower back, the

hind end, and proximal pelvic limbs.(15) Coats may take on an unkempt or ratty appearance. Medium- and long-haired coats are also likely to become matted.

10. After history-taking, the next step in the diagnostic plan is to perform a thorough physical exam.(6)

Returning to Case 16: Feline Weight Loss

You examine Figaro and document the following abnormal findings in his medical record:

- bilaterally symmetrical epaxial and caudal thigh muscle atrophy
- grade 2/6 systolic heart murmur
- palpable thyroid slip.

Based upon Figaro's history, systolic BP, and physical examination findings, you suspect that Figaro has hyperthyroidism.

Round Two of Questions for Case 16: Feline Weight Loss

1. Define hypertension in cats.
2. Based upon Figaro's systolic BP reading at today's visit, is he hypertensive?
3. Figaro has never had hypertension on past physical exams. Kat asks if he could have developed white coat syndrome. Describe this condition.
4. Other than white coat syndrome, what causes hypertension in cats?
5. What are the potential health-related concerns for Figaro if his hypertension persists?
6. If systolic BP is not routinely measured on physical examination, what presenting complaint is often the first sign that the veterinary patient is hypertensive?
7. On physical examination today, you palpated a thyroid slip. Where is the thyroid located in the cat?
8. Should you be able to feel a NORMAL (i.e. non-enlarged) thyroid gland in a healthy cat on routine physical exam?
9. How do you feel for an enlarged thyroid gland?
10. Which hormones does an enlarged thyroid gland overproduce if the patient is hyperthyroid?
11. Is a palpable thyroid slip diagnostic for hyperthyroidism?
12. If a patient does not have a thyroid slip, can s/he still be hyperthyroid?
13. What are possible causes of hyperthyroidism?
14. Of the causes that you identified in Question #13 (above), which is the most likely cause in cats?
15. How common is thyroid cancer in cats?
16. What constitutes the minimum database to obtain a definitive diagnosis of hyperthyroidism?
17. What test results do you expect to see on your minimum database if Figaro is in fact hyperthyroid?
18. If Figaro's test results are equivocal, what additional test(s) might you need to perform?
19. What additional tests might you perform to identify any comorbidities prior to treatment?
20. What are treatment options for hyperthyroidism?
21. What are the advantages of each treatment option that you outlined in Question #20 (above)?
22. What are potential complications of each treatment option that you outlined in Question #20 (above)?

Answers to Round Two of Questions for Case 16: Feline Weight Loss

1. Hypertension is the medical term for elevated BP. In cats, hypertension is characterized as having persistently elevated, indirect systolic BP at greater than 160–170 mmHg and/or elevated diastolic pressures greater than 100 mmHg.(4, 16–21)

2. Based upon Figaro's systolic BP reading at today's visit, yes, he is hypertensive.

3. White coat syndrome occurs when stress in a clinical setting activates the sympathetic nervous system in some, but not all patients.(4) This results in situational tachycardia and hypertension.(4)

4. Hypertension may be primary or secondary to underlying disease.(16, 18, 19, 22–24) Primary systemic hypertension occurs more frequently in dogs than cats, but may be more common in cats than was once believed.(18, 25–29)

    Secondary systemic hypertension often results from renal disease.(16, 18–22, 30–33) Other causes of secondary systemic hypertension in cats include:(16, 18–20, 24, 31, 34–37)

    - acromegaly
    - chronic anemia
    - diabetes mellitus
    - erythropoietin treatments
    - hyperthyroidism
    - hyperadrenocorticism
    - pheochromocytomas
    - primary hyperaldosteronism
    - high-salt diets.

5. Sustained hypertension is likely to damage one or more of the so-called target organs: the eyes, kidneys, heart, and brain.(4, 6, 16) These organs are impacted by hypertension before other tissues in the body because they have a rich arterial supply.(4, 16)

    In cats, target organ damage to one or both eyes is common.(4, 6, 19, 20, 38) In the early stages of hypertensive retinopathy, the retina will appear swollen during fundic exam.(16) If hypertension persists, then retinal hemorrhages may also be observed.(16, 19, 20, 24, 26, 33) Hemorrhages may be focal or extensive.(39) In severe cases, hypertensive retinopathy progresses to detachment of one or both retinas.(4)

6. If systolic BP is not routinely measured on physical examination, the presenting complaint of blindness (due to retinal detachment) is often the first sign that the veterinary patient is hypertensive.(16)

7. The paired thyroid gland is seated along the ventral neck in close apposition to the trachea, distal to the cricoid cartilage.(6) Its right and left lobes are connected by a bridge of tissue called the isthmus.

8. Given its location in the ventral neck, the thyroid gland of a normal cat is typically too deep to palpate.(40, 41) The same is true in dogs.

9. To feel for the thyroid gland, the clinician may stand directly behind the patient or immediately in front. I prefer the former approach. The patient can be seated or standing.

    Standing behind the patient, I use my non-dominant hand to gently extend the cat's head and neck. The thumb and index finger of the dominant hand are pinched together as if I were crimping pie crust. Together, the thumb and index finger are then placed in the jugular furrows such that they straddle the trachea. Beginning at the larynx, the thumb and index finger are then progressively slid down the throat, applying firm and constant pressure all the way to the thoracic inlet.

    If there are one or more thyroid nodules, the nodule(s) will "slip" through the fingers as a subcutaneous "pop" of tissue that is not typically present on palpation.(6)

    Some clinicians prefer to turn the cat's elevated head and neck 45 degrees to the left from the vertical to palpate the right lobe of the thyroid, and 45 degrees to the right from the vertical to palpate the left lobe of the thyroid.(42, 43)

    Other clinicians prefer to stand face-to-face with the cat and repeat the procedure outlined above.

10. Hyperthyroidism is a condition in which thyroxine (T4) and triiodothyronine (T3) are overproduced.(44–48)

11. A palpable thyroid slip is supportive of, but not diagnostic of hyperthyroidism.(6) Not all cats with palpable thyroid glands are hyperthyroid (43). For reasons yet to be understood, some cats with enlargement of the thyroid are euthyroid: their total thyroxine (TT4) is normal, if not low.(49)

12. If a patient does not have a palpable thyroid slip, then s/he could still be hyperthyroid. This is because developmentally, the thyroid gland arises from the pharyngeal floor and may have ectopic tissue that extends through the thoracic inlet into the thoracic cavity.(50–52) The patient may therefore have an enlarged thyroid that is out of reach. Just because you may not feel an enlarged thyroid in the cervical region does not rule out hyperthyroidism.

13. Hyperthyroidism can result from three broad categories of disease:(4, 6)
    - a primary disorder, meaning that it originates from the thyroid gland itself
    - a secondary disorder, meaning that it originates from overstimulation of the thyroid gland by the pituitary gland via overproduction of thyroid-stimulating hormone (TSH)
    - a tertiary disorder, meaning that it originates from overstimulation of the thyroid gland indirectly by the hypothalamus via overproduction of thyrotropin-releasing hormone, TRH. TRH then acts on the pituitary gland to cause it to overproduce TSH, which then causes an overproduction of T4 and fT4.

14. In cats, hyperthyroidism is usually a primary disease.(4, 41) There is pathology within the thyroid itself. The enlarged thyroid is neoplastic.(4, 41)

15. Primary malignant tumors of the thyroid, such as carcinoma, are rare in cats.(41, 48, 53, 54) The majority of thyroid tumors in the cat that cause hyperthyroidism are benign.(41, 53, 54) There are different terms in the medical literature to describe this overactive neoplastic thyroidal tissue. Most textbooks refer to it as adenomatous hyperplasia, adenomas, or multinodular adenomatous goiter.(41, 46, 48, 55)

16. The following items constitute the minimum database to obtain a definitive diagnosis of hyperthyroidism:(4, 6, 56)
    - complete blood count (CBC)
    - chemistry profile
    - total thyroxine (TT4).

    In an academic setting, note that the diagnosis of hyperthyroidism may also be confirmed by demonstrating increased thyroidal uptake of radioactive iodine isotopes, 131I or 123I.(57) Quantitative thyroid studies are rarely performed in clinical practice because of the expense. (57) More often, qualitative thyroid scans are performed to determine if the thyroid is unilaterally or bilaterally involved and/or if there is a site of functional ectopic thyroid tissue.(57)

17. If Figaro is hyperthyroid, then I would expect to see the following clinicopathologic data:(8, 13, 56, 57)
    - RBC:
        - increased PCV (57)
        - increased mean corpuscular volume (MCV) (57)
        - mild erythrocytosis:
            - anemia is more likely if concurrent renal dysfunction, in which case anemia results from decreased renal production of erythropoietin

- +/– macrocytosis
  - +/– Heinz body formation.(13, 57, 59)
- WBC:
  - non-specific changes, if any, most often indicative of a stress response:(57)
    - leukocytosis
    - lymphopenia
    - eosinopenia
    - neutrophilia
- chemistry profile:
  - elevated serum aspartate aminotransferase (AST)(57)
  - elevated serum alanine transferase (ALT)
  - elevated serum alkaline phosphatase (ALK PHOS or ALP)
  - decreased creatinine, in the absence of renal dysfunction, due to reduced muscle mass(57)
  - mild to moderate azotemia if concurrent renal dysfunction:(57)
    - elevated blood urea nitrogen (BUN)
    - elevated creatinine
  - +/– hyperglycemia(56)
  - +/– hyperphosphatemia in the absence of azotemia due to altered bone metabolism in hyperthyroid patients(56)
  - +/– mild hypokalemia:(56)
    - unknown etiology
    - rarely clinically significant
- TT4:
  - elevated TT4.

18. If Figaro's TT4 is at the high end of the normal range or borderline, then you may elect to proceed with an additional test that measures free T4 (fT4) by equilibrium dialysis (ED).(8) Free T4 represents the non-protein bound thyroxine in circulation.(9, 10) An elevation in Figaro's value for fT4 would support the diagnosis of hyperthyroidism even if his TT4 were equivocal.(8)

19. Hyperthyroidism may mask underlying renal disease.(8) If patients receive treatment for hyperthyroidism, then pre-existing renal dysfunction may worsen.(8) It is therefore critical to screen patient for renal disease prior to managing hyperthyroidism.(8)

    An assessment of renal function includes evaluation of BUN and creatinine, as measured in the patient's blood chemistry profile.(8) Patients with renal disease develop azotemia, that is, elevations in both BUN and creatinine.(4, 6, 9, 10) Unfortunately, both BUN and creatinine are later markers of renal disease.(4, 6, 9, 10) Creatinine does not increase until 75% of renal function has been lost.(4, 6, 9, 10) Therefore, neither BUN nor creatinine is an effective measure of early renal dysfunction.(4, 6, 9, 10)

    A urinalysis offers a different approach to assessing renal health.(4, 6, 9, 10) Measurement of urine specific gravity (USG) allows us to evaluate the patient's concentrating ability as a measure of renal health.(4, 6) Loss of concentrating ability in renal disease occurs sooner than azotemia.(10) Therefore, urinalysis offers a means by which to diagnose renal disease earlier than hematology-based diagnostics. USG varies immensely in hyperthyroid cats (1.009–1.050; mean: 1.031), depending upon the presence or absence of renal dysfunction and, when present, to what degree.(56, 57)

A newer test for renal function evaluates the patient's symmetric dimethylarginine (SDMA), a methylated arginine amino acid.(60–64) SDMA is a renal biomarker.(60–64) It is excreted by the kidneys and more accurately reflects glomerular filtration rate (GFR).(60–64) In addition, SDMA is not influenced by age, body condition, and lean body mass, unlike creatinine. (60–64) As a result, SDMA is both more reliable and more sensitive.(60–64) SDMA increases when 40% of renal function is lost as compared to 75%, which is required to see a spike in creatinine.(60–64)

20. Treatment options for hyperthyroidism include:(8, 57, 65, 66)

   - administration of radioactive iodine as 131I
   - medical management with methimazole or carbimazole
   - surgical thyroidectomy
   - iodine-restriction using prescription diet.

Other means of management have been reported, including percutaneous ultrasound-guided radiofrequency heat ablation or percutaneous ethanol injection into the thyroid.(57, 67–69) However, these are rarely if ever performed considering the alternatives because of the high risk of complications.(57)

21. Each treatment option for hyperthyroidism carries its own set of advantages. These have been outlined below:(8)

   - radioactive iodine:***

     - kills overproducing thyroid cells while sparing those with normal function
     - requires one injection or capsule
     - curative in 95% of cases
     - low relapse rate of 5%
     - risk of inducing a hypothyroid state is low

   - medical management with methimazole or carbimazole:(65, 66)

     - response rate is 95% or greater
     - does not require hospitalization
     - can be discontinued if renal function declines

   - surgical thyroidectomy:

     - relatively quick procedure
     - can be performed by generalist without needing special equipment
     - curative in 90% of cases if both glands are removed
     - 35–60% curative if one gland is removed

   - iodine-restriction using prescription diet:

     - does not require daily medicating via the oral or transdermal routes
     - response rate is 82% or higher
     - does not worsen renal function.

Note: ***Considered to be the gold standard treatment.(8) Historically, it was administered intravenously; however, it is equally effective when given subcutaneously, so much so that this is now the preferred route.(57)

22. The treatment options for hyperthyroidism are not without risk. The following list outlines potential complications of each.(8, 57)

   - Radioactive iodine:

- costly
- can only be performed at certain facilities that have special licensing and/or certification
- can only be performed as inpatient procedure
- patient must be hospitalized for days to weeks following the procedure
- after the patient goes home, there is risk of client exposure to radioactive substances for up to 2 weeks:
    - caution must be exercised when cleaning up cat waste
    - cuddling with the cat is not advised during this period.

- Medical management with methimazole or carbimazole:(65, 66)
    - up to one in four cats develop adverse reactions, which may be severe:(57)
        - hepatopathy:
            - increased ALT
            - increased ALK PHOS
            - increased bilirubin
            - hepatic necrosis and degeneration
        - blood dyscrasias:
            - immune-mediated hemolytic anemia
            - aplastic anemia (rare)
            - thrombocytopenia
            - neutropenia
        - gastrointestinal upset:
            - anorexia
            - vomiting
        - facial pruritus
        - renal decompensation
        - coagulopathy (rare, but possible)
    - medication must be given for life
    - relapse occurs in 100% of cases if medication is discontinued
    - tumor growth is not inhibited
    - tumor transformation into malignancy is possible.

- Surgical thyroidectomy:
    - requires hospitalization and general anesthesia
    - hypocalcemia in the post-operative period may be life-threatening if both parathyroid glands are damaged intraoperatively
    - patients may require medication in the post-operative period
    - cannot be reversed
    - may alter vocalizations
    - may alter the sound of the cat's purr or the cat's ability to purr
    - can result in Horner's syndrome or laryngeal paralysis post-operatively.

- Iodine-restriction using prescription diet:
    - the cat cannot eat anything else ever (unless treats are also low in iodine)
    - 100% relapse rate if diet is discontinued.

Returning to Case 16: Feline Weight Loss

Kat authorizes you to proceed with a diagnostic work-up, which confirms that Figaro's TT4 is significantly elevated (see Figure 16.2).

Kat elects to start Figaro on methimazole therapy at a dose of 2.5 mg per os (PO) per cat every 12 hours.

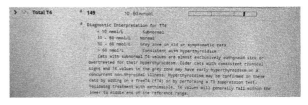

Figure 16.2 TT4 results. Courtesy of Jule Schweighoefer.

Round Three of Questions for Case 16: Feline Weight Loss

1. What is the mechanism of action for methimazole?
2. Not all cats develop side effects. How soon are side effects likely to occur if they are going to?
3. How long after starting treatment is Figaro likely to be euthyroid?
4. At what point should you recheck Figaro's TT4?
5. At the next check-up, Kat acknowledges that Figaro is getting wise to her at/around medication time and it is becoming increasingly difficult to pill him. Her friend told her about transdermal methimazole. Kat would like to hear more about it.

    A. Do you sell this product?
    B. How does it work?
    C. Is it safe for Kat to apply?
    D. Where would Kat apply it?
    E. Is it effective?
    F. Does it have fewer side effects? If so, which ones have reduced risk of occurring?

Answers to Round Three of Questions for Case 16: Feline Weight Loss

1. Methimazole blocks the production of thyroid hormones by inhibiting the enzyme, thyroid peroxidase.(5, 8)

2. Not all cats develop side effects. If side effects occur, they are likely to develop within the first month and a half of initiating treatment.(8, 70) If Figaro can successfully make it through the first two to three months of treatment without seeing any adverse effects, then he is unlikely to experience facial pruritus or vomiting secondary to methimazole administration.(70)

3. Figaro should be euthyroid within two to three weeks of initiating methimazole treatment.(8, 57)

4. Most clinicians recheck Figaro's TT4 within the first two to three weeks of initiating methimazole treatment and again between 4 and 6 weeks.(8, 65, 66) At minimum, the following parameters are rechecked at those times:(65, 66)

    - CBC
    - BUN
    - creatinine
    - ALT
    - ALK PHOS.

5.   A) No, you do not carry transdermal methimazole, but you can prescribe it through specialty pharmacies. It must be compounded.

B) Methimazole is added to a formulation that contains pluronic lecithin organogel (PLO). (65, 66) This enhances drug absorption across the outermost layer of skin.(65, 66)

C) The transdermal formulation of methimazole can also be absorbed through human skin, so Kat would need to apply it wearing examination gloves or finger cots.(65, 66) This would keep her safe.

D) Kat would need to apply the medication to Figaro's inner pinna.(65, 66) Usually one pinna is used for dose one, and the other pinna is used for dose two.(65, 66) Owners need to be instructed to remove the excess crust of old medication prior to applying the next dose.(65, 66)

E) The transdermal formulation has lower bioavailability than oral methimazole.(65, 66) This means that transdermal application of methimazole is less effective than if the patient takes it orally.(65, 66) Even so, approximately two-thirds of cats that receive the transdermal formulation will become euthyroid within a month of treatment – so it is a worthwhile endeavor to try for those who cannot administer the oral version.(66)

Note that efficacy also varies depending upon manufacturer and how the drug is stored.(65, 66) Clients should be instructed not to refrigerate the product.(65, 66) Clients should also be instructed that the product needs to be replaced if at any point its components separate out of suspension.(65, 66)

F) There is reduced frequency of vomiting when cats are given transdermal methimazole as opposed to oral methimazole.(65, 66)

CLINICAL PEARLS

- There is no substitute for a comprehensive patient history. Open-ended questions and clarifying questions are essential.

- If an older cat presents with a history of weight loss despite a normal-to-increased appetite, there are at least five differential diagnoses to consider. History-taking provides you with an initial screening tool to assist with prioritizing differentials.

- As you brainstorm your list of differential diagnoses, consider what you might expect to find on physical examination. Although you plan to perform a comprehensive physical exam on every patient, brainstorming helps you to think of what you are looking for to determine your wants versus your needs. For example, an older cat with weight loss that is eating well is highly suspicious for hyperthyroidism. It is essential for you to palpate the ventral neck to feel for a thyroid slip.

- The presence of a palpable thyroid slip is not enough to make a definitive diagnosis of hyperthyroidism; however, it is supportive of this endocrinopathy.

- Likewise, the absence of a palpable thyroid slip cannot rule out hyperthyroidism. Ectopic tissue may be present and out of reach.

- On physical exam, hyperthyroid cats often have muscle atrophy, tachycardia, a systolic heart murmur, and/or a gallop rhythm.

- Hyperthyroid cats are often hypertensive. Persistent hypertension causes target organ damage. Retinopathy is common, and ranges from mild retinal edema to retinal hemorrhage and, ultimately, retinal detachment.

- Cats that do not routinely have their BP checked may present with the chief complaint of blindness.

- Definitive diagnosis of hyperthyroidism in clinical practice typically involves bloodwork to confirm that the patient has an elevated total thyroxine (TT4).

- If the patient has a high-end normal TT4 and/or TT4 is borderline, then an add-on free T4 (fT4) by ED can be run. An elevation in fT4 is consistent with hyperthyroidism.

- Treatment options include medication, surgery, diet, and radioactive iodine. Client education is key to exploring pros and cons of each treatment modality.

References

1. MacMartin C, Wheat HC, Coe JB, Adams CL. Effect of question design on dietary information solicited during veterinarian-client interactions in companion animal practice in Ontario, Canada. J Am Vet Med Assoc 2015;246(11):1203–14.
2. Coe JB, editor. Practical communication tips for partnering with clients in framing their nutrition truths. Hill's global symposium: harnessing the power of the microbiome; July 14–15, 2019. Toronto, Canada.
3. Englar R. Writing skills for veterinarians. Sheffield: 5M Publishing; 2019.
4. Englar RE. Common clinical presentations in dogs and cats. Hoboken, NJ: Wiley/Blackwell; 2019. pages cm p.
5. Plumb DC Stockholm W, ed. Plumb's veterinary drug handbook. 8th ed. Ames, Iowa: PharmaVet Inc.; 2015.
6. Englar RE. Performing the small animal physical examination. Hoboken, NJ: Wiley/Blackwell; 2017.
7. Gunn-Moore D, Miller JB. The cat with weight loss and a good appetite. In: Rand J, editor. Problem-based feline Medicie. New York: Elsevier; 2006. p. 301–29.
8. Carney HC, Ward CR, Bailey SJ, Bruyette D, Dennis S, Ferguson D, et al. 2016 AAFP guidelines for the management of feline hyperthyroidism. J Feline Med Surg 2016;18(5):400–16.
9. Côté E. Clinical veterinary advisor. Dogs and cats. 3rd ed. St. Louis, MO: Elsevier Mosby; 2015.
10. Ettinger SJ, Feldman EC, Côté E. Textbook of veterinary internal medicine: diseases of the dog and the cat. 8th ed. St. Louis, MO: Elsevier; 2017.
11. Tilley LP, Smith FWK, Tilley LP. Blackwell's five-minute veterinary consult: canine and feline. 4th ed. Ames, IA: Blackwell; 2007.
12. Wooten SJ. The feline facets of Cushing's disease. 2018. DVM. Available from: https://www.dvm360.com/view/feline-facets-cushings-disease.
13. Ward CR. Feline thyroid storm. Vet Clin North Am Small Anim Pract 2007;37(4):745–54.
14. Xenoulis PG, Zoran DL, Fosgate GT, Suchodolski JS, Steiner JM. Feline exocrine pancreatic insufficiency: A retrospective study of 150 cases. J Vet Intern Med 2016;30(6):1790–7.
15. Williams K, Downing R. How to recognize pain in aging cats. VCA Hospitals. Available from: https://vcahospitals.com/know-your-pet/behavior-changes-and-pain-in-aging-cats.
16. Maggio F, DeFrancesco TC, Atkins CE, Pizzirani S, Gilger BC, Davidson MG. Ocular lesions associated with systemic hypertension in cats: 69 cases (1985–1998). J Am Vet Med Assoc 2000;217(5):695–702.
17. Sansom J, Rogers K, Wood JL. Blood pressure assessment in healthy cats and cats with hypertensive retinopathy. Am J Vet Res 2004;65(2):245–52.
18. Henik RA. Systemic hypertension and its management. Vet Clin North Am Small Anim Pract 1997;27(6):1355–72.
19. Littman MP. Spontaneous systemic hypertension in 24 cats. J Vet Intern Med 1994;8(2):79–86.
20. Morgan RV. Systemic hypertension in four cats: ocular and medical findings. J Am Anim Hosp Assoc 1986;22:615–21.
21. Stiles J, Polzin DJ, Bistner SI. The prevalence of retinopathy in cats with systemic hypertension and chronic-renal-failure or hyperthyroidism. J Am Anim Hosp Assoc 1994;30(6):564–72.
22. Henik RA, Snyder PS, Volk LM. Treatment of systemic hypertension in cats with amlodipine besylate. J Am Anim Hosp Assoc 1997;33(3):226–34.

23. Komáromy AM, Andrew SE, Denis HM, Brooks DE, Gelatt KN. Hypertensive retinopathy and choroidopathy in a cat. Vet Ophthalmol 2004;7(1):3–9.

24. Turner JL, Brogdon JD, Lees GE, Greco DS. Idiopathic hypertension in a cat with secondary hypertensive retinopathy associated with a high-salt diet. J Am Anim Hosp Assoc 1990;26(6):647–51.

25. Brown SA, Henik RA. Diagnosis and treatment of systemic hypertension. Vet Clin North Am Small Anim Pract 1998;28(6):1481–94.

26. Sansom J, Barnett KC, Dunn KA, Smith KC, Dennis R. Ocular disease associated with hypertension in 16 cats. J Small Anim Pract 1994;35(12):604–11.

27. Bovée KC, Littman MP, Saleh F, Beeuwkes R, r Pn W, Kinter LB. Essential hereditary hypertension in dogs: a new animal model. J Hypertens Suppl 1986;4(5):S172–1.

28. Tippett FE, Padgett GA, Eyster G, Blanchard G, Bell T. Primary hypertension in a colony of dogs. Hypertension 1987;9(1):49–58.

29. Littman MP, Robertson JL, Bovée KC. Spontaneous systemic hypertension in dogs: five cases (1981–1983). J Am Vet Med Assoc 1988;193(4):486–94.

30. Ross LA. Hypertension and chronic renal failure. Semin Vet Med Surg Small Anim 1992;7(3):221–6.

31. Kobayashi DL, Peterson ME, Graves TK, Lesser M, Nichols CE. Hypertension in cats with chronic renal failure or hyperthyroidism. J Vet Intern Med 1990;4(2):58–62.

32. Jensen J, Henik RA, Brownfield M, Armstrong J. Plasma renin activity and angiotensin I and aldosterone concentrations in cats with hypertension associated with chronic renal disease. Am J Vet Res 1997;58(5):535–40.

33. Snyder PS. Amlodipine: a randomized, blinded clinical trial in 9 cats with systemic hypertension. J Vet Intern Med 1998;12(3):157–62.

34. Peterson ME, Taylor RS, Greco DS, Nelson RW, Randolph JF, Foodman MS, et al. Acromegaly in 14 cats. J Vet Intern Med 1990;4(4):192–201.

35. Cowgill LD, James KM, Levy JK, Browne JK, Miller A, Lobingier RT, Egrie JC. Use of recombinant human erythropoietin for management of anemia in dogs and cats with renal failure. J Am Vet Med Assoc 1998;212(4):521–8.

36. Chun R, Jakovljevic S, Morrison WB, DeNicola DB, Cornell KK. Apocrine gland adenocarcinoma and pheochromocytoma in a cat. J Am Anim Hosp Assoc 1997;33(1):33–6.

37. Flood SM, Randolph JF, Gelzer AR, Refsal K. Primary hyperaldosteronism in two cats. J Am Anim Hosp Assoc 1999;35(5):411–6.

38. Littman MP. Hypertension. In: Ettinger SJ, editor. Textbook of veterinary internal medicine. 5th ed. Philadelphia: W. B. Saunders; 2000. p. 179–82.

39. Crispin SM, Mould JR. Systemic hypertensive disease and the feline fundus. Vet Ophthalmol 2001;4(2):131–40.

40. Rijnberk A, van Sluijs FS. Medical history and physical examination in companion animals. The Netherlands: Elsevier Limited; 2009.

41. Feldman EC, Nelson RW. Canine and feline endocrinology and reproduction. 3rd ed. St Louis, MO: Saunders; 2004.

42. Norsworthy GD, Adams VJ, McElhaney MR, Milios JA. Palpable thyroid and parathyroid nodules in asymptomatic cats. J Feline Med Surg 2002;4(3):145–51.

43. Norsworthy GD, Adams VJ, McElhaney MR, Milios JA. Relationship between semi-quantitative thyroid palpation and total thyroxine concentration in cats with and without hyperthyroidism. J Feline Med Surg 2002;4(3):139–43.

44. Peterson ME, Kintzer PP, Cavanagh PG, Fox PR, Ferguson DC, Johnson GF, Becker DV. Feline hyperthyroidism: pretreatment clinical and laboratory evaluation of 131 cases. J Am Vet Med Assoc 1983;183(1):103–10.

45. Hoenig M, Goldschmidt MH, Ferguson DC, Koch K, Eymontt MJ. Toxic nodular goitre in the cat. J Small Anim Pract 1982;23(1):1–12.

46. Peterson ME, Ward CR. Etiopathologic findings of hyperthyroidism in cats. Vet Clin North Am Small Anim Pract 2007;37(4):633–45.

47. Baral R, Peterson ME. Thyroid gland disorders. In: Little SE, editor. The Cat: clinical medicine and management. Philadelphia, PA: Elsevier Saunders; 2012. p. 571–92.

48. Mooney CT. Pathogenesis of feline hyperthyroidism. J Feline Med Surg 2002;4(3):167–9.

49. Chaitman SJ, Hess R, Senz R, Van Winkle T, Ward C. Thyroid adenomatous hyperplasia in euthyroid cats. J Vet Intern Med 1999;13:242.

50. Gilbert SG. Pictorial anatomy of the cat. Seattle: University of Washington Press; 1968. vii, 120 p. p.
51. Dyce KM, Sack WO, Wensing CJG. Textbook of veterinary anatomy. 2nd ed. Philadelphia: Saunders; 1996. xiii, 856 p. p.
52. Eiler H. Endocrine glands. In: Reece WO, editor. Dukes' physiology of domestic animals. 12th ed. Ithaca, NY: Comstock Pub. Associates; 2004.
53. Turrel JM, Feldman EC, Nelson RW, Cain GR. Thyroid carcinoma causing hyperthyroidism in cats: 14 cases (1981–1986). J Am Vet Med Assoc 1988;193(3):359–64.
54. Hibbert A, Gruffydd-Jones T, Barrett EL, Day MJ, Harvey AM. Feline thyroid carcinoma: diagnosis and response to high-dose radioactive iodine treatment. J Feline Med Surg 2009;11(2):116–24.
55. Carpenter JL. Tumors and tumorlike lesions. In: Holzworth J, editor. Diseases of the cat: medicine and surgery. Philadelphia, PA: Saunders; 1987.
56. Shiel RE, Mooney CT. Testing for hyperthyroidism in cats. Vet Clin North Am Small Anim Pract 2007;37(4):671–91.
57. Mooney CT. Feline hyperthyroidism. Diagnostics and therapeutics. Vet Clin North Am Small Anim Pract 2001;31(5):963–83.
58. Gough A, Thomas A, O'Neill D Hoboken NJ, ed. Breed predispositions to disease in dogs and cats. 3rd ed. Hoboken, NJ: Wiley; 2018.
59. Christopher MM. Relation of endogenous Heinz bodies to disease and anemia in cats: 120 cases (1978–1987). J Am Vet Med Assoc 1989;194(8):1089–95.
60. Nabity MB, Lees GE, Boggess MM, Yerramilli M, Obare E, Yerramilli M, et al. Symmetric dimethylarginine assay validation, stability, and evaluation as a marker for the early detection of chronic kidney disease in dogs. J Vet Intern Med 2015;29(4):1036–44.
61. Hall JA, Yerramilli M, Obare E, Yerramilli M, Jewell DE. Comparison of serum concentrations of symmetric dimethylarginine and creatinine as kidney function biomarkers in cats with chronic kidney disease. J Vet Intern Med 2014;28(6):1676–83.
62. Hall JA, Yerramilli M, Obare E, Yerramilli M, Yu S, Jewell DE. Comparison of serum concentrations of symmetric dimethylarginine and creatinine as kidney function biomarkers in healthy geriatric cats fed reduced protein foods enriched with fish oil, L-carnitine, and medium-chain triglycerides. Vet J 2014;202(3):588–96.
63. Hall JA, Yerramilli M, Obare E, Yerramilli M, Almes K, Jewell DE. Serum concentrations of symmetric dimethylarginine and creatinine in dogs with naturally occurring chronic kidney disease. J Vet Intern Med 2016;30(3):794–802.
64. Hall JA, Yerramilli M, Obare E, Yerramilli M, Melendez LD, Jewell DE. Relationship between lean body mass and serum renal biomarkers in healthy dogs. J Vet Intern Med 2015;29(3):808–14.
65. Trepanier LA. Medical management of hyperthyroidism. Clin Tech Small Anim Pract 2006;21(1):22–8.
66. Trepanier LA. Pharmacologic management of feline hyperthyroidism. Vet Clin North Am Small Anim Pract 2007;37(4):775–88.
67. Goldstein RE, Long C, Swift NC, Hornof WJ, Nelson RW, Nyland TG, Feldman EC. Percutaneous ethanol injection for treatment of unilateral hyperplastic thyroid nodules in cats. J Am Vet Med Assoc 2001;218(8):1298–302.
68. Mallery KF, Pollard RE, Nelson RW, Hornof WJ, Feldman EC. Percutaneous ultrasound-guided radiofrequency heat ablation for treatment of hyperthyroidism in cats. J Am Vet Med Assoc 2003;223(11):1602–7.
69. Wells AL, Long CD, Hornof WJ, Goldstein RE, Nyland TG, Nelson RW, Feldman EC. Use of percutaneous ethanol injection for treatment of bilateral hyperplastic thyroid nodules in cats. J Am Vet Med Assoc 2001;218(8):1293–7.
70. Peterson ME, Kintzer PP, Hurvitz AI. Methimazole treatment of 262 cats with hyperthyroidism. J Vet Intern Med 1988;2(3):150–7.

Case 17

Canine Weight Gain

It has been a year and a half since Baguette visited the clinic. At that last consult with Nora Parsons, you had outlined the following weight management plan.

- Goal body weight: 58 lb = 26.4 kg.
- Ideal rate of weight loss: 0.5–2% of her body weight each week.(1–4)
- For Baguette to lose weight initially, she should consume between 859–1057 kcal day.
- Nora had elected to stick with Brubaker's Adult Large Breed dry (340 kcal/cup). Instructions:
- Weigh out all food on a digital scale.
- Feed 3/4 cup TID (three times per day) for a total of 765 calories.
- Feed 100–150 calories per day as various snacks:

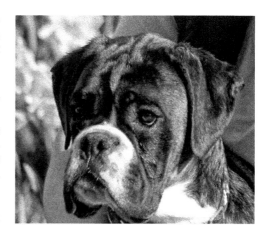

Figure 17.1 Your patient, Baguette, returns. She is now 6 years old. Courtesy of Jayne Regan.

  - after taking a comprehensive diet history, it was apparent that treats were how Nora best showed her love to Baguette
  - removing treats from the daily agenda would have set Nora up for success.

- Walk Baguette for 30–45 minutes every day (minimum).
- Reassess her progress at weekly weigh-ins.
- After 1 month of progress, can switch to bi-monthly weigh-ins.

Baguette was supposed to return 2 weeks later for a weigh-in progress check. Nora never scheduled the appointment. You telephoned twice that first week and your team did the same, but despite best efforts, Baguette was lost to follow-up.

When Nora arrives at the clinic, she apologizes to the technician who greets her in the waiting area. "I should have come back sooner," she acknowledges. "It's just that, well, life got in the way." Nora then explains that both parents passed away within 12 months of each other, and as their chosen executor, she was stuck in the middle of an ugly sibling battle about the estate. It was too much to bear. Ultimately, she did right by her parents, but now neither her brother nor her sister were speaking to her. All she had in life was Baguette.

True to her word, Nora rationed Baguette's food and managed to make all of the proposed changes. Despite her best efforts, Baguette retained the weight that she had gained. If anything, she looked even rounder. The technician confirms this at weigh-in today: At her last visit, Baguette weighed 72.4 lb (32.9 kg). Today, she weighs 80.2 lb (36.5 kg) and her vital signs are as follows.

BCS: 8/9
Mentation: BAR

TPR

T: 100.7°F (38.2°C)
P: 56 beats per minute
R: 24 breaths per minute

Nora is embarrassed about Baguette's weight. "I don't understand," she says. "I did everything you said."

The technician validates how frustrating it must be, given that Nora has worked so hard to change Baguette's lifestyle. He assures her that "we will figure it out." Consider the following list of questions to help you work through this clinical case.

Round One of Questions for Case 17: Canine Weight Gain

1. Identify broad mechanisms by which weight gain occurs.
2. Of the broad mechanisms that you listed in Question #1 (above), which is LEAST likely in this patient. Explain why.
3. What are additional questions that you would like to ask Nora to investigate if one or more of the other mechanisms that you listed in Question #1 could be at play?
4. Which differential diagnoses are consistent with a canine history of weight gain despite appropriate caloric restriction?
5. For each differential diagnosis that you listed in Question #4 (above), what are the primary historical and/or physical examination features that you would expect to hear and/or see (in addition to weight gain)?
6. After history-taking, what is your next step in the diagnostic plan?

Answers to Round One of Questions for Case 17: Canine Weight Gain

1. Broad mechanisms by which weight gain occurs include:

   - decreased metabolic requirements:

     - decreased metabolic activity
     - decreased metabolic rate

   - increased consumption of food:

     - increased appetite (and therefore increased caloric intake) – change in brand, protein source, carbohydrate source, texture or consistency; new food is more palatable
     - increased access to food (and therefore increased caloric intake):

       - not weighing food / "eyeballing" food measurements instead – 1 cup of food turns out to be >1 cup, this may seem minor, but over time the extra adds up
       - increased number of meals fed
       - change in feeding routine from being meal-fed to being free-fed
       - increased number of people in the home who are feeding the pet

     - increased quality of energy-dense food.

2. Assuming that Nora is telling the truth and that she has adhered to the weight loss management plan then it is LEAST likely that Baguette is continuing to gain weight because of increased consumption of food.

3. I would like to investigate the possibility that Baguette has decreased metabolic requirements. To be thorough, we need to ask the following questions.

   - How is Baguette's energy level as compared to the last visit?
   - Do you have to push Baguette to exercise?
   - Is Baguette exercise intolerant?

- Is Baguette sedentary in her home environment?
- Does she appear lethargic?
- Does Baguette seem weak?

I would also want to take a comprehensive patient health history so that I do not approach the case with blinders on. Patients that have metabolic imbalances often do not operate in a closed system in which only metabolism seems "off." More often, they may exhibit other changes concurrently that suggest systemic illness.

Refer to a veterinary communication text, such as *Writing Skills for Veterinarians*(5) or *A Guide to Oral Communication in Veterinary Medicine*(6) to refresh your understanding of history-taking. Recall that, in addition to querying Nora about Baguette's activity level, a comprehensive patient history should include the following.(7–11)

- Travel history:

    - Has Baguette travelled in the past year and a half?
    - Nora mentioned having to plan and attend two parents' funerals. Did Baguette journey with her? If so, is it possible that others were in her life at that time that gave her extra and/or fed her more than her assigned rations?

- Current medications:

    - Over-the-counter products
    - Prescriptions:

        - Has Baguette been seen by anyone else since her last visit to your clinic?
        - If so, has anyone else dispensed prescription medication?
        - If yes, was she prescribed glucocorticoids? (Glucocorticoids, such as prednisolone, cause polyphagia.(12, 13))

    - Vitamins
    - Supplements

- History of preventative care at other clinics:

    - Has Baguette been seen by anyone else since her last visit to your clinic?

- Past medical history:

    - Has Baguette had any medical issues since her last visit to your clinic that you should be aware of?
    - If so, how were these issues addressed and medically managed?

- Past pertinent diagnostic tests and test results, including laboratory and imaging:

    - Has Baguette received any testing by any other clinic in her absence from yours?
    - If so, what were these tests and what did they reveal?

- Past pertinent therapeutic trials and outcomes:

    - What, if anything else, has Nora tried to manage Baguette's weight?

4. The following differential diagnoses are consistent with a canine history of weight gain despite appropriate caloric restriction:

- hyperadrenocorticism (Cushing's syndrome; Cushing's disease)
- hypothyroidism.

5. Considering each differential diagnosis that I have outlined in Question #4, I would expect to see the following historical and/or physical exam features, in addition to weight gain.

- Hyperadrenocorticism:(12, 14–16)

  - expected historical features:

    - age predisposition: middle-aged to older dogs
    - breed predisposition:(17, 18)

      - Poodles, especially miniature poodles
      - Dachshunds
      - Boxers
      - Boston terriers
      - Yorkshire terriers
      - Staffordshire terriers

    - polyuria (PU)
    - polydipsia (PD)
    - polyphagia (PP)
    - history may be suggestive of urinary tract infection (UTI), which is a common sequela of this endocrinopathy. Clients may report urinary accidents (house-soiling), pollakiuria, straining to urinate, etc.

  - anticipated physical exam findings:(12, 16, 19–21)

    - bilaterally symmetrical truncal hypotrichosis that may or may not progress to alopecia,(22) the head and limbs are classically spared(19)
    - calcinosus cutis, that is, deposits of calcium within the dermis:
    - these deposits may be generalized
    - these deposits often increase in number over cervical, axillary, and inguinal regions(19)
    - coat that has not shed out properly(19)
    - comedones(19)
    - delayed wound healing
    - dull coat
    - excessive panting because glucocorticoids influence the respiratory center
    - hyperpigmentation of the skin if chronic secondary bacterial and fungal infections are present(22)
    - muscle atrophy, especially around the head and face
    - thin ventral abdominal skin(22)
    - the skin may feel paper-thin(19)
    - the skin is also easily bruised due to the increased fragility of dermal vessels(19)
    - increased tendency to bruise
    - pot-bellied appearance
    - palpable hepatomegaly
    - weak.

- Hypothyroidism:(12, 14–16, 21, 23)

  - expected historical features:(12, 14–16, 21, 23–25)

    - middle-aged to older – however, hypothyroid patients that have a breed predisposition for this condition may present with clinical signs as early as 2 to 3 years of age(19, 20)
    - breed predispositions:(19)

      - Doberman Pinschers
      - Golden Retrievers
      - Old English Sheepdogs

- Irish Setters
- Great Danes

- client may report that the patient is sluggish
- client may report that the patient is exercise intolerant
- client may report that the patient seems mentally dull or depressed
- client may report that the patient is cold-intolerant:(19) +/– shivering(23)
- client may report seizure activity

- anticipated physical exam findings:(12, 16, 19, 21, 23–25)

  - +/– anterior uveitis
  - +/– bradycardia
  - +/– central nervous system (CNS) abnormalities: ataxia, head tilt, and seizure disorders
  - +/– constipation
  - +/– corneal lipid deposits
  - +/– CN deficits(23)
  - facial nerve paralysis
  - dermatologic changes:(19, 26)
  - bilaterally symmetrical truncal alopecia(21)
  - ceruminous otitis
  - coats may also fail to regrow post-clipping, or the loss of guard hairs may give the illusion that the "puppy coat" has been retained(19, 27)
  - +/– nasal hypopigmentation(23)
  - other common sites of alopecia include pressure points, such as over the elbows and hips,(19) callus formation may be quite pronounced
  - poor wound healing
  - pruritus if secondary bacterial and/or fungal infections are present(19)
  - "rat tail" – alopecic tail
  - "ring around the collar"
  - an alopecic patch outlining the neck
  - seborrhea oleosa or sicca
  - Superficial pyoderma
  - muscle weakness
  - paresis
  - paraparesis
  - quadriparesis
  - +/– PNS abnormalities – knuckling
  - "Tragic face,"(24) which results from myxedema (cutaneous mucinosis), a rare condition that is associated with hypothyroidism:(21)
  - lack of thyroid hormone reduces the breakdown of glycosaminoglycans
  - hyaluronic acid is deposited in the dermis
  - the skin appears thickened, particularly over the eyelids and cheeks – edema is nonpitting
  - urogenital abnormalities:
  - testicular atrophy and infertility in male patients
  - irregular cycles and infertility in female patients.

6. After history-taking, the next step in the diagnostic plan is to perform a thorough physical exam.(16)

Returning to Case 17: Canine Weight Gain

You take a thorough history to discern the following details, which round out your clinical picture.

- Baguette stayed at home with a pet sitter when Nora had to travel out of state twice to be with families during the funerals of both of her parents. The pet sitter was given strict feeding instructions and Nora was only gone for a week each time.
- Nora remains the only person in the home to feed Baguette.
- Baguette is not allowed outdoors without supervision, so Nora knows for sure that Baguette is not getting into a stash of treats elsewhere (i.e. neighbor's trash).
- Baguette is hard to motivate to do anything. She used to be excited to go on walks. Now, she balks at them.
- Baguette started to lose fur at/around her collar. Nora thought it was from her having to tug constantly at Baguette to motivate her to walk, so she switched to a harness about three months ago. The "ring around the collar" never went away. She still looks "bald" in that location.
- At around the same time, her fur started to thin out at/around both flanks. Boxers don't have a ton of fur as it is, so this was quite apparent. A couple of friends joked that Baguette had a bad haircut . . . except that it wasn't funny anymore. The fur loss seemed to be worsening.
- Baguette does not appear to be itchy. Nora has not seen any fleas.
- Baguette's skin looks "normal" to Nora, other than that there appears to be a lot of dandruff.
- Nora has not taken Baguette anywhere else for evaluation. She only trusts your clinic. Accordingly, Baguette is not receiving any new medications.
- Nora ran out of heartworm prophylaxis about 6 months ago.
- Baguette's appetite is normal: she still loves to eat. That's about all she wants to do these days.
- Baguette's thirst is unchanged.
- Baguette's urinary and bowel habits have not changed.
- Baguette has otherwise appeared to be in good health were it not for the weight gain.

You evaluate Baguette and confirm the following features on physical exam:

- dull, brittle coat
- dry, flaky skin
- ceruminous otitis au
- truncal alopecia

    - "rat tail"
    - "ring around the collar."

Based upon Baguette's history and physical examination findings, you suspect that Baguette has hypothyroidism.

Round Two of Questions for Case 17: Canine Weight Gain

1. You didn't mention anything about Baguette's thyroid on physical exam. Should you be able to feel a NORMAL (i.e. non-enlarged) thyroid gland in a healthy dog on routine physical exam?
2. Should you be able to feel a thyroid gland in a dog that is hypothyroid? Why or why not?
3. Which hormones does the thyroid gland UNDERproduce if the patient is hypothyroid?
4. What causes hypothyroidism in dogs?
5. Of the causes that you identified in Question #4 (above), which is the most likely cause in dogs?
6. How common is thyroid cancer in dog?
7. What is the incidence of thyroid tumors in dogs? (This encompasses both benign tumors as well as those that are malignant?)
8. Are there breed or sex predispositions for thyroid tumors in dogs?

9. If a thyroid tumor develops in a dog, is it more likely to be benign or malignant?
10. If a thyroid tumor develops in a dog, how likely is it to be functional, that is, capable of influencing thyroid hormone secretion?
11. What clinicopathologic features on complete blood count (CBC) and serum chemistry profile are supportive of a diagnosis of hypothyroidism?
12. In addition to clinicopathologic data that you outlined in Question #11 (above), what is a useful screening tool for the diagnosis of hypothyroidism?
13. What additional test(s) might you need to perform to assist you with a definitive diagnosis?
14. If the patient is truly hypothyroid, what test results do you expect to see for those that you outlined in Question #13 (above)?
15. Other than hypothyroidism, what can potentially cause levels of thyroxine to fall below the normal reference range?
16. It is essential to take a complete history concerning what (if any) other medications the patient is taking when you elect to run a thyroid panel because many drugs can affect testing. Which drugs are known to alter canine thyroid hormone test results?
17. How is hypothyroidism treated in dogs?
18. How do you know you have selected the appropriate dose for your patient?
19. How quickly does the patient respond to treatment?
20. What are potential adverse effects of the treatment option(s) that you outlined in Question #17 (above)?

Answers to Round Two of Questions for Case 17: Canine Weight Gain

1. Given its location in the ventral neck, the thyroid gland of a normal dog is typically too deep to palpate.(16, 28–30) The same is true in cats.

2. No, you do not typically feel a thyroid gland in a dog that is hypothyroid. This is because the gland is UNDERproducing hormones, meaning that it has not hypertrophied (enlarged).(12, 16)

3. Hypothyroidism is a condition in which thyroxine (T4) and triiodothyronine (T3) are UNDERproduced.(12, 14–16)

4. Hypothyroidism can result from three broad categories of disease:(12, 16, 19)

   - a primary disorder, meaning that it originates from the thyroid gland itself
   - a secondary disorder, meaning that it originates from lack of stimulation of the thyroid gland by the pituitary gland via UNDERproduction of thyroid stimulating hormone (TSH)
   - a tertiary disorder, meaning that it originates from lack of stimulation of the thyroid gland indirectly by the hypothalamus via UNDERproduction of thyrotropin-releasing hormone (TRH). Because there is less TRH to act upon the pituitary gland to trigger the release of TSH, there is an UNDERproduction of T4.

5. In dogs, hypothyroidism is usually a primary disease.(12, 15, 21) There are two main causes of primary hypothyroidism in dogs:(21, 31)

   - lymphocytic thyroiditis
   - idiopathic thyroid atrophy.

6. Thyroid cancer is a much less common cause of primary hypothyroidism in the dog.

7. Thyroid tumors (both benign and malignant) represent 1.1–3.8% of all canine neoplasia.(32–35)

8. Neither sex is predisposed to thyroid neoplasia.(36–42) However, the Beagle, Boxer, Golden retriever, and Husky breeds appear to be at increased risk within the US.(36, 37, 41–43) By contrast, the breeds that are overrepresented in Scotland are the Shetland Collie, Old English Sheepdog, and the Cairn terrier.(44)

9. When thyroid tumors develop in the dog, they are more likely to be malignant.(30, 33, 36, 37) Only 9% are adenomas.(32)

10. Canine thyroid tumors are UNLIKELY to be functional.(12, 16, 30, 45) Less than 25% of canine patients with thyroid tumors have clinical presentations and/or clinicopathologic data that suggest a hyperthyroid state.(33, 37, 38, 46, 47) This is in stark contrast to what is seen in clinical practice in cats.(12, 16)

11. If Baguette is hypothyroid, then I would expect to see the following clinicopathologic data:(12, 14, 15, 23, 48)
   - CBC – normocytic, normochromic, non-regenerative anemia
   - chemistry profile:
     - elevated cholesterol
     - elevated triglycerides
     - mild increase in liver enzymes
     - +/– mild increase in creatinine kinase.

12. Testing for total thyroxine (TT4) is an appropriate screening tool in that its sensitivity is relatively high: it falls between 89% and 100%.(49–52) Patients are unlikely to be hypothyroid if TT4 falls within the normal reference range and is not borderline.
    If TT4 is low, then the patient *may* be hypothyroid. Additional tests are indicated.

13. Additional confirmatory tests for hypothyroidism are usually lumped together in a so-called thyroid panel, which tests for the following hormones, in addition to TT4:(14, 15, 53)
   - free T4 (fT4)
   - TSH
   - +/– thryoglobulin autoantibodies – up to 50% of hypothyroid dogs have autoantibodies to thyroglobulin.(19)

   Measuring serum T3 is usually not helpful in making the diagnosis.(14)

14. If the patient is truly hypothyroid, then you would expect to see a LOW fT4 and a HIGH TSH. (14, 15)

15. Hypothyroidism is not the only cause of low TT4. TT4 experiences diurnal variation. This may cause TT4 to be lower than normal at certain points throughout the day.
    Other causes of low TT4 include:(14, 15)
   - breed-specific lower-than-normal reference range for thyroxine, in which case the "low" value is actually normal for the patient:(14)
     - Alaskan sled dogs
     - Chinese Shar-peis
   - Sighthounds
   - certain drugs(13, 19, 54–61)
   - non-thyroidal illness.

Non-thyroidal illness can be associated with so-called sick euthyroid syndrome. This means that the patient is truly euthyroid; however, illness has suppressed the concentration of circulating thyroid hormones.(14, 15) Most typically, TT4 is impacted by non-thyroidal illness.(54, 62) Free T4 may be impacted, although if so, it is usually to a lesser degree.(54, 62)

16. The following drugs may influence canine thyroid function test results:(13, 19, 54–61)

   - clomipramine
   - high-dose aspirin
   - high-dose prednisone
   - phenobarbital
   - thyroxine supplementation
   - trimethoprim-sulfamethoxazole.

17. Hypothyroidism is typically treated in dogs by providing life-long supplementation by means of oral levothyroxine (L-thyroxine) sodium.(14, 15, 63) This is a synthetic drug.(14) It is usually administered every 12 hours.(14, 64)

18. It is important to monitor the effects of the initial dose by re-examining the patient and having the patient submit to serum TT4 testing 4 to 6 weeks after initiating therapy.(14) Note that timing of the blood draw is critical to obtaining a test result that will be of diagnostic value.(14) You want to schedule the blood draw to take place 4 to 6 hours after the medication has been administered.(14, 63) Dose adjustments are made as needed.

19. Response to treatment varies depending upon the system that has been impacted by this endocrinopathy.(14) Mental alertness is usually quick to improve.(14) Clients with dull dogs often report that they have brightened in terms of awareness within 1 to 2 weeks following initiation of treatment. Skin and other neurologic abnormalities may take several months to resolve.(14)

20. Treatment is relatively safe because you are simply giving the patient what his/her body would have produced. In that respect, you are providing replacement therapy rather than adding on a compound that is unfamiliar to the system.

Returning to Case 17: Canine Weight Gain

You prescribe levothyroxine sodium at a dose of 0.01 mg/kg. You round up such that Baguette is dispensed a 45-day supply of 0.4 mg to be given per os (PO) BID (every 12 hours), with instructions to return in 30 days.

Baguette returns in 2 weeks to evaluate her progress and to recheck her TT4. Nora acknowledges that she's 2 weeks early, but that this was the only day/time that worked for her schedule. As requested, she planned ahead and gave Baguette her medication 5 hours prior to her scheduled blood draw.

At today's visit, Baguette has (finally!) lost weight. Nora cheers when the scale reads 76.4 lb!

Nora is also excited to share that Baguette is back to her bouncy, cheerful, active self! She's so eager to go for walks that now she almost pulls Nora down the street!

Baguette's blood is drawn uneventfully and is sent off to the lab for analysis. You receive the finalized results in your inbox the following day:

Initial reading (TT4): 9 nmol/L (reference range: 13–51 nmol/L)

Reading at re-check exam (TT4): 76 nmol/L (reference range: 13–51 nmol/L)

Round Three of Questions for Case 17: Canine Weight Gain

1. If lab error is not to blame, what is the most likely explanation for this reading?
2. If this value is real and it were to remain this high, unchecked, what could be potential consequences for Baguette?
3. Assuming that you dispensed the tabs of the correct size to the client, meaning that there's not a pharmacy error to blame, what is the next question that you will ask the client?

Answers to Round Three of Questions for Case 17: Canine Weight Gain

1. The most likely explanation is iatrogenic hyperthyroidism.(14) Either I calculated the dose wrong or the client is administering the medication incorrectly.

2. If this value is real and it were to remain this high, unchecked, then Baguette is likely to experience tachycardia, hypertension, hyperexcitability, nervousness, and/or panting.(64)

3. I need to confirm the dosing instructions with the client.

    • Take me through how many tabs of medication you are giving to Baguette.
    • How often are you giving that number of tabs to Baguette?

Returning to Case 17: Canine Weight Gain

You telephone Nora to discuss Baguette's test results. When you ask her to confirm the dosing of levothyroxine, she tells you that she has been giving Baguette two tabs morning and night. Nora is embarrassed to find that this dose is twice what had been prescribed! No wonder Baguette is bouncy. It's like her whole body has been revved! She agrees to cut back to the originally prescribed dose and return in another month to repeat blood testing.

CLINICAL PEARLS

• Weight gain typically results from a combination of overindulgence (i.e. too high of a caloric intake) and inactivity.

• Most obese dogs are not hypothyroid.

• Hypothyroidism is over-diagnosed.

• Comprehensive dietary histories are essential to quantify caloric intake to the best of your ability before automatically assuming that the patient must be hypothyroid.

• Hypothyroid dogs are often middle-aged to older, although dogs of breeds that are predisposed to endocrinopathy may present as early as two or three years of age.

• Hypothyroid dogs may present with a history of being mentally dull and exercise intolerant.

• On physical exam, hypothyroid dogs often have truncal alopecia, +/− "ring around the collar", +/− "rat tail".

- Hypothyroid dogs are predisposed to secondary bacterial and fungal skin infections.

- When hypothyroidism is suspected, screening bloodwork is performed. Anemia may be present on the CBC. Hypercholesterolemia and hypertriglyceridemia are supportive of the diagnosis.

- Serum total thyroxine (TT4) is an important screening tool for hypothyroidism. If the patient has a normal TT4, then hypothyroidism is unlikely.

- If the patient's TT4 is low, then additional diagnostic tests are required.

- Low TT4 is not pathognomonic for hypothyroidism. Non-thyroidal illness and medications can also suppress TT4.

- Know that certain breeds have a lower-than-normal TT4. These dogs will fall below the "normal" reference range, but their values are considered to be normal for them. Sighthounds are the most commonly used example.

References

1. Linder D, Mueller M. Pet obesity management: beyond nutrition. Vet Clin North Am Small Anim Pract 2014;44(4):789–806.
2. Butterwick RF, Hawthorne AJ. Advances in dietary management of obesity in dogs and cats. J Nutr 1998;128(12);Suppl:2771S–5S.
3. Laflamme DP, Kuhlman G, Lawler DF. Evaluation of weight loss protocols for dogs. J Am Anim Hosp Assoc 1997;33(3):253–9.
4. Linder DE, Parker VJ. Dietary aspects of weight management in cats and dogs. Vet Clin North Am Small Anim Pract 2016;46(5):869–82.
5. Englar R. Writing skills for veterinarians. Sheffield: 5M Publishing; 2019.
6. Englar R. A guide to oral communication in veterinary medicine. Sheffield: 5M Publishing; 2020.
7. Cameron S, Turtle-song I. Learning to write case notes using the SOAP format. J Couns Dev 2002;80(3): 286–92.
8. Rockett J, Lattanzio C, Christensen C. The veterinary technician's guide to writing SOAPS: A workbook for critical thinking. Heyburn, ID: Rockett House Publishing LLC; 2013.
9. Borcherding S. Documentation manual for writing SOAP notes in occupational therapy. 2nd ed. Thorofare, NJ: Slack Incorporated; 2005.
10. Kettenbach G, Kettenbach G. Writing patient/client notes: ensuring accuracy in documentation. 4th ed. Philadelphia, PA: F. A. Davis; 2004.
11. Kettenbach G. Writing SOAP notes: with patient/client management formats. 3rd ed. Philadelphia, PA: F. A. Davis Company; 2004.
12. Englar RE. Common clinical presentations in dogs and cats. Hoboken, NJ: Wiley/Blackwell; 2019.
13. Plumb DC. Plumb's veterinary drug handbook. 8th ed. Ames, IA: PharmaVet Inc.; 2015.
14. Côté E. Clinical veterinary advisor. Dogs and cats. 3rd ed. St. Louis, MO: Elsevier Mosby; 2015.
15. Ettinger SJ, Feldman EC, Côté E. Textbook of veterinary internal medicine: diseases of the dog and the cat. 8th ed. St. Louis, MO: Elsevier; 2017.
16. Englar RE. Performing the small animal physical examination. Hoboken, NJ: Wiley/Blackwell; 2017.
17. Merck Vet Man. Whitehouse Station, NJ: Merck & Co. Inc. 2016.
18. Gough A, Thomas A, O'Neill D Hoboken NJ, ed. Breed predispositions to disease in dogs and cats. 3rd ed. Hoboken, NJ: Wiley; 2018.
19. Frank LA. Comparative dermatology--canine endocrine dermatoses. Clin Dermatol 2006;24(4):317–25.
20. Feldman EC, Nelson RW. Canine and feline endocrinology and reproduction. St. Louis, MO: W. B. Saunders; 2004.

21. Scott-Moncrieff JC. Clinical signs and concurrent diseases of hypothyroidism in dogs and cats. Vet Clin North Am Small Anim Pract 2007;37(4):709–22.

22. Zur G, White SD. Hyperadrenocorticism in 10 dogs with skin lesions as the only presenting clinical signs. J Am Anim Hosp Assoc 2011;47(6):419–27.

23. Dixon RM, Reid SW, Mooney CT. Epidemiological, clinical, haematological and biochemical characteristics of canine hypothyroidism. Vet Rec 1999;145(17):481–7.

24. Panciera DL. Conditions associated with canine hypothyroidism. Vet Clin North Am Small Anim Pract 2001;31(5):935–50.

25. Beaver BV, Haug LI. Canine behaviors associated with hypothyroidism. J Am Anim Hosp Assoc 2003;39(5):431–4.

26. Baker K. Hormonal alopecia in dogs and cats. Pract 1986;8(2):71–8.

27. Credille KM, Slater MR, Moriello KA, Nachreiner RF, Tucker KA, Dunstan RW. The effects of thyroid hormones on the skin of beagle dogs. J Vet Intern Med 2001;15(6):539–46.

28. Rijnberk A, van Sluijs FS. Medical history and physical examination in companion animals. Amsterdam: Elsevier; 2009.

29. Feldman EC, Nelson RW. Canine and feline endocrinology and reproduction. 3rd ed. St. Louis, MO: Saunders; 2004.

30. Barber LG. Thyroid tumors in dogs and cats. Vet Clin North Am Small Anim Pract 2007;37(4):755–73.

31. Graham PA, Refsal KR, Nachreiner RF. Etiopathologic findings of canine hypothyroidism. Vet Clin North Am Small Anim Pract 2007;37(4):617–31.

32. Wucherer KL, Wilke V. Thyroid cancer in dogs: an update based on 638 cases (1995–2005). J Am Anim Hosp Assoc 2010;46(4):249–54.

33. Page RL. Tumors of the endocrine system. In: Withrow SJ, MacEwen EG, editors. Small animal clinical oncology. 3rd ed. Philadelphia, PA: Saunders; 2001. p. 423–7.

34. Capen CC. Tumors of the endocrine glands. In: Meuten DJ, editor. Tumors in domestic animals. 4th ed. Ames, IA: Iowa State Press; 2002. p. 638–64.

35. Mooney CT. Hyperthyroidism. Textbook of veterinary internal medicine: diseases of the dog and cat. 6th ed. St. Louis, MO: Elsevier Saunders; 2005. p. 1544–60.

36. Brodey RS, Kelly DF. Thyroid neoplasms in the dog. A clinicopathologic study of fifty-seven cases. Cancer 1968;22(2):406–16.

37. Leav I, Schiller AL, Rijnberk A, Legg MA, DER, der Kinderen PJ. Adenomas and carcinomas of the canine and feline thyroid. Am J Pathol 1976;83(1):61–122.

38. Carver JR, Kapatkin A, Patnaik AK. A comparison of medullary thyroid carcinoma and thyroid adenocarcinoma in dogs: a retrospective study of 38 cases. Vet Surg VS 1995;24(4):315–9.

39. Patnaik AK, Lieberman PH. Gross, histologic, cytochemical, and immunocytochemical study of medullary thyroid carcinoma in sixteen dogs. Vet Pathol 1991;28(3):223–33.

40. Birchard SJ, Roesel OF. Neoplasia of the thyroid-gland in the dog – a retrospective study of 16 cases. J Am Anim Hosp Assoc 1981;17(3):369–72.

41. Harari J, Patterson JS, Rosenthal RC. Clinical and pathologic features of thyroid tumors in 26 dogs. J Am Vet Med Assoc 1986;188(10):1160–4.

42. Hayes HM, Jr., Fraumeni JF, Jr. Canine thyroid neoplasms: epidemiologic features. J Natl Cancer Inst 1975;55(4):931–4.

43. Scott-Moncrieff JC. Thyroid disorders in the geriatric veterinary patient. Vet Clin North Am Small Anim Pract 2012;42(4):707–25.

44. Sullivan M, Cox F, Pead MJ, McNELL P. Thyroid tumours in the dog. J Small Anim Pract 1987;28(6):505–12.

45. Liptak JM. Canine thyroid carcinoma. Clin Tech Small Anim Pract 2007;22(2):75–81.

46. Marks SL, Koblik PD, Hornof WJ, Feldman EC. 99mTc-pertechnetate imaging of thyroid tumors in dogs: 29 cases (1980–1992). J Am Vet Med Assoc 1994;204(5):756–60.

47. Kent MS, Griffey SM, Verstraete FJ, Naydan D, Madewell BR. Computer-assisted image analysis of neovascularization in thyroid neoplasms from dogs. Am J Vet Res 2002;63(3):363–9.

48. Panciera DL. Hypothyroidism in dogs: 66 cases (1987–1992). J Am Vet Med Assoc 1994;204(5):761–7.

49. Nelson RW, Ihle SL, Feldman EC, Bottoms GD. Serum free thyroxine concentration in healthy dogs, dogs with hypothyroidism, and euthyroid dogs with concurrent illness. J Am Vet Med Assoc 1991;198(8):1401–7.

50. Peterson ME, Melián C, Nichols R. Measurement of serum total thyroxine, triiodothyronine, free thyroxine, and thyrotropin concentrations for diagnosis of hypothyroidism in dogs. J Am Vet Med Assoc 1997;211(11):1396–402.

51. Scott-Moncrieff JC, Nelson RW, Bruner JM, Williams DA. Comparison of serum concentrations of thyroid-stimulating hormone in healthy dogs, hypothyroid dogs, and euthyroid dogs with concurrent illness. Vet Med Assoc 1998;212(3):387–91.

52. Dixon RM, Mooney CT. Evaluation of serum free thyroxine and thyrotropin concentrations in the diagnosis of canine hypothyroidism. J Small Anim Pract 1999;40(2):72–8.

53. Ferguson DC. Testing for hypothyroidism in dogs. Vet Clin North Am Small Anim Pract 2007;37(4):647–69, v, v.

54. Gulikers KP, Panciera DL. Evaluation of the effects of clomipramine on canine thyroid function tests. J Vet Intern Med 2003;17(1):44–9.

55. Hall IA, Campbell KL, Chambers MD, Davis CN. Effect of trimethoprim/sulfamethoxazole on thyroid function in dogs with pyoderma. J Am Vet Med Assoc 1993;202(12):1959–62.

56. Daminet S, Croubels S, Duchateau L, Debunne A, van Geffen C, Hoybergs Y, et al. Influence of acetylsalicylic acid and ketoprofen on canine thyroid function tests. Vet J 2003;166(3):224–32.

57. Daminet S, Paradis M, Refsal KR, Price C. Short-term influence of prednisone and phenobarbital on thyroid function in euthyroid dogs. Can Vet J 1999;40(6):411–5.

58. Gaskill CL, Burton SA, Gelens HC, Ihle SL, Miller JB, Shaw DH, et al. Effects of phenobarbital treatment on serum thyroxine and thyroid-stimulating hormone concentrations in epileptic dogs. J Am Vet Med Assoc 1999;215(4):489–96.

59. Frank LA, Hnilica KA, May ER, Sargent SJ, Davis JA. Effects of sulfamethoxazole-trimethoprim on thyroid function in dogs. Am J Vet Res 2005;66(2):256–9.

60. Müller PB, Wolfsheimer KJ, Taboada J, Hosgood G, Partington BP, Gaschen FP. Effects of long-term phenobarbital treatment on the thyroid and adrenal axis and adrenal function tests in dogs. J Vet Intern Med 2000;14(2):157–64.

61. Williamson NL, Frank LA, Hnilica KA. Effects of short-term trimethoprim-sulfamethoxazole administration on thyroid function in dogs. J Am Vet Med Assoc 2002;221(6):802–6.

62. Kantrowitz LB, Peterson ME, Melián C, Nichols R. Serum total thyroxine, total triiodothyronine, free thyroxine, and thyrotropin concentrations in dogs with nonthyroidal disease. J Am Vet Med Assoc 2001;219(6):765–9.

63. Dixon RM, Reid SW, Mooney CT. Treatment and therapeutic monitoring of canine hypothyroidism. J Small Anim Pract 2002;43(8):334–40.

64. Plumb DC. Plumb's veterinary drug handbook. 9th ed. Hoboken, NJ: Pharma Vet Inc.; 2018.

Case 18

The Cat with Hematuria

Pita was purchased by her current owner, Don Pasquel, from a local breeder at 12 weeks of age. Since then, Pita has been the apple of Don's eye. She has never lived with anyone other than Don, so she isn't used to housemates, and she has not had to share Don's attention until recently.

Ten days ago, Don's girlfriend, Penelope Branson, moved into the one-bedroom apartment. Pita wasn't keen on Penelope. In truth, she only liked Don. However, Pita was particularly irritated by two new arrivals that came with Penelope, her two cats, BJ and PT. Both were indoor-only neutered male domestic shorthaired (DSM) cats. As far as Pita was concerned, they shared her age and that was it.

Space came at a premium. There was no way to escape overcrowded living arrangements. On top of that, their introductions to one another had not gone smoothly. BJ and PT were bold and had approached her long before she was willing to welcome them into the home. Whether their approach was to offer peace or to challenge her, she couldn't be sure. She gave a warning hiss. They were undaunted. One even raised a paw to swat at the air between them.

Pita had a lot of attitude, yes, but the one attribute she lacked was courage. She hightailed it under the bed and refused to come out until well after dinner. Even then, she sulked. Despite

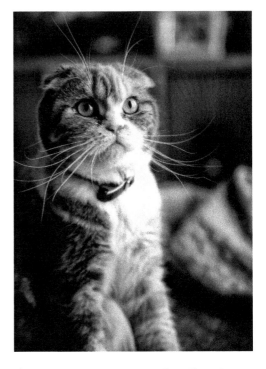

Figure 18.1 Meet your next patient, Pita, a 3-year-old spayed female Scottish Fold cat. Courtesy of Victoria Stone.

the other two cats not being in her direct line of sight, her nose told her that they were still there. As far as she was concerned, this gift of "brothers" needed to be returned. Yet day after day, it was becoming apparent that BJ and PT were here to stay.

Three days ago, Penelope found what appeared to be cat pee around the drain in the bottom of the bathtub. No one had caught the culprit, so it was anyone's guess as to how the urine got there.

Two days ago, Penelope stepped in something wet on the bathroom tile when she was brushing her teeth. At first, she thought it was leftover water from Don's shower earlier that morning, but when she checked the bottom of her sock, it was stained a peach color and smelled strong, like urine. Penelope told Don that Pita was peeing all over the house out of spite.

Today, Don heard a cry coming from the litter room. He witnessed Pita climbing into the box and squatting, but she only produced a few drops of urine. This failed attempt to produce urine of any substantial amount repeated itself several times. When Pita finally gave up, her tail quivered. She was restless. She couldn't get settled. She fluctuated between velcroing herself to Don and sitting on her haunches, grooming incessantly under her tail in between mournful cries.

This turn of events concerns Don greatly. In the past 3 years, Pita has never been sick, and he's never seen her this uncomfortable. Despite Penelope's claims that Pita is playing him, he scoops her up and presents her to your clinic as a walk-in emergency.

A technician walks Don and Pita to the nearest examination room so that her vitals can be taken. The technician documents her findings in the chart and alerts you right away that your next patient is here.

Consider the following questions to help you prepare for this consultation.

Weight: 8.5 lb (3.9 kg)
BCS: 4/9
Mentation: QAR

TPR

T: 100.5°F (38.1°C)
P: 194 beats per minute
R: 26 breaths per minute

Round One of Questions for Case 18: The Cat with Hematuria

1. Define the following terms, which describe clinical signs that result from pathology of the urinary tract:

   - anuria
   - dysuria
   - oliguria
   - pigmenturia

   - pollakiuria
   - polyuria
   - stranguria.

2. Which of the terms listed in Question #1 (above) might you use in the medical record to document Don's description of Pita?
3. What is the expected color of urine? How does this color vary?
4. What are abnormal colors of urine and how might they arise?
5. What additional questions might you need to ask Don to expand upon the urinary history that has been provided above?
6. Diminished urine production can be physiologic. Provide two examples of how this is so.
7. Identify the most common causes of pathologic oliguria.
8. After history-taking, what is your next step in the diagnostic plan?
9. What will you be looking for when you perform the next step in your diagnostic plan?

Answers to Round One of Questions for Case 18: The Cat with Hematuria

1. The following terms describe clinical signs that result from pathology of the urinary tract. Their definitions have been provided below:(1–3)

   - anuria: lack of urination; inability to urinate
   - dysuria: painful or difficult urination
   - oliguria: reduced urine output; lower-than-normal urine production
   - pigmenturia: the presence of something in urine that imparts an abnormal color
   - pollakiuria: increased frequency of urination; increased attempts to urinate
   - polyuria: increased volume of urine; higher-than-normal urine production
   - stranguria: straining to urinate.

2. Based upon Don's description of Pita over the past few days, culminating in her activities in the litterbox this morning, I would document that Pita appears to be exhibiting dysuria, oliguria, pigmenturia, pollakiuria, and stranguria.

3. Normal urine is yellow because it contains urobilinogen, a byproduct of bilirubin metabolism that is excreted by the kidney.(1, 4, 5) There is not one shade of yellow to describe normal urine.(1) Which shade of yellow urine is varies depending upon how concentrated the urine is.(1, 4, 5)

   Because the first urine sample of the morning is typically more concentrated, it tends to be a stronger shade of yellow, as compared to samples that are taken later in the day.(1, 5) (See **Plate 4** and Figure 18.2)

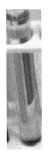

4. Abnormal urine color typically stems from pathology. The most commonly seen abnormal colors of urine in clinical practice include the following.(1, 5)

   Figure 18.2
   Dilute urine.

   - Brown:

     - Myoglobin is a protein in muscle.
     - When damaged muscle is broken down, myoglobin is released into the bloodstream. This results in myoglobinuria.

   - Cream or milky:

     - This color and corresponding opacity is caused by an abundance of leukocytes in the urine.
     - Leukocytes may be present in urine secondary to bacterial urinary tract infections (UTIs) or prostatic abscesses (which, of course, Pita doesn't have!).
     - Leukocytes may also be present in cases of sterile cystitis, in which the lower urinary tract is inflamed, rather than infected.

   - Orange:

     - Orange discoloration of the urine may indicate extreme dehydration.
     - Orange discoloration of the urine may also result from an abundance of bilirubin in the urine, as occurs with hepatobiliary dysfunction.

   - Peach-to-Pink, ranging all the way up to red:

     - Red discoloration of the urine is caused by an abundance of erythrocytes in the urine.
     - Erythrocytes may be present due to:

       - UTIs
       - urolithiasis, which abrades the lining of the lower urinary tract
       - sterile cystitis, secondary to inflammation of the lower urinary tract.

   (See **Plates 5a–5f.**)

5. I would want to expand upon the history as follows.

   - Describe the apartment set-up.

     - Where does Pita spend her day relative to where BJ and PT hang out?
     - Where does Pita eat relative to where BJ and PT are fed?
     - Where does Pita sleep relative to where BJ and PT sleep?
     - What have the interactions between Pita, BJ, and PT been like since that first night when introductions went south?

       - Can they be in the same room together?
       - How close (physically) can they be to one another?
       - Describe Pita's body language during interactions with BJ and PT:
       - body posture
       - ear carriage

- pupil size and shape
- tail position
- Describe BJ and PT's body language using the same descriptors as above.
- Do the cats hiss/spit/growl/vocalize at one another?
- Do the cats physically attack one another?

- Is there vertical space (cat trees, furniture/shelves)?
- Other than vertical space, what are prime resources in the house?
- Does each cat have their own resource or are resources required to be shared?
- Are there escape routes in the house for one or more cats to get away from the aggressor?
- Have any altercations led to redirection aggression?

  - BJ to PT?
  - PT to BJ?
  - Pita to Don?

  - Pita to Penelope?
  - BJ or PT to Don?
  - BJ or PT to Penelope?

- Litter box set-up:

  - How many litter boxes were present when only Pita lived with Don?

    - Where were the boxes located?
    - What kind of litter was used? Clay or clumpable? Scented or unscented? Regular or lightweight? Brand?
    - Has anything about the litter itself changed?

  - How many litter boxes are present now that there are three cats in the household?

    - If there are additional boxes, where are they located? Are all the boxes now together? Are the boxes spaced throughout the house?
    - If there are additional boxes, where did they come from? Are they new? Or are they old boxes from BJ/PT's house, which carry their scent?

  - How often was the litter scooped when only Pita lived with Don?
  - How often is the litter scooped now that three cats live in the household?

- Has Pita ever exhibited house-soiling before?
- Do BJ and PT have a history of house-soiling?
- What, if anything, has Don or Penelope done to facilitate interactions between the cats? E.g. have they tried synthetic feline pheromone?

Based upon clinical acumen, the introduction of two new cats is likely linked to Pita's chief complaint, particularly given the timeline that Don has provided. For this reason, most of these clarifying questions concentrate on the inter-cat relationships and the spatial arrangement of the apartment relative to cat-specific resources.

However, as clinicians we do not want to wear blinders and limit our inspection to what appears to be most obvious. Therefore, it is also important to keep in mind other potential causes of oliguria, including acute kidney injury (AKI), as from exposure to nephrotoxins. For this reason, I would want to ask Don if Pita has had any exposure to:(1, 6)

- ethylene glycol
- heavy metals
- lilies.

Note that not all lilies are nephrotoxic. Those within the genera *Lilium* and *Hemerocallis* are and include:(7, 8)

- Asiatic lilies
- day lilies
- easter lilies

- stargazer lilies
- tiger lilies.

As clinicians, we often forget to ask about houseplants during history-taking or about accessible vases that contain flowers in the home environment. It is essential that we include these questions when we take a comprehensive history on a patient that presents with altered urine output. We do not want to miss out on diagnosing nephrotoxins that are life-threatening.

Sometimes owners will acknowledge the presence of nephrotoxic plants in the home but claim that the pet never eats them. Recognize that, although the mechanism of lily toxicosis is unknown, it is not necessary for a cat to ingest a leaf or stem to developing toxicosis. Ingestion of pollen alone or water that contains lily pollen is sufficient to induce nephrotoxicity.(7)

As an extension of a line of questioning that targets nephrotoxins, I would want to inquire as to whether Pita has been vomiting. I would also ask about appetite: Is Pita eating?

6. Physiologic oliguria occurs when the body needs to conserve water, as when the patient is dehydrated.(1) The rise in plasma osmolality and reduced circulating blood volume trigger anti-diuretic hormone (ADH) to be released from the hypothalamus.(1, 4, 9, 10) ADH "tells" the kidney to reabsorb water.(1, 4, 9) This is achieved through the insertion of aquaporin-2 water channels into the membranes of the distal tubules and collecting ducts.(1, 11) Water is now able to re-enter systemic circulation.(1) A byproduct of this is that the urine becomes more concentrated.(1, 4, 9)

    Physiologic oliguria also occurs as a compensatory mechanism when the body is faced with hypotension.(1) In this case, reabsorption of water back into circulation counters hypotension by raising blood volume.(1)

    Note that physiologic oliguria is temporary.(1) It will resolve as soon as the inciting factor is corrected.(12) Consider the dehydrated patient. When euhydration is restored, normal urine production will resume.(1)

7. Pathologic oliguria may result from:(1, 12–15)

    *   increased resistance to blood flow at the level of the afferent glomerular vessels
    *   loss of nephrons
    *   macroscopic obstruction of urinary flow:

        *   inflammation of the lower urinary tract
        *   neoplasia of the urinary bladder or prostate
        *   urethral plug (cats > dogs)
        *   urinary stricture
        *   urolithiasis

    *   microscopic obstruction of urinary flow

        *   obstruction of the lumens of nephrons

    *   reduced permeability of the glomerulus
    *   rupture of the urinary tract
    *   toxins

        *   ethylene glycol
        *   grapes and raisins
        *   lily toxicosis.

8. After history-taking, the next step in the diagnostic plan is to perform a comprehensive physical exam.(16)

9. Although my physical exam will be comprehensive, I will concentrate on assessing the urogenital tract for the following features.(1, 16)

- Renal palpation:(14, 17)

  - Size:

    - In a patient with oliguria, I am particularly concerned about kidney size. I want to rule out renomegaly because renomegaly has been associated with oliguria in patients that have AKI.
    - Renal size is estimated by abdominal palpation, comparing renal length to finger width.(14)
    - The clinician starts by measuring the width of his second through fourth fingers, in centimeters, when they are adjacent to each other, as if wearing mittens.
    - Next, the clinician palpates the patient's kidneys.
    - If, for instance, the clinician notes that the length of the cat's left kidney spans the width of three of his fingers, and he knows in advance how wide his fingers are, he can estimate the length, in centimeters, of that kidney.(14)
    - Renal size estimates as obtained through palpation are imperfect, but they are a starting point.(14)
    - If based on palpation, renal size is much too small or much too large, then palpation estimates can be confirmed through imaging.(14, 18–32)
    - Abdominal radiographs allow kidney length to be compared to the length of the body of the second lumbar vertebra (L2). This establishes the patient's renal length ratio.(14, 20) Normal renal length ratios in the cat have been cited as 2.0–3.0.(19, 21–24)
    - Abdominal ultrasonography allows for a direct measurement of renal length and therefore improves accuracy. Renal length in the cat, for instance, is typically between 3.8–4.4 cm, but can reach as high as 5.3 cm.(18, 21, 25, 28, 29)

  - Shape – normal kidneys are shaped like kidney beans.(14)
  - Surface contour – normal kidneys should have smooth surfaces rather than undulated.
  - Presence or absence of pain – renal palpation should not be painful to the patient.(14, 17)

- Urinary bladder palpation:

  - Is the urinary bladder palpable?
  - What is the relative size of the urinary bladder?
  - Is the urinary bladder rock hard? This presentation is more typical of male cats with urinary tract obstruction (UTO).
  - Is the urinary bladder compressible?
  - Does the wall of the urinary bladder appear to be thickened?
  - Does palpation of the urinary bladder cause discomfort?
  - Does palpation of the urinary bladder cause the patient to strain? In male cats with urinary tract obstruction (UTO) one might witness pulsing of the penis as the patient unsuccessfully attempts to void.
  - Does palpation of the urinary bladder cause the patient to void?

    - If so, what is the color of the urine that is produced?
    - Is there macroscopic particulate matter in the urine that is produced (i.e. blood clots, plugs, stones)?
    - What is the apparent turbidity of the urine that is produced?

- Visual inspection of the perineum:

  - Is there vulvar discharge?
  - Is there staining of the peri-vulvar fur? Rust-brown discoloration of peri-vulvar fur raises our index of suspicion that the patient might have hematuria or may be excessively grooming that region of the body

- Visual inspection of the ventral abdomen:

  - Some, but not all, cats with chronic cystitis may overgroom the ventrum overlaying the urinary bladder, causing them to develop hypotrichosis or alopecia
  - Based upon the clinical history, Pita does not sound as though she has chronic cystitis, but it is important to be thorough.

Returning to Case 18: The Cat with Hematuria

You expand upon the patient history before evaluating Pita. When you elicit Don's perspective, he expresses concern that Pita is sick, but that Penelope (who is not present at today's visit) remains unconvinced. According to Don, Penelope believes that Pita's house-soiling is rooted in behavior. She says that Pita is just being "spiteful." Don needs answers today because Penelope has put her foot down. She says that she will not tolerate cat pee in "her" home. You validate Don's frustration and reassure him that you will work together to get to the bottom of Pita's chief complaint.

You then examine Pita and make note of the following physical examination features.

- Pita is euhydrated.
- Pita's peri-vulvar fur is stained rust-brown.
- Pita's kidneys are appropriately sized and shaped.
- Pita does not appear to react to renal palpation.
- Pita's urinary bladder is small.
- Pita reacts with reproducible abdominal tensing and vocalizes when you palpate her urinary bladder.
- You do not palpate any obvious bladder stones.

Round Two of Questions for Case 18: The Cat with Hematuria

1. Given Pita's signalment and history, what is the likelihood of a UTI?
2. How might the likelihood of a UTI change if Pita were a senior cat instead of a 3-year-old?
3. How might the likelihood of a UTI change if Pita were a dog instead of a cat?
4. What are the body's inherent defense mechanisms to reduce the chance of developing a UTI?
5. Which risk factors increase the chance of UTI development?
6. How will you rule in or rule out a UTI?
7. If a patient has a UTI, what do you expect to find when you perform the diagnostic test(s) that you indicated in Question #6 (above)?
8. Which add-on test may be required as part of your diagnostic plan to rule in or rule out a UTI?
9. How do you collect a urine sample from a cat?
10. Outline the advantages and disadvantages of each method of urine collection that you outlined in Question #9 (above). Include potential risks for each method of collection.

Answers to Round Two of Questions for Case 18: The Cat with Hematuria

1. Given Pita's signalment and history, what is the likelihood of a UTI?

    Pita is a 3-year-old spayed female cat. Because of her age, it is unlikely that she has developed a UTI. UTIs represent less than 2% of lower urinary tract disease in cats that are less than 10 years old.(1, 33)

2. Age is a definite risk factor for cats. Cats that are greater than 10 years old are more likely to develop UTIs.(33)

3. UTIs are relatively common occurrences in dogs as compared to cats.(1, 34–36) Fourteen percent of dogs develop at least one UTI in their lifetime.(34, 37) Persistent and/or recurrent UTIs also occur in a subset of the canine population.(34, 37–39)

4. The body has several mechanisms to protect against UTI, including:(1, 35, 40–43)

   • commensal flora
   • glycosaminoglycan layer
   • tissue folds along the length of the proximal urethra to trap bacterial invaders
   • unidirectional flow of urine
   • urethral length
   • urine composition – high levels of urea and organic acids deter bacteria
   • urine concentrating ability, urine specific gravity (USG) – high osmolality deters bacteria. Cat urine is particularly concentrated.(35) Feline USG typically exceeds 1.045.(35, 43)

5. The following risk factors increase the likelihood of UTI development:(1, 33–35, 44–49)

   • abnormal urinary tract anatomy:

       • ectopic ureter
       • recessed vulva

   • bladder atony
   • bladder mucosa abnormalities
   • endocrinopathies:

       • diabetes mellitus
       • hyperadrenocorticism
       • hyperthyroidism
       • hypoadrenocorticism

   • glycosuria
   • immunosuppression
   • indwelling urinary catheters
   • neoplasia of the urinary tract
   • peri-vulvar dermatitis
   • pharmacologic therapy:

       • chemotherapy
       • corticosteroids

   • prostatitis
   • recent antibiotic therapy
   • urinary surgery:

       • cystotomy
       • perineal urethrostomy.

6. Urinalysis is the primary diagnostic test for diagnosis of bacterial UTI.(33) Urinalysis includes:(1, 5, 35)

   • gross observation of the urine:

       • color

- • volume of urine
- • clarity of urine
- • presence/absence of macroscopic particulate matter
- measurement of USG
- dipstick analysis:(1, 5, 35, 50–52)
  - • bilirubin:
    - • normal to see trace to +1 in concentrated canine urine, particularly males
    - • never normal to see bilirubinuria in cats(50)
  - • glucose:
    - • when glucose exceeds 180–220 mg/dL in the dog and 260–280 mg/dL in the cat, glucose will spill into the urine(53)
    - • glycosuria may be due to stress hyperglycemia, particularly in cats
    - • glycosuria may also be due to true pathology, such as diabetes mellitus or renal tubular disease
  - • heme, or occult blood:
    - • detects heme protein in the urine (intact erythrocytes, hemoglobin, myoglobin)

(Note that a false positive reaction can occur if cystocentesis resulted in microscopic hematuria.)

  - • ketones:
    - • dipsticks detect acetoacetate >>> acetone
    - • dipsticks do not detect β-hydroxybutyrate
  - • pH:
    - • ranges from 5.0–7.5 in dogs and cats
    - • varies based upon the patient's diet:
    - • meat-based diets will cause aciduria
    - • plant-based diets will cause alkalinuria
    - • other causes of alkalinuria include post-prandial alkaline tide and urease-containing bacterial UTI
  - • protein:
    - • albumin is the primary protein that is detected
    - • proteinuria may be physiologic (exercise, fever, stress)
    - • proteinuria may be pathologic:
    - • congestive heart failure
    - • glomerular disease
    - • hemorrhage
    - • lower urinary tract inflammation
    - • upper urinary tract inflammation
    - • false negatives are common if urine is dilute or acidic
    - • false positives are common if urine is concentrated or alkaline
    - • false positives are more likely to occur in cats

(Note: readings for bilirubin and ketones may be inaccurate if urine is discolored. The following measurements are unreliable in dogs and cats: leukocyte esterase, nitrate, urobilinogen.)

- examination of the urine sediment using light microscopy:

• amorphous debris	• epithelial cells
• bacteria	• erythrocytes

- fat droplets
- leukocytes
- urinary casts

- urinary crystals
- yeast.

7. If a patient has a UTI, common findings on urinalysis include:(1, 33)

- macroscopic or microscopic hematuria
- macroscopic or microscopic pyuria
- proteinuria.

8. Bacteria can be missed on examination of the urine sediment, particularly if the urine is dilute. (54) It is prudent to perform a urine culture to obtain a definitive diagnosis.(1, 35) When you perform a urine culture, it is essential that you pair it with a so-called sensitivity report. Sometimes this is referred to as susceptibility testing. Susceptibility testing occurs in vitro with the hopes that it can predict antibiotic efficacy in vivo. It is an imperfect science because it is dependent upon a variety of factors that are outside of your control, including the following.

- Which pathogen is being tested for.
- Which media is being used to grow the pathogen(s).
- How is the culture plate incubated?
- How bacterial growth is assessed?

Despite these potential flaws, susceptibility testing is the best tool we have to help us select an appropriate antibiotic choice for our patient in the event that s/he has a UTI.(33, 47, 55)

Repeat testing may also be used to augment clinical response to therapy in guiding treatment decisions, including when to discontinue antibiotic therapy.(1, 33)

9. Urine is typically collected from a cat by:(1, 5)

- "free catch," that is, the patient voided
- cystocentesis.

Urinary catheterization is not a routine means by which urine is collected in healthy cats. However, indwelling catheters that have been placed to manage UTO may be sampled continuously during case management to evaluate urine samples and response to therapy.

10. There are advantages and disadvantages to each method of urine collection.

- Free catch:

  - Advantages:

    - Can be performed by the client at home.
    - Does not require special training/technique or machinery (i.e. ultrasound machine).
    - Does not require restraint.
    - Is non-invasive.
    - Is inexpensive.
    - It avoids iatrogenic hematuria that may result from cystocentesis or catheterization.

  - Disadvantages:

    - In dogs, marking behavior may make it difficult to collect an ideal sample size (6 mL).
    - Unlike leashed dogs, which we can follow closely and strategically place a urine collection tool beneath, cats are a bit trickier to collect from in this manner.
    - We can't follow most of our cats around with a collection cup and expect for them to urinate.

- Most of our cats eliminate when we are out of sight.
- To collect a "free catch" sample, we often need to empty out the litterboxes and replace them with special beads (NOSORB) or hydrophobic sand (Kit4Cat).
- Cats may refuse to eliminate in the box once its substrate has been swapped out.
- Owners of multi-cat households may struggle with having to isolate the cat of interest, particularly if multiple cats share a single box in the household.
- Cats can hold their bladders for a long time, so they may wait us out for 12–24 hours. This will delay results and treatment.
- If a sterile container is not used at home, there is the potential for contamination with residues, microbes, and other items that may be lining the container.
- There is the potential for contamination of the sample with epithelial cells, WBCs, bacteria, debris, etc. from the distal urethra, vagina/vulva, penis/prepuce, skin or fur.
- Because of this, free catch samples are not ideal samples for culturing.
- Samples are rarely fresh. After collection, clients often must refrigerate them for hours before they are able to hand-deliver them to the clinic.

- Risks:

  - False positive result:
  - Free catch samples often contain debris and bacterial contaminants that imply a UTI is present when it is not.(5)
  - Refrigeration of samples may result in artifacts that suggest a UTI is present when it is not.

- Cystocentesis:

  - Advantages:

    - Requires minimal restraint.
    - Usually does not require sedation.
    - There is little to no contamination of the sample from the lower urinary tract.
    - Less risk (than urinary catheterization) of causing iatrogenic infection.

  - Disadvantages:

    - Requires experience, regardless of whether this procedure is performed blindly or is ultrasound-guided.
    - This technique is expected to cause microscopic hematuria (<50 RBCs/HPF).
    - This technique is contraindicated if:

      - you cannot palpate the urinary bladder and you do not have access to ultrasound
      - the patient has confirmed neoplastic disease of the urinary bladder
      - the patient has presumptive neoplastic disease of the urinary bladder
      - the patient has confirmed coagulopathy
      - the patient has presumptive coagulopathy.

  - Risks:

    - This technique could lacerate the urinary bladder if the patient thrashes mid-procedure.
    - You may inadvertently aspirate the intestinal tract or major abdominal vessels.

Returning to Case 18: The Cat with Hematuria

After discussing the advantages and disadvantages of various urine collection techniques, Don consents to having Pita's urine sampled via ultrasound-guided cystocentesis. Gross appearance of urine is documented below.

Color: peach-pink

Volume: 3.0 mL

Clarity of urine: slightly cloudy

No overt macroscopic particulate matter

USG: 1.055

>	pH	7.0	
>	Urine Protein	neg	
>	Glucose	neg	
>	Ketones	neg	
>	Blood / Hemoglobin	250	Ery/µL
>	Bilirubin	neg	
>	Urobilinogen	norm	
>	White Blood Cells	6 /HPF	
>	Red Blood Cells	29 /HPF	

Figure 18.3 Key urinalysis findings for Pita. Note the presence of both hematuria and pyuria.

Key features of Pita's urinalysis are described in Figure 18.3. Pita's urine is negative for bacteriuria, crystalluria, and casts.

Don also consents to two-view orthogonal radiographs to rule out urolithiasis. This imaging study is unremarkable.

Round Three of Questions for Case 18: The Cat with Hematuria

1. Pita's urinalysis confirms hematuria. What causes hematuria?
2. True or false: UTIs in cats are commonly linked to urolithiasis.
3. Even though urine sediment exam did not demonstrate bacteriuria, you elect to submit a urine culture to rule out UTI definitively. Which bacteria are most frequently cultured in UTIs in cats and dogs?
4. If the urine culture is negative, what is the most likely diagnosis?
5. What are risk factors for the condition that you identified in Question #4 (above)?
6. If Pita has the condition that you named in Question #4 (above), what is your therapeutic plan for case management?

Answers to Round Three of Questions for Case 18: The Cat with Hematuria

1. Pathological causes of hematuria, include:(1, 5, 34, 35, 42, 46–49, 55–62)

    * bleeding disorders
    * glomerulopathy
    * heat stroke
    * infection of the urogenital tract
    * inflammation of the urogenital tract
    * neoplasia of the urogenital tract
    * urethral tear
    * urolithiasis
    * trauma.

2. False. UTIs in cats are not commonly linked to urolithiasis. However, UTIs in dogs are.(63–66)

3. Most UTIs are bacterial and are caused by aerobes.(33) The most common bacterial isolates in both dogs are cats include:(33–36, 38, 39, 47, 67, 68)

   - *Enterococcus* spp. (*E. faecalis*)
   - *Escherichia coli*
   - *Streptococcus* spp.

   Other genera that are routinely cultured include:(33, 35, 47, 67, 69, 70)

   - Enterobacter
   - Klebsiella
   - Pasteurella
   - *Proteus*
   - *Pseudomonas*
   - *Staphylococcus* spp.

     - *S. aureus*
     - *S. bovis*
     - *S. intermedius.*

4. If the urine culture is negative, the most likely diagnosis is feline idiopathic cystitis (FIC).(1) This condition is also referred to as feline urologic syndrome (FUS), the most common cause of feline lower urinary tract disease (FLUTD).(33, 45, 59, 60, 71–74) FIC is a self-limiting, but recurring syndrome of sterile, hemorrhagic cystitis.(33, 59, 71, 75–78)

5. Risk factors for FIC include:(1, 33, 60)

   - inactivity
   - indoor lifestyle
   - inter-cat conflict
   - long-haired

   - multi-cat household
   - purebred
   - obesity
   - stress.

6. If Pita has FIC, then case management requires the prescription of an analgesic agent to improve patient comfort.(1, 33) Antispasmodic drugs may also be prescribed along with amitriptyline for its anti-inflammatory and analgesic properties.(1, 33) Stress management will also play an important role in speeding resolution of this bout and in reducing recurrence.(33)

CLINICAL PEARLS

- House-soiling cannot be assumed to be behavioral unless all medical causes have been ruled out.

- History-taking plays an essential role in evaluating a patient that presents for inappropriate urination. When that patient is a cat, it is critical to investigate the following:

  - changes in household
  - relocation (new home)
  - additions to household (people, other pets)
  - subtractions to household (people, other pets)
  - changes in litter box quantity, location, substrate, or hygiene (i.e. frequency of scooping).

- In cases that involve potential urinary tract pathology, history-taking should include questions about:

    - whether urination seems difficult: is there straining? is there pain?
    - urination frequency
    - urine output (volume)
    - urine color (when observed)
    - urine particulate matter (when observed).

- When taking a patient history, it is critical not to wear blinders. When a patient presents with oliguria, be sure to ask about potential exposure to toxins that could be nephrotoxic.

- Physical examination for feline patients that present with a urinary complaint should emphasize renal and urinary bladder palpation. Examination of perineal (peri-vulval or peri-preputial) fur can also provide clues.

- UTIs are relatively uncommon in young cats. However, urinalysis +/– culture and susceptibility should be performed to rule in or rule out UTI as a possible diagnosis. Imaging is performed to rule out urolithiasis.

- The most common cause of FLUTD is feline idiopathic cystitis (FIC). This is a sterile, recurrent condition with self-limiting flare-ups that are often triggered by stress. Resolution can be expedited by managing patient stress and discomfort with analgesia.

References

1. Englar RE. Common clinical presentations in dogs and cats. Hoboken, NJ: Wiley/Blackwell; 2019.
2. Côté E. Clinical veterinary advisor. Dogs and cats. 3rd ed. St. Louis, MO: Elsevier Mosby; 2015.
3. Ettinger SJ, Feldman EC, Côté E. Textbook of veterinary internal medicine: diseases of the dog and the cat. 8th ed. St. Louis, MO: Elsevier; 2017.
4. Reece WO. Kidney function in mammals. In: Dukes HH, Reece WO, editors. Dukes' physiology of domestic animals. 12th ed. Ithaca, NT: Comstock Pub. Associates; 2004. p. 73–106.
5. Grauer GF, Pohlman LM. Urinalysis interpretation. NAVC Clin's Brief 2016 (March):93–101.
6. Balakrishnan A, Drobatz KJ. Management of urinary tract emergencies in small animals. Vet Clin North Am Small Anim Pract 2013;43(4):843–67.
7. Fitzgerald KT. Lily toxicity in the cat. Top Companion Anim Med 2010;25(4):213–7.
8. Stokes JE, Forrester SD. New and unusual causes of acute renal failure in dogs and cats. Vet Clin North Am Small Anim Pract 2004;34(4):909–22.
9. Nichols R. Polyuria and polydipsia – diagnostic approach and problems associated with patient evaluation. Vet Clin N Am. Small 2001;31(5):833.
10. Marks SL, Taboada J. Hypernatremia and hypertonic syndromes. Vet Clin North Am Small Anim Pract 1998;28(3):533–43.
11. Agarwal SK, Gupta A. Aquaporins: The renal water channels. Indian J Nephrol 2008;18(3):95–100.
12. Tilley LP, Smith FWK. The 5-minute veterinary consult: canine and feline. 3rd ed. Baltimore, MD: Lippincott Williams & Wilkins; 2004.
13. Fulkerson CM, Knapp DW. Management of transitional cell carcinoma of the urinary bladder in dogs: a review. Vet J 2015;205(2):217–25.
14. Englar RE. Performing the small animal physical examination. Hoboken, NJ: Wiley; 2017.
15. Cain DT, Battersby I, Doyle R. Response of dogs with urinary tract obstructions secondary to prostatic carcinomas to the alpha-1 antagonist prazosin. Vet Rec 2016;178(4):96.

16. Englar RE. Performing the small animal physical examination. Hoboken, NJ: Wiley/Blackwell; 2017.

17. Evans HE, Christensen GC. The urogenital system. In: Evans HE, Miller ME, editors. Miller's anatomy of the dog. 3rd ed. Philadelphia, PA: W. B. Saunders; 1993. p. 494–558.

18. Barrett RB, Kneller SK. Feline kidney mensuration. Acta Radiol Suppl 1972;319:279–80.

19. Lee R, Leowijuk C. Normal parameters in abdominal radiology of the dog and cat. J Small Anim Pract 1982;23(5):251–69.

20. Scherk M. The upper urinary tract. In: Little SE, editor. The cat: clinical medicine and management. St. Louis, MO: Saunders Elsevier; 2012.

21. Walter PA, Feeney DA, Johnston GR, Fletcher TF. Feline renal ultrasonography: quantitative analyses of imaged anatomy. Am J Vet Res 1987;48(4):596–9.

22. Shiroma JT, Gabriel JK, Carter RL, Scruggs SL, Stubbs PW. Effect of reproductive status on feline renal size. Vet Radiol Ultrasound 1999;40(3):242–5.

23. Owens J. The genitourinary system. In: Biery D, editor. Radiographic interpretation for the small animal clinician. St. Louis: Ralston Purina, Co.; 1982. p. 175.

24. Biery D. Upper urinary tract. In: O'Brien T, editor. Radiographic diagnosis of abdominal disorders in the dog and cat. Davis, CO: Covel Park Vet; 1981. p. 484–5.

25. Debruyn K, Paepe D, Daminet S, Combes A, Duchateau L, Peremans K, Saunders JH. Renal dimensions at ultrasonography in healthy Ragdoll cats with normal kidney morphology: correlation with age, gender and bodyweight. J Feline Med Surg 2013;15(12):1046–51.

26. Walter PA, Feeney DA, Johnston GR, Fletcher TF. Feline renal ultrasonography: quantitative analyses of imaged anatomy. Am J Vet Res 1987;48(4):596–9.

27. Barr FJ. Evaluation of ultrasound as a method of assessing renal size in the dog. J Small Anim Pract 1990;31(4):174–9.

28. Yeager AE, Anderson WI. Study of association between histologic features and echogenicity of architecturally normal cat kidneys. Am J Vet Res 1989;50(6):860–3.

29. Park IC, Lee HS, Kim JT, Nam SJ, Choi R, Oh KS, et al. Ultrasonographic evaluation of renal dimension and resistive index in clinically healthy Korean domestic short-hair cats. J Vet Sci 2008;9(4):415–9.

30. Hoey SE, Heder BL, Hetzel SJ, Waller KR. Use of computed tomography for measurement of kidneys in dogs without renal disease. J Am Vet Med Assoc 2016;248(3):282–7.

31. Finco DR, Stiles NS, Kneller SK, Lewis RE, Barrett RB. Radiologic estimation of kidney size of the dog. J Am Vet Med Assoc 1971;159(8):995–1002.

32. Lobacz MA, Sullivan M, Mellor D, Hammond G, Labruyère J, Dennis R. Effect of breed, age, weight and gender on radiographic renal size in the dog. Vet Rad Ultrasound Off J Am Coll Vet Rad Int Vet Rad Assoc 2012;53(4):437–41.

33. Filippich LJ. Cat with urinary tract signs. In: Rand J, editor. Problem-based feline medicine. Edinburgh. New York: Saunders; 2006. p. 173–92.

34. Thompson MF, Litster AL, Platell JL, Trott DJ. Canine bacterial urinary tract infections: new developments in old pathogens. Vet J 2011;190(1):22–7.

35. Litster A, Thompson M, Moss S, Trott D. Feline bacterial urinary tract infections: an update on an evolving clinical problem. Vet J 2011;187(1):18–22.

36. Bartges J, Barsanti JA. Bacterial urinary tract infections in cats. In: Bonagura JD, editor. Current veterinary therapy. Philaldelphia, PA: W.B. Saunders; 2000. p. 880–2.

37. Ling GV. Therapeutic strategies involving antimicrobial treatment of the canine urinary tract. J Am Vet Med Assoc 1984;185(10):1162–4.

38. Norris CR, Williams BJ, Ling GV, Franti CE, Johnson RAL, Ruby AL. Recurrent and persistent urinary tract infections in dogs: 383 cases (1969–1995). J Am Anim Hosp Assoc 2000;36(6):484–92.

39. Seguin MA, Vaden SL, Altier C, Stone E, Levine JF. Persistent urinary tract infections and reinfections in 100 dogs (1989–1999). J Vet Intern Med 2003;17(5):622–31.

40. Blanco LJ, Bartges JW. Understanding and eradicating bacterial urinary tract infections. Vetmed-US 2001;96(10):776.

41. Bartges JW. Bacterial urinary tract infections – simple and complicated. Vetmed-US 2005;100(3):224.

42. Bartges J, Burns KM. Lower urinary tract signs in a cat. NAVC Clin's Brief 2017 (September):35–9.

43. Lees GE, Rogers KS. Treatment of urinary tract infections in dogs and cats. J Am Vet Med Assoc 1986;189(6):648–52.
44. Gregory CR, Vasseur PB. Long-term examination of cats with perineal urethrostomy. Vet Surg 1983;12(4):210–2.
45. Lekcharoensuk C, Osborne CA, Lulich JP. Epidemiologic study of risk factors for lower urinary tract diseases in cats. J Am Vet Med Assoc 2001;218(9):1429–35.
46. Dowling PM. Bacterial urinary tract infections. Merck Vet Man 2018. Available from: https://www.merckvetmanual.com/pharmacology/systemic-pharmacotherapeutics-of-the-urinary-system/bacterial-urinary-tract-infections.
47. Olin SJ, Bartges JW. Urinary tract infections: treatment/comparative therapeutics. Vet Clin North Am Small Anim Pract 2015;45(4):721–46.
48. Ogeer-Gyles J, Mathews K, Weese JS, Prescott JF, Boerlin P. Evaluation of catheter-associated urinary tract infections and multi-drug-resistant Escherichia coli isolates from the urine of dogs with indwelling urinary catheters. J Am Vet Med Assoc 2006;229(10):1584–90.
49. Adams LG. Diagnosing and managing recurrent urinary tract infections DVM. 360 [Internet]; 2010. Available from: http://veterinarycalendar.dvm360.com/diagnosing-and-managing-recurrent-urinary-tract-infections-proceedings.
50. Wamsley H, Alleman R. Complete urinalysis. In: Elliott J, Grauer GF, editors. BSAVA manual of canine and feline nephrology and urology. Quedgeley: British Small Animal Veterinary Association; 2007.
51. Lefebvre HP. Renal function testing. In: Bartges J, Polzin DJ, editors. Ames, IA: Wiley-Blackwell; 2011. p. 91–6.
52. Fry MM. Urinalysis. In: Bartges J, Polzin DJ, editors. Nephrology and urology of small animals. Ames, IA: Wiley/Blackwell; 2011. p. 91–6.
53. Osborne CA, Stevens JB, Lulich JP. A clinician's analysis of urinalysis. In: Osborne CA, Finco DR, editors. Canine and feline nephrology and urology. Baltimore, MD: Williams & Wilkins; 1995. p. 136–205.
54. Behrend EN, editor. Diagnosis of polyuria/polydipsia: case-based approach. Proceedings of the North American Veterinary Conference (NAVC); 2005; Orlando, FL.
55. Jessen LR, Sørensen TM, Bjornvad CR, Nielsen SS, Guardabassi L. Effect of antibiotic treatment in canine and feline urinary tract infections: a systematic review. Vet J 2015;203(3):270–7.
56. Daniel G, Labato MA. Hematuria in dogs. NAVC Clin's Brief 2017 (November):32–3.
57. Rebar AH. Hematuria in a dog. NAVC Clin's Brief 2008.
58. Galemore E, Labato MA. Recurrent hematuria in a dog. NAVC Clin's Brief 2016(December):86–9.
59. Kruger JM, Osborne CA, Lulich JP. Changing paradigms of feline idiopathic cystitis. Vet Clin North Am Small Anim Pract 2009;39(1):15–40.
60. Defauw PA, Van de Maele I, Duchateau L, Polis IE, Saunders JH, Daminet S. Risk factors and clinical presentation of cats with feline idiopathic cystitis. J Feline Med Surg 2011;13(12):967–75.
61. Callens A, Bartges J. Update on feline urolithiasis. In: Little SE, editor. Consultations in feline internal medicine. St. Louis, MO: Elsevier, Inc.; 2016. p. 499–508.
62. White JD, Norris JM, Bosward KL, Fleay R, Lauer C, Malik R. Persistent haematuria and proteinuria due to glomerular disease in related Abyssinian cats. J Feline Med Surg 2008;10(3):219–29.
63. Okafor CC, Pearl DL, Lefebvre SL, Wang MS, Yang MY, Blois SL, et al. Risk factors associated with struvite urolithiasis in dogs evaluated at general care veterinary hospitals in the United States. Vet Med A 2013;243(12):1737–45.
64. Bartges JW, Callens AJ. Urolithiasis. Vet Clin North Am Small Anim Pract 2015;45(4):747–68.
65. Seaman R, Bartges JW. Canine struvite urolithiasis. Comp Cont Educ Pract 2001;23(5):407.
66. Palma D, Langston C, Gisselman K, McCue J. Canine struvite urolithiasis. Compendium 2013;35(8):E1.
67. Ling GV, Norris CR, Franti CE, Eizele PH, Johnson DL, Ruby AL, et al. Interrelations of organism prevalence, specimen collection method, and host age, sex, and breed among 8,354 canine urinary tract infections (1969–1995). J Vet Intern Med 2001;15(4):341–7.
68. Cohn LA, Gary AT, Fales WH, Madsen RW. Trends in fluoroquinolone resistance of bacteria isolated from canine urinary tracts. J Vet Diagn Invest 2003;15(4):338–43.
69. Listster A, Moss SM, Honnery M, Rees B, Trott DJ. Prevalence of bacterial species in cats with clinical signs of lower urinary tract disease: recognition of Staphylococcus felis as a possible feline urinary tract pathogen. Vet Microbiol 2007;121(1–2):182–8.

70. Barsanti JA. Genitourinary infections. In: Greene CE, editor. Infectious diseases of the dog and cat. St. Louis, MO: Elsevier Saunders; 2012. p. 1013–31.
71. Kruger JM, Osborne CA, Goyal SM, Wickstrom SL, Johnston GR, Fletcher TF, Brown PA. Clinical-evaluation of cats with lower urinary-tract disease. J Am Vet Med Assoc 1991;199(2):211–6.
72. Buffington CA, Chew DJ, Kendall MS, Scrivani PV, Thompson SB, Blaisdell JL, Woodworth BE. Clinical evaluation of cats with nonobstructive urinary tract diseases. J Am Vet Med Assoc 1997;210(1):46–50.
73. Osborne CA, Kruger JM, Lulich JP. Feline lower urinary tract disorders. Definition of terms and concepts. Vet Clin North Am Small Anim Pract 1996;26(2):169–79.
74. Gerber B, Eichenberger S, Reusch CE. Guarded long-term prognosis in male cats with urethral obstruction. J Feline Med Surg 2008;10(1):16–23.
75. Barsanti JA, Finco DR, Shotts EB, Blue J, Ross L. Feline urologic syndrome – further investigation into etiology. J Am Anim Hosp Assoc 1982;18(3):391–5.
76. Kruger JM, Conway TS, Kaneene JB, Perry RL, Hagenlocker E, Golombek A, Stuhler J. Randomized controlled trial of the efficacy of short-term amitriptyline administration for treatment of acute, nonobstructive, idiopathic lower urinary tract disease in cats. J Am Vet Med Assoc 2003;222(6):749–58.
77. Markwell PJ, Buffington CAT, Chew DJ, Kendall MS, Harte JG, DiBartola SP. Clinical evaluation of commercially available urinary acidification diets in the management of idiopathic cystitis in cats. J Am Vet Med Assoc 1999;214(3):361–5.
78. Gunn-Moore DA, Shenoy CM. Oral glucosamine and the management of feline idiopathic cystitis. J Feline Med Surg 2004;6(4):219–25.

Case 19

The Cat Who Can't Pee

Barnaby is one of three Sphynx that are owned by Jay Catsby. Jay is a stockbroker who first discovered this exotic breed when he visited the home of one of his clients. He had never seen a hairless cat but was sold on the breed as soon as he held one in his lap. Jay was surprised to find how smooth and velvety the skin felt – and how warm, too! He appreciated the Sphynx's unusual appearance. The breed seemed stately and regal. Sphynx cats also appeared to be remarkably dog-like in terms of their desire for affection. Jay appreciated that his client's Sphynx sought him out rather than the other way around. Jay was drawn to the social nature of the Sphynx breed. He had previously owned aloof cats of the barnyard variety and was looking for companionship to come home to after logging long hours at the office. Sphynx cats seemed like a perfect fit.

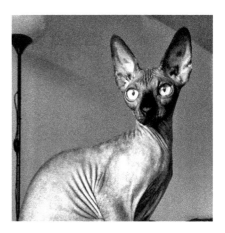

Figure 19.1 Meet your next patient, Barnaby, a 5-year-old, castrated male Sphynx cat.

To start his collection, Jay purchased full-blooded sisters, Triscuit and Mango. When the sisters were 6 years old, Jay elected to add a third to the household. Jay purchased Barnaby as a 4-month-old kitten. The transition from a two-cat to three-cat household was seamless. Triscuit mothered Barnaby and Mango was Barnaby's favorite playmate. Together, the trio lived full days with no shortage of love.

Other than keeping on top of routine skin care that is typical for the breed, Jay has not encountered any health scares, that is, until this morning. Barnaby was not on Jay's bed when he awoke. That was the first sign that something was wrong. When Jay searched the house, he found Barnaby in the laundry room, sitting on his rump, looking at his perineum intently. Despite Jay calling to him, Barnaby continued to groom.

Jay ignored him at first and headed to the kitchen. By this time, Triscuit and Mango were practically climbing the cabinets to be fed. Jay put their bowls in the usual spot, but Barnaby did not join them to eat. That's when Jay heard a mournful cry coming from the mud room. Jay found Barnaby in the litter box trying to eliminate, but no urine or stool was produced. Jay observed Barnaby squeeze his belly repeatedly as if trying to relieve himself, but the litter remained dry. Barnaby exited the box, sat on his haunches, and again tried to groom before repeating the cycle all over again.

After three failed attempts, Jay was on the telephone with your clinic. At your recommendation, the customer care representative instructed Jay to bring Barnaby in right away. Barnaby threw up in transit once. This was unusual for him. He travelled often by vehicle and never got car sick.

When he arrives, Barnaby is rushed to the treatment area for triage. His vital signs are documented below.

Weight: 10.2 lb (4.6 kg)
BCS: 4/9
Mentation: Depressed

TPR

T: 98.6°F (37°C)
P: 148 beats per minute
R: 27 breaths per minute

Round One of Questions for Case 19: The Cat Who Can't Pee

1. Given Barnaby's history, which diagnosis concerns you most at this time?
2. If Barnaby has the condition that you identified in Question #1 (above), what do you expect to find on your triage examination?
3. How does Barnaby's temperature at initial presentation compare to the normal reference range?
4. Is Barnaby's temperature consistent with the diagnosis that you proposed in Question #1 (above)?
5. How does Barnaby's heart rate (HR) at initial presentation compare to the normal reference range?
6. Is Barnaby's HR consistent with the diagnosis that you proposed in Question #1 (above)?
7. What is the most likely cause of Barnaby's HR?

Answers to Round One of Questions for Case 19: The Cat Who Can't Pee

1. In a male cat that has an acute history of anuria and stranguria, I am most concerned about urinary tract obstruction (UTO). Patients with UTO are said to be "blocked".

2. If Barnaby is in fact "blocked," then I would expect to feel a distended, non-compressible, rock-hard urinary bladder that is tender on abdominal palpation.(1)

   On physical examination, you might also expect to see Barnaby's penis extruded from the prepuce.(1) The penile tip is often discolored. It may be red due to self-mutilation, or purple-black from ischemic changes.(1, 2)

   I might even observe Barnaby's penis pulsing due to urethral spasms.(1)

3. The normal reference range for feline rectal temperature is 100.5°F – 102.5°F, although this range varies somewhat depending upon your choice of reference text.(3, 4) Barnaby is therefore considered to be mildly hypothermic on initial presentation.

4. Yes, Barnaby's temperature is consistent with a diagnosis of UTO.(1, 2)

5. HR for a cat is largely dependent upon sympathetic tone.(1) The resting HR of an adult cat in its home environment is 120–140 beats per minutes.(5) The HR of an adult cat in a clinic setting tends to be much greater, averaging 180–220 beats per minute. Stress activates the sympathetic nervous system, causing the heart to beat faster and with greater force.(1) This pathway is particularly accentuated in cats.(1) This physiologic change is mediated through the fight-or-flight hormone, epinephrine.(6–12)

   Barnaby's HR is lower than it is in most cats that present to the clinic.(1, 4) I would therefore consider him to be bradycardic at initial presentation.

6. Yes, Barnaby's HR is consistent with a diagnosis of UTO.(1, 2, 13)

7. I suspect that Barnaby's bradycardia is caused by hyperkalemia.(2, 13) Hyperkalemia is a common finding in cats with UTO.(2, 13–15) It results from reduced glomerular filtration rate (GFR).(1) When GFR is adequate, potassium is excreted from the kidneys.(1) When GFR is compromised, potassium remains in the bloodstream and concentrations build.(14) The body attempts to compensate by pushing potassium intracellularly.(14, 16–18) This action makes the inside of each cell less negative.(1) This less negative resting potential makes depolarization of each cell more challenging.(18) One adverse effect is difficulty regulating HR.(14, 18) Affected patients are bradycardic.(1)

Returning to Case 19: The Cat Who Can't Pee

Your triage examination confirms your suspicions that Barnaby is "blocked." When you communicate this to Jay, he has several questions that he would like you to address before you proceed with case management.

Round Two of Questions for Case 19: The Cat Who Can't Pee

1. What caused this to occur?
2. How will you definitively diagnose the causes that you identified in Question #1 (above)?
3. What are risk factors for the development of UTO in cats?
4. Is UTO a medical emergency? Why or Why not?
5. What are your proposed next steps in Barnaby's diagnostic plan?
6. What are you looking for in each diagnostic test that you selected in Question #5 (above)
7. What are your proposed treatment goals to resolve Barnaby's UTO?
8. Can UTO recur?

Answers to Round Two of Questions for Case 19: The Cat Who Can't Pee

1. I would need to answer this question with transparency: "At this point, I don't know what caused Barnaby's obstruction, but we are going to work together to get to the root of this."
    I would then explain that there are several causes of UTO. UTO may result from:(13)

   • urethral plugs
   • urolithiasis
   • urinary tract neoplasia
   • "other."

   Urethral plugs are protein-rich accumulations of inflammatory cells and urinary crystals.(19–21) These are a common cause of UTO in cats.(2, 13, 14, 19, 20)
    Uroliths are a fancy way to describe urinary stones.(1, 4) These stones may develop anywhere in the upper and lower urinary tracts:(1)

   • nephroliths (kidney stones)
   • ureteroliths (stones in one or both ureters)
   • cystoliths (bladder stones)
   • urethral stones.

   Not all uroliths are obstructive, but they certainly can be.(22)
    Urinary tract neoplasia is uncommon in dogs and cats.(23–29) When it occurs, it is typically malignant transitional cell carcinoma (TCC) involving the trigone of the urinary bladder.(23–27, 29–34) Dogs are more frequently affected than cats, and females are at greater risk than males for development of this disease.(1)
    I would need to inform Jay that despite our best efforts, as many of half of all cases of feline UTO are idiopathic.(1, 13, 35) That is, we never determine a cause.

2. Urethral plugs may be identified during the "unblocking" procedure. These may be submitted to an outside laboratory for structural analysis to determine composition.
    Most uroliths go undetected on physical examination so abdominal imaging in the form of radiography or ultrasonography is essential to confirm urolithiasis.(22, 36)

Ultrasonography can also be used to confirm the presence of a mass within the lumen of the urinary bladder.(22, 23) Note that ultrasound-guided fine-needle aspirates (FNAs) through the bladder wall, as through cystocentesis, to obtain samples of neoplastic tissue are not advised. (23) There is concern that you might seed neoplastic cells throughout the abdomen.(23) If neoplastic tissue is suspected, then samples should be obtained through urinary catheterization.(23) Urine can be collected in this manner, with the hope that exfoliated abnormal cells may end up in the sample.(23) An alternate approach is surgical biopsy; however, that represents the most invasive of all staging modalities presented here.

3. Risk factors for the development of UTO in cats include:(1)

    •   bacterial UTIs increase the risk for development of feline UTO, but the majority of cases do not involve active infection(13, 20, 37–40)
    •   being fed an exclusively dry food diet(2, 37)
    •   crystalluria
    •   indoor-only lifestyle(2)
    •   sex: male cats are more commonly affected than females because the male urethra is very narrow(2, 13, 14, 41)
    •   stress.

4. Yes, UTO is a medical emergency.(2, 13) Electrolyte and acid-base abnormalities that result from UTO are life-threatening, particularly when the obstruction is complete and protracted. (2, 13–15)

    Cardiovascular stabilization is a priority.(2, 13) Hyperkalemia must be addressed first because this imbalance has the potential to kill the cat before the blockage does.(2, 13) Hyperkalemia is life-threatening because it induces arrhythmias.(1) Many blocked cats also become hypocalcemic.(1) This also potentiates arrhythmias.(14)

5. Proposed next steps in my diagnostic plan include:

    •   baseline bloodwork:

        •   complete blood count (CBC)
        •   chemistry profile
        •   acid-base status

    •   electrocardiogram (ECG)
    •   two-view abdominal radiograph and/or abdominal ultrasound
    •   urinalysis and culture with susceptibility results.

6. Bloodwork is advised to establish a baseline, both for establishing treatment protocols and for developing an anesthetic plan in preparation for unblocking. I would expect to see the following clinicopathologic abnormalities on baseline bloodwork:(1, 2, 13–15)

    •   azotemia:

        •   blood urea nitrogen (BUN)
        •   creatinine

    •   hyperkalemia
    •   +/– hypocalcemia
    •   metabolic acidosis.

    An ECG is advised to evaluate the heart for signs of hyperkalemic cardiomyopathy. As potassium levels rise in the bloodstream of a patient with UTO, the patient develops characteristic changes on the ECG that include:(2, 13, 18, 42–51)

- decreased to flattened P wave amplitude
- prolonged P-R and Q-T intervals
- so-called "tented," meaning tall, T waves
- widened QRS complexes.

Note that the progression of ECG changes is proportional to the degree to which serum potassium climbs.(42, 43) If serum potassium exceeds 7.5 mEq/L and medical management is not instituted, then patient fatality is likely.(18, 43)

Patients that are hypocalcemic also experience characteristic ECG changes. These include prolongation of the S-T and Q-T intervals.(14, 16, 18) Development of any of these changes on ECG signal that intervention is required urgently. Two-view abdominal radiographs and/or ultrasonography are advised to evaluate the patient for obstructive urolithiasis. Urinalysis with culture and susceptibility testing is advised to evaluate the patient for UTI.

7. My proposed treatment goals for Barnaby are as follows.(1, 52, 53)

- Stabilize the patient.
- Provide pain control (analgesia).
- Place an intravenous (IV) catheter.(2, 13)
- Correct electrolyte imbalances.(2, 13)
- Anesthetize the patient.
- Unblock the patient to relieve the urinary obstruction.
- Maintain patency of the urethra with a temporary, but indwelling, urinary catheter.
- Monitor ins and outs.
- Provide IV fluid therapy to correct hydration and post-renal azotemia, to flush out the lower urinary tract.(2, 13)

8. Yes, UTO can recur.(1, 14, 21, 35, 54)

Returning to Case 19: The Cat Who Can't Pee

After answering Jay's questions, you provide him with an estimate for your proposed diagnostic plan, general anesthesia, the unblocking procedure, post-unblocking radiographs, and inpatient care. Jay bristles at the high-end of the quote ($2250), but he ultimately signs on the dotted line. You and your team get started on Barnaby's care right away.

Round Three of Questions for Case 19: The Cat Who Can't Pee

1. When you return from obtaining informed consent, your technician asks you to evaluate Barnaby's ECG (see Figure 19.2).
    How will you address what you see on Barnaby's ECG?

2. While you are addressing Barnaby's ECG, you ask your technician to gather supplies for the unblocking procedure. At your request, she gathers two different types of urinary catheters (see **Plates 6a and 6b**).

    a. What is the appropriate name for urinary catheter option A?
    b. What is the appropriate name for urinary catheter option B?
    c. Which material is each catheter, A and B, made from?
    d. Which urinary catheter, A or B, will you use first and why?
    e. Which option, A or B, is an appropriate choice for an indwelling urinary catheter?

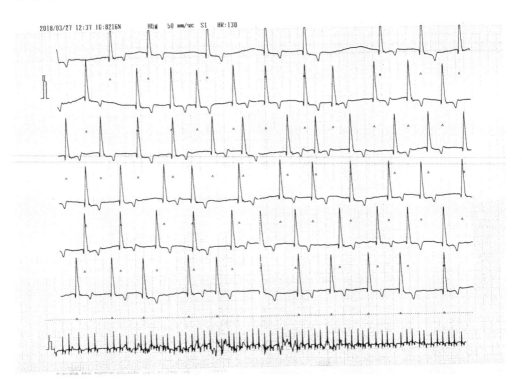

Figure 19.2 ECG demonstrating significant changes in the electrical rhythm of Barnaby's heart. Courtesy of Drs Yuichu Miyagawa and Naoyuki Takemura, Nippon Veterinary and Life Science University, Tokyo, Japan.

3. How are urinary catheters that are displayed in **Plate 6a** sized?
4. Which size(s) of urinary catheter is/are typically placed in a male cat during unblocking?
5. Is placement of an indwelling urinary catheter a sterile procedure? Why or why not?
6. What personal protective equipment (PPE), if any, will you use when placing the indwelling urinary catheter?
7. You will make use of lubricant to facilitate passage of the urinary catheter. Your technician hands you a multi-use tube of lubricant. Is this an appropriate choice. Why or why not?
8. Are there additional types of feline urinary catheters other than the two that have been depicted in **Plates 6a and 6b**?
9. Walk me through the unblocking procedure in broad terms.
10. Outline post-procedural treatment goals.
11. Are antibiotics warranted?

Answers to Round Three of Questions for Case 19: The Cat Who Can't Pee

1. Hyperkalemia secondary to UTO will resolve as soon as you unblock the patient. However, time is of the essence and you may need to address ECG changes before you are able to physically alleviate the obstruction. This requires one of three approaches.(55)

- Calcium gluconate (10%) can be administered IV slowly at 0.5–1.0 mL/kg.

  - This is cardioprotective.
  - It does not actually reduce serum potassium levels. Its administration simply buys time for you to unblock the patient.

- Dextrose (50%) is administered IV in diluted form to trigger the body to release insulin. Insulin drives potassium into the cell, thereby reducing hyperkalemia. You may also elect to administer 1 unit of regular insulin along with a dextrose bolus to speed the process by which potassium moves intracellularly.
- Sodium bicarbonate can be administered slowly IV.(56) This works by changing the blood pH so that it is more alkaline.(56) Alkalemia drives potassium intracellularly.(56)

2. Your technician has gathered two different types of urinary catheters:

   a. Urinary catheter A is commonly referred to as a "red rubber." Other names include a feeding tube, after its other common function.
   b. Urinary catheter B is a "tom cat catheter."
   c. Red rubber catheters are made from natural latex. This is a softer material than silicone and vinyl. The tom cat urinary catheter is made out of polypropylene, which makes it rigid and inflexible.
   d. You will first make use of urinary catheter B (the tom cat catheter) because its rigidity facilitates dislodging the obstruction. By contrast, urinary catheter A (the red rubber) is too flexible and will not be able to alleviate the urethral obstruction.
   e. For this reason, the tom cat catheter is typically placed first. Once the obstruction is relieved, it is removed and replaced with a red rubber catheter, which may stay in place for 2–5 days.
   f. Urinary catheter A (the red rubber) is an appropriate choice for an indwelling urinary catheter because its flexibility and softer feel will improve patient comfort. By contrast, catheter B is not a good choice for use as an indwelling catheter because its rough edges are likely to cause traumatic injury to the urethra.

3. The relative size of red rubber catheters is described using French (Fr) units.
   The size in French divided by 3 is the tube's external diameter in millimeters.
   For example, a 3.5 Fr catheter is approximately 1.2 mm in diameter.
   Please do *not* memorize this number.
   Most red rubbers range in size from 8 French (8 Fr) to 18 French (18 Fr)

   $$\ldots < 8 \text{ Fr} < 10 \text{ Fr} < 12 \text{ Fr} < 14 \text{ Fr} \ldots$$

   The smaller the number, the smaller the tube; the larger the number, the larger the tube.

4. Two sizes of red rubber tubes are routinely placed in male cats during the unblocking process:

   - 3.5 Fr
   - 5 Fr.

   Placement of the 5 Fr is preferred to the 3.5 Fr because of its larger lumen.

5. Placement of an indwelling urinary catheter is intended to be a sterile procedure. You do not want to introduce bacteria into the urinary tract. Doing so will cause an ascending UTI.

6. Because placement of an indwelling urinary catheter is a sterile procedure, you should practice aseptic technique. This means that you need to don sterile gloves using open gloving.
   In the case of feline UTO, gloves are there primarily to protect the patient. However, keep in mind that gloves also protect you from zoonotic diseases that may be transmitted in the urine. For

instance, urine of patients with leptospirosis is infectious to people. Patients that are leptospirosis suspects should prompt additional consideration concerning personal protective equipment (PPE). For example, when working with patients that may have leptospirosis, I routinely don eyewear to protect against inadvertent splashes of urine into the eye that could transmit infection.

7. You should use sterile single-use packs of lubricant rather than a multi-use vial to reduce the risk of introducing bacteria into the lower urinary tract.

8. Yes, there are other types of urinary catheters available for purchase other than the tom cat catheter and the red rubber.

   For instance, MILA has devised an "upgraded" feline urinary catheter that replaces the need for two. In this model, the same tool is used to unblock the patient and leave in the patient as an indwelling catheter. Because one catheter is used instead of two (the tom cat catheter, followed by the red rubber), there should be LESS trauma to the urethra and reduced risk of infection.

   Another option is a polytetrafluorethylene (PTFE) catheter, which is sometimes referred to as a Slippery Sam. This has suture holes built into the silicone hub to facilitate securing the catheter to the prepuce. The Slippery Sam is also radiopaque, which makes it easier to achieve radiographic confirmation post-unblocking that the catheter is correctly placed.

9. The patient is anesthetized and placed in either dorsal or lateral recumbency, depending upon the clinician's preference.(56) The patient is clipped and prepped for the procedure.

   The penis is then extruded from the prepuce.(56) The penis is maintained in this position by grasping the base of the prepuce.(56) To facilitate insertion and passage of the urinary catheter, the urethra must be straightened out.(56) To achieve this, firm pressure is applied to the prepuce to direct the penis in a caudal direction so that it lays parallel to the spine.(56)

   Select an open-ended 3.5 Fr polypropylene tom cat catheter.(56) Flush the catheter with sterile 0.9% saline or a mixture of saline and sterile lubricant.

   Attach a syringe containing sterile saline or a mixture of saline and sterile lubricant to the urinary catheter. Now insert the catheter tip into the distal urethra.(56) Advance the tom cat catheter retrograde into the urethra slowly while pulsing the plunger of the syringe at regular intervals. Ideally this will flush the obstruction out of the urethra and into the bladder.(56)

   Once the obstruction has been relieved, you may flush the urinary bladder and empty it several times, using 0.9% sterile saline.(56) Once flushing has been performed, the tom cat catheter is removed and replaced with a red rubber catheter or a Slippery Sam, an alternate product.(56) This will stay in place as an indwelling urinary catheter until the patient's urethral inflammation subsides.

   Stay sutures should be placed in the prepuce on either side.(56) Wrap waterproof adhesive tape around the red rubber catheter adjacent to the prepuce, taking care to leave room for tabs. (56) Secure the white tape to the stay sutures using suture.(56)

10. Post-procedural treatment goals include:(56)

    - resolution of obstruction to reestablish flow of urine
    - confirming proper placement of the urinary catheter via a lateral abdominal radiograph
    - pain management – buprenorphine and butorphanol are common choices
    - management of urethral spasms – phenoxybenzamine and prazosin are common choices
    - IV fluid therapy to maintain hydration and electrolyte balance:
      - requires measurement of ins and outs
      - requires bloodwork to be repeated every 12–24 hours or as needed.

11. Because few cats have a UTI at time of presentation, blanket antibiotic use in all UTO cats is discouraged.(56) Administering antibiotics when unnecessary may promote drug resistance.(56)

Antibiotics should be prescribed only in the face of bacteriuria and pyuria. Even then, antibiotic selection should be determined ultimately by culture and susceptibility testing.

Returning to Case 19: The Cat Who Can't Pee

You successfully place an indwelling urinary catheter and Barnaby is recovered from anesthesia without event. Consider the following questions as you prepare for his inpatient stay.

Round Four of Questions for Case 19: The Cat Who Can't Pee

1. What are general rules for management of indwelling urinary catheters in inpatients?
2. Skin adjacent to the urinary catheter should be monitored for signs of infection. What are you looking for that might indicate infection?
3. When a patient has an indwelling urinary catheter, it is important for us to measure urine outflow. How do you measure that?
4. We need to compare how much urine the patient is producing to that which is considered normal.

    a. What is normal urine output in mL/kg/day for a companion animal patient?
    b. What is normal urine output in mL/kg/hour for a companion animal patient?

5. What if urine output is zero? What does that mean? What do you do?
6. Post-obstructive diuresis is common.(2, 13, 14, 57, 58) How do you manage this?
7. When is it appropriate to discharge the patient?
8. If UTO recurs more than once, which surgery may be indicated?

Answers to Round Four of Questions for Case 19: The Cat Who Can't Pee

1. General rules for management of indwelling urinary catheters in inpatients are as follows.

    *   Always wash hands and don disposable gloves before handling urinary catheters and lines to protect patients and personnel from contamination during examination.
    *   New gloves should be used with each patient.
    *   Use a closed collection system to prevent external contamination of the urinary catheter.
    *   Consider the purchase of sterile single-use collection bags with one-way valves to prevent urine reflux back into the patient.
    *   Place the collection bag and tubing at a level lower than the patient to encourage urine flow and to minimize urine pooling. Pooling in collection lines can lead to sediment build up and occlusion.

2. Skin adjacent to the urinary catheter should be monitored for signs of infection. These include:(59)

    *   redness
    *   inflammation
    *   hemorrhage
    *   discharge
    *   odor.

    Check also for urine leakage around the catheter. Also assess urine color and turbidity. If urine that was becoming clear suddenly relapses to a cloudy or hemorrhagic state, then the potential for iatrogenic infection should be considered.(59) Cystocentesis can be performed to rule out UTI.(59)

3. Urine should be poured into a measuring beaker at regular intervals to accurately read and report volume. Hourly readings or every-other-hour readings are typical.

4. Urine production in the average canine or feline patient ranges from 20–40 mL/kg/day or 1–2 mL/kg/hour.(60)

5. Urine output volume should never be zero.
    If no urine is noted, then the collection system and the bladder size should be assessed. Possible issues leading to an empty urine collection bag include occlusion within the system, a leak between connections in the system, or a displaced catheter.
    If the urine output is in fact zero, then oliguria or anuria must be addressed immediately. This could indicate acute kidney injury (AKI), otherwise known as acute renal failure (ARF).

6. Post-obstructive diuresis is managed with aggressive fluid therapy to prevent hypovolemia.(13) Measuring ins and outs facilitates making adjustments concerning rate of IV fluid administration. Simply put, if more fluid is lost than is put into the patient, then the patient needs to receive an increased rate of IV fluids.

7. The patient can be discharged from the hospital once the following conditions have been met.(1)

    • The patient is now euhydrated.
    • The urinary catheter has been pulled.
    • The patient has been observed to urinate on its own.

8. Patients that routinely re-obstruct may benefit from PU.(13)

CLINICAL PEARLS

• UTO is a life-threatening medical emergency.

• Male cats are at greater risk of UTO because urethral diameter is reduced in size as compared to females.

• UTO is often idiopathic but can also result from urethral plugs or urolithiasis. Neoplastic disease involving the urinary bladder or urethra can also be obstructive to urine output, but rarely occurs in cats.

• Patients present for acute onset of:

  • dysuria, stranguria, oliguria, and/or anuria
  • excessive grooming at/around perineum
  • recumbency
  • anorexia or vomiting
  • rock-hard, non-compressible, painful urinary bladder
  • penis extruded from prepuce
  • discolored penile tip
  • pulsing penis due to non-productive urethral spasms.

- Classic UTO findings on physical exam include:

  - rock-hard, non-compressible, painful urinary bladder
  - penis extruded from prepuce
  - discolored penile tip
  - pulsing penis due to non-productive urethral spasms.

- Patients with UTO are often hypothermic and bradycardic on presentation.

- Bradycardia results from hyperkalemia.

- Hyperkalemia is due to decreased GFR.

- Hyperkalemia is associated with ECG abnormalities:

  - decreased to absent P waves
  - prolonged P-R and Q-T intervals
  - "tented" (tall) T waves
  - widened QRS complexes.

- Hyperkalemia can induce life-threatening arrhythmias. Because it can be fatal, hyperkalemia needs to be addressed urgently, often before the patient is unblocked.

- UTO resolution involves anesthetizing the patient to relieve the obstruction, followed by placement of an indwelling urinary catheter. Urinary catheter size and material impact patient comfort.

- Placement of a urinary catheter allows you to monitor your patient's ins and outs and adjust intravenous (IV) fluid therapy accordingly.

- Post-obstruction diuresis is common and often requires aggressive fluid therapy to prevent hypovolemia.

- Pain management and anti-spasmodic agents are typically prescribed.

- Antibiotics are not indicated unless urinalysis confirms UTI, in which case antibiotic selection should be guided by culture and susceptibility results.

References

1. Englar RE. Common clinical presentations in dogs and cats. Hoboken, NJ: Wiley/Blackwell; 2019. pages cm p.
2. George CM, Grauer GF. Feline urethral obstruction: diagnosis and management. Today's. Vet Pract 2016 (July/August):36–46.
3. Rijnberk A, Stokhof AA. General examination. In: Rijnberk A, van Sluijs FJ, editors. Medical history and physical examination in companion animals. New York: Elsevier; 2009.
4. Englar RE. Performing the small animal physical examination. Hoboken, NJ: Wiley/Blackwell; 2017.
5. Merck Vet Man. Whitehouse Station, NJ: Merck & Co., Inc. 2016.
6. Levine ED. Feline fear and anxiety. Vet Clin North Am Small Anim Pract 2008;38(5):1065–79, vii, vii.
7. Fear Free L. Module 1: fear free behavior modification basics. Denver, CO; 2018.
8. Cunningham JG, Klein BG. Cunningham's textbook of veterinary physiology. 5th ed. St. Louis, MO: Elsevier/Saunders; 2013.
9. Currie WB. Structure and function of domestic animals. Boston, MA: Butterworths; 1988.
10. Reece WO, Erickson HH, Goff JP, Uemura EE. Dukes' physiology of domestic animals. Ames, IA: John Wiley & Sons, Inc.; 2015.

11. Nibblett BM, Ketzis JK, Grigg EK. Comparison of stress exhibited by cats examined in a clinic versus a home setting. Appl Anim Behav Sci 2015;173:68–75.

12. Quimby JM, Smith ML, Lunn KF. Evaluation of the effects of hospital visit stress on physiologic parameters in the cat. J Feline Med Surg 2011;13(10):733–7.

13. Balakrishnan A, Drobatz KJ. Management of urinary tract emergencies in small animals. Vet Clin North Am Small Anim Pract 2013;43(4):843–67.

14. Thomovsky EJ. Managing the common comorbidities of feline urethral obstruction. DVM. 360 [Internet]; 2011. Available from: http://veterinarymedicine.dvm360.com/managing-common-comorbidities-feline-urethral-obstruction.

15. Sabino CV. Urethral obstruction in cats. Vet Team Brief 2017 (April):37–41.

16. DiBartola SP, de Morais HA. Disorders of potassium: hypokalemia and hyperkalemia. In: DiBartola SP, editor. Fluid, electroyte, and acid base disorders in small animal medicine. St. Louis, MO: Elsevier; 2006. p. 91–121.

17. Giebisch G, Windhager E. Transport of potassium. In: Boron WF, Boupaep EL, editors. Medical physiology: a cellular and molecular approach. Philadelphia, PA: Elsevier; 2005. p. 814–27.

18. Tag TL, Day TK. Electrocardiographic assessment of hyperkalemia in dogs and cats. J Veter Emer Crit 2008;18(1):61–7.

19. Gerber B, Boretti FS, Kley S, Laluha P, Müller C, Sieber N, et al. Evaluation of clinical signs and causes of lower urinary tract disease in European cats. J Small Anim Pract 2005;46(12):571–7.

20. Kruger JM, Osborne CA, Goyal SM, Wickstrom SL, Johnston GR, Fletcher TF, Brown PA. Clinical evaluation of cats with lower urinary tract disease. J Am Vet Med Assoc 1991;199(2):211–6.

21. Sumner JP, Rishniw M. Urethral obstruction in male cats in some Northern United States shows regional seasonality. Vet J 2017;220:72–4.

22. Filippich LJ. Cat with urinary tract signs. In: Rand J, editor. Problem-based feline medicine. New York: Saunders; 2006. p. 173–92.

23. Knapp DW, McMillan SK. Tumors of the urinary system. In: Withrow SJ, Vail DM, Page RL, editors. Withrow and MacEwen's small animal clinical oncology. 5th ed. St. Louis, MO: Elsevier; 2013. p. 572–82.

24. Valli VE, Norris A, Jacobs RM, Laing E, Withrow S, Macy D, et al. Pathology of canine bladder and urethral cancer and correlation with tumour progression and survival. J Comp Pathol 1995;113(2):113–30.

25. Mutsaers AJ, Widmer WR, Knapp DW. Canine transitional cell carcinoma. J Vet Intern Med 2003;17(2):136–44.

26. Knapp DW, Glickman NW, Denicola DB, Bonney PL, Lin TL, Glickman LT. Naturally-occurring canine transitional cell carcinoma of the urinary bladder A relevant model of human invasive bladder cancer. Urol Oncol 2000;5(2):47–59.

27. Norris AM, Laing EJ, Valli VE, Withrow SJ, Macy DW, Ogilvie GK, et al. Canine bladder and urethral tumors: a retrospective study of 115 cases (1980–1985). J Vet Intern Med 1992;6(3):145–53.

28. Nikula KJ, Benjamin SA, Angleton GM, Lee AC. Transitional cell carcinomas of the urinary tract in a colony of beagle dogs. Vet Pathol 1989;26(6):455–61.

29. Capasso A, Raiano V, Sontuoso A, Olivero D, Greci V. Fibrosarcoma of the urinary bladder in a cat. JFMS Open Rep 2015;1(1):2055116915585019.

30. Osborne CA, Low DG, Perman V, Barnes DM. Neoplasms of the canine and feline urinary bladder: incidence, etiologic factors, occurrence and pathologic features. Am J Vet Res 1968;29(10):2041–55.

31. Strafuss AC, Dean MJ. Neoplasms of the canine urinary bladder. J Am Vet Med Assoc 1975;166(12):1161–3.

32. Tarvin G, Patnaik A, Greene R. Primary urethral tumors in dogs. J Am Vet Med Assoc 1978;172(8):931–3.

33. Wilson GP, Hayes HM, Casey HW. Canine urethral cancer. J Am Anim Hosp Assoc 1979;15(6):741–4.

34. Fulkerson CM, Knapp DW. Management of transitional cell carcinoma of the urinary bladder in dogs: a review. Vet J 2015;205(2):217–25.

35. Gerber B, Eichenberger S, Reusch CE. Guarded long-term prognosis in male cats with urethral obstruction. J Feline Med Surg 2008;10(1):16–23.

36. Bartges JW, Callens AJ. Urolithiasis. Vet Clin North Am Small Anim Pract 2015;45(4):747–68.

37. Segev G, Livne H, Ranen E, Lavy E. Urethral obstruction in cats: predisposing factors, clinical, clinicopathological characteristics and prognosis. J Feline Med Surg 2011;13(2):101–8.

38. Kruger JM, Osborne CA, Lulich JP. Changing paradigms of feline idiopathic cystitis. Vet Clin North Am Small Anim Pract 2009;39(1):15–40.

39. Lee JA, Drobatz KJ. Characterization of the clinical characteristics, electrolytes, acid–base, and renal parameters in male cats with urethral obstruction. J Veter Emer Crit 2003;13(4):227–33.
40. Lekcharoensuk C, Osborne CA, Lulich JP. Epidemiologic study of risk factors for lower urinary tract diseases in cats. J Am Vet Med Assoc 2001;218(9):1429–35.
41. Little SE. The lower urinary tract. In: Little SE, editor. The cat: clinical medicine and management. St. Louis, MO: Elsevier; 2012.
42. DiBartola SP. Fluid, electrolyte, and acid–base disorders in small animal practice. 4th ed. St. Louis, MO: Saunders/Elsevier; 2012.
43. Odunyano A. Management of potassium disorders. NAVC Clin's Brief 2014 (March):69–72.
44. Tilley LP, Smith FWK, Tilley LP. Blackwell's five-minute veterinary consult: canine and feline. 4th ed. Ames, IA: Blackwell; 2007.
45. Schaer M. Hyperkalemia in cats with urethral obstruction. Electrocardiographic abnormalities and treatment. Vet Clin North Am 1977;7(2):407–14.
46. Parks J. Electrocardiographic abnormalities from serum electrolyte imbalance due to feline urethral obstruction. J Am Anim Hosp Assoc 1975;11:101–9.
47. Surawicz B. Relationship between electrocardiogram and electrolytes. Am Heart J 1967;73(6):814–34.
48. Dreifus LS, Pick A. A clinical correlative study of the electrocardiogram in electrolyte imbalance. Circulation 1956;14(5):815–25.
49. Ettinger PO, Regan TJ, Oldewurtel HA. Hyperkalemia, cardiac conduction, and the electrocardiogram: a review. Am Heart J 1974;88(3):360–71.
50. Cote E. Feline arrhythmias: an update. Vet Clin N am. Small 2010;40(4):643.
51. Tilley LP. Essentials of canine and feline electrocardiography. Philadelphia, PA: Lea & Febiger; 1993.
52. Côté E. Clinical veterinary advisor. Dogs and cats. 3rd ed. St. Louis, MO: Elsevier Mosby; 2015.
53. Ettinger SJ, Feldman EC, Côté E. Textbook of veterinary internal medicine: diseases of the dog and the cat. 8th ed. St. Louis, MO: Elsevier; 2017.
54. Ruda L, Heiene R. Short- and long-term outcome after perineal urethrostomy in 86 cats with feline lower urinary tract disease. J Small Anim Pract 2012;53(12):693–8.
55. George CM, Grauer GF. Feline urethral obstruction: diagnosis and management: today's veterinary practice. Available from: https://todaysveterinarypractice.com/feline-urethral-obstruction-diagnosis-management/#.
56. Pachtinger G. Urinary catheter placement for feline urethral obstruction. Clinician's. Brief 2014 (July).
57. Francis BJ, Wells RJ, Rao S, Hackett TB. Retrospective study to characterize post-obstructive diuresis in cats with urethral obstruction. J Feline Med Surg 2010;12(8):606–8.
58. Baum N, Anhalt M, Carlton CE, Scott R. Post-obstructive diuresis. J Urol 1975;114(1):53–6.
59. O'Neill KE, Labato MA. Urinary catheters and infection. Clinician's. Brief 2015 (November).
60. Schoeman JP, editor. Approach to polyuria and polydipsia in the dog. Proceedings of the 33rd world small animal veterinary congress; 2008; Dublin, Ireland. World Small Animal Veterinary Association (WSAVA).

Case 20

The Dog That Is Straining to Urinate

Sookie was adopted by James and Jasmine Watson 6 weeks ago from the local humane society. The couple had recently become empty nesters when their last daughter of three graduated from college. Although James and Jasmine were proud that they had raised their children to be independent, they had to admit that the house was far too quiet these days. At the advice of a friend, they decided to foster a dog or two. They never imagined adopting one for good. Then they met Sookie.

According to her medical records, which the shelter kept on file, Sookie had belonged to an elderly man who was moving out of state into his son's home. Although the gentleman had wished to keep Sookie; his son already had a full house, complete with a wife, four children, and a dog of his own. As a terrier mix, Sookie did not take up much space. However, the son's dog was reportedly aggressive towards other dogs and would not tolerate four-legged house guests. The only way for the gentleman to make the move permanent,

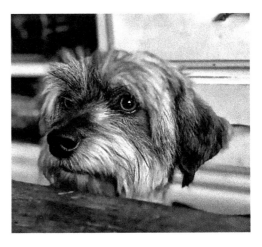

Figure 20.1 Meet your new patient, Sookie, a 6-year-old spayed female mixed breed dog. Courtesy of Keleigh Schettler.

which was required on account of his health, was to find Sookie a good home. He did his research and handpicked who he thought would be the perfect family, but at the last minute the arrangement fell through. It broke his heart to leave Sookie behind, but the shelter promised to find her forever home.

Sookie had difficulty transitioning to life at the shelter. For the first few days, she held onto hope that her owner would return. When it became apparent that he was not coming back, she sunk into a deep decline. Sookie stopped trying to come to the cage front when visitors walked by. For the most part, Sookie just existed. Nothing more. Nothing less.

It wasn't until the Watsons stopped by one sunny afternoon that her spirits lifted. She heard James' voice before she saw him. He sounded familiar, like an old friend. One ear pricked forward, then the other and her tail automatically fell into a slow wag. When James stopped in front of her cage and said hello, something inside willed her into action. For reasons that she didn't quite understand, she was motivated to get up and give it a go.

Jasmine fell in love with her eyes first. Her eyes told a story of heartbreak and rebirth, as if she had been hurt before but was open to the next chapter, a new beginning.

"Look, James," Jasmine remarked. "I think she needs us." And just like that, the trio became family.

Sookie settled into her new home with ease and had not once given the Watsons any reason for alarm. Perhaps that is why it was so startling for Jasmine and James to wake up this morning to find an accident on their kitchen tile (see **Plate 7**).

Sookie had not had any accidents over the past 6 weeks, so this was very out of character! Even more concerning was that her urine looked bloody. Sookie had also asked to go outside three times already this morning and it wasn't even noon. Something was definitely wrong. The Watsons scheduled an appointment with you to investigate.

They have just arrived at the clinic. Sookie's vital signs are taken by one of your technicians and documented in her record below.

You examine Sookie and find that:

Weight: 24.6 lb (11.2 kg)
BCS: 4/9
Mentation: QAR

TPR

T: 101.6°F (38.7°C)
P: 108 beats per minute
R: Panting

- her peri-vulvar fur is stained rust-brown
- she reacts with reproducible abdominal tensing and vocalizes when you palpate her urinary bladder
- her bladder wall feels thickened
- you feel hard structures grinding against one another within the lumen of the urinary bladder.

Review the following questions to guide your consultation with the Watsons as you consider her diagnosis, urolithiasis (urinary stones).

Round One of Questions for Case 20: The Dog That Is Straining to Urinate

1. True or false? All uroliths are obstructive.
2. True or false? All uroliths are palpable on physical exam.
3. When there is more than one stone in the bladder, you can feel them scrape against one another. What is this sensation called?
4. True or false? All patients with uroliths present with clinical signs.
5. In addition to urinary accidents (inappropriate urination), what are common clinical signs that patients exhibit when they have uroliths?
6. What causes hematuria in a patient that has one or more uroliths?
7. What might owners of male dogs comment on during history-taking that may clue you in to the fact that the dog has uroliths?
8. If you already know, based upon abdominal palpation, that Sookie has bladder stones, why is it still important to perform an imaging study?
9. Radiographic interpretation is based upon analysis of different opacities on a radiograph. What causes different opacities to form?
10. Five opacities are visible on radiographs. Name these and identify the color (black/white/shades of grey) with which they are associated.
11. What do we call objects that appear black on radiographs?
12. What do we call objects that appear white on radiographs?
13. Urinary stones are which opacity?
14. Can you identify the composition of urinary stones based upon their size or shape as they appear on radiographs?
15. How big must a radiodense stone be to show up on a radiograph?
16. How does the patient's breed help you to predict the mineral content of urinary stones in any given patient?
17. Why do urinary stones form?
18. In which sex and species are we most concerned about the potential for urinary tract obstruction (UTO) when stones are present and why?

Answers to Round One of Questions for Case 20:
The Dog That Is Straining to Urinate

1. False. All uroliths have the potential to become obstructive, but not all uroliths are obstructive.(1, 2)

2. False. Not all uroliths are palpable on physical exam.(2) Uroliths are only palpable in one out of every five dogs that have them.(3)

3. When there is more than one stone in the bladder, you can feel them scrape against one another. This sensation is called crepitation.(4)

4. False. Not all patients with uroliths present with clinical signs. In fact, for many patients, urolithiasis is an incidental finding, either on abdominal palpation or abdominal imaging.(1)

5. When patients are symptomatic for urolithiasis, owners may report one or more of the following clinical signs:(2)
   - abdominal straining
   - dysuria
   - stranguria
   - pollakiuria
   - hematuria
   - excessive grooming:
      - perineum in cats and female dogs
      - prepuce in male dogs
   - guarding the abdomen
   - increased respiratory rate (RR), secondary to pain.

6. Hematuria typically occurs in patients that have one or more uroliths because the stone(s) roll(s) around and scrape(s) the bladder wall.(5)

7. Owners of male dogs may report that the patient's stream is "off."(2) Patients may posture to urinate, without producing the expected volume of urine.(2)

8. Even though you know that Sookie has bladder stones, cystoliths, based upon abdominal palpation, it is still important to perform an imaging study. This is because the urinary bladder is not the only location where stones may form. Urinary stones may also occur at the following locations:(2, 4)
   - kidney(s) – when they form here, they are called nephroliths
   - ureter(s) – when they form here, they are called ureteroliths
   - urethra – when they form here, they are called urethroliths.

   It is critical to know where stones are in the urinary tract to predict where obstruction(s) may occur and/or to plan appropriate medical or surgical interventions. It is equally important to image the abdomen to know approximately how many stones you may be dealing with and their approximate size. Size helps to gauge the likelihood of stone passage through the urinary tract and/or if an obstruction is likely to develop.

9. Radiographic interpretation is based upon analysis of different opacities on a radiograph.(6) Opacities are formed by the penetration of tissue by X-rays, invisible high energy waves.(6) X-rays pass through body tissues to expose radiographic film that sits on the other side of the

patient.(6) Not all tissues absorb X-rays to the same degree.(6) The greater the amount of tissue absorption, the fewer X-rays reach the film.(6) The fewer the X-rays that reach the film, the whiter the image appears.(6)

10. Five opacities are visible on radiographs.(6)

   - Metal
      - Metal absorbs THE MOST X-rays and will appear as bright white.
   - Bone
      - Bone absorbs A LOT of X-rays and will appear as grey-white.
   - Soft tissue
      - Soft tissue (i.e. muscle) absorbs SOME X-rays and will appear grey.
   - Fat
      - Fat absorbs a SMALL number of X-rays and so will appear dark grey.
   - Air
      - Air absorbs the LEAST number of X-rays and so will appear black.

11. Objects that appear black on radiographs are called radiolucent.(6)

12. Objects that appear white on radiographs are called radiopaque.(6) Sometimes this quality is referred to as being radiodense.(6)

13. The radiopacity of uroliths depends upon their mineral composition.(6, 7)

   - Calcium oxalate and silica uroliths appear as radiopaque on radiographic images.(1, 5, 8, 9)
      - The false-negative detection rate is 5%.(10)
   - If they contain sufficient calcium phosphate, then magnesium ammonium phosphate (struvite) stones will also appear as radiopaque.(10, 11)
      - The false-negative detection rate is 2%.(10)
   - Urate and cystine uroliths appear as radiolucent on radiographic images.(1, 5)
      - Because of their radiolucency, these stones often go undetected on standard radiographic films: the false-negative detection rate is 25%. (10)
      - If you wish to detect radiolucent stones, then you must make use of advanced imaging techniques, such as double-contrast cystography, or abdominal ultrasound.(1, 5)

14. No, you cannot determine the mineral composition of each urolith based upon the way it appears in terms of radiographic size or shape.(10, 12) There is no standard size for uroliths based upon mineral composition. Judging stones by their shape is equally erroneous. For instance, even though the majority of magnesium ammonium phosphate stones are ovoid in terms of radiographic appearance, one in five will be misidentified.(13)

15. A radiodense stone must be at least three millimeters in diameter in order for it to show up on a radiograph.(6)

16. The patient's breed can help you to make an educated guess as to type(s) of stone(s) that is/are most likely to be present.(2)

- Calcium oxalate stones tend to be associated with small breeds of dogs:(3, 9, 14)

  - Miniature Schnauzer
  - Lhasa Apso
  - Shih Tzu
  - Yorkshire terrier
  - Bichon Frize.

- Dalmatians and English Bulldogs are at increased risk of developing urate stones.(15)

  - The chance that a urolith will be urate-based in a Dalmatian is 228.9 times greater than in any other breed, with males being 16.4 times more at risk than females.
  - The chance that a urolith will be urate-based in an English Bulldog is 43 times greater than in any other breed, with males being 14.3 times more at risk than females.

- English Bulldogs are also at increased risk of developing cystine stones.(15)

  - The chance that a urolith will be cystine-based in an English Bulldog is 32.3 times greater than in any other breed, with only males represented in a 1994 study by Bartges et al.

17. Urinary stones formation is multifactorial. Contributing factors include:

- an abundance of inorganic protein in the urine to form a matrix upon which uroliths may form
- presence of crystallization promotors:

  - urine solutes:

    - solubility
    - saturation concentration
    - urine ph:
    - aciduria promotes formation of calcium oxalate crystals(2)
    - alkalinuria promotes formation of struvite crystals(2)

- presence of UTI

  - struvite stones are often the result of urinary tract infections (UTIs)(1, 2)
  - females less than one year old or greater than 10 are most at risk of developing UTIs(9, 16–18)
  - certain types of bacteria – *Staphylococcus*, *Enterococcus*, and *Proteus* spp. – produce the enzyme, urease
  - urease catalyzes the hydrolysis of urea to produce ammonia(9, 19)
  - ammonia makes the urine more alkaline(2)
  - alkaline urine promotes the formation of struvites.(2, 20)

18. Male cats are at increased risk of UTO due to the narrow diameter of their urethra.(1)

    Stones are also more likely to cause urethral obstruction in male dogs because of the os penis. The os penis, or baculum, is a bone that accompanies the penile urethra.(21–23) This mineralization is scant by comparison to the macroscopic os penis of the dog, and it does not appear to be present in all cats.(22, 24–26) When the os penis is present, it is seated dorsal to the canine urethra and ventral to the feline urethra within the glans. In dogs, the os penis is grooved to accommodate the urethra.(21, 25, 26) Stones are likely to get trapped in the urethra at the level of the os penis, making them difficult to pass.(2)

Returning to Case 20: The Dog That Is Straining to Urinate

You convince the Watsons that you need to perform orthogonal abdominal radiographs. One of the two views has been provided in Figure 20.2.

Review the following questions as you prepare to consult with the Watsons concerning next steps for Sookie's case management.

Round Two of Questions for Case 20: The Dog That Is Straining to Urinate

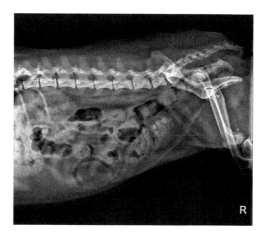

Figure 20.2 Right lateral abdominal radiograph that is diagnostic for urolithiasis.

1. Uroliths can be surgically excised. What is the appropriate medical term for the surgical procedure that involves cutting stones out of the urinary bladder?

2. Other than for the purpose of excising, why else might we perform the surgery that you identified in Question #1 (above)?

3. Bladder surgery makes use of stay sutures. What are stay sutures? Why are they used?

4. What are measures that you take to reduce the risk of peritoneal contamination when you cut into the urinary bladder?

5. What are measures that you can take to reduce the risk of damaging the ureteral openings when incising the urinary bladder during surgery?

6. False-negative urine cultures often occur in dogs with urolithiasis. What can you do during surgery to confirm the accuracy of the culture findings?

7. Why and how might you place a urinary catheter intraoperatively in a male dog to facilitate the procedure?

8. Why and how might you place a urinary catheter intraoperatively in cats or in a female dog like Sookie, to facilitate the procedure?

9. Which suture qualities are most important when selecting the material with which you will close the urinary bladder?

10. During closure of the urinary bladder, which layer of the bladder wall must you include in your suture pattern and why?

11. When suturing the urinary bladder, what do you need to avoid doing to reduce the chance of calculus formation?

12. Following closure, it is critical that the urinary bladder be watertight. How do you assess this?

13. What should you do before you recover the patient from general anesthesia?

14. What is the purpose of continuing intravenous (IV) fluids in the post-operative period?

15. How long does it take after surgery for the urinary bladder to regain its strength?

16. What are anticipated clinical signs in the postoperative period following this surgical procedure?

17. How common is recurrence of uroliths following surgical excision?

18. Surgery is not the only approach to urolithiasis management. Which canine urolith(s) can be managed medically via a dissolution protocol?

19. Describe your understanding of the dissolution protocol for the urolith that you identified in Question #17 (above).

20. How long, on average, does it take for uroliths to dissolve using the protocol that you outlined in Question #18 (above)?

21. In which sex and species would you be most concerned about the time it takes for the dissolution protocol to be effective?

22. What is lithotripsy? Could it be an alternative to surgical excision of cystoliths and/or dissolution therapy with diet?

Answers to Round Two of Questions for Case 20: The Dog That Is Straining to Urinate

1. Cystoliths are excised from the urinary bladder in a surgical procedure that is called a cystotomy. (27–29)

2. Other than for the purpose of excising, a cystotomy might be performed to biopsy a mass within the urinary bladder or to resect a portion of the bladder wall that contains a mass.(28, 29) That is the extent to which most general practitioners will operate on the urinary bladder. Board-certified surgeons may perform cystotomies to facilitate advanced techniques, such as ureteral reimplantation, or to correct intramural ectopic ureters.(29)

3. Bladder surgery makes use of stay sutures.(28) Stay sutures are temporarily placed intraoperatively to allow the surgeon to manipulate the urinary bladder without repeatedly having to grasp the organ itself.(28) Bladder mucosa is quick to swell, and you want to minimize unnecessary trauma.(28, 29)

4. To reduce the risk of peritoneal contamination when you cut into the urinary bladder, you should pack off the bladder by surrounding it with moistened laparotomy pads.(29)

5. To reduce the risk of damaging the ureteral openings when incising the urinary bladder during surgery, you should make your incision along the ventral aspect of the bladder apex.(28, 29)

6. False-negative urine cultures often occur in dogs with urolithiasis. To confirm the accuracy of the culture findings, you can use surgical scissors to take a sliver of the bladder wall at the site of your incision and submit that sample for histopathology.(29)

7. To assess the patency of the urethra in a male dog, you can ask a technician to insert a urinary catheter into the urethral orifice at the tip of the penis and pass it retrograde into the urinary bladder during the cystotomy.(29) You can also flush the urethra as you pass the catheter to dislodge smaller stones and grit from within the lower urinary tract.(29)

8. To assess the patency of the urethra in cats or in a female dog, like Sookie, you can insert a urinary catheter through the incision into the urinary bladder and pass the catheter antegrade into the urethra.(29) You can also flush the urethra as you pass the catheter to dislodge smaller stones and grit from within the lower urinary tract.(28, 29)

9. The suture that you use to close the urinary bladder should be both monofilament and absorbable.(27, 29)

    Monofilaments are less likely to harbor bacteria at surgical sites as compared to braided suture.(27) Therefore, monofilaments are less likely to be a nidus for infection than braided suture.

    The urinary bladder is also delicate. Using monofilament suture causes less tissue drag than the braided variety.(27)

    Suture should be absorbable because suture removal is not an option for cystotomy. Additionally, non-absorbable suture provides a matrix that may encourage stones to recur.(27)

10. During closure of the urinary bladder, you must take care to include the submucosa in your suture pattern because it is the holding layer.(27, 30–32) It is what will give the closure strength.

11. When suturing the urinary bladder, avoid full-thickness passage of the suture through the bladder wall into the bladder lumen.(29) Having the suture enter the lumen of the bladder increases the chance that new stones will form.(29–33)

12. Following closure, it is critical that the urinary bladder be watertight.(33) To assess this, you can use your fingers to gently "clamp" off the outflow tract, the neck of the bladder. You then insert a sterile needle, attached to a syringe filled with sterile 0.9% sodium chloride, into the lumen of the bladder. You fill up the bladder and watch the suture line. The bladder should expand as saline is introduced into the lumen, but the suture line should remain dry. This is a way to leak test the urinary bladder.(28) If any leaks are present, then they should be sealed by strategic placement of additional simple interrupted or cruciate sutures.(34)

13. On average, it takes 2 to 3 weeks for the urinary bladder to regain its original strength after surgery.(27–29, 31, 33)

14. You should repeat an abdominal imaging study to be sure that you have removed all visible (radiopaque) uroliths.(28) You may think that you got them all, but very often there are ones that are missed that require extraction and/or additional flushing of the urinary tract.(29) In one published study, residual uroliths were identified in as many as one out of every five cats at a teaching hospital.(35)

15. It is beneficial to continue intravenous (IV) fluids in the postoperative period because these add to urine volume, which helps to flush out the urinary tract.(28) Blood clots may form at the incision site in the immediate postoperative period.(29) It is important to flush these out so that they do not accumulate to a size that then might lead to a UTO.(29)

16. In the first 24–48 hours following surgery, it is typical for the urine to take on a pink hue from mild hematuria.(28, 29) The patient may also experience dysuria, stranguria, and pollakiuria for the first few days following this procedure.(28, 29) However, these should improve daily.(28)

17. Recurrence of uroliths is common in canine patients. Recurrence may occur in as many as one in four dogs within the first year following cystotomy. This relapse is frustrating to the client and veterinary team alike.

18. Surgery is not the only approach to managing bladder stones. Magnesium ammonium phosphate (struvite) stones may resolve with diet and antibiotic therapy, when indicated.(1)

19. Recall that struvite stones often result from UTIs.(1) Certain bacteria produce the enzyme, urease. Urease catalyzes the hydrolysis of urea to produce ammonia.(9, 19) Ammonia makes the urine more alkaline. Alkaline urine promotes struvite stone development.(20)

    Dissolution of struvite stones therefore requires you to both address underlying UTI (if present) and acidify the urine. Urine pH must consistently drop below 6.0–6.5. This is usually achieved by feeding a prescription diet that contains:

    • high sodium
    • reduced phosphorus
    • reduced magnesium
    • reduced protein.

Sodium promotes osmotic diuresis. Precipitation of urinary crystals and the formation of uroliths is less likely to occur in dilute urine, that is, urine with a USG <1.025. Dilute urine also contains less urea, which means that ammonia-producing bacteria have fewer substrates to feed upon. Lower levels of ammonia, in combination with reduced dietary phosphorus and magnesium, limit struvite development.

20. On average, it takes 8–12 weeks for uroliths to dissolve using the protocol outlined above. Some patients require 20 weeks of diet management for radiopaque stones to disappear on radiographs.

21. I would be reluctant to enroll male cats in dissolution trials for fear that they might develop UTO, given the narrow diameter of their urethras.

22. Lithotripsy is an alternative to surgical excision of uroliths. It uses pulses of energy to break urinary stones into pieces small enough to pass through the outflow tract without causing UTO.(36, 37) In people, this procedure is frequently used to treat nephroliths and cystoliths. Lithotripsy is not routinely available in companion animal practice due to lack of training and equipment, but it offers a practical alternative to surgery and may become more prevalent as the veterinary profession evolves.

Returning to Case 20: The Dog That Is Straining to Urinate

The Watsons elect to take Sookie to surgery to speed resolution of urolithiasis. Pre-anesthetic blood work is within normal limits. Urine is collected via cystocentesis. Urinalysis results have been provided (see Figures 20.3a–20.3c). Urine culture is pending.

Sookie undergoes cystotomy without intraoperative complications and a significant number of stones are removed from Sookie (see Figure 20.4).

Sookie is discharged to the care of her owners the following day.

>	Color	Pale Yellow	
>	Clarity	Slightly Cloudy	
>	Specific Gravity	1.035	
>	pH	7.0	
>	Urine Protein	30	mg/dL
>	Glucose	neg	
>	Ketones	neg	
>	Blood / Hemoglobin	neg	
>	Bilirubin	neg	
>	Urobilinogen	4	mg/dL
	Leukocyte Esterase	100	Leu/µL
>	White Blood Cells	3 /HPF	
>	Red Blood Cells	>50 /HPF	
>	Bacteria, Cocci	None to rare	
>	Bacteria, Rods	Present	
>	Squamous Epithelial Cells	None to rare	
>	Non-Squamous Epithelial Cells	1 - 2 /HPF	
>	Hyaline Casts	None to rare	
>	Non-Hyaline Casts	None to rare	

Figure 20.3a Urinalysis results for Sookie.

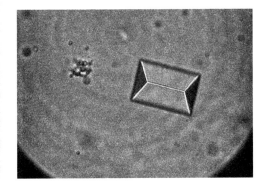

Figure 20.3b Photomicrograph of urinalysis: Crystal "A." Courtesy of Brad Minson.

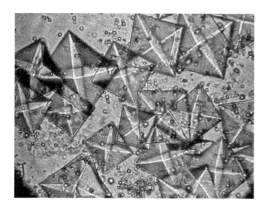

Figure 20.3c Photomicrograph of urinalysis: Abundance of Crystals of Subtype "B." Courtesy of Brad Minson.

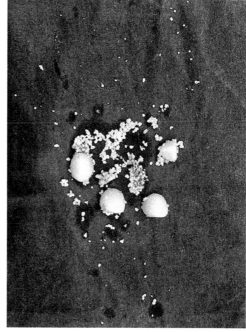

Figure 20.4 Post-operative urolith collection from Sookie. Courtesy of Joseph Onello.

Round Three of Questions for Case 20: The Dog That Is Straining to Urinate

1. Identify the urinary crystal in Figure 20.3b.
2. Identify the urinary crystals in Figure 20.3c.
3. Can you identify the crystals based upon their appearance in Figure 20.4? If yes, what are they? If not, what do you need to do to confirm their composition?

Answers to Round Three of Questions for Case 20: The Dog That Is Straining to Urinate

1. The urinary crystal in Figure 20.3b is a struvite.

2. The urinary crystals in Figure 20.3c are calcium oxalates.

3. No, you cannot determine the type(s) of stone(s) that you are dealing with based upon surgical appearance (size or shape). In order to determine the mineral composition, you will need to submit the stone(s) to an outside laboratory. It is essential to establish mineral composition because this dictates how case management should proceed.

CLINICAL PEARLS

- Uroliths can develop at any point along the urinary tract: kidney (nephrolith), ureter (ureterolith), bladder (cystolith), urethra (urethrolith).

- Not all uroliths are obstructive. Not all cause patients to exhibit clinical signs. When patients are symptomatic, clients typically report one or more of the following:

  - abdominal guarding
  - abdominal straining
  - dysuria
  - hematuria
  - increased grooming at perineum and/or prepuce
  - increasing RR / panting (pain)
  - pollakiuria
  - stranguria
  - "change in urine stream" (male dogs).

- Some, but not all, cystoliths are palpable on abdominal exam. Even if cystoliths are palpable, imaging studies of the abdomen are indicated to rule out concurrent uroliths elsewhere.

- Whether or not a urolith is visible on radiographs depends upon its size and radiopacity.

  - Uroliths must be 3 mm or more to be visible.
  - Uroliths must be radiopaque/radiodense in order to show up on film as white.
  - Radiopaque/radiodense uroliths include calcium oxalate, silica, and most magnesium ammonium phosphate, also known as triple phosphate or struvite.
  - Radiolucent uroliths, such as urate and cystine, do not show up on standard abdominal radiographs.
  - Contrast cystography or abdominal ultrasound are typically used to visualize radiolucent stones.

- Cystoliths are often surgically excised. Stones are then submitted for mineral composition analysis in the immediate post-operative period to guide medical management for prevention. Stone recurrence is common.

- Dissolution therapy is an option for struvite stones and involves acidification of the urine. However, it does not offer an immediate resolution. The patient's sex and species must be taken into consideration. Male cats, for instance, are at increased risk of UTO.

References

1. Filippich LJ. Cat with urinary tract signs. In: Rand J, editor. Problem-based feline medicine. Edinburgh. New York: Saunders; 2006. p. 173–92.
2. Englar RE. Common clinical presentations in dogs and cats. Hoboken, NJ: Wiley/Blackwell; 2019.
3. Bartges JW, Kirk C, Lane IF. Update: management of calcium oxalate uroliths in dogs and cats. Vet Clin North Am Small Anim Pract 2014;34(4):969–87, vii, vii.
4. The Merck Veterinary Manual. Whitehouse Station, NJ: Merck & Co., Inc.; 2016.
5. Englar RE. Performing the small animal physical examination. Hoboken, NJ: Wiley; 2017.
6. Thrall DE. Textbook of veterinary diagnostic radiology. 7th edition. St. Louis, MO: Elsevier; 2018.
7. Ettinger SJ, Feldman EC, Côté E. Textbook of veterinary internal medicine: diseases of the dog and the cat. 8th edition. St. Louis, MO: Elsevier; 2017.

8. Park RD, Wrigley RH. The urinary bladder. In: Thrall DE, editor. Textbook of veterinary diagnostic radiology. 4th edition. Philadelphia, PA: Saunders; 2002. p. 571–92.

9. Bartges JW, Callens AJ. Urolithiasis. Vet Clin North Am Small Anim Pract 2015;45(4):747–68.

10. Feeney DA, Weichselbaum RC, Jessen CR, Osborne CA. Imaging canine urocystoliths – detection and prediction of mineral content. Vet Clin N Am Small 1999;29(1):59.

11. Grauer GF. Ammonium urate urolithiasis. Clinician's Brief 2014:51–5.

12. Weichselbaum RC, Feeney DA, Jessen CR, Osborne CA, Koehler L, Ulrich L. Evaluation of the morphologic characteristics and prevalence of canine urocystoliths from a regional urolith center. American Journal of Veterinary Research 1998;59(4):379–87.

13. Englar RE. Performing the small animal physical examination. Hoboken, NJ: Wiley/Blackwell; 2017.

14. Lekcharoensuk C, Lulich JP, Osborne CA, Pusoonthornthum R, Allen TA, Koehler LA, et al. Patient and environmental factors associated with calcium oxalate urolithiasis in dogs. Journal of the American Veterinary Medical Association 2000;217(4):515–9.

15. Bartges JW, Osborne CA, Lulich JP, Unger LK, Koehler LA, Bird KA, et al. Prevalence of cystine and urate uroliths in bulldogs and urate uroliths in dalmatians. Journal of the American Veterinary Medical Association 1994;204(12):1914–8.

16. Okafor CC, Pearl DL, Lefebvre SL, Wang MS, Yang MY, Blois SL, et al. Risk factors associated with struvite urolithiasis in dogs evaluated at general care veterinary hospitals in the United States. Vet Med A 2013;243(12):1737–45.

17. Seaman R, Bartges JW. Canine struvite urolithiasis. Comp Cont Educ Pract 2001;23(5):407–+.

18. Palma D, Langston C, Gisselman K, McCue J. Canine struvite urolithiasis. Compendium 2013;35(8):E1; quiz E1.

19. Osborne CA, Polzin DJ, Abdullahi SU, Leininger JR, Clinton CW, Griffith DP. Struvite urolithiasis in animals and man: formation, detection, and dissolution. Advances in Veterinary Science and Comparative Medicine 1985;29:1–101.

20. Tarttelin MF. Feline struvite urolithiasis: factors affecting urine pH may be more important than magnesium levels in food. The Veterinary Record 1987;121(10):227–30.

21. Aspinall V. Anatomy and physiology of the dog and cat II. The male reproductive system. Veterinary Nursing Journal 2004;19(6):200–4.

22. Evans HE, Miller ME. Miller's anatomy of the dog. 4th edition. St. Louis, MO: Elsevier; 2013.

23. Singh B, Dyce KM. Dyce, Sack, and Wensing's textbook of veterinary anatomy. St. Louis, MO: Saunders; 2018.

24. Piola V, Posch B, Aghte P, Caine A, Herrtage ME. Radiographic characterization of the os penis in the cat. Vet Radiol Ultrasound 2011;52(3):270–2.

25. Tobon Restrepo M, Altuzarra R, Espada Y, Dominguez E, Mallol C. Novellas R. CT characterization of the feline os penis. J Feline Med Surg 2019:X19873195:http://www.ncbi.nlm.nih.gov/pubmed/1098612.

26. Osborne CA, Caywood DD, Johnston GR, Polzin DJ, Lulich JP, Kruger JM, Ulrich LK. Feline perineal urethrostomy: a potential cause of feline lower urinary tract disease. Vet Clin North America. Small Anim Pract 1996;26(3):535–49.

27. Lipscomb VJ. Bladder. In: Tobias KM, Johnston SA, editors. Veterinary surgery: small animal. Two. St. Louis, MO: Saunders; 2012.

28. Little JP, Hardie RJ. Bladder. In: Langley-Hobbs SJ, Demetriou J, Ladlow JF, editors. Feline soft tissue and general surgery. New York: Saunders/Elsevier; 2014.

29. Tobias KM. Cystotomy. In: Tobias KM, editor. Manual of small animal soft tissue surgery. Ames, IA: Wiley/Blackwell; 2010.

30. Cornell KK. Cystotomy, partial cystectomy, and tube cystostomy. Clin Tech Small Anim Pract 2000;15(1):11–6.

31. Thieman-Mankin KM, Ellison GW, Jeyapaul CJ, Glotfelty-Ortiz CS. Comparison of short-term complication rates between dogs and cats undergoing appositional single-layer or inverting double-layer cystotomy closure: 144 cases (1993–2010). Journal of the American Veterinary Medical Association 2012;240(1):65–8.

32. Stone EA, Kyles AE. Cystotomy and partial cystectomy. In: Bojrab MJ, Waldron DR, and Toombs JP, editors. Current Techniques in Small Animal Surgery. 5th edition. Jackson, WY: Teton New Media; 2014. p. 481–482.

33. Radasch RM, Merkley DF, Wilson JW, Barstad RD. Cystotomy closure. A comparison of the strength of appositional and inverting suture patterns. Veterinary Surgery 1990;19(4):283–288.

34. Pope ER. Cystotomy. Clinician's. Brief 2016 (March):28–34.
35. Lulich JP, Osborne CA. Changing paradigms in the diagnosis of urolithiasis. Vet Clin North Am. Small Anim Pract 2009;39(1):79–91.
36. Adams LG, Berent AC, Moore GE, Bagley DH. Use of laser lithotripsy for fragmentation of uroliths in dogs: 73 cases (2005–2006). Journal of the American Veterinary Medical Association. 2008;232(11):1680–7.
37. Davidson EB, Ritchey JW, Higbee RD, Lucroy MD, Bartels KE. Laser lithotripsy for treatment of canine uroliths. Vet Surg 2004;33(1):56–61.

Case 21

The Cat That Is Peeing a Lot

Dorito is an established patient of yours. He belongs to Miss Frita Lay, who has been coming to your clinic since she accompanied her parents on visits with her childhood pets. Twenty years later, she's still entrusting the care of her loved ones to you and your associates.

Dorito is one of three neutered male cats in an indoor-only household. Dorito is the eldest, followed by 7-year-old Cheeto, and 4-year-old Tostito. Other than routine dental prophylaxis under general anesthesia as needed, Dorito has been healthy.

Dorito lives in a two-story home that contains two litter boxes per floor. Frita scoops all four boxes every evening. Over the year, this has given her a sense of what is typical in terms of urine and fecal quantity. Over the past month, Frita has noticed that the boxes are getting fuller sooner. She scoops more clumps than she used to, and some of the clumps seem larger. At first, it was inconsistent, so no alarm bells were triggered. But now she's finding that the number of clumps has doubled, as has the size of some, but not all.

Once Frita realized that more urine was being produced than normal, it took some serious detective work to figure out who was responsible. None of her three cats particularly enjoyed being watched in the bathroom. Most of the time they waited until she was out of sight, if not out of the house. Privacy was valued at a premium in the Lay household.

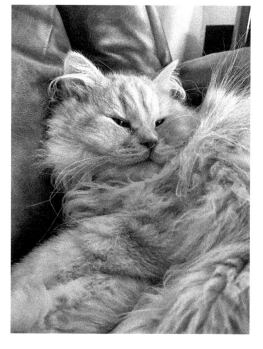

Figure 21.1 Meet your next patient, Dorito, a 9-year-old castrated male cat. Courtesy of Jennifer Lang.

However, twice now in the past week, Frita has caught Dorito coming out of the spare bedroom, where the litter boxes are kept, during the lunch hour, whereas in the past he used to be sound asleep. On both occasions, she checked out the litter and found a large, fresh clump. This led her to believe that Dorito was the one responsible for the change in urine volume and frequency.

To her knowledge, Dorito does not seem to be in any discomfort or pain. However, he does appear to be drinking significantly more than he used to. In the past, Frita rarely witnessed any of the three cats quenching their thirst. Lately, every time she turns around, Dorito is at the water dish.

Dorito's appetite also seems "off." He will eat, but less than usual, and only if coaxed. Frita has also noticed that Dorito has vomited three times in the past week!

Dorito has presented today for evaluation to see if there is any underlying medical reason for his apparent increase in both thirst and urination. Your technician meets Dorito and Frita in the exam room and takes his vitals. These have been outlined below.

Weight: 9.6 lb (4.4 kg) – down by 0.8lb or 0.36 kg since his last visit, four months ago
BCS: 3/9
Muscle Condition Score: Moderate muscle loss
Mentation: QAR

TPR

T: 101.3°F (38.5°C)
P: 187 beats per minute
R: 26 breaths per minute

Round One of Questions for Case 21: The Cat That Is Peeing a Lot

1. What is the appropriate medical term for "increased thirst?"
2. Fill in the blank:

    If thirst exceeds _____mL/kg/day in a CAT, then it is considered excessive.

3. Fill in the blank:

    If thirst exceeds _____mL/kg/day in a DOG, then it is considered excessive.

4. Based upon your answer for Question #2 (above), how much would Dorito need to drink each day to be considered excessive?
5. What is the appropriate medical term for "increased urination?"
6. Fill in the blank:

    If urine output exceeds _____mL/kg/day in a CAT, then it is considered excessive.

7. Fill in the blank:

    If urine output exceeds _____mL/kg/day in a DOG, then it is considered excessive.

8. Based upon your answer for Question #6 (above), how much would Dorito need to urinate each day for the volume to be considered excessive?
9. In health, thirst and urination are linked processes. If renal function is adequate, a dehydrated patient will maximally concentrate urine to conserve water and will be driven to drink.

    a. Which hormone is responsible for conserving water?
    b. Where in the body is this hormone produced?
    c. How is water conserved when this hormone is released?

10. The nephron is the functional unit of the kidney. Fill in the blank with a fraction:

    The kidneys' ability to concentrate urine is significantly impaired when _____ of the nephrons are not functioning appropriately.

11. Polyuric patients lose excessive amounts of water in the urine. What do polyuric patients do to compensate for this?

12. What happens when the compensatory mechanism that you identified in Question #11 (above) is inadequate?
13. What are key features on physical examination that will alert you to the fact that the compensatory mechanism in Question #11 (above) is inadequate?
14. Prior to her visit, Frita has done some research online. Her google search, "cat peeing more than normal," suggested that Dorito might have diabetes mellitus. How does diabetes mellitus contribute to polyuria?
15. Prior to her visit, Frita has done some research online. Her google search, "cat peeing more than normal," suggested that Dorito might have diabetes insipidus. How does diabetes insipidus contribute to polyuria?
16. Frita's google search also suggested that you check Dorito's calcium levels. Frita is concerned because she's been giving Dorito one cat vitamin every day. She purchased these online and wants to know if they are to blame. "I was only trying to keep him healthy," she says. "Please tell me I didn't make him sick."
    Tell Frita what causes hypercalcemia.
17. How does hypercalcemia contribute to polyuria?
18. What additional clinical signs might you expect to see in a patient with hypercalcemia?
19. Which malignant neoplasia(s) has/have been associated with hypercalcemia?
20. Other than endocrinopathies and hypercalcemia, what are additional causes of polyuria?
21. Consider the role of history-taking: what questions do you need to ask the client when taking the history of a patient who presents for presumptive polyuria and/or polydipsia?
22. After quantifying water consumption and/or polyuria, what is the next step in the diagnostic plan?

Answers to Round One of Questions for Case 21: The Cat That Is Peeing a Lot

1. The appropriate medical term for "increased thirst" is polydipsia.(1–4)

2. If thirst exceeds 45 mL/kg/day in a CAT, then it is considered excessive.(5)

3. If thirst exceeds 90 mL/kg/day in a DOG, then it is considered excessive.(5)

4. Dorito weighs 4.4 kg today. He would need to drink 4.4 kg × 45 mL/kg/day to be considered polydipsic. This amounts to 198 mL (6.7 oz; 0.84 cups).

5. The appropriate medical term for "increased urination" is polyuria.(1–4)

6. If urine output exceeds 40 mL/kg/day in a CAT, then it is considered excessive.(5)

7. If urine output exceeds 45 mL/kg/day in a DOG, then it is considered excessive.(5)

8. Dorito weighs 4.4 kg today. He would need to urinate more than 4.4 kg × 40 mL/kg/day to be considered polydipsic. This amounts to 176 mL (5.95 oz; 0.74 cups)

9. In health, thirst and urination are linked processes. If renal function is adequate, a dehydrated patient will maximally concentrate urine to conserve water and will be driven to drink.

   a. Antidiuretic hormone (ADH), otherwise known as vasopressin, is responsible for conserving water.(3, 5–12)
   b. ADH is produced by the hypothalamus.(6, 7)

    c.   When plasma osmolality increases ADH is secreted.(6, 7, 12) ADH causes water in the filtrate to be reabsorbed from the distal tubules and collecting ducts of the nephrons.(6, 7) This is achieved through the upregulation of aquaporin channels.(13) These channels allow water that would have ended up in the urine to instead return to systemic circulation.(3) Urine volume is thus reduced.(6, 7) The urine that is produced is more concentrated.(6, 7) Concentration of urine is only possible when kidneys are both functional and responsive to ADH.(3, 6)

Note that concentration of urine also requires maintenance of medullary hypertonicity.(3, 6) This concentration gradient is established and maintained by the movement of sodium, chloride, and urea out of nephrons' lumens and into the renal medullary interstitium.(14) In the absence of this gradient, osmotic forces are diminished.(14) There is less pull to draw water out of the nephron, and back into the bloodstream.(14) Urine is therefore inadequately concentrated.(14) This state is referred to as medullary washout.(6, 14)

10. The nephron is the functional unit of the kidney. Fill in the blank with a fraction:
     The kidneys' ability to concentrate urine is significantly impaired when 2/3 of the nephrons are not functioning appropriately.

11. Polyuric patients lose excessive amounts of water in the urine. To compensate for this, polyuric patients increase water intake. Their thirst rises and they drink more water. We call this compensatory polydipsia.(3)

12. At a certain point, compensatory polydipsia is inadequate. The patient cannot physically drink enough water to maintain water balance, and the patient becomes dehydrated.(15)

13. Dehydration is apparent on physical exam. Depending upon the degree to which the patient is dehydrated, you may see changes in the following physical exam features:(3, 15, 16)

- capillary refill time (CRT)
- eye position within the orbits
- heart rate (HR)
- mucous membrane moistness
- peripheral pulse quality
- skin turgor.

Five percent is the smallest percentage at which dehydration is clinically detectable.(15) A patient that is 5% dehydrated has a subtle loss in skin elasticity.(15–17)

    Six to eight percent dehydration results in a delayed return of skin to normal positioning following an attempt to tent the skin.(17) The oral mucous membranes are beginning to get dry and CRT may be slightly prolonged.(16, 17) The eyes may be positioned slightly back in the orbits as if sunken; however, this is subtle.(17)

    A patient is said to be 10–12% dehydrated when there is persistent skin tenting and the oral mucous membranes are so dry that the veterinarian's fingers stick to them.(15) At this level of dehydration, the eyes appear sunken.(15) This makes the nictitans appear prominent bilaterally. (16) CRT is definitively prolonged.(17)

    A patient that is 10–12% dehydrated may experience signs of shock.(17) These include:(17)

- tachycardia
- weak pulses
- cool extremities.

Beyond 12% dehydration, survival is unlikely.(17)

14. Diabetes mellitus is an endocrinopathy in which the patient develops hyperglycemia with subsequent glucosuria.(3, 5, 18, 19) The condition was named using the Latin word, mellitus, to reflect that the urine is honeyed or sweet.(5, 6)

This results from either insulin deficiency or insulin resistance.(3, 5, 18–20) Cells need insulin in order to be able to make use of circulating glucose in the bloodstream.(18) If insulin is deficient or if cells are resistant to its effects, then glucose is incapable of entering tissues.(18) This causes blood levels of glucose to rise.

In health, glucose that is filtered by the kidneys is reabsorbed.(20) This requires glucose to bind to transport proteins in the proximal convoluted tubules.(7) The limiting factor for glucose transport is the number of transport proteins.(7) If these become saturated, as is true of a patient that is hyperglycemic, some glucose will remain behind in the filtrate.(7, 20)

Glucose within the filtrate sets the stage for osmotic diuresis.(3) Water is drawn into the urine. (7, 20, 21) This creates large quantities of urine that is glucose-rich. Thus the patient becomes polyuric. To compensate for hypovolemia, the patient develops compensatory polydipsia.

15. Diabetes insipidus is a different kind of endocrinopathy in which the patient passes large quantities of dilute urine that contains very little, if any, glucose.(6, 11, 22) The condition was named because the urine is so dilute that it is said to be insipid, that is, tasteless.(5, 6)

There are two forms of diabetes insipidus, central and nephrogenic.(5, 6, 11, 22)

• Central diabetes insipidus (CDI) occurs when ADH is not produced or released.(5, 6, 11, 22) If the hypothalamus fails to produce ADH, then the kidneys are not directed to reabsorb water from the filtrate. Water is wasted, despite the body's need to conserve it. Hence, the urine remains dilute. In fact, it cannot be concentrated. This sets the stage for hypovolemia and compensatory polydipsia.(3)
• Nephrogenic diabetes insipidus (NDI) occurs when the body produces ADH, yet the kidneys are insensitive to it.(6, 9, 10, 23–25) Renal response may be blunted because of an inherent defect, or the kidneys may be unable to respond to ADH because of medullary washout.(6, 8–10, 26)

16. Hypercalcemia often occurs secondary to renal failure, primary hyperparathyroidism, hypoadrenocorticism (Addison's) or neoplasia.(5, 27–29) Hypercalcemia may be idiopathic.(28)

17. Different mechanisms have been proposed to explain how polyuria results from hypercalcemia, including:(28, 30–35)

• antagonism of ADH
• downregulation of aquaporin channels
• hypercalcemia-induced thirst
• impairment of the sodium-potassium pump in the loop of henle
• medullary washout.

18. Dogs with hypercalcemia are often polyuric.(5) They also frequently present to the clinic for gastrointestinal upset. Anorexia, vomiting, and constipation are common complaints.(5) Hypercalcemic cats tend to display less clinical signs than dogs.(28, 35) However, they may present for general malaise, lethargy, or weakness.(5, 35)

19. When hypercalcemia has a neoplastic origin, it is referred to as hypercalcemia of malignancy. The most common causes of hypercalcemia of malignancy in dog and cat are:(5, 27–29)

• anal sac apocrine gland adenocarcinoma
• lymphosarcoma
• multiple myeloma.

20. Other than endocrinopathies and hypercalcemia, causes of polyuria include:(5, 6, 11, 12, 14, 19–22, 27, 36–40)

- diet

  - high sodium
  - low protein

- electrolyte imbalance:

  - hypokalemia
  - hyponatremia

- encephalopathy

- Fanconi's syndrome
- hepatopathy
- infectious disease

  - pyometra – *Escherichia coli* endotoxins interfere with the nephron's ability to reabsorb sodium(41)

- medullary washout
- neoplasia
- pharmaceutical agents:

  - anticonvulsants (phenobarbital, phenytoin, primidone)
  - diuretics
  - glucocorticoids

- post-obstructive diuresis
- psychogenic polydipsia
- pyelonephritis
- urinary tract pathology

  - chronic kidney disease (CKD).

21. When a patient presents for polyuria, history-taking is a critical piece of the diagnostic puzzle. (3, 6)

    Lead with an open-ended question to allow the client to share a detailed description of what it is that s/he is noticing at home.(4, 42)

- Tell me . . .
- Share with me . . .
- Describe for me . . .

It is important that you ask the client to clarify what s/he considers to be excessive thirst or urination.(3) This is often easier to discern in dogs than cats because a dog that is peeing more is often having accidents in the home, whereas a cat that is peeing more often just makes more frequent trips to the litter box. If the client is not scooping the litter daily and/or if the client has multiple cats, then s/he may miss out on the fact that there is a urination issue.

When considering new additions to the household, such as puppies, it is important that you clarify the client's expectations.

- How long does the client feel that the pup should be able to hold its bladder?
  Compare the client's expectations with the reality of the situation:
- How long *should* a puppy of that age be able to hold its bladder.

Are the client's expectations reasonable?

Keep in mind that what is considered "normal" for the patient often varies based upon its life stage. Again, consider puppies. A 3-month-old puppy cannot typically hold its bladder overnight. It is expected that a pup of this age will have urinary accidents. In this case, urination is

THE CAT THAT IS PEEING A LOT

not excessive or inappropriate, although the client may view it as such. Rather, urinary accidents are expected if the client does not wake up in the middle of the night to take the pup outside.

On the other hand, a fully housetrained adult that has started to urinate in the house raises a red flag, particularly if frequency of urination is increased.(3)

Clients of patients that present for presumptive polyuria/polydipsia (PU/PD) should be queried about:(3, 4, 42)

- activity level
- concurrent medications
- concurrent metabolic or endocrine diseases
- dietary history
- environment:

  - indoor
  - outdoor (ambient temperature, humidity)

- thirst:

  - how much water is the patient offered per day?
  - how much water does the patient drink per day?
  - does the patient seek out unusual sources of water (e.g. bathtub, toilet bowl, pool, spa)?

- urination habits:

  - amount of urine
  - frequency of urination
  - other urinary signs:

- change in urine color – hematuria
- change in urine odor – glucosuria, pyuria
- dysuria
- hematuria
- stranguria.

It is helpful if your client can quantify water consumption.(6) This data may be compared to measurements of urine specific gravity (USG) at various points in time.(6) If the patient is drinking more than 90 mL/kg/day (dog) or 45 mL/kg/day (cat), then polydipsia is confirmed, and a work-up is indicated.(5, 6)

22. After history-taking, the next step in the diagnostic plan is to perform a thorough physical exam. (15)

Returning to Case 21: The Cat That Is Peeing a Lot

After taking a complete patient history, you perform a physical exam. You make note of the following findings:

- halitosis
- decreased skin turgor
- pallor
- caudal thigh muscle atrophy
- epaxial muscle atrophy
- bilaterally small kidneys:

  - nonpainful on palpation
  - normal contours.

319

Round Two of Questions for Case 21: The Cat That Is Peeing a Lot

1. Define halitosis.
2. Define pallor.
3. What might contribute to Dorito's physical exam finding, halitosis?
4. What might contribute to Dorito's physical exam finding, pallor?
5. On physical exam, Dorito has atrophy of the epaxials and caudal thigh muscles. What causes one or more muscle groups to atrophy?
6. Differentiate sarcopenia and cachexia.
7. Which common clinical conditions tend to cause cachexia?
8. Why do we need to address cachexia in our patients?
9. You were able to palpate Dorito's kidneys on physical exam. Where are the kidneys located within the abdomen? Is renal palpation part of the routine examination in cats or does the fact that Dorito's kidneys were palpable reflect underlying pathology?
10. You discerned that Dorito's kidneys are bilaterally small. What is the typical length of a kidney in a cat (in centimeters)?
11. After you have made a baseline assessment concerning kidney size on physical exam, how is kidney size typically confirmed?
12. What is the medical term for an enlarged kidney?
13. Which are the primary differential diagnoses that cause ENLARGED kidneys?
14. Which are the primary differential diagnoses that cause SMALL kidneys?
15. Putting it all together – Dorito's signalment, history, and physical exam findings – what is the most likely differential diagnosis? Why?
16. You need to continue your diagnostic investigation into Dorito's presenting complaint. What constitutes a minimum database when testing for causes of polyuria and polydipsia (PU/PD)?
17. Which clinicopathologic findings will support your suspicion that Dorito does in fact have the condition that you identified in Question #15 (above)?

Answers to Round Two of Questions for Case 21: The Cat That Is Peeing a Lot

1. Halitosis is the medical term for bad breath.(1, 3, 5)

2. Pallor refers to generalized paleness.(3) In human patients, pallor may be used to describe unusual lightness of the skin as compared to one's normal complexion. Patients with pallor may look "ghost white" as if all the color has been drained from one's face. Pallor is the opposite of appearing flushed.

   By contrast, in veterinary medicine, pallor typically refers to paleness of mucous membranes because most of our companion animal species and breeds have skin that is covered with fur.(3) Mucous membranes are epithelial linings of body cavities and organ surfaces.(43, 44) Mucous membranes that are examined routinely in cats and dogs are the gums.(45–47) In health, non-pigmented gingiva should appear pink.(46–50) Some patients have naturally pigmented gums, mottled or black.(47) These pigments make it challenging to use mucous membranes as indicators of general wellness.(47) In these situations, it is easier to examine alternate mucous membranes, such as the vulva and the prepuce.(45–47, 51)

3. Periodontal disease is the most common cause of halitosis.(1, 5) Other causes include:(1, 5, 52–65)

   - abnormal ingestive behavior or pica, as occurs with coprophagy
   - extra-oral factors:

- dirty or wet "beards" of dogs with abundant facial fur
- gastrointestinal obstruction (foreign body, neoplasia, stricture)
- hepatopathy
- inflammatory bowel disease (IBD)
- lip fold dermatitis
- megaesophagus
- metabolic dysfunction:

    - ketones in diabetic ketoacidosis (DKA)
    - uremia due to renal disease

- rhinitis
- sinusitis
- small intestinal bacterial overgrowth (SIBO).

- oral factors

    - abscess (soft tissue, tooth root)
    - cleft palate
    - malocclusion, causing food material to be trapped between teeth
    - neoplasia and associated tissue necrosis
    - oro-nasal fistula
    - pathologic bleeding, hemorrhage, as is associated with coagulopathy or oral tumors
    - physiologic bleeding associated with teething
    - retained teeth, causing overcrowding with food material trapped between teeth
    - stomatitis.

4. Pale mucous membranes typically result from either anemia or vasoconstriction.(47, 66)
   Anemia refers to a state in which the blood contains fewer red blood cells than normal, or those red blood cells contain subnormal levels of hemoglobin.(3)
   Broadly, anemia results from one of three pathways.(3, 47, 66, 67)

- The bone marrow does not produce enough erythrocytes.
- Excessive numbers of erythrocytes are lost as hemorrhage.
- Too many erythrocytes are destroyed, as from immune-mediated disease.

Vasoconstriction is the process by which vessel walls contract to narrow their lumens.(3) In particular, this affects arteries and arterioles.(68) Vasoconstriction is often a physiologic response to an assault on the body's homeostasis, such as shock or hypothermia.(3) The purpose of vasoconstriction as a reaction to shock is to raise systemic BP.(3) The purpose of vasoconstriction as a reaction to hypothermia is to shunt blood away from the extremities to retain heat at the body's core.(69)
   Anemic or vasoconstricted patients both are likely to present with pale mucous membranes.

5. Muscle atrophy can result from:(3, 15)

- age
- malnutrition
- neoplasia
- neurologic dysfunction at the level of the spinal cord or peripheral nerve – muscles that are capable of movement do not activate because they no longer receive the appropriate signals from nerves
- orthopedic injury that limits physical activity.

6. Both sarcopenia and cachexia refer to loss of lean body mass.(3, 15) They differ as to what causes it.(3, 15) Sarcopenia is age-related muscle atrophy.(3, 15) Cachexia refers to loss of muscle mass due to disease.(70)

7. Common diseases that cause patients to become cachexic include:(70)

   - CKD
   - congestive heart failure
   - neoplasia.

8. Cachexia is associated with increased rates of morbidity and mortality in both people(70–73) and veterinary patients.(74–76) It is critical that clinicians detect loss of lean muscle mass early in disease processes because early interventions may improve both quality and quantity of life.(15)

9. The kidneys are in the retroperitoneal space, ventral to the sublumbar muscles.(15) The right kidney is cranial to the left.(15) The right kidney sits opposite the first three lumbar vertebrae compared to the left kidney, which spans the second through fifth.(15) The right kidney is cupped cranially by the caudate process of the liver.(15)

   Both kidneys are much more mobile in cats as compared to dogs.(15) Both kidneys should be palpable in cats on routine physical examination.(77–79)

10. Normal kidney length in cats varies between 3.8–4.4 cm, but can reach as long as 5.3 cm (80–84).

11. After you have ballparked kidney size on physical exam, abdominal imaging is a useful tool to confirm renal length with improved accuracy than one's fingertips.(15) Size measurements can be taken from radiographs or ultrasonographic studies.(3, 15, 82, 85) When evaluated on radiographs, the kidneys are compared to the length of the second lumbar vertebra to establish the patient's renal length ratio.(77) Depending upon which study is referenced, normal renal length ratios in the cat have been cited as 2.0–3.0.(81, 85–88)

    More recently, abdominal ultrasonography has become a preferred imaging modality because in addition to confirming renal length, it can provide information about renal architecture.(80, 89, 90)

12. Renomegaly is the appropriate medical term for an enlarged kidney.(3, 15, 91)

13. Renomegaly is often the sign of pathology, including, but not limited to:(3, 15, 92, 93)

    - acute kidney injury (AKI), otherwise known as acute renal failure (ARF):

        - often linked to toxins – ethylene glycol, grapes and raisins (some dogs), heavy metals, lily toxicosis (cats) (93)
        - also seen in certain types of infectious disease – leptospirosis, Lyme nephritis, Rocky Mountain spotted fever (RMSF) (93)

    - other causes include:(93–99)

• anaphylaxis	• hydronephrosis
• heatstroke	• infarcts
• sepsis	• polycystic kidney disease (PKD)
• severe dehydration	• pyelonephritis
• severe hypotension	• renal neoplasia
• amyloidosis	• ureteral obstruction.

    Larger than normal kidney size also appears to be linked in cats to sexual status.(3, 15) Testosterone stimulates renal hypertrophy.(100, 101) Therefore, intact tomcats have a larger renal length ratio of 2.1–3.2 as compared to 1.9–2.6 in neutered males.(86, 100, 102, 103)

14. CKD is the most common cause of bilaterally small kidneys.(92, 104, 105)

15. Putting it all together – the patient's signalment, history, and physical exam findings – Dorito most likely has CKD.

CKD is a common condition in older cats.(3, 15, 104, 105)

The patient's history is consistent with PU/PD, as caused by CKD:

- increased thirst
- increased urination frequency
- increased urine volume.

Decreased appetite and vomiting are non-specific, but supportive of CKD.(3) In cases of CKD, these clinical signs result from the accumulation of uremic toxins.(91, 104, 106) Uremic toxins are compounds that ordinarily would be filtered and excreted by the kidneys. Cats with CKD have dysfunctional kidneys, so these compounds build up in the bloodstream. In addition, renal dysfunction causes gastrin excretion by the kidney to be reduced. The resultant hypergastrinemia causes gastric pH to drop.(104) This promotes upper gastrointestinal acidity, which can contribute to nausea and gastric ulceration.(104) These in turn suppress appetite.(104)

The patient's physical exam findings can also be explained by CKD.

- Recall that CKD is the most common cause of bilaterally small kidneys.(92, 104, 105)
- Halitosis results from uremic toxins. Halitosis may also result from gastric bleeding and/or bleeding associated with oral ulcers.
- Decreased skin turgor reflects clinical dehydration, which results from the patient's PU/PD status.
- In cases of CKD, pallor is caused by anemia, which is due to impaired renal production of erythropoietin. Erythropoietin is essential because it stimulates the bone marrow to produce new erythrocytes. When erythropoietin concentrations are sub-normal, red blood cell populations are not replenished at the anticipated rate. Affected patients become anemic. The anemia is non-regenerative because the key stimulator of bone marrow, erythropoietin, is not present.
- Caudal thigh and epaxial muscle atrophy most probably reflect a combination of sarcopenia and cachexia in cats with CKD. As CKD progresses, proteinuria increases. Protein loss in the urine means that less protein is retained by the body and available for use as building blocks to repair and regenerate muscle.

16. A minimum database for a diagnostic work-up of polyuria and polydipsia typically includes:(3, 6, 14)
    - complete blood count (CBC)
    - serum biochemistry profile
    - urinalysis.

17. Based upon my presumptive diagnosis, CKD, I would expect to see the following clinicopathologic findings in Dorito's diagnostic work-up:(91, 104, 105)

    - blood pressure (BP) – many CKD patients are hypertensive(104)
    - CBC – nonregenerative anemia
    - Serum biochemistry profile:

        - azotemia:

            - elevated blood urea nitrogen (BUN)
            - elevated creatinine

        - +/– hyperphosphatemia
        - +/– hypocalcemia
        - +/– hypokalemia

- urinalysis:

  - active urine sediment
  - inappropriately dilute urine
  - +/– proteinuria
  - +/– concurrent UTI.

Returning to Case 21: The Cat That Is Peeing a Lot

You convince Frita to proceed with a minimum database that includes a CBC, chemistry profile, and urinalysis. Dorito's results are as follows:

- CBC – moderate anemia
- chemistry profile – azotemia, hyperphosphatemia, hypokalemia
- urinalysis – USG 1.015.

Round Three of Questions for Case 21: The Cat That Is Peeing a Lot

1. Frita wants to know what USG measures. What do you tell her?
2. How is USG measured in clinical practice?
3. Which patient-specific factors influence USG?
4. Which value(s) for USG is/are considered normal in a dog versus a cat?
5. How does Dorito's USG compare with that which is considered normal?
6. Are Dorito's test results consistent with your presumptive diagnosis?
7. Which additional test(s) do you need to run and why?
8. Which organization guides staging of Dorito's condition?
9. Treatment for this condition is multifactorial, but largely depends upon staging. What does staging this condition involve?
10. Treatment for this presumptive condition is multifactorial. Outline your proposed treatment plan (in broad terms, i.e. no doses of medications are necessary).

Answers to Round Three of Questions for Case 21: The Cat That Is Peeing a Lot

1. USG is a measure of how concentrated the urine is.(3) How concentrated the urine is tells us about the function of the kidneys.(3) As kidneys become dysfunctional, they progressively lose the ability to concentrate the urine and the urine becomes increasingly dilute.

2. USG is measured in clinical practice using a refractometer. The refractometer compares the density of the urine against the density of pure water (1.00).

3. Proteinuria and glycosuria increase USG. Therefore, the actual USG for a patient that spills a significant amount of protein and/or glucose into its urine will be lower than what the refractometer reports.

4. In health, USG varies widely depending upon several factors, including hydration status and water intake.(107) The expected range for most dogs is 1.015–1.045; the expected range for most cats is 1.035–1.060.(107) When urine falls below the low end of this revised normal range for each of the two species, it is said to be dilute.(107)

5. Dorito's USG is below normal.

6. Yes, Dorito's test results are consistent with a diagnosis of CKD.

7. Many patients with CKD are hypertensive, so I would want to measure Dorito's BP.(104)
   I would also recommend that Dorito's urine be cultured. This diagnostic test is essential when urine is dilute because bacteria may be present in such low numbers that it is missed on routine urinalysis.(37)
   Cats like Dorito, with CKD, are at increased risk of developing UTIs.(108) Having dilute urine in fact predisposes them to infection.(108) Recall that urine concentration is an inherent defense mechanism against UTI.(109–113) Without high levels of urea and organic acid, bacteria are undeterred and are more likely to take up residence.

8. Guidance with regards to staging of CKD is provided by the International Renal Interest Society (IRIS).(104, 106)

9. Staging of CKD is based upon the following factors:(104, 106)

   • serum or plasma creatinine concentration
   • urine protein to creatinine ratios (UPCs).

   Substages are determined based upon whether the patient is proteinuric and/or hypertensive. (104, 106)

10. Treatment is multifactorial and aims to address the following:(91, 104, 106)

    • blood pH – CKD is associated with metabolic acidosis
    • electrolytes – CKD is often associated with hypokalemia and hyperphosphatemia
    • hydration – CKD is often associated with dehydration
    • nutrition – CKD is often associated with decreased appetite and vomiting.

CLINICAL PEARLS

• Polyuria with compensatory polydipsia (PU/PD) is a common clinical presentation. In companion animal practice, it may result from the following:

  • altered electrolytes, i.e. hypercalcemia, hyponatremia, hypokalemia
  • CKD
  • diabetes insipidus
  • diabetes mellitus
  • diet
  • hyperadrenocorticism
  • infectious disease
  • pharmaceutical agents.

• Cats that drink more than 45 mL/kg/day and produce more than 40 mL/kg/day of urine are PU/PD.

• Dogs that drink more than 90 mL/kg/day and produce more than 45 mL/kg/day of urine are PU/PD.

• It is difficult for owners to quantify thirst and urine production, particularly in cats.

- At a certain point, polyuric patients cannot possibly drink enough water to maintain their hydration status. At this point, they become dehydrated.

  - Dehydration can be clinically detected at 5%.
  - Patients that are 6–8% dehydrated have reduced skin turgor, somewhat dry mucous membranes, and a potentially sluggish CRT.
  - Patients that are 10–12% dehydrated have a skin tent that persists, and mucous membranes are tacky. Both eyes will appear sunken into their respective orbit. This makes both nictitating membranes prominent.

- Because so many different conditions are associated with PU/PD, history-taking and physical examination are essential diagnostic tools to narrow down your list of top differentials.

- A diagnosis of CKD can be made based upon history, physical exam findings, CBC, chemistry profile and urinalysis (UA).

- Staging of CKD is done based upon guidelines from the IRIS.

- Staging facilitates treatment planning, which is multifactorial and addresses dehydration, metabolic acidosis, hypokalemia, hyperphosphatemia, and nutrition.

References

1. Côté E. Clinical veterinary advisor. Dogs and cats. 3rd ed. St. Louis, MO: Elsevier Mosby; 2015.
2. Ettinger SJ, Feldman EC, Côté E. Textbook of veterinary internal medicine: diseases of the dog and the cat. 8th ed. St. Louis, MO: Elsevier; 2017.
3. Englar RE. Common clinical presentations in dogs and cats. Hoboken, NJ: Wiley/Blackwell; 2019.
4. Englar R. Writing skills for veterinarians. Sheffield: 5M Publishing; 2019.
5. Tilley LP, Smith FWK. The 5-minute veterinary consult: Canine and feline. 3rd ed. Baltimore, MD: Lippincott Williams & Wilkins; 2004.
6. Nichols R. Polyuria and polydipsia – diagnostic approach and problems associated with patient evaluation. Vet Clin N Am Small 2001;31(5):833
7. Reece WO. Kidney function in mammals. In: Dukes HH, Reece WO, editors. Dukes' physiology of domestic animals. 12th ed. Ithaca, NY: Comstock Pub. Associates; 2004. p. 73–106.
8. DiBartola SP. Disorders of sodium and water: Hypernatremia and hyponatremia. In: DiBartola SP, editor. Fluid therapy in small animal practice. Philadelphia, PA: W.B. Saunders; 1992.
9. Feldman EC, Melson RW. Water metabolism and diabetes insipidus. In: Feldman EC, Melson RW, editors. Canine and feline endocrinology and reproduction. Philadelphia, PA: W.B. Saunders; 1996.
10. Hardy RM. Disorders of water metabolism. Vet Clin North Am Small Anim Pract 1982;12(3):353–73.
11. Verbalis JG. Disorders of water metabolism. In: Hall JE, Nieman LK, editors. Contemporary endocrinology: handbook of diagnostic endocrinology. Totowa, NJ: Humana Press Inc.; 2003. p. 23–53.
12. Marks SL, Taboada J. Hypernatremia and hypertonic syndromes. Vet Clin North Am Small Anim Pract 1998;28(3):533–43.
13. Agarwal SK, Gupta A. Aquaporins: the renal water channels. Indian J Nephrol 2008;18(3):95–100.
14. Schoeman JP, editor. Approach to polyuria and polydipsia in the dog. Proceedings of the 33rd world small animal veterinary congress; 2008; Dublin, Ireland. World Small Animal Veterinary Association (WSAVA).
15. Englar RE. Performing the small animal physical examination. Hoboken, NJ: Wiley/Blackwell; 2017.
16. DiBartola SP, Bateman S. Introduction to fluid therapy. In: DiBartola SP, editor. Fluid, electrolyte, and acid–base disorders in small animal practice. 3rd ed. St. Louis, MO: Saunders/Elsevier; 2006. p. 325–44.
17. DiBartola SP, Bateman S. Introduction to fluid therapy. In: DiBartola SP, editor. Fluid, electrolyte, and acid–base disorders in small animal practice. 3rd ed. St. Louis, MO: Saunders/Elsevier; 2006.

18. Goff JP. Disorders of carbohydrate and fat metabolism. In: Dukes HH, Reece WO, editors. Dukes' physiology of domestic animals. 12th ed. Ithaca, NY: Comstock Pub. Associates; 2004.

19. Reusch CE. Feline diabetes mellitus. In: Feldman EC, Nelson RW, Reusch C, Scott-Moncrieff JCR, editors. Canine and feline endocrinology. 4th ed. St. Louis, MO: Elsevier Saunders; 2015. p. 258–314.

20. Feldman EC, Nelson RW. Diagnostic approach to polydipsia and polyuria. Vet Clin North Am Small Anim Pract 1989;19(2):327–41.

21. Gordon J. Clinical approach to polyuria (Proceedings). DVM 360 [Internet]; 2011. Available from: http://veterinarycalendar.dvm360.com/clinical-approach-polyuria-proceedings-0.

22. Leroy C, Karrouz W, Douillard C, Do Cao C, Cortet C, Wémeau JL, Vantyghem MC. Diabetes insipidus. Ann Endocrinol (Paris) 2013;74(5–6):496–507.

23. Breitschwerdt EB. Clinical abnormalities of urine concentration and dilution. Compend Contin Educ Pract Vet 1981;3:412–4.

24. Robertson GL. Differential diagnosis of polyuria. Annu Rev Med 1988;39:425–42.

25. Swartz-Porsche D. Diabetes insipidus. In: Kirk RW, editor. Current veterinary therapy VII. Philadelphia, PA: W.B. Saunders; 1980. p. 1005–11.

26. Barsanti JA, DiBartola SP, Finco DR. Diagnostic approach to polyuria and polydipsia. In: Bonagura JD, editor. Kirk's current veterinary therapy. Philadelphia, PA: W.B. Saunders; 2000. p. 831–5.

27. Cone F. Polyuria, polydipsia, and hypercalcemia. NAVC Clin's Brief 2009 (June);46.

28. Cook AK. Guidelines for evaluating hypercalcemic cats. DVM 360 [Internet]; 2008. Available from: http://veterinarymedicine.dvm360.com/guidelines-evaluating-hypercalcemic-cats.

29. Savary KC, Price GS, Vaden SL. Hypercalcemia in cats: a retrospective study of 71 cases (1991–1997). J Vet Intern Med 2000;14(2):184–9.

30. Levi M, Peterson L, Berl T. Mechanism of concentrating defect in hypercalcemia. Role of polydipsia and prostaglandins. Kidney Int 1983;23(3):489–97.

31. Suki WN, Eknoyan G, Rector FC, Jr., Seldin DW. The renal diluting and concentrating mechanism in hypercalcemia. Nephron 1969;6(1):50–61.

32. Vanherweghem JL, Ducobu J, d'Hollander A, Toussaint C. Effects of hypercalcemia on water and sodium excretion by the isolated dog kidney. Pflug Arch 1976;363(1):75–80.

33. Brunette MG, Vary J, Carrière S. Hyposthenuria in hypercalcemia. A possible role of intrarenal blood-flow (IRBF) redistribution. Pflug Arch 1974;350(1):9–23.

34. Goldfarb S, Agus ZS. Mechanism of the polyuria of hypercalcemia. Am J Nephrol 1984;4(2):69–76.

35. Schenck PA, Chew DJ, Behrend EN. Update on hypercalcemic disorders. In: August J, editor. Consultations in feline internal medicine. St. Louis, MO: Elsevier; 2005. p. 157–68.

36. Osborne CA. The ins and outs of polyuria and polydipsia. DVM 360 [Internet]; 2003. Available from: http://veterinarynews.dvm360.com/ins-and-outs-polyuria-and-polydipsia.

37. Behrend EN, editor. Diagnosis of polyuria/polydipsia: Case-based approach. Proceedings of the north American veterinary conference (NAVC); 2005; Orlando, FL.

38. Nolan B, Labato MA. Polyuria and polydipsia in a dog. NAVC Clin's Brief 2013 (November):66–9.

39. de Brito Galvão JF, Parker V, Schenck PA, Chew DJ. Update on feline ionized hypercalcemia. Vet Clin North Am Small Anim Pract 2017;47(2):273–92.

40. de Brito Galvão JF, Schenck PA, Chew DJ. A quick reference on hypercalcemia. Vet Clin North Am Small Anim Pract 2017;47(2):241–8.

41. Bruyette DS. Diagnostic approach to polyuria and polydipsia. DVM 360 [Internet]; 2008. Available from: http://veterinarycalendar.dvm360.com/diagnostic-approach-polyuria-and-polydipsia-proceedings-0.

42. Englar R. A guide to. Oral Communication in Veterinary Medicine. Sheffield: 5M Publishing; 2020.

43. Evans HE, Miller ME. Miller's anatomy of the dog. 4th ed. St. Louis, MO: Elsevier; 2013.

44. Singh B, Dyce KM. Dyce, Sack, and Wensing's textbook of veterinary anatomy. 5th ed. St. Louis, MO: Saunders; 2018.

45. Rozanski E. Quiz: Mucous membrane evaluation in dogs. NAVC Clin's Brief 2017 (August).

46. Rudolph LW. Assessing patient hydration. Vet Team Brief 2016 (August):18–22.

47. Englar RE. Performing the small animal physical examination. Hoboken, NJ: Wiley; 2017. pages cm p.

48. Rudloff E. Assessment of hydration. In: Crit Care Med Silverstein DC, Hopper K, editors. Small Animal. St. Louis, MO: Elsevier 2015:307–10.
49. Donohoe C. Fluid therapy. In: Battaglia A, Steele A, editors. Small animal emergency and critical care for veterinary technicians. St. Louis, MO: Elsevier; 2016. p. 61–77.
50. Boag A, Hughes D. Fluid therapy. In: King LG, Boag A, editors. BSAVA manual of canine and feline emergency and critical care. Gloucester: BSAVA; 2007. p. 30–45.
51. Cave C. High dependency nursing. In: Aspinall V, editor. The complete textbook of veterinary nursing. St. Louis, MO: Elsevier; 2011. p. 421–38.
52. Bellows J. Halitosis. NAVC Clin's Brief 2012 (April):24–5.
53. Tabor B. Understanding and treating diabetic ketoacidosis. Vet Tech 2008;29(4). Available from: http://www.vetfolio.com/internal-medicine/understanding-and-treating-diabetic-ketoacidosis.
54. Sherding RG. Regurgitation, dysphagia, and esophageal dysmotility. DVM 360 [Internet]; 2011. Available from: http://veterinarycalendar.dvm360.com/regurgitation-dysphagia-and-esophageal-dysmotility-proceedings.
55. Mace S, Shelton GD, Eddlestone S. Megaesophagus. Compend Contin Educ Vet 2012;34(2):E1.
56. Eubanks DL. Canine oral malodor. J Am Anim Hosp Assoc 2006;42(1):77–9.
57. Eubanks DL. 'Doggy breath': What causes it, how do I evaluate it, and what can I do about it? J Vet Dent 2009;26(3):192–3.
58. Ehrhart N. Common oral tumors in dogs and cats. NAVC Clin's Brief 2013 (January).
59. Perrone JR. Top 5 feline Oral Health concerns. Vet Team Brief 2016 (January/February).
60. Reiter A. Oral inflammatory and ulcerative disease in small animals. Merck veterinary manual [Internet]. Available from: https://www.merckvetmanual.com/digestive-system/diseases-of-the-mouth-in-small-animals/oral-inflammatory-and-ulcerative-disease-in-small-animals.
61. Pellin M, Turek M. A review of feline oral squamous cell carcinoma. Today's Vet Pract 2016 (November/December):24–33.
62. Bilgic O, Duda L, Sánchez MD, Lewis JR. Feline oral squamous cell carcinoma: Clinical manifestations and literature review. J Vet Dent 2015;32(1):30–40.
63. Garrett LD, Marretta SM. Feline oral squamous cell carcinoma: An overview. DVM 360 [Internet]; 2007. Available from: http://veterinarymedicine.dvm360.com/feline-oral-squamous-cell-carcinoma-overview.
64. Soltero-Rivera MM, Krick EL, Reiter AM, Brown DC, Lewis JR. Prevalence of regional and distant metastasis in cats with advanced oral squamous cell carcinoma: 49 Cases (2005–2011). J Feline Med Surg 2014;16(2):164–9.
65. Oral cavity tumors. Available from: https://www2.vet.cornell.edu/departments-centers-and-institutes/cornell-feline-health-center/health-information/feline-health-topics/oral-cavity-tumors.
66. Campbell VL. Critical care triage. DVM 360 [Internet]; 2011. Available from: http://veterinarycalendar.dvm360.com/critical-care-triage-proceedings.
67. Harvey JW. What type of anemia? NAVC Clin's Brief 2010 (April):34–8.
68. Pachtinger GE. Hypovolemic shock. NAVC Clin's Brief 2014 (October):13–6.
69. Reuss-Lamky H. Hypothermia overview. NAVC Clin's Brief 2015 (November):12–6.
70. Freeman LM. Cachexia and sarcopenia: Emerging syndromes of importance in dogs and cats. J Vet Intern Med 2012;26(1):3–17.
71. Anker SD, Ponikowski P, Varney S, Chua TP, Clark AL, Webb-Peploe KM, et al. Wasting as independent risk factor for mortality in chronic heart failure. Lancet 1997;349(9058):1050–3.
72. Anker SD, Negassa A, Coats AJ, Afzal R, Poole-Wilson PA, Cohn JN, Yusuf S. Prognostic importance of weight loss in chronic heart failure and the effect of treatment with angiotensin-converting-enzyme inhibitors: an observational study. Lancet 2003;361(9363):1077–83.
73. Freeman LM, Roubenoff R. The nutrition implications of cardiac cachexia. Nutr Rev 1994;52(10):340–7.
74. Baez JL, Michel KE, Sorenmo K, Shofer FS. A prospective investigation of the prevalence and prognostic significance of weight loss and changes in body condition in feline cancer patients. J Feline Med Surg 2007;9(5):411–7.
75. Scarlett JM, Donoghue S. Associations between body condition and disease in cats. J Am Vet Med Assoc 1998;212(11):1725–31.
76. Doria-Rose VP, Scarlett JM. Mortality rates and causes of death among emaciated cats. J Am Vet Med Assoc 2000;216(3):347–51.

77. Scherk M. The upper urinary tract. In: Little SE, editor. The cat: Clinical medicine and management. St. Louis, MO: Saunders Elsevier; 2012.

78. van Dongen AM, L'Eplattenier HF. Kidneys and urinary tract. In: Rijnberk A, van Sluijs FJ, editors. Medical history and physical examination in companion animals. 2nd ed. St. Louis, MO: Saunders Elsevier; 2009.

79. Dyce KM, Sack WO, Wensing CJG. Textbook of veterinary anatomy. 2nd ed. Philadelphia, PA: Saunders; 1996.

80. Debruyn K, Paepe D, Daminet S, Combes A, Duchateau L, Peremans K, Saunders JH. Renal dimensions at ultrasonography in healthy Ragdoll cats with normal kidney morphology: Correlation with age, gender and bodyweight. J Feline Med Surg 2013;15(12):1046–51.

81. Walter PA, Feeney DA, Johnston GR, Fletcher TF. Feline renal ultrasonography: Quantitative analyses of imaged anatomy. Am J Vet Res 1987;48(4):596–9.

82. Barrett RB, Kneller SK. Feline kidney mensuration. Acta Radiol Suppl 1972;319:279–80.

83. Yeager AE, Anderson WI. Study of association between histologic features and echogenicity of architecturally normal cat kidneys. Am J Vet Res 1989;50(6):860–3.

84. Park IC, Lee HS, Kim JT, Nam SJ, Choi R, Oh KS, et al. Ultrasonographic evaluation of renal dimension and resistive index in clinically healthy Korean domestic short-hair cats. J Vet Sci 2008;9(4):415–9.

85. Lee R, Leowijuk C. Normal parameters in abdominal radiology of the dog and cat. J Small Anim Pract 1982;23(5):251–69.

86. Shiroma JT, Gabriel JK, Carter RL, Scruggs SL, Stubbs PW. Effect of reproductive status on feline renal size. Vet Radiol Ultrasound 1999;40(3):242–5.

87. Owens J. The genitourinary system. In: Biery D, editor. Radiographic interpretation for the small animal clinician. St. Louis, MO: Ralston Purina Co.; 1982. p. 175.

88. Biery D. Upper urinary tract. In: O'Brien T, editor. Radiographic diagnosis of abdominal disorders in the dog and cat. Davis, CO: Covel Park Vet; 1981. p. 484–5.

89. Walter PA, Feeney DA, Johnston GR, Fletcher TF. Feline renal ultrasonography – Quantitative-analyses of imaged anatomy. Am J Vet Res 1987;48(4):596–9.

90. Barr FJ. Evaluation of ultrasound as a method of assessing renal size in the dog. J Small Anim Pract 1990;31(4):174–9.

91. Tilley LP, Smith FWK. The 5-minute veterinary consult: Canine and feline. 3rd ed. Baltimore, MD: Lippincott Williams & Wilkins; 2004.

92. Gough A, Murphy KF Chichester, ed. Differential diagnosis in small animal medicine. 2nd ed. Ames, IA: John Wiley & Sons Inc.; 2015.

93. Balakrishnan A, Drobatz KJ. Management of urinary tract emergencies in small animals. Vet Clin North Am Small Anim Pract 2013;43(4):843–67.

94. Greco DS. Feline acromegaly. Top Companion Anim Med 2012;27(1):31–5.

95. Powell LL. Canine heatstroke. NAVC Clin's Brief 2008 (August):13–6.

96. Sullivant A, Archer T. Anuric renal and hepatic failure in a dog. NAVC Clin's Brief 2016 (August):68–72.

97. Smith KR. Easter lily toxicosis. NAVC Clin's Brief 2006(March):81–2.

98. Linklater A. Human medication intoxications. NAVC Clin's Brief 2013 (May):69–73.

99. Harkin KR. Canine leptospirosis. NAVC Clin's Brief 2005 (June):15–9.

100. Selye H. The effect of testosterone on the kidney. J Urol 1939;42(4):637–41.

101. Jean-Faucher C, Berger M, Gallon C, de Turckheim M, Veyssière G, Jean C. Sex-related differences in renal size in mice: Ontogeny and influence of neonatal androgens. J Endocrinol 1987;115(2):241–6.

102. Huang KC, McIntosh BJ. Effect of sex hormones on renal transport of p-aminohippuric acid. Am J Physiol 1955;183(3):387–90.

103. Freudenberger CB, Howard PM. Effects of ovariectomy on body growth and organ weights of the young albino rat. Proc Soc Exp Biol Med 1937;36(2):144–8.

104. Bartges JW. Chronic kidney disease in dogs and cats. Vet Clin North Am Small Anim Pract 2012;42(4): 669–92.

105. Langston CE, Eatroff AE. Chronic kidney disease. In: Silverstein DC, Hopper K, editors. Small animal critical care medicine. St. Louis, MO: Saunders/Elsevier; 2015. p. 661–6.

106. Polzin DJ. Chronic kidney disease in small animals. Vet Clin North Am Small Anim Pract 2011;41(1):15–30.

107. (IRIS) Iris. Urine specific gravity. 1.035 to 1.060 for cats; 2019. Available from: http://www.iris-kidney.com/education/urine_specific_gravity.html#:~:text=What%20USG%20values%20are%20considered.

108. Filippich LJ. Cat with urinary tract signs. In: Rand J, editor. Problem-based feline medicine. New York: Saunders; 2006. p. 173–92.

109. Litster A, Thompson M, Moss S, Trott D. Feline bacterial urinary tract infections: An update on an evolving clinical problem. Vet J 2011;187(1):18–22.

110. Blanco LJ, Bartges JW. Understanding and eradicating bacterial urinary tract infections. Vetmed-US 2001;96(10):776.

111. Bartges JW. Bacterial urinary tract infections – Simple and complicated. Vetmed-US 2005;100(3):224–+.

112. Bartges J, Burns KM. Lower urinary tract signs in a cat. NAVC Clin's Brief 2017 (September):35–9.

113. Lees GE, Rogers KS. Treatment of urinary tract infections in dogs and cats. J Am Vet Med Assoc 1986;189(6):648–52.

Case 22

The Dog That Is Straining to Defecate

Owen may have been a part of your practice since he was a pup, but he's been in Emmett Parker's life since the day he was born. Owen was the biggest of six pups from the first and only litter that Emmett had planned. Emmett didn't fancy himself to be a dog breeder. The only reason he'd bred Owen's mom, Tess, was because she was the best hunter he had ever owned, and he was reluctant to lose that genetic line when she passed.

Owen was the spitting image of Tess and took after her in every way. When he wasn't treeing raccoons, he was off exploring the five-acre property that he and Emmett called home. The property backed up to a reservoir, and between swimming and racing through the woods, there was never a shortage of something to do. Emmett and Owen often took weekend getaways. Owen never tired of the chase, but these days, Emmett hunted for sport far less than he used to. While Owen

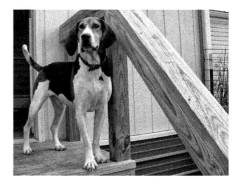

Figure 22.1 Meet your new patient, Owen, an 8-year-old intact male Treeing Coonhound dog. Courtesy of Jayne Regan.

was off catching the latest scent trail, Emmett was invested in his own pursuit: getting married. Over the years, he had chased a handful of women. None were keepers. Then Chelsea came along. Chelsea was adventurous and daring and fond of the outdoors. All their hobbies aligned, except, of course, for hunting. The longer Chelsea remained in his life, the less Emmett worked Owen and the more Owen was left to his own devices.

You had met Chelsea at Owen's last visit and had congratulated her and Emmett on their recent engagement. At that visit Emmett had shared that he'd be doing a lot more traveling in the coming months on account of work, leaving Chelsea in charge of Owen's healthcare.

Chelsea is here today, presenting Owen for evaluation of a 2-day history of straining to defecate. When Emmett departed last weekend for an international business trip, Owen was fine. Shortly after, he developed an urgency to go outside. At first Chelsea chalked it up to him being stir crazy without Emmett. At times, the two seemed glued at the hip. It wasn't until Chelsea witnessed Owen's protracted attempts at unproductive squatting that she grew concerned. The more he tried to defecate, the more frantic he seemed to be about having to go. He would circle and circle and squat, only to repeat the process. At one point, he yelped. That's when Chelsea knew Owen needed your help.

Your technician takes Owen's vital signs and documents them into his medical record before loading Chelsea and Owen into the next available consultation room.

Weight: 78.5 lb (35.7 kg)
BCS: 6/9
Mentation: BAR

TPR

T: 101.6°F (38.7°C)
P: 100 beats per minute
R: panting

As Chelsea waits for you to enter to initiate the consultation, she googles Owen's symptoms out of desperation, wondering what they could possibly mean.

Round One of Questions for Case 22: The Dog That Is Straining to Defecate

1. Which noun is the appropriate medical term to describe a patient's difficulty with defecating?
2. Which noun is the appropriate medical term to describe straining to defecate?
3. Based upon the patient history, it is evident that Owen is exhibiting both difficulty defecating and straining to produce stool. Which additional questions would you like to ask Chelsea to better understand the patient's clinical presentation?
4. After taking a comprehensive patient history, you ask Chelsea what concerns her most about Owen. She shares what she read online: "Male dogs that strain to produce stool have enlarged prostates." "If that's the case," she says, "then can't we just neuter him?"

   - Which condition is she referring to?
   - What causes this condition?
   - What is the link between this condition and difficulty defecating?
   - How do you confirm this condition in the dog?
   - Does neutering resolve this issue?

5. Chelsea is particularly interested in neutering Owen because "He is marking everywhere, even in the house. Emmett overlooks it, but I live there now, too, and I just can't."
   Will neutering Owen resolve his marking behavior?
6. You reassure Chelsea that you will evaluate Owen's prostate; however, there are other conditions that you need to consider. Aside from prostatomegaly, what can contribute to constipation in dogs?
7. In addition to what you outlined in Question #6 (above), are there any additional conditions that could contribute to constipation in cats?
8. After taking a comprehensive patient history, what is the next step in the diagnostic plan?

Answers to Round One of Questions for Case 22: The Dog That Is Straining to Defecate

1. Dyschezia is the appropriate medical term to describe a patient's difficulty defecating.(1, 2)

2. Tenesmus is the appropriate medical term to describe straining to defecate.(1, 2)

3. Based upon the patient history, it is evident that Owen is exhibiting both difficulty defecating and straining to produce stool. You might want to ask Chelsea about the following content areas to better understand Owen's clinical presentation.

   - Open-ended statements, such as "Describe your patient's bowel habits," provide an expanded opportunity for Chelsea to share her observations with you.(3) Although she provided an abbreviated history in response to the technician's query, she may not have shared all the essential details with you. She may not have known precisely what kind of information would be helpful, so you will likely need to ask follow-up clarifying questions to extract those details from Chelsea's description.
   - Have these episodes ever happened before?
   - How long do these episodes go on?

- How often do these episodes recur?
- What, if anything, is produced when Owen appears to be straining?

  - Is any stool at all passed?
  - What does the stool look like?
  - What is the stool's shape and has it changed? (Dogs with prostate disease often develop ribbon-like stools.)
  - Is the stool coated with mucous?
  - Is the stool coated with fresh red blood?
  - What is the color of the stool?

    - Is the stool black and tarry?

  - What is Owen's fecal score today?

    - What is Owen's "usual" fecal score?
    - How, if at all, has his fecal score changed?

A fecal score is a numerical value that attempts to classify stool by its shape and consistency. (3) (See Figure 22.2.)

There is no universal fecal scoring system.(2) Many nutritional companies have developed their own scoring system and promotional handouts to encourage dialogue between clients and the veterinary team.(3) Scores facilitate communication about stool quality so that participants in the consultation are on the same page. What one person calls hard stool may be "normal" according to someone else.(3) Using a fecal score provides consistency in clinical dialogues by defining key terms and allowing clients to identify more specifically how their pets' stool has changed.

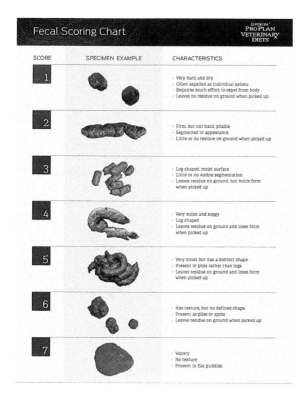

Figure 22.2 Fecal scoring system. Courtesy of Nestlé-Purina.

Diet contributes to fecal output so it is important that we look beyond the description of Owen's stool and ask very specific questions about what it is that he is consuming.(2)

- How is Owen's appetite?

  - Is he still eating?
  - Is his appetite unchanged?
  - Is his appetite increased?
  - Is his appetite decreased?

- What does Owen eat in terms of dog food?
- What does Owen eat in terms of people food, including snacks?
- What else does Owen eat?
- Has Owen's diet changed?
- Is Owen unsupervised outdoors?
- Does Owen have a history of eating items (plants, dirt, other animals, other animals' stool) outdoors?
- Does Owen have a history of eating non-food items?
- Could he have gotten into anything?
- What could he have gotten into?

It is also important to ask about vomiting. If Owen is having difficulty having feces pass through his digestive tract, could there be an obstruction to the flow? If so, that might cause him to be backed up and/or vomit stomach contents because, simply put, there's nowhere for them to go. I would ask the following.

- Is Owen vomiting?
- If so:

  - Describe the vomiting:
  - Is he really vomiting?
  - Or is he regurgitating?
  - When does vomiting occur relative to eating?
  - When did the vomiting start?
  - What is the frequency? How many times has he vomited?
  - Is vomiting productive? Does anything come up?
  - What are the contents of the vomitus?
  - What is the color of the vomitus?
  - Does the vomitus contain blood?

I might also ask about whether Owen is scooting or grooming his perineum excessively.

I might ask if Chelsea has noticed any blood or unusual discharge at sites where he has previously been seated. If so, that might clue me into the possibility that he has an anal sac abscess.

I would also want to inquire about his overall orthopedic health. Past orthopedic disease, such as limb dislocations or pelvic fractures, and present orthopedic disease, including osteoarthritis, may make posturing to defecate challenging. This, in turn, may lead to incomplete evacuation of feces and constipation. Because I have known Owen since a pup, I would know about past orthopedic disease, of which he has none. However, it is possible that he may have developed osteoarthritis since I last examined him, in which case it is important to ask about his activity level:

- Describe Owen's activity level:

  - Is Owen as active as he normally is or is Owen slowing down?
  - If he appears to be slowing down, in what way?
  - How has his activity level changed?

- • What has Chelsea noticed at home?
- • Are there activities that he still does, but for shorter stretches of time?
- • Are there now activities that he seems reluctant to do?

- • How is Owen in terms of jumping?

  - • Is Owen allowed to get up onto furniture (i.e. bed, couch)?
  - • If yes, does he still do it or has there been a change?
  - • Does it seem more challenging for Owen to get in and out of the car?

- • Does it seem more challenging to motivate Owen to be active?
- • How is his energy level? Does he tire easily?
- • Has his gait changed?
- • Does he seem painful when walking?
- • Does he exhibit generalized or focal weakness?
- • Is he ever lame?

  - • If yes, which limb(s)?
  - • Is/are the affected limb(s) consistent or does he exhibit shifting leg lameness?
  - • Is lameness intensified by activity?
  - • Is lameness reduced by activity?
  - • Is lameness worse immediately after rest?
  - • Does he ever walk out of being lame, meaning, does lameness resolve as the day progresses?

Dogs with prostatic disease may change the way that they walk. Some of my colleagues describe them as "walking on eggshells."

Because prostatic disease has not yet been ruled out in Owen, I would also want to ask a few related questions.

- • How are Owen's urinary habits?
- • Have there been any changes with regards to his urine output?
- • Have there been any changes with regards to his urine stream?
- • Does he appear to have bloody urine?
- • Does he have discharge from his penis? If so, is this typical or has something changed?

4. After taking a comprehensive patient history, you ask Chelsea what concerns her most about Owen. She shares what she read online: "Male dogs that strain to produce stool have enlarged prostates." "If that's the case," she says, "then can't we just neuter him?"

- • Chelsea has likely read about enlarged prostates in older male dogs. Prostatic hypertrophy or benign prostatic hyperplasia (BPH) is a common clinical finding in dogs as they age.(4–8)
- • BPH is a normal age-related change that is mediated by dihydrotestosterone (DHT).(9) Testosterone is converted into DHT within the prostate itself with the help of the enzyme, 5-alpha-reductase.(9, 10) DHT promotes growth of the prostate through hyperplasia and hypertrophy.(10)
- • Let's consider how BPH impacts stool passage. When a dog is in the standing position, the prostate is ventral to the rectal canal.(6) As the prostate enlarges, it pushes against the rectum.(6) Although the rectum itself is normal, its lumen is narrowed by the enlarged prostate, which has, in a sense, outgrown its space in the body and is now impinging upon other structures.

As stool passes through the digestive tract, it encounters this "kink" in the rectum. Depending upon the patient's fecal consistency – for instance, if the stool is relatively firm and therefore less compressible – dogs may have to work harder to evacuate the feces because now they must squeeze the stool through a smaller-than-anticipated tube. It's as if an artificial stricture is present within the rectum. It takes force (straining to defecate) to overcome that. For this reason, dogs with prostatomegaly often present with dyschezia and tenesmus.(2, 6)

- The prostate is palpable in health in most dogs by rectal examination.(6) Although the prostate is more prominent in intact, sexually mature dogs, it can still be appreciated in those that are castrated.(4–6)

Recall from anatomy that the prostate is a bi-lobed structure that typically sits one to two centimeters caudal to the neck of the bladder, along the cranial aspect of the pubic symphysis.(6) As dogs age, the prostate may sink out of the pelvic canal, cranially, making it more difficult to feel, particularly in large-breed dogs.(6) To facilitate palpation in these patients, the clinician's free hand can cup the ventral abdomen cranial to the pelvis. When the clinician hikes the ventral abdomen up in this manner, the prostate tends to be lifted and raised back into the pelvic canal, where it is palpable digitally per rectum.

Palpation of the prostate should not elicit pain.(4, 5) Both the right and left lobes can be felt and along the prostate's dorsal midline, a sulcus is palpable.(6) This divides the right side from the left.(6)

On rectal palpation, dogs with BPH will have prostatomegaly.(2, 6) Affected prostates will be uniformly enlarged, with smooth surfaces. They will be non-painful.(7)

Physical exam findings are noteworthy because they are key to differentiating dogs with BPH from dogs with prostatitis. Prostatitis is exceedingly painful. In addition, dogs with prostatitis often present with clinical signs of systemic illness, including fever, lethargy, depression, and/or anorexia.(7)

Prostatic neoplasia is also palpable per rectum, but tends to result in multinodular, asymmetrical lesions.(7)

- Because BPH is fueled by testosterone, bilateral orchiectomy is curative.(9) Prostate size will reduce by 50% within three weeks of surgical castration.(9)

5. Although neutering may reduce Owen's marking behavior, it is unlikely to resolve it. Owen is now eight years old and marking has become a learned behavior. Chelsea may be able to implement changes in the home environment that successfully modify Owen's marking, but I would not expect her to be able to extinguish it. For example, Chelsea can make marking sites less attractive to Owen by thoroughly cleaning them with enzymatic cleaners to remove pet odors and stains.

6. There are many causes of constipation in dogs, other than prostatomegaly. These include: (2, 11–21)

- decreased exercise
- dietary factors:

  - decreased water intake
  - excess fiber
  - foreign body ingestion

- drugs:

  - anticholinergics
  - Kaolin pectin or Kaopectate®
  - opioids

- mechanical obstruction:

  - neoplasia of the colon, prostate, or rectum (see Figure 22.3)
  - pelvic canal narrowing, as from pelvic fracture

- perineal hernia
- polyp
- rectal prolapse (See Figure 22.4)
- sublumbar lymphadenopathy

- metabolic disease:
  - hypercalcemia
  - hyperparathyroidism
  - hypokalemia secondary to chronic kidney disease (CKD)
  - hypothyroidism

- neuromuscular disease:
  - intervertebral disc disease (IVDD)
  - paraplegia
  - spinal cord disease
  - tail pull injury, causing sacral nerve damage

- painful evacuation of stool:
  - anal sacculitis
  - anal stricture
  - peri-anal fistula

- painful posturing during defecation
- supplements, such as iron
- toxins, such as lead.

7. Smooth muscle dysfunction can contribute to idiopathic megacolon in cats.(2)

8. After history-taking, the next step in the diagnostic plan is to perform a comprehensive physical exam.(6)

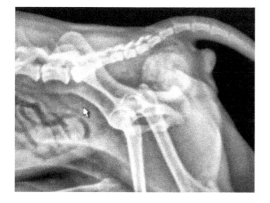

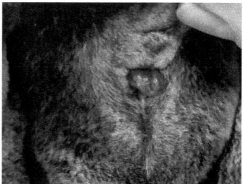

Figure 22.3 Lateral abdominal radiograph with a space-occupying mass caudal to the pelvic canal. This mass was palpable on physical exam. Courtesy of Pamela Mueller.

Figure 22.4 Partial rectal prolapse in a puppy.

Returning to Case 22: The Dog That Is Straining to Defecate

Your clarifying questions during history-taking contribute the following information to Owen's patient profile:

- To Chelsea's knowledge, these episodes have never happened to Owen before.
- Chelsea has only seen Owen produce a tiny nugget of hard stool this morning (Fecal Score of 1 using the Nestlé-Purina scale).
- The color of this stool was normal (dark brown).
- The stool was not coated in mucous or blood.
- Chelsea has not observed diarrhea.
- Chelsea has not observed vomiting.
- Owen's urine stream, volume, and frequency of urination appear normal.
- Owen's activity level seems normal.
- His gait is normal.
- He does not appear to have any trouble jumping.
- Owen does tend to experience the world through taste. Anything he can put his mouth on, he will be tempted to sample.
- To Chelsea's knowledge, Owen has never ingested non-food items in the house, but he does tend to find (and ingest!) all sorts of carcasses, including fur, skin, and bones.
- Owen's appetite may be slightly off, but that's not unusual for him when Emmett is away.
- Owen's diet is unchanged (commercially available, non-name brand senior kibble).
- Owen is still meal-fed; the numbers of feedings per day (two) and the meal volume are unchanged.
- Owen is not receiving any medication other than monthly, year-round preventative products: oral heartworm/endoparasite and topical flea/tick prophylaxis.

After taking a thorough patient history, you examine Owen. Physical examination discloses the following findings:

- Owen has iris atrophy and what appears to be nuclear sclerosis bilaterally.
- Owen's ears contain a moderate amount of ceruminous debris.

  - There is no appreciable aural odor.
  - Ear canals are non-stenotic, non-erythematous, and non-painful.
  - Both tympanic membranes are visible via otoscopy.

- There is mild caudal thigh muscle atrophy.
- Owen has mildly decreased range of motion on bilateral hip extension. You subjectively consider this to be normal for his age.
- The prostate is palpably enlarged, but not to the degree that you would consider it to be obstructing the lumen of the rectal canal.

  - Both lobes of the prostate are bilaterally symmetrical, with smooth contours.
  - Owen is non-reactive on prostatic palpation, which leads you to believe that the prostate is not painful.

Rectal examination is negative for:

- anal sac enlargement and/or impaction
- narrowed pelvic canal
- peri-anal fistula
- perineal hernia
- rectal prolapse
- rectal masses
- sublumbar lymphadenopathy.

Round Two of Questions for Case 22: The Dog That Is Straining to Defecate

1. Now that you have taken a thorough history and performed a physical examination, which differential diagnoses are still viable?
2. How will you investigate the differentials that you outlined in Question #1 (above)? What are your next steps in the diagnostic plan?

Answers to Round Two of Questions for Case 22: The Dog That Is Straining to Defecate

1. The following differential diagnoses are still on the table as potential causes of Owen's dyschezia and tenesmus:

   • mechanical obstruction:

     • bowel stricture
     • foreign body ingestion
     • neoplasia of the colon, prostate, or rectum

   • metabolic disease
   • neuromuscular disease.

2. An appropriate initial diagnostic plan for Owen is to run baseline bloodwork (complete blood count [CBC] and chemistry profile) and urinalysis to collect a minimum database and an abdominal imaging study.

   Bloodwork and urinalysis collectively screen for general wellbeing and may make certain types of metabolic disease more or less likely. For example, if Owen were hypothyroid, then I might expect to see the following clinicopathologic data:(2, 9, 10, 22, 23)

   • CBC:

     • normocytic, normochromic, non-regenerative anemia

   • chemistry profile:

     • elevated cholesterol
     • elevated triglycerides
     • mild increase in liver enzymes
     • +/– mild increase in creatinine kinase.

Seeing these findings on Owen's bloodwork may prompt me to pursue yet another screening test to assess his total thyroxine (TT4).

Abdominal imaging may involve radiographs and/or ultrasonography to evaluate internal structures. Each modality has both advantages and disadvantages. Abdominal radiographs are a common starting point for survey imaging, particularly in patients that are suspicious for foreign body obstruction.(2, 24, 25) Although radiographs lack the detail that can be obtained by ultrasound and computed tomography (CT), they offer rapid turnaround time in terms of diagnostic results.(26) This is valuable when determining if patients require immediate intervention.

Abdominal radiographs may also highlight one or more masses that may require additional investigation. Sometimes, the masses themselves are not visible on radiographs, but they displace organs, which is apparent. This so-called "mass effect" may make the clinician perform follow-up sonography with or without ultrasound-guided fine-needle aspirate.

Neither baseline bloodwork/urinalysis nor abdominal imaging is the best approach to diagnose neuromuscular disease, but they are essential steps in the rule-out process. If both studies are negative for mechanical obstruction and metabolic disease, then Owen would need to be reassessed. I might at that point be inclined to recommend advanced imaging in the form of CT or magnetic resonance imaging (MRI) to evaluate Owen for IVDD or other forms of spinal disease. However, I would have expected to find neurologic deficits on physical exam, which I did not. For this reason, I am prioritizing mechanical obstruction or metabolic disease as likelier diagnoses.

Returning to Case 22: The Dog That Is Straining to Defecate

At your recommendation, Chelsea elects to proceed with a minimum database (CBC, chemistry profile, and urinalysis) as well as two-view abdominal radiographs. Bloodwork and urinalysis are unremarkable. Both radiographs have been provided for you to review (see Figures 22.5 and 22.6).

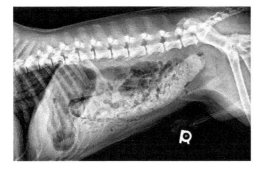

Figure 22.5 Right lateral radiograph of canine abdomen. Courtesy of Nicole Johnson.

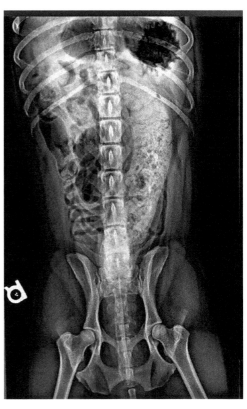

Figure 22.6 Ventro-dorsal (V/D) abdominal radiograph of the same dog that is imaged in Figure 22.5. Courtesy of Nicole Johnson.

Round Three of Questions for Case 22: The Dog That Is Straining to Defecate

1. Why is it important that you perform a systematic approach when evaluating radiographs?
2. When you evaluate abdominal radiographs, what broad structures are you looking for?
3. When you evaluate abdominal organs, what (broadly) are you examining them for?
4. One of our differential diagnoses for Owen was mechanical obstruction, as from ingestion of a foreign body. Which radiological findings are associated with intestinal obstruction?

5. How might we use small intestinal diameter as a predictor of obstruction in the dog?
6. Does dilated bowel always signify mechanical obstruction?
7. If radiological findings are ambiguous concerning intestinal obstruction, what next step(s) might you take to investigate further?
8. Describe what you see: what are Owen's radiographic findings?
9. Based upon what you see in the radiograph, what is Owen's diagnosis?
10. How will you manage Owen in the short-term to address his diagnosis?
11. When you manually sift through his impacted feces, you find an assortment of bony fragments, rock-like shards, and grit. It appears that Owen has a propensity to ingest non-food items, a condition called pica.(27–32) What causes pica?
12. How can you manage Owen's pica in the future?

Answers to Round Three of Questions for Case 22: The Dog That Is Straining to Defecate

1. It is important that you evaluate radiographs the same way every time so that you do not miss lesions that are clinically relevant, particularly those that are incidental findings and/or those that are not in the organ system of interest. For example, let's consider a different case in which you may have taken abdominal radiographs as part of the diagnostic work-up for a dog with vomiting. However, you need to be certain that you examine systems outside of the digestive tract because non-digestive problems can also cause and/or contribute to the presenting complaint. If we examine radiographs using a systematic approach, then we are less likely to have tunnel vision and miss something important.

2. When you evaluate abdominal radiographs, you should examine the following components:

   - diaphragm
   - gastrointestinal tract:

     - stomach
     - small bowel
     - large bowel
     - accessory organs, such as the pancreas*
   - hepatobiliary tract:

     - liver
     - gall bladder*

   - urinary tract:

     - kidneys
     - ureter*
     - urinary bladder
     - urethra*

   - genital tract:

     - prostate (males)
     - uterus (intact females)*
     - penis (males)

   - abdominal serosal detail
   - musculoskeletal system:

     - vertebral column

- os penis (males)
- pelvis
- proximal hind limbs.

Note that the items that are starred (*) are not typically visible in abdominal radiographs of healthy patients; however, we still need to train our eye to get in the habit of examining the region where they would be located if there were an issue. For instance, our trained eye still needs to follow the expected path of the urethra, because it is possible to identify radiopaque urethroliths upon careful inspection. If we are not in the habit of looking for them, they are easily missed.

3. When you examine abdominal organs, be sure to note the following.

- Location:
    - Is each organ where it is supposed to be or is it displaced?
- Number:
    - If it is a paired organ, can you see both (i.e. two kidneys)?
- Opacity:
    - Which radiopacity is the organ supposed to be?
    - How does its current radiopacity compare against that which you expected?
- Shape:
    - What is the appropriate shape of this organ?
    - How does its current shape compare against that which you expected?
- Size:
    - What is the expected size of this organ?
    - How does its current size compare against that which you expected?

4. One of the diagnoses for Owen was mechanical obstruction, as from ingestion of a foreign body. The following radiological findings are supportive of intestinal obstruction:(33–36)

- a foreign body that is identified within the digestive tract
- increased peritoneal fluid
- intestinal dilation, in particular, segmental intestinal dilation
- plication of loops of bowel.

5. Small intestinal diameter is often used as a predictor of obstruction in the dog, although how this is measured on radiographs depends largely upon which reference you use.(33) The following measures have historically been considered to represent the normal upper limit of intestinal diameter in dogs.

- A ratio of small intestinal diameter (SI): the height of the body of the fifth lumbar vertebra (L5) that is less than or equal to 1.6.(33)
- A ratio of SI maximal diameter : SI minimal diameter that is less than or equal to 2.0.(36)
- A ratio of SI maximal diameter : an estimated average of small intestinal diameters that is less than or equal to 1.3.(36)
- The height of one lumbar vertebra.(37)
- Three widths of the 12th rib.(35)

Beyond these measurements, small bowel is considered to be pathologically dilated in dogs.(33) Dilation is more likely to be due to obstruction in dogs that have a ratio of:(36)

- SI maximal diameter : the height of L5 that is greater than or equal to 2.4
- SI maximal diameter : SI minimal diameter that is greater than or equal to 3.4
- SI maximal diameter : an estimated average of small intestinal diameters that is greater than or equal to 1.9.

6. No, dilated bowel does not always signify mechanical obstruction. Gas within the bowel can occur simply due to aerophagia. Consider, for instance, a panting dog that takes part in an imaging study. This patient is likely to have a significant amount of air in the digestive tract, just because of its increased respiratory activity. Likewise, gas may be formed by microflora within the colon. This can reflux into the distal small bowel and appear on abdominal films. Finally, patients may present with ileus, that is, a true nonmechanical obstruction of gut peristalsis without having an actual physical blockage. Ileus may result from electrolyte imbalance, drugs, or other underlying pathology. In and of itself, dilation does not confirm mechanical obstruction. It may, however, support mechanical obstruction when concurrent with other clinical (i.e. projectile, persistent vomiting) or radiological signs (i.e. plication of bowel loops) that suggest a physical blockage.

7. If radiological findings are ambiguous concerning intestinal obstruction, then the following diagnostic steps may be considered:(35)

   - contrast radiography (i.e. a barium study)
   - abdominal ultrasonography.

   Sonography more accurately diagnoses intestinal obstruction than radiography.(38, 39) However, abdominal ultrasound is not always readily available in clinical practice as a diagnostic tool and its accuracy relies heavily upon user skill.(36)

8. Owen's stomach contains a fair amount of gas. Some loops of small bowel contain gas, but these do not appear to be distended. There also does not appear to be an obstructive pattern within the small bowel.

   The descending colon is appreciably distended with granular content that resembles fecal matter. On the V/D view, there are what appear to be a few fragments within this granular content that are more radiopaque.

9. Based upon the radiographic study, Owen appears to be constipated. The radiopaque fragments could be bone or other grit from ingesta. It is unclear at this point what has caused Owen to develop constipation.

10. In the short-term, Owen may be medically managed by administering an enema to loosen the retained stool and ease its passage. Once the impacted feces have been evacuated, they may be manually explored with gloved fingers to determine if the contents include one or more foreign bodies. This may clue you in on how to prevent recurrence. For example, I once administered an enema to a Dachshund that produced a scrunchie, a fabric-covered elastic hair tie. This foreign body could have precipitated a surgical emergency had it become obstructed within the stomach or small bowel. Knowing that this was ingested by the dog allowed me to customize aftercare instructions that included keeping the laundry out of reach and the floor free and clear of scrunchies.

    If there is no obvious foreign body within the impacted fecal matter, then you may have to consider whether this is a one-time event or whether it is likely to recur. If there are concerns about potential recurrence, then dietary therapy may be employed. Patients may be prescribed either a low- or high-fiber diet depending upon the presumptive cause of constipation.

11. Pica may result from medical or behavioral issues.(2, 30)

Medical causes of pica include, but are not limited to:(2, 30, 40–45)

- anemia
- dietary or nutrient deficiency
- gastrointestinal parasites
- malabsorptive and/or maldigestion syndromes:
    - exocrine pancreatic insufficiency (EPI)
    - inflammatory bowel disease (IBD)
- metabolic disease:
    - diabetes mellitus
    - hyperadrenocorticism
    - hyperthyroidism
- neuropathy:
    - abnormal hunger and satiety signals within the CNS
- poor plane of nutrition
- portosystemic shunt (PSS)
- structural disease:
    - esophageal stricture
    - megaesophagus.

Behavioral causes of pica include, but are not limited to:(2, 29–32, 43, 46–56)

- age-related – teething in puppies
- anxiety
- attention-seeking
- early weaning
- lack of enrichment
- maternal nesting behavior
- obsessive-compulsive disorder (OCD)
- play solicitation
- response to stress
- taste preference – feces from animals that eat meat-rich diets may be savory to certain dogs.

12. A basket muzzle can be placed to prevent abnormal ingestive behaviors, including pica. This muzzle is bulky to wear, but achieves its function (preventing pica) while allowing the patient to pant freely and drink water as needed.(6)

CLINICAL PEARLS

- Dyschezia and tenesmus are clinical signs that may be suggestive of:
    - dysfunction at the level of the intestinal tract:
        - in particular: increased intestinal transit time, as caused by constipation, space-occupying mass, stricture
    - dysfunction at the level of the urogenital tract:
        - in particular: the accessory sex glands (the prostate).

- Comprehensive history-taking is essential to guide your prioritization of differential diagnoses. In particular, clarifying questions should concentrate on:

  - activity level
  - appetite
  - attitude
  - changes in gait or mobility
  - current history of access to non-food items, unsupervised time outdoors, etc. – what could the patient have gotten into?
  - diet history
  - is the patient vomiting?
  - past history of pica – what has the patient gotten into?
  - urinary habits:

    - frequency
    - volume
    - steady stream (males)

  - urogenital discharge.

- Rectal examination is an essential part of the physical in any patient that presents for dyschezia and/or tenesmus to evaluate the patient for:

  - masses in the rectal canal
  - pelvic canal narrowing
  - perineal hernia
  - prostatomegaly (males)
  - strictures in the rectal canal
  - sublumbar lymphadenopathy.

- Baseline bloodwork (CBC, chemistry profile), urinalysis, and imaging studies often constitute the minimum database.

- In this clinical scenario, radiographs are important screening tools for mechanical obstruction, organomegaly, abnormal changes in organ shape, margins, and/or radiopacity. Follow-up studies with contrast and/or abdominal ultrasonography may be indicated.

- Constipation may be resolved in the short-term via enema. However, finding and addressing the underlying cause is critical to prevent recurrence.

References

1. Englar R. Writing skills for veterinarians. Sheffield: 5M Publishing; 2019.
2. Englar RE. Common clinical presentations in dogs and cats. Hoboken, NJ: Wiley/Blackwell; 2019.
3. Greco DS. Diagnosis and dietary management of gastrointestinal disease: purina veterinary diets. Available from: https://www.purinaproplanvets.com/media/1202/gi_quick_reference_guide.pdf.
4. de Gier J, van Sluijs FJ. Male reproductive tract. In: Rijnberk A, Sluijs FJv, editors. Medical history and physical examination in companion animals. 2nd ed. New York: Saunders/Elsevier; 2009. p. 117–22.
5. van Dongen AM, L'Eplattenier HF. Kidneys and urinary tract. In: Rijnberk A, van Sluijs FJ, editors. Medical history and physical examination in companion animals. 2nd ed. St Louis, MO: Saunders Elsevier; 2009.
6. Englar RE. Performing the small animal physical examination. Hoboken, NJ: Wiley/Blackwell; 2017.
7. Foster RA. Common lesions in the male reproductive tract of cats and dogs. Vet Clin North Am Small Anim Pract 2012;42(3):527–45, vii, vii.

8. Krawiec DR. Canine prostate disease. J Am Vet Med Assoc 1994;204(10):1561–4.

9. Côté E. Clinical veterinary advisor. Dogs and cats. 3rd ed. St. Louis, MO: Elsevier Mosby; 2015.

10. Ettinger SJ, Feldman EC, Côté E. Textbook of veterinary internal medicine: diseases of the dog and the cat. 8th ed. St. Louis, MO: Elsevier; 2017.

11. Tilley LP, Smith FWK. The 5-minute veterinary consult: canine and feline. 3rd ed. Baltimore, MD: Lippincott Williams & Wilkins; 2004.

12. Rothuizen J, Schrauwen E, Theyse LFH, Verhaert L. Digestive tract. In: Rijnberk A, van Sluijs FJ, editors. Medical history and physical examination in companion animals. Philadelphia, PA: Elsevier; 2009. p. 86–100.

13. Trevail T, Gunn-Moore D, Carrera I, Courcier E, Sullivan M. Radiographic diameter of the colon in normal and constipated cats and in cats with megacolon. Vet Radiol Ultrasound 2011;52(5):516–20.

14. Washabau R. Feline constipation, obstipation, and megacolon: prevention, diagnosis, and treatment. World small animal veterinary association world congress [Internet]; 2001. Available from: https://www.vin.com/VINDBPub/SearchPB/Proceedings/PR05000/PR00118.htm.

15. Washabau R. Constipation, obstipation, and megacolon. In: August JR, editor. Consultations in feline internal medicine. 3rd ed. Philadelphi, PAa: Saunders; 1997. p. 104–12.

16. Bredal WP, Thoresen SI, Kvellestad A. Atresia-coli in a 9-week-old kitten. J Small Anim Pract 1994;35(12):643–5.

17. Broek AHM, Else RW, Hunter MS. Atresia ani and urethrorectal fistula in a kitten. J Small Anim Pract 1988;29(2):91–4.

18. Yam P. Decision making in the management of constipation in the cat. Pract 1997;19(8):434–40.

19. Hudson EB, Farrow CS, Smith SL. Acquired megacolon in a cat. Mod Vet Pract 1979;60(8):625–7.

20. Washabau R, Holt D. Feline constipation and idiopathic megacolon. In: Bonagura JD, editor. Kirk's current veterinary therapy. 13th ed. Philadelphia, PA: W.B. Saunders; 2000. p. 648–52.

21. Freiche V, Houston D, Weese H, Evason M, Deswarte G, Ettinger G, et al. Uncontrolled study assessing the impact of a psyllium-enriched extruded dry diet on faecal consistency in cats with constipation. J Feline Med Surg 2011;13(12):903–11.

22. Dixon RM, Reid SW, Mooney CT. Epidemiological, clinical, haematological and biochemical characteristics of canine hypothyroidism. Vet Rec 1999;145(17):481–7.

23. Panciera DL. Hypothyroidism in dogs: 66 cases (1987–1992). J Am Vet Med Assoc 1994;204(5):761–7.

24. Boag A, Hughes D. Emergency management of the acute abdomen in dogs and cats 1. Investigation and initial stabilization. Pract 2004;26(9):476–83.

25. Twedt DC. Differential diagnosis and therapy of vomiting. Vet Clin North Am Small Anim Pract 1983;13(3):503–20.

26. Heeren V, Edwards L, Mazzaferro EM. Acute abdomen: Diagnosis. Comp Cont. Educ Pract 2004;26(5):350.

27. Nijsse R, Mughini-Gras L, Wagenaar JA, Ploeger HW. Coprophagy in dogs interferes in the diagnosis of parasitic infections by faecal examination. Vet Parasitol 2014;204(3–4):304–9.

28. Bamberger M, Houpt KA. Signalment factors, comorbidity, and trends in behavior diagnoses in cats: 736 cases (1991–2001). J Am Vet Med Assoc 2006;229(10):1602–6.

29. Houpt K. Ingestive behavior problems of dogs and cats. Vet Clin North Am Small Anim Pract 1982;12(4):683–92.

30. Tilley LP, Smith FWK. The 5-minute veterinary consult: canine and feline. 3rd ed. Baltimore, MD: Lippincott Williams & Wilkins; 2004.

31. Stepita ME. Feline anxiety and fear-related disorders. In: Little S, editor. Consultations in Feline Internal medicine. St. Louis, MO: Elsevier; 2016. p. 900–10.

32. Demontigny-Bédard I, Beauchamp G, Bélanger MC, Frank D. Characterization of pica and chewing behaviors in privately owned cats: a case-control study. J Feline Med Surg 2016;18(8):652–7.

33. Graham JP, Lord PF, Harrison JM. Quantitative estimation of intestinal dilation as a predictor of obstruction in the dog. J Small Anim Pract 1998;39(11):521–4.

34. O'Brien TR. The small intestine. Radiographic Diagnosis of Abdominal Disorderes in the Dog and the Cat. Philadelphia: W. B. Saunders; 1978. p. 279–320.

35. Thrall DE. Textbook of veterinary diagnostic radiology. 7th ed. St. Louis, MO: Elsevier; 2018.

36. Finck C, D'Anjou MA, Alexander K, Specchi S, Beauchamp G. Radiographic diagnosis of mechanical obstruction in dogs based on relative small intestinal external diameters. Vet Radiol Ultrasound 2014;55(5):472–9.

37. Kantrowitz B, Biller D. Using radiography to evaluate vomiting in dogs and cats. Vet Med 1992;87:806–13.

38. Sharma A, Thompson MS, Scrivani PV, Dykes NL, Yeager AE, Freer SR, Erb HN. Comparison of radiography

and ultrasonography for diagnosing small-intestinal mechanical obstruction in vomiting dogs. Vet Radiol Ultrasound 2011;52(3):248–55.

39. Tyrrell D, Beck C. Survey of the use of radiography vs. ultrasonography in the investigation of gastrointestinal foreign bodies in small animals. Vet Radiol Ultrasound 2006;47(4):404–8.

40. Kvitko-White HL, Cook AK. Managing iron deficiency anemia. DVM360 [Internet]; 2014. Available from: http://veterinarymedicine.dvm360.com/managing-iron-deficiency-anemia.

41. Bécuwe-Bonnet V, Bélanger MC, Frank D, Parent J, Hélie P. Gastrointestinal disorders in dogs with excessive licking of surfaces. J Vet Behav 2012;7(4):194–204.

42. Wells DL. Comparison of two treatments for preventing dogs eating their own faeces. Vet Rec 2003;153(2):51–3.

43. Hart BL, Hart LA. Canine and feline behavioral therapy. Philadelphia, PA: Lea & Febiger; 1985.

44. Overall KL. Clinical behavioral medicine for small animals. London: Mosby Year Book; 1997.

45. McKeown D, Luescher A, Machum M. Coprophagia: food for thought. Can Vet J 1988;29(10):849–50.

46. Neville PF. Treatment of behaviour problems in cats. Pract 1991;13(2):43–50.

47. Neville PF, editor. Treatment of fabric-eating disorder in cats. North American Veterinary Conference (NAVC); 1996; Orlando, FL. Eastern States Veterinary Association.

48. Houpt KA. Feeding and drinking behavior problems. Vet Clin North Am Small Anim Pract 1991;21(2):281–98.

49. Sawyer LS, Moon-Fanelli AA, Dodman NH. Psychogenic alopecia in cats: 11 cases (1993–1996). J Am Vet Med Assoc 1999;214(1):71–4.

50. Beaver BVG. Canine behavior: insights and answers. 2nd ed. St Louis, MO: Saunders/Elsevier; 2009.

51. Horwitz DF. Chewing in dogs. NAVC Clin's Brief 2007 (November):15–6.

52. Crowell-Davis SL. Stereotypic behavior and compulsive disorder. Comp Cont Educ Pract 2007;29(10):625–8.

53. Landsberg G, Hunthausen W, Ackerman L. Stereotypic and compulsive disorders. In: Landsberg G, Hunthausen W, editors. Handbook of behavior problems of the dog and the cat. Edinburgh: Saunders; 2003. p. 195–225.

54. Frank D. Repetitive behaviors in cats and dogs: are they really a sign of obsessive–compulsive disorders (OCD)? Can Vet J 2013;54(2):129–31.

55. Overall KL, Dunham AE. Clinical features and outcome in dogs and cats with obsessive–compulsive disorder: 126 cases (1989–2000). J Am Vet Med Assoc 2002;221(10):1445–52.

56. Morgan JA, Moore LE. A quick review of canine exocrine pancreatic insufficiency. DVM360 [Internet]; 2009. Available from: http://veterinarymedicine.dvm360.com/quick-review-canine-exocrine-pancreatic-insufficiency.

Case 23

The Adult Diarrheic Dog

Alec Rainey and his husband Xavier are long-term clients of your practice. This past weekend, their daughter, Tiffany, graduated from Oxford University with an undergraduate bachelor's in Fine Art degree. Tiffany is a jack-of-all-trades in the studio and her forte is oil painting. She has a prestigious job lined up as a curator of a private collection in the UK and there is much to celebrate. Alec and Xavier decided to throw her a graduation party in honor of her accomplishments and to wish her well on this next chapter of her professional life. They decided to host the get-together at their home. Weather permitted them to spend much of Saturday afternoon on the terrace. Tiffany was excited to see her professors and closest friends. The only one who was more enthused than Tiffany was Yahtzee, whose

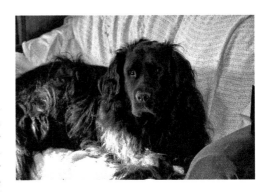

Figure 23.1 Meet your patient, Yahtzee, a 6-year-old spayed female Newfoundland dog. Courtesy of Kathy Knowles.

passion in life was making new acquaintances. Yahtzee was a gentle giant and the life of any party. She could make her way in any crowd, but it was hard to say whether she enjoyed the people more or being a mooch. It had been a long time since they'd had this many people over, and Yahtzee made the most of it.

By Saturday evening, everyone was spent. It was nearly midnight when the last guest drove away, and Alec knew that they'd have a long day ahead of them by way of clean-up. Yahtzee uncharacteristically woke them in the middle of the night to go outside. Alec was too tired to think anything of it, and he didn't follow her outside to see what all the fuss was about. Instead, he let her out and headed back to bed. In the morning, she was bright and cheerful, peering through the sliding glass door. Yahtzee ate some, but not all of her breakfast. She seemed more interested in "helping" Xavier put away the courtyard chairs. Helping really meant standing in the way. Every time he wanted to tote something to the garage, he had to make a full semi-circle around her.

The morning sped by. It wasn't until early afternoon, when everyone had settled back indoors, that something seemed off about Yahtzee. She wanted back out. Again. And again. By the third time, Alec's attention was piqued, and he followed her. She ran with urgency to the shrubbery border alongside the house and produced semi-formed stool after what seemed like an inordinate amount of straining. About an hour later, Yahtzee again squatted, this time in the house. (See **Plate 8**.)

BCS: 6/9
Mentation: QAR

TPR

T: 100.2°F (37.9°C)
P: 86 beats per minute
R: 24 breaths per minute

Since then, Yahtzee has had four more episodes of jelly like, foul-smelling diarrhea. Each time, she reacts explosively, with urgency. She can't always hold it in until she gets outside. After two more accidents in the house, Alec calls the clinic. You are on call. You instruct him to meet you there. About a half-hour later, he arrives. You take Yahtzee's vital signs and record them below.

Round One of Questions for Case 23: The Adult Diarrheic Dog

1. Case #22 introduced the concept of fecal scoring. Using the Nestlé-Purina fecal system, does Yahtzee rank nearer to a 1/7 or a 7/7?
2. Why is it helpful to ask the client to score the feces?
3. What are broad mechanisms by which diarrhea occurs? (Hint: this is not intended to be a list of the specific differential diagnoses for diarrhea.)
4. Loose fecal matter can be classified as small or large bowel diarrhea based upon where it originates within the gut. What are common causes of small bowel diarrhea in dogs?
5. What is the medical term for inflammation of the colon, which may result in large bowel diarrhea?
6. In addition to the term that you identified in Question #5 (above), what are common causes of large bowel diarrhea?
7. Is the patient's history consistent with small bowel or large bowel diarrhea? Explain your answer.
8. Based upon your localization of Yahtzee's diarrhea, if she were to have blood in her stool, would you expect her to exhibit hematochezia or melena? Explain your answer.
9. After taking a comprehensive patient history, what is the next step in the diagnostic plan?

Answers to Round One of Questions for Case 23: The Adult Diarrheic Dog

1. Using the Nestlé-Purina fecal system, Yahtzee would score nearer to a 7/7. As the fecal score increases toward the high end of the scale, the feces become increasingly wet due to high water content. When fecal matter scores a seven out of seven, it has no shape and forms flat puddles.

    Comparing **Plate 8** (Yahtzee's feces) to Figure 22.2 (the Nestlé-Purina fecal scale), I would score Yahtzee's fecal matter as a 6/7. It forms piles instead of spreading out over the ground in puddles, like water, and it has texture, although it lacks a definitive shape.

2. Fecal scoring ascribes more uniform descriptors to the language surrounding defecation so that the client and the veterinary team are on the same page. Not everyone's idea of diarrhea is the same. One client may say that his/her pet has "diarrhea" when in actuality the stool is formed, just a bit softer and/or easier to deform than is typical. Another client may say that his/her pet has "soft stool" when in fact the stool is liquified. In both circumstances, the visual that the client provided may paint a different picture in the mind of the veterinary team than what the client had intended. Inaccurate descriptors may alter the clinician's approach to the case. I am less inclined, for instance, to prescribe an anti-diarrheal drug to a dog that truly has soft stool, whereas I am more likely to reach for one to medically manage a dog with liquid diarrhea.

    Fecal scoring is imperfect, but it provides a starting point. It also helps the client to consider (and put a number to!) what is typical for the patient as compared to what the fecal score is at today's visit. Those kinds of comparisons are very helpful in understanding what is "normal" for a given patient.(1) This helps the clinician to understand what it is that s/he and the client are collectively working toward getting back to.

3. Diarrhea may result from the following broad mechanisms:(1–4)

    *   hypermotility within the gut
    *   increased gut wall permeability, as from intestinal inflammation
    *   osmotic forces that draw water into the gut:

        *   food may be ingested that is osmotically active, but poorly digested – high-fiber diets
        *   medications may be administered that are osmotically active:

- lactulose
- magnesium sulfate
- sugar alcohols (mannitol, sorbitol, xylitol)

- active secretion into the gut may be triggered by:

  - bacterial toxins
  - luminal secretagogues
  - bile acids
  - non-osmotic laxatives

- overstimulation of the parasympathetic nervous system

  - reduced absorption by the gut, for instance, due to gut resection.

4. Loose fecal matter can be classified as small or large bowel diarrhea based upon where it originates within the gut. Common causes of small bowel diarrhea include:(1, 5–17)

- dietary indiscretion
- exocrine pancreatic insufficiency (EPI)
- food allergy
- food intolerance
- hypoadrenocorticism
- infectious enteritis:

  - bacterial
  - fungal:

    - histoplasmosis
    - phycomycosis
    - pythiosis

  - parasitic:

    - hookworms
    - protozoa
    - roundworms
    - tapeworms

  - viral:

    - canine parvovirus type 1 (CPV-1, minute virus)
    - canine parvovirus type 2 (CPV-2)
    - coronavirus

- pancreatitis
- portosystemic shunt
- protein-losing enteropathy (PLE):

  - inflammatory bowel disease (IBD):

    - eosinophilic IBD
    - granulomatous enteritis
    - lymphocytic-plasmacytic IBD

  - intestinal lymphangiectasia
  - intestinal neoplasia

- small intestinal bacterial overgrowth (SIBO) as from malabsorptive small bowel disease
- toxicosis.

Refer to Case #7 if you would like to review one common cause of small bowel diarrhea in pediatric patients, canine parvovirus.

5. The medical term for inflammation of the colon, which may result in large bowel diarrhea, is colitis.(1, 16–18)

6. Common causes of large bowel diarrhea include:(1, 2, 11, 12, 19–21)

    *   dietary indiscretion
    *   infectious colitis:

        *   *Campylobacter* spp.
        *   *Clostridium* spp.
        *   *Cryptosporidium* spp.
        *   *Entamoeba histolytica*
        *   *Escherichia coli*
        *   *Giardia* spp.
        *   *Histoplasma capsulatum*
        *   *Salmonella* spp.
        *   Prototheca

    *   endoparasitism:

        *   hookworms
        *   tritrichomonas
        *   whipworms

    *   food allergy
    *   food intolerance
    *   histiocytic ulcerative colitis
    *   IBD
    *   neoplasia.

7. The patient's history is most consistent with large bowel diarrhea because Yahtzee is exhibiting the following clinical signs:(1, 5, 16, 17)

    *   gelatinous appearance of fecal matter due to high mucous content
    *   increased frequency of defecation
    *   increased urgency of defecation
    *   semi-formed stool
    *   tenesmus.

8. Large bowel diarrhea is more likely to be associated with hematochezia as opposed to melena. (1, 22) Hematochezia signifies a lower bowel bleed.(1, 22) Fresh blood from the lower bowel mixes with stool to form red streaks that coat the outside of the stool.(1, 22) (See **Plate 9**.)

    By contrast, melena refers to stool that has taken on the appearance of black tar.(1, 22) This signifies an upper gastrointestinal bleed, as from the esophagus or stomach. When blood from the upper gastrointestinal tract is digested, it mixes with the stool to create the classic black appearance of melena.(1, 22) (See **Plate 10**.)

9. After history-taking, the next step in the diagnostic plan is to perform a comprehensive physical exam.(22)

Returning to Case 23: The Adult Diarrheic Dog

You examine Yahtzee. Her examination is unremarkable except for:

- mild discomfort on palpation of her abdomen
- erythematous skin surrounding her anus
- frank red blood and gelatinous mucus noted on your gloved fingers following rectal examination.

You tell Alec that you suspect colitis secondary to dietary indiscretion; however, you recommend that fecal examination be performed.

Round Two of Questions for Case 23: The Adult Diarrheic Dog

1. Alec asks you to clarify what is involved in a "fecal examination."
2. What causes the normal brown color of healthy stool?
3. What can the color of stool tell the examiner?
4. What are abnormal colors of stool?
5. The estimate that you provided Alec lists fecal cytology as an in-house diagnostic test. Alec asks you what specifically you are looking for when you perform this test.
6. Differentiate Campylobacter-like organisms (CLOs) from *Clostridium* spp. based upon appearance when viewed under light microscopy.
7. Is the shape of CLOs that you described in Question #6 (above) pathognomonic for *Campylobacter*?
8. Although fecal cytology may be suggestive of CLOs or *Clostridium* spp., which diagnostic test should you do to confirm either diagnosis?
9. Are *Campylobacter* spp. always pathologic?
10. Are either *Campylobacter* spp. or *Clostridium* spp. zoonotic?
11. You also explain to Alec that you wish to rule out common endoparasites that could cause colitis. What are the clinically relevant hookworms in dogs and cats?
12. If this patient had a significant hookworm burden, then what clinical sign(s) might you have expected to see on presentation?
13. What are clinically relevant whipworms in dogs and cats?
14. If this patient had a significant whipworm burden, then what clinical sign(s) might you have expected to see on presentation?
15. Differentiate hookworm from whipworm ova based upon appearance when viewed under light microscopy after routine fecal flotation for cytology.
16. Is the whipworm ova shape pathognomonic?
17. Are either hookworms or whipworms zoonotic?
18. How would you treat hookworms or whipworms?
19. In addition to drug name and dose, what do you need to know in order to clear an infection with hookworms or whipworms?
20. If you do not see endoparasites on fecal flotation, can you definitively rule them out as differential diagnoses?
21. If infectious causes of colitis are not identified, how will you address Yahtzee's presenting complaint?
22. If infectious causes of colitis are not identified, is the administration of metronidazole indicated? Why or why not?
23. If Yahtzee were a cat, what are potential consequences of administering high-dose metronidazole?

Answers to Round Two of Questions for Case 23: The Adult Diarrheic Dog

1. A "fecal examination" typically involves one or more of the following procedures:(1, 12)

    - gross inspection of fecal matter
    - direct fecal smear with saline
    - fecal flotation
    - fecal cytology with Diff-Quik staining.

    Gross inspection of fecal matter requires the examiner to assess the consistency of the sample (preferably using the Nestlé-Purina fecal scoring scale) as well as its color, mucous content, and whether fresh red blood (or melena) appears to be present.(1)

2. Stool color predominantly comes from bile.(1) Bile is made up of water, bile salts, and pigments that result from the breakdown of erythrocytes.(23) Erythrocytes contain hemoglobin, a protein that is responsible for transporting oxygen.(23) When hemoglobin is broken down, degradation products include bilirubin and biliverdin.(23) The former is yellow-red in color; the latter is green.(23) Within the intestinal lumen, biliverdin is converted into stercobilin.(23) Stercobilin is what gives stool its characteristic brown color.(23)

3. Fecal color provides important information regarding gastrointestinal and systemic health.(1) For example, fecal color depends upon:

    - diet
    - function/dysfunction within the hepatobiliary tract
    - functional/dysfunctional pancreas
    - hydration status
    - mucosal integrity:

        - presence/absence of inflammation
        - presence/absence of erosions or ulcers, masses, and/or mucosal tears
        - presence/absence of gastrointestinal bleeding.

4. Grossly abnormal colors of stool include:(1, 12)

    - black tar
    - fresh red streaks
    - pale or colorless
    - yellow
    - gray-white.

    We have already discussed black tar (melena) and fresh red streaks (hematochezia) in the first round of questions that is paired with this clinical vignette.

    When stool appears pale or colorless, it is referred to as acholic feces.(1, 12) Acholic feces result from either EPI or a bile duct obstruction.(1)

    Yellowish or mustardy colored stool is often associated with diarrhea.(1) It can result from infection, such as coccidiosis, or it may develop secondary to antibiotic use.(17)

    If stool is clay-yellow in color, then it could indicate biliary dysfunction.(17)

    Gray-white stool is usually iatrogenic and due to administration of oral contrast agents, for instance, as part of a barium series.

    Just as we need to get in the habit of asking the client to use fecal scoring as a descriptor to compare today's stool to what is the pet's "norm," we need to ask about fecal color. We need to ask specifically what the feces used to look like in terms of color compared to what it does now. This provides us with a baseline. This information, combined with the historical timeline of when color changed, may facilitate diagnosis.

5. The estimate that you provided Alec lists fecal cytology as an in-house diagnostic test. Alec asks you what specifically you are looking for when you perform this test. You tell him that fecal cytology examines the feces under the microscope to identify the presence of infectious organisms.

    Fecal cytology is varied in its approach based upon organisms you are suspecting and/or searching for.

    - If you are looking for *Giardia trophozoites* or *T. foetus*, then you may perform what's called a direct fecal smear with saline.(1, 12) This allows you to see the organisms live and differentiate them from one another based upon their motion. *Giardia* is a flagellate protozoan parasite that has a "falling leaf" type of movement when viewed by light microscopy.(24) *T. foetus* is similar in size to *Giardia*, but has an undulating membrane that spans its entire body length.(24) This changes the movement of *T. foetus* such that it appears to roll rather erratically.(24)
    - If you are interested in identifying the eggs of roundworms, hookworms, whipworms, tapeworms, and coccidia, then fecal cytology is more likely to involve centrifugation followed by fecal flotation to concentrate ova before examining the sample under the microscope. (1, 12) One may also identify *Giardia* cysts using this approach; however, this ability is very much dependent upon the experience of the examiner.(12)
    - If you are interested in identifying bacterial populations, then you are more likely to use Diff-Quik, gram staining, or acid-fast stains on a thin layer of dried fecal matter to differentiate, for instance, *Clostridium* spp. from *Cryptosporidium* spp.(12)
    - Depending upon your index of suspicion and how comprehensive you wish to be in terms of your diagnostic work-up, you may choose to perform all three methods of fecal cytology.

6. When viewed under light microscopy, *Campylobacter* spp. take on a seagull wing S-shape.(1) (See Figure 23.2.)

    By contrast, when viewed under light microscopy, *Clostridium* spp. take on a characteristic safety pin shape.(1) (See Figure 23.3.)

7. It is important to recognize that, no, the gull wing shape is not pathognomonic for *Campylobacter* spp.(1, 25) Other bacteria that exhibit this shape include *Helicobacter* spp., *Arcobacter* spp., and *Anaerobiospirillum* spp.(25)

8. Although fecal cytology may be suggestive of CLOs or *Clostridium* spp., it is important to perform a fecal culture to confirm either diagnosis.(1, 25)

9. No, the presence of *Campylobacter* spp. within the gut is not necessarily pathologic.(1, 25) These organisms can be part of the normal flora.(25)

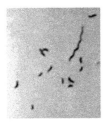

Figure 23.2 Campylobacter-like organisms on fecal examination. Note the characteristic gull wing or S-shape.

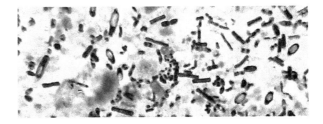

Figure 23.3 *Clostridium* spp. on fecal examination. Note the characteristic safety pin shape of the purple-staining organisms.

10. *Campylobacter* spp. are zoonotic.(25–31) Whether or not *Clostridium* spp. are zoonotic remains unclear.(25) However, it is thought that there is the potential for transmission of *Clostridium* spp. (25) Therefore, caution should be exerted, particularly in those households with one or more immunosuppressed individuals.(25)

11. Clinically important hookworms in dogs and cats include:(11)

    * *Ancylostoma caninum*
    * *Ancylostoma tubaeforme*
    * *Uncinaria stenocephala.*

12. Hookworms drain their hosts of blood so I would have expected this patient to present with pallor on physical exam if she had a significant hookworm burden.(32) I might also have expected this patient to have dark, tarry diarrhea, which was not described in the vignette.

13. The clinically relevant whipworm in dogs is *Trichuris vulpes*.(11)

14. Patients with whipworms may break with diarrhea and hematochezia, like this patient; however, in the long-term these patients often present with non-specific signs and weight loss.(19)

15. Hookworm and whipworm ova can be differentiated based upon appearance when viewed under light microscopy (see Figures 23.4–23.6).

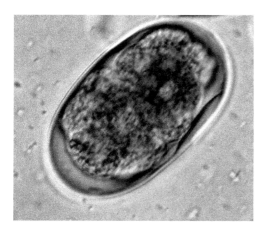

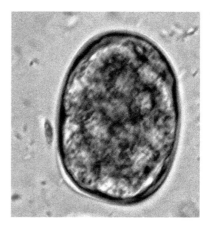

Figure 23.4 Hookworm ova (Uncinaria) on fecal examination, using light microscopy. Courtesy of Dr. Araceli Lucio-Forster, Cornell University College of Veterinary Medicine.

Figure 23.5 Hookworm ova (Ancylostoma) on fecal examination, using light microscopy. Courtesy of Dr. Araceli Lucio-Forster, Cornell University College of Veterinary Medicine.

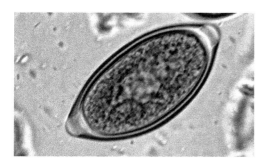

Figure 23.6 Whipworm egg, 20×. Note the football shape with plugs at both ends. Courtesy of Dr. Araceli Lucio-Forster, Cornell University College of Veterinary Medicine.

16. No, the shape of whipworm ova is not pathognomonic for *Trichuris*.(1) Other parasites, in particular the respiratory capillarids, *Eucoleus (Capillaria) aerophila* and *Eucoleus (Capillaria) boehmi*, are similarly shaped, but smaller in size.(19)

17. Hookworms are zoonotic.(1, 32, 33) They infect people by penetrating their skin, usually when people walk barefoot through wet sand or soil.(33) Once infected, larvae tunnel through the skin over a protracted course of weeks to months.(1) Larvae may remain in the skin, causing cutaneous larval migrans, or they may migrate beneath the skin to deeper tissues.(1) This results in so-called visceral larval migrans.(1) The liver and gut are most often involved.(32, 33)

    Canine whipworms, on the other hand, are not believed to be infectious to people.(1, 34) People can become infected with their own species of whipworm.

18. Hookworms or whipworms are treated with anthelmintic medications. The following medications are typically prescribed to treat hookworms: fenbendazole, pyrantel, and milbemycin. (35, 36)

    Febantel, fenbendazole, milbemycin, and moxidectin are often prescribed to manage whipworms.(34, 35)

19. In addition to drug name and dose, you need to know the life cycle of the parasite that you are dealing with in order to clear an infection. If you only treat hookworms or whipworms once, then an infection may not be cleared because all life stages have not been addressed. You also need to consider environmental decontamination or else the patient will become re-infected. Because environmental contamination is prevalent and difficult to address, it is advised that clients administer year-round broad-spectrum parasite control for coverage against animal infection as well as zoonotic disease.(34, 36) Drug resistance will need to be monitored to determine if deworming agents need to be rotated. Only time will tell.

20. Even if infectious causes of colitis are not identified using the in-house diagnostic tests that I've described, I cannot definitively rule out endoparasitism. Just because I have not recovered ova from fecal flotation does not guarantee that the patient is negative for endoparasites; it just means that none were seen on exam today. It may be that only a handful of worms are present, or the worms that are present are immature.(34) Alternatively, the patient may have a same-sex infection, in which case ova will never be produced.(34)

    Even when eggs are produced by endoparasites, it may be challenging to detect them on fecal flotation. In particular, false-negative examinations are common with whipworm infections. (34) False negatives occur in these cases because of the following three reasons.(34)

    - Whipworms have a long prepatent period. This means that eggs have not typically been shed in the feces at the time of initial presentation. Clinical signs often precede detection of ova.
    - Whipworm eggs are not shed continuously. They may be absent today, but present tomorrow. Unless serial fecal exams are performed, ova may be missed.
    - Whipworm eggs are dense. If adequate centrifugation is not performed, then they may not be recovered.

21. For the reasons that I outlined in the answer to Question #20 (above), I would be inclined to treat the patient with a broad-spectrum dewormer even if I fail to identify infectious organisms (including endoparasites) on in-house diagnostic tests. Even though the patient history makes me prioritize dietary indiscretion as a differential diagnosis over endoparasites, I would not want to overlook an easily treated diagnosis that could have potential health consequences for the humans in the home.

    In addition to prescribing a broad-spectrum dewormer, I would converse with the client about potential short-term changes to the diet that may facilitate resolution of colitis. These include:(16, 17, 21, 37–39)

- fasting for 24–48 hours (this is a treatment option that I am more likely to ascribe to when the patient presents not only with diarrhea, but also nausea or vomiting)
- feeding a low residue diet:
    - home-cooked boiled chicken breast (no skin, no bones) and cooked rice
    - home-cooked boiled chicken breast (no skin, no bones) and cooked plain pasta
    - lean boiled hamburger and cooked rice
    - lean boiled hamburger and cooked plain pasta
    - prescription diets, including, but not limited to:
        - Hill's Prescription Diet I/D
        - Purina ProPlan Veterinary Diet EN
        - Royal Canin Veterinary Diet Gastrointestinal Low Fat
        - hypoallergenic dietary trial (an elimination diet)
- increasing soluble dietary fiber, i.e. supplementing the diet with psyllium hydrophilic mucilloid (Metamucil®):
    - soluble fiber adsorbs water, thus drying out feces
    - soluble fiber is fermented by colonic bacteria
- Increasing insoluble dietary fiber, increases fecal bulk, distending the colon and thereby improving motility
- +/– probiotics
- +/– antimicrobial drugs.

22. If infectious causes of colitis are not identified, some clinicians choose to administer a trial of metronidazole.(16, 17) Metronidazole may or may not be indicated.

    Metronidazole is an antibiotic with anti-inflammatory effects.(35) Because of the latter, it is often prescribed as an anti-diarrheal agent.(35) In clinical practice, there is a saying that every case of diarrhea has a "metronidazole deficiency." Anecdotally, this refers to the fact that metronidazole tends to be over-prescribed in clinical practice.

    It is true that metronidazole can be effective at managing clinical signs (diarrhea) and clinical diagnoses (IBD).(35) It is also effective against Clostridial diarrhea.(35)

    However, a primary cause of colitis is rarely bacterial.(40)

    Furthermore, administration of metronidazole does not always speed resolution of diarrhea. (40–42) If it does, it may only hasten it by a short period of time (of the order of 1–5 days).

    One also worries about the development of antimicrobial resistance(40, 43–46), and the potential for metronidazole to adversely impact the normal flora of the gut.(47)

    Because metronidazole administration is associated with pros and cons, it is important to weigh the decision to treat in every patient rather than treating all patients with the same protocol.

23. If Yahtzee were a cat, then she would be at increased risk of developing neurotoxicity secondary to high-dose metronidazole.(35) Clinical signs might include nystagmus and seizure activity.(35)

CLINICAL PEARLS

- Fecal scoring plays an important role as a descriptor of stool consistency, shape, and texture. Different scoring systems are available. Stool that scores a 7/7 on the Nestlé-Purina scale is essentially liquified.

- Diarrhea results from one or more of the following mechanisms:
  - hypermotility of the gut
  - increased gut wall permeability
  - osmotic forces that draw water into the gut
  - active secretion into the gut.

- Loose stool can be classified as small bowel or large bowel based upon its characteristics.
  - Large bowel diarrhea, which was the clinical presentation for this chapter, is characterized by:
    - gelatinous semi-forced stool
    - high mucous content
    - increased frequency of defecation
    - increased urgency of defecation
    - tenesmus
    - +/– hematochezia.

- Large bowel diarrhea often results from dietary indiscretion, but can also be due to infectious colitis, endoparasitism, food allergies and/or intolerance, IBD, and neoplasia.

- History, physical examination, and rectal examination play essential roles in prioritizing differential diagnoses and in developing the diagnostic plan.

- Thorough fecal examination is an important step in the diagnostic process and should include one or more of the following tests:
  - gross observation of the fecal sample
  - direct fecal smear with saline
  - fecal flotation
  - stained fecal cytology.

- Not observing ova on fecal flotation cannot definitively rule out endoparasitism. There are many reasons for false negatives.

- Because of the potential for false negatives, patients with colitis are often dewormed. Dietary therapy is frequently used to speed resolution of clinical signs. Antimicrobial therapy can be considered on an individual patient basis.

References

1. Englar RE. Common clinical presentations in dogs and cats. Hoboken, NJ: Wiley/Blackwell; 2019.
2. Tilley LP, Smith FWK. The 5-minute veterinary consult: canine and feline. 3rd edition. lviii. Baltimore, MD: Lippincott Williams & Wilkins; 2004.
3. Schiller LR. Secretory diarrhea. Curr Gastroenterol Rep 1999;1(5):389–97.
4. Thiagarajah JR, Donowitz M, Verkman AS. Secretory diarrhoea: mechanisms and emerging therapies. Nat Rev Gastroenterol Hepatol 2015;12(8):446–57.

5. Allenspach K. Diagnosis of small intestinal disorders in dogs and cats. Vet Clin North Am Small Anim Pract 2013;43(6):1227–40.
6. Englar RE. Performing the small animal physical examination. Hoboken, NJ: Wiley; 2017.
7. Marks SL, Kather EJ. Bacterial-associated diarrhea in the dog: a critical appraisal. Vet Clin North Am Small Anim Pract 2003;33(5):1029–60.
8. Greene CE. Enteric bacterial infections. In: Greene CE, editor. Infectious diseases of the dog and cat. St Louis, MO: Saunders/Elsevier; 1998. p. 243–5.
9. Cave NJ, Marks SL, Kass PH, Melli AC, Brophy MA. Evaluation of a routine diagnostic fecal panel for dogs with diarrhea. J Am Vet Med Assoc 2002;221(1):52–9.
10. Guilford WG, Strombeck DR. Gastrointestinal tract infections, parasites, and toxicosis. In: Guilford WG, Center SA, editors. Stromback's Small animal gastroenterology. 3rd edition. Philadelphia, PA: W. B. Saunders; 1996. p. 411–32.
11. Magne ML. Selected topics in pediatric gastroenterology. Vet Clin North Am Small Anim Pract 2006;36(3): 533–48, vi, vi.
12. Greco DS. Diagnosis and dietary management of gastrointestinal disease: purina veterinary diets. Available from: https://www.purinaproplanvets.com/media/1202/gi_quick_reference_guide.pdf.
13. Gaschen F, editor. Small intestinal diarrhea – causes and treatment. WSAVA World Congress; 2006.
14. Matz ME. Chronic diarrhea in a dog. NAVC Clin's Brief 2006 (April):75–7.
15. Sokolow SH, Rand C, Marks SL, Drazenovich NL, Kather EJ, Foley JE. Epidemiologic evaluation of diarrhea in dogs in an animal shelter. Am J Vet Res 2005;66(6):1018–24.
16. Côté E. Clinical veterinary advisor. Dogs and cats. 3rd ed. St. Louis,. MO: Elsevier Mosby; 2015.
17. Ettinger SJ, Feldman EC, Côté E. Textbook of veterinary internal medicine: diseases of the dog and the cat. 8th ed. St. Louis, MO: Elsevier; 2017.
18. Englar R. Writing skills for veterinarians. Sheffield: 5M Publishing; 2019.
19. Zajac AM. A case of canine diarrhea. NAVC Clin's Brief 2003 (April):13–4.
20. German AJ. Large bowel diarrhea. NAVC Clin's Brief 2006 (February):54–5.
21. Lecoindre P, Gaschen FP. Chronic idiopathic large bowel diarrhea in the dog. Vet Clin North Am Small Anim Pract 2011;41(2):447–56.
22. Englar RE. Performing the small animal physical examination. Hoboken, NJ: Wiley/Blackwell; 2017.
23. Reece WO, Erickson HH, Goff JP, Uemura EE. Dukes' physiology of domestic animals. 13th ed. Ames, IA: Wiley/Blackwell; 2015.
24. Leib MS. Giardia and Tritrichomonas foetus: an update (Proceedings). DVM360 [Internet]; 2010. Available from: https://www.dvm360.com/view/giardia-and-tritrichomonas-foetus-update-proceedings.
25. Weese JS. Bacterial enteritis in dogs and cats: diagnosis, therapy, and zoonotic potential. Vet Clin North Am Small Anim Pract 2011;41(2):287–309.
26. Adak GK, Cowden JM, Nicholas S, Evans HS. The Public Health Laboratory Service national case-control study of primary indigenous sporadic cases of campylobacter infection. Epidemiol Infect 1995;115(1): 15–22.
27. Damborg P, Olsen KE, Møller Nielsen E, Guardabassi L. Occurrence of Campylobacter jejuni in pets living with human patients infected with C. jejuni. J Clin Microbiol 2004;42(3):1363–4.
28. Fullerton KE, Ingram LA, Jones TF, Anderson BJ, McCarthy PV, Hurd S, et al. Sporadic campylobacter infection in infants: a population-based surveillance case-control study. Pediatr Infect Dis J 2007;26(1):19–24.
29. Gillespie IA, O'Brien SJ, Adak GK, Tam CC, Frost JA, Bolton FJ, et al. Point source outbreaks of Campylobacter jejuni infection--are they more common than we think and what might cause them? Epidemiol Infect 2003;130(3):367–75.
30. Tam CC, Higgins CD, Neal KR, Rodrigues LC, Millership SE, O'Brien SJ, Campylobacter Case-Control Study Group. Chicken consumption and use of acid-suppressing medications as risk factors for Campylobacter enteritis, England. Emerg Infect Dis 2009;15(9):1402–8.
31. Tenkate TD, Stafford RJ. Risk factors for campylobacter infection in infants and young children: a matched case-control study. Epidemiol Infect 2001;127(3):399–404.
32. Guidelines for veterinarians: prevention of zoonotic transmission of ascarids and hookworms. Available from: https://www.cdc.gov/parasites/zoonotichookworm/resources/prevention.pdf.

33. Schantz PM. Zoonotic parasitic infections contracted from dogs and cats: how frequent are they? DVM; 2007. Available from: http://veterinarymedicine.dvm360.com/zoonotic-parasitic-infections-contracted-dogs-and-cats-how-frequent-are-they.

34. Trichuris Vulpis Trichuris: Companion Animal Parasite Council; 2020. Available from: https://capcvet.org/guidelines/trichuris-vulpis/#.

35. Plumb DC Stockholm, ed. Plumb's veterinary drug handbook. 9th ed. Hoboken, NJ: Pharma Vet Inc.; 2018.

36. Hookworms: Companion Animal Parasite Council; 2020. Available from: https://capcvet.org/guidelines/hookworms/#.

37. Leib MS. Chronic large bowel diarrhea in dogs: what's new? Proceedings. DVM360 [Internet] 2008. Available from: https://www.dvm360.com/view/chronic-large-bowel-diarrhea-dogs-whats-new-proceedings-0.

38. White R, Atherly T, Guard B, Rossi G, Wang C, Mosher C, et al. Randomized, controlled trial evaluating the effect of multi-strain probiotic on the mucosal microbiota in canine idiopathic inflammatory bowel disease. Gut Microbes 2017;8(5):451–66.

39. Jensen AP, Bjørnvad CR. Clinical effect of probiotics in prevention or treatment of gastrointestinal disease in dogs: A systematic review. J Vet Intern Med 2019;33(5):1849–64.

40. Grimes M. Antibiotics in canine GI disease: when to use and when to ditch. DVM360 [Internet]; 2020. Available from: https://www.dvm360.com/view/antibiotics-in-canine-gi-disease-when-to-use-and-when-to-ditch.

41. Sharma A, Thompson MS, Scrivani PV, Dykes NL, Yeager AE, Freer SR, Erb HN. Comparison of radiography and ultrasonography for diagnosing small-intestinal mechanical obstruction in vomiting dogs. Vet Radiol Ultrasound 2011;52(3):248–55.

42. Langlois DK, Koenigshof AM, Mani R. Metronidazole treatment of acute diarrhea in dogs: A randomized double blinded placebo-controlled clinical trial. J Vet Intern Med 2020;34(1):98–104.

43. Lappin MR, Blondeau J, Boothe D, Breitschwerdt EB, Guardabassi L, Lloyd DH, et al. Antimicrobial use guidelines for treatment of respiratory tract disease in dogs and cats: antimicrobial Guidelines Working Group of the International Society for Companion Animal Infectious Diseases. J Vet Intern Med 2017;31(2):279–94.

44. Marks SL, Kather EJ. Antimicrobial susceptibilities of canine Clostridium difficile and Clostridium perfringens isolates to commonly utilized antimicrobial drugs. Vet Microbiol 2003;94(1):39–45.

45. Schmidt VM, Pinchbeck G, McIntyre KM, Nuttall T, McEwan N, Dawson S, Williams NJ. Routine antibiotic therapy in dogs increases the detection of antimicrobial-resistant faecal Escherichia coli. J Antimicrob Chemother 2018;73(12):3305–16.

46. Weese JS, Blondeau J, Boothe D, Guardabassi LG, Gumley N, Papich M, et al. International Society for Companion Animal Infectious Diseases (ISCAID) guidelines for the diagnosis and management of bacterial urinary tract infections in dogs and cats. Vet J 2019;247:8–25.

47. Suchodolski JS, Olson E, Honneffer J. Effects of hydrolyzed protein and metronidazole on the fecal microbiome and metabolome in healthy dogs. J Vet Intern Med 2016;30(4):1407–519.

Case 24

The Dog That Can't Keep Food Down

Draco is a long-term patient of yours. You have known him since his adoption by Lenny Chisum from a local humane organization at 2 years of age. Draco is the prototypical Boxer: overexuberant in every way. There aren't enough hours in the day to burn off his excess energy. Although a doggie door makes it possible for him to come and go from the home whenever he pleases, Draco spends most of his days roaming the property, unsupervised. Lenny inherited a significant amount of land, and although he does not use it as a working ranch, that does not stop Draco from finding distractions with which to occupy his time. There is always something to dig up, chase, or ingest.

Draco samples everything he can get his mouth on, so it isn't surprising that on occasion he upchucks something that doesn't quite go down right. Yet, for the past month or so, Lenny has noticed an upswing in these episodes. Instead of once a month, Lenny now finds piles of ingested food scattered around the house, two

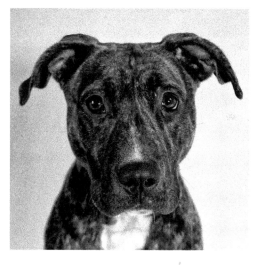

Figure 24.1 Meet your new patient, Draco, an 8-year-old, castrated male Boxer Cross. Courtesy of John Schwartz.

to three times a week. It is rare that Lenny catches Draco in the act, but because the dog is the only pet in the home, there is no one else to blame.

Lenny is presenting Draco to you for evaluation of increased frequency of vomiting. The technician takes his vital signs before loading Draco into the next available consultation room. She notes that Draco has lost six pounds since his last visit eight months ago. Lenny is surprised by this weight loss. It's definitely not because of increased activity. If anything, Draco tires out more quickly and his energy seems 'off'. Lenny had blamed Draco's slowing down on age, but now he's concerned that there's something more insidious brewing.

Weight: 62 lb (28.2 kg)
BCS: 4/9
Mentation: BAR

TPR

T: 101.7°F (38.7°C)
P: 86 beats per minute
R: panting

361

Round One of Questions for Case 24: The Dog That Can't Keep Food Down

1. Draco is presenting for evaluation of vomiting. What is the appropriate medical term for vomiting? What is the appropriate medical term for the contents of the material that has been thrown up?
2. Vomiting is a reflex. Where is the vomiting center located within Draco's brain?
3. The vomiting center in Draco's brain receives inputs from other parts of the body. Where are the four primary sources of input located that tell Draco's brain it's time to vomit?
4. Keeping in mind the sources that you identified in Question #3 (above), what are common triggers of vomiting at each location?
5. Which sensation precedes vomiting?
6. Which clinical signs typically precede vomiting?
7. Is vomiting an active or passive process?
8. If Lenny witnessed Draco vomiting, describe what you would expect him to see.
9. How sure are you that Draco is in fact vomiting?
10. What other process could explain his purging of food?
11. What additional information do you need from Lenny to be certain?
12. Using an open-ended question or statement, how will you ask Lenny for the information that you expressed a need for in Question #10 (above)?
13. What are essential closed-ended follow-up questions that you could ask Lenny to clarify the patient history?

Answers to Round One of Questions for Case 24: The Dog That Can't Keep Food Down

1. Draco is presenting for evaluation of vomiting. The appropriate medical term for vomiting is emesis.(1) The product of emesis is vomitus.

2. The vomiting center is located within Draco's brain at the level of the lateral reticular formation of the medulla oblongata.(2–6)

3. The vomiting center within Draco's medulla oblongata receives inputs from four primary sources:(2–5, 7–11)

   - cerebral cortex
   - chemoreceptor trigger zone (CRTZ)
   - peripheral sensory receptors
   - vestibular apparatus.

   These four sources of information pass on essential messages to the vomiting center to initiate vomiting.(4, 9)

4. Stress, anxiety, and excitement are processed within the cerebral cortex and can trigger vomiting reflex.(3) This so-called psychogenic vomiting is relatively common in people and is thought to be possible in animals, although the mechanism by which this occurs has not yet been established.(2, 3)

   The CRTZ sits along the floor of the medulla's fourth ventricle, where the blood-brain barrier is incomplete, allowing the CRTZ to screen the bloodstream for chemical red flags.(2–4, 7, 12) In addition to bacterial toxins, the presence of the following drugs and toxins in the bloodstream may trigger alarm:(2, 3, 8)

- drugs
  - antibiotics
  - apomorphine
  - cardiac glycosides
  - chemotherapeutic agents
  - morphine
  - non-steroidal anti-inflammatory drugs (NSAIDs)
  - salicylates
  - select antibiotics
- uremic toxins.

The abdominal viscera contains the greatest concentration of peripheral sensory receptors in the entire body.(2, 3) As visceral organs distend, their degree of stretch is translated into an electrical impulse that messages the vomiting center.(2, 3) Inflammation in these organs, without distension, can also trigger sensory receptors to message the vomiting center.(2) Organs outside of the digestive tract also contain sensory receptors that report to the vomiting center. The urinary bladder, for instance, communicates with the vomiting center through the vagus and sympathetic nerve trunk.(2, 7)

The vestibular system, which coordinates the body's posture and balance, also relays information to the vomiting center.(13–19) A functional vestibular system requires both central and peripheral components.(14) The central vestibular system is composed of the brainstem, the cerebellum, and two caudal cerebellar peduncles.(20, 21) The peripheral vestibular system is composed of the middle ear and inner ear, including the semicircular canals, the utricle and saccule, and the eighth cranial nerve (CN VIII), the vestibulocochlear nerve.(20–22)

It is the peripheral vestibular system that communicates with the vomiting center through CN VIII.(3) This explains how motion sickness causes emesis.(2–4)

5. Vomiting is preceded by nausea.(2, 3)

6. Dogs or cats that are about to vomit typically demonstrate one or more of the following signs: (3, 4, 10)

- frequent swallowing
- licking their lips
- ptyalism (drooling).

7. It is an active process to initiate emesis.(3, 23) It requires force to bring material up and out of the digestive tract.(13)

8. If Lenny witnessed Draco vomiting, then I would have expected him to see Draco having abdominal contractions and heaving.(13)

9. We are not certain that Draco is vomiting because Lenny has not actually witnessed this. Lenny has only found the aftermath.

10. We cannot rule out regurgitation based upon the clinical vignette and the patient history. Unlike vomiting, regurgitation is a passive process by which food is evacuated from the upper digestive tract.(23–25) There is no effort involved.(13) There are no abdominal contractions.(13) Regurgitation is also not typically preceded by nausea.(24, 25)

11. Ideally, I would want to hear a description from Lenny himself of the actual act of Draco evacuating food. Since we can't get that level of detail (Lenny hasn't been present during an episode), I would want to ask more questions about the actual material that was brought up by Draco.

Regurgitated material comes from the esophagus, so it is typically tubular in shape.(24) The food is in its undigested form because it has yet to reach the stomach to mix with gastric acid to form chyme.(13) The undigested material may be mixed with water and frothy saliva, but not bile.(24)

On the other hand, bile is frequently seen in vomitus.(13) Bile is a greenish to yellow-brown slurry of acids, salts, pigments, and other compounds that are made by the liver and stored in the gall bladder.(13) Bile is typically released by the gall bladder to facilitate digestion, but is often evacuated with stomach contents during emesis.(13)

I would therefore question Lenny about the shape of the vomitus. Although this is a subjective line of questioning, a tubular shape is more consistent with regurgitation. So is undigested food and the absence of bile.

12. I could make use of the following open-ended statement: "Lenny, tell me about Draco's vomit." I could also rephrase that statement into a question: "Lenny, what does Draco's vomit look like?" or "Lenny, how would you describe Draco's vomit?"

For more information on open-ended questions or statements, please refer to either *Writing Skills for Veterinarians* or *A Guide to Oral Communication in Veterinary Medicine*.(1, 12)

13. I may need to ask the following closed-ended clarifying questions to gain additional details that will help me to differentiate vomiting from regurgitation.

- What color is Draco's vomit?
- Does Draco vomit food?
- Is the food that comes up in his vomit digested?

Although Lenny has not witnessed Draco "vomiting," he may have witnessed what happens in the immediate period before each event. So, it is worth asking the following.

- Before each episode, do you notice Draco licking his lips a lot?
- Before each episode, do you notice Draco drooling a lot?
- Before each episode, do you notice Draco swallowing a lot?

These questions will help us to establish whether Draco is nauseous. If he is, then he is more likely to be vomiting than regurgitating.

For more information on closed-ended questions, please refer to either *Writing Skills for Veterinarians* or *A Guide to Oral Communication in Veterinary Medicine*.(1, 12)

Returning to Case 24: The Dog That Can't Keep Food Down

You ask Lenny to describe the "vomit." Lenny shares that episodes are sporadic. When episodes occur, they are usually within an hour or so of eating. Food that comes up is undigested. The bolus is tubular in shape and smells sour. Often, the contents are slimy. Lenny does not think that any bile comes up.

As you're examining Draco, Lenny recalls that he did happen to observe one episode yesterday morning. The event occurred about 20 minutes after eating breakfast. Lenny heard what sounded like an isolated gag. He looked up. He saw Draco open his mouth, and food literally fell out. He did not observe retching or heaving. It seemed easy, like he didn't have to work at it at all.

Lenny is not sure if the two are related, but lately Draco's breath has an unusual odor. This surprises Lenny because Draco's teeth look clean, not like they usually do just before a dental cleaning. You agree with Lenny that, on physical examination, Draco's teeth look spotless. Other than caudal thigh muscle atrophy, his evaluation is unremarkable.

Round Two of Questions for Case 24: The Dog That Can't Keep Food Down

1. Based upon the new details that have been provided in the patient history, is Draco more likely to be vomiting or regurgitating?
2. What could account for the unusual odor that Lenny is smelling on Draco's breath?

Answers to Round Two of Questions for Case 24: The Dog That Can't Keep Food Down

1. Based upon the expanded patient profile, Draco is more likely to be regurgitating. The client has witnessed a passive process and the tubular contents suggest that they came from the esophagus rather than the stomach.

2. If Draco is regurgitating, then undigested food is retained within the esophagus. If this sequestration of food within the esophagus is protracted, then the ingesta essentially decays. This creates an unpleasant odor.(26)

Returning to Case 24: The Dog That Can't Keep Food Down

You share your concerns with Lenny that Draco is likely to be regurgitating rather than vomiting. Consider the following questions as you work through the case and the implications of your presumptive diagnosis.

Round Three of Questions for Case 24: The Dog That Can't Keep Food Down

1. Fill in the blank: Regurgitation is the hallmark of disease within the _____.
2. The esophagus is the conduit between the mouth and the stomach. Define dysphagia.
3. Outline where dysphagia may arise along the pathway of transporting food from the mouth to the stomach.
4. Outline the broad causes of esophageal dysphagia.
5. Which cause(s) of esophageal dysphagia is/are LEAST likely in Draco?
6. Which cause(s) of esophageal dysphagia is/are most likely in Draco?
7. In addition to performing a physical exam, how might you investigate esophageal dysphagia further? What will you include in your diagnostic plan?

Answers to Round Three of Questions for Case 24: The Dog That Can't Keep Food Down

1. Regurgitation is the hallmark of disease within the esophagus.(24, 27)

2. Dysphagia is defined as difficulty transporting food from the mouth to the stomach.

3. There are four main types of dysphagia.(13)

- Oral dysphagia – patients with this condition struggle with prehension of food, that is, getting food into the mouth.
- Pharyngeal dysphagia – patients with this condition struggle to move a bolus of food from the entrance of the mouth to the base of the tongue.
- Cricopharyngeal dysphagia – patients with this condition are unable to successfully swallow.(28–31)
- Esophageal dysphagia – patients with this condition struggle to transport the bolus of food from the esophagus to the stomach.(28, 32)

4. Causes of esophageal dysphagia include:(13, 28, 32, 33)

- esophageal "mass":
    - esophageal stricture
    - foreign body
    - extraluminal compression of the esophagus:
        - significant cardiomegaly
        - hilar lymphadenopathy
        - mediastinal mass
        - vascular ring abnormalities
    - intraluminal mass that occludes the lumen of the esophagus
- esophagitis
- megaesophagus:
    - primary
    - secondary.

5. Vascular ring anomalies, such as persistent right aortic arch (PRAA), are least likely in Draco. (28, 34, 35) Affected patients tend to present for evaluation of regurgitation as weanlings, as they switch from a milk-based to solid-food diet. The esophagus essentially becomes strangled by an encircling branch of the aorta that has failed to regress.(34) Draco is well past the weanling stage of life. At 8 years old, I would have expected this to have presented before today.

   An esophageal foreign body is also less likely to explain Draco's clinical presentation because his history of regurgitation has been ongoing for approximately a month.

   Esophageal masses are rare in dogs.(36) They represent less than 0.5% of canine cancer.(36)

   Significant cardiomegaly is unlikely in Draco without being associated with abnormalities on physical exam. If Draco does in fact have heart disease to the degree necessary to cause esophageal dysfunction, then I would expect him to demonstrate one or more of the following physical exam findings at today's visit:

- heart murmur
- +/– increased bronchovesicular lung sounds
- +/– mild crackles on auscultation of the caudodorsal lung fields.
   Instead, Draco's cardiovascular exam was within normal limits.

6. Of the remaining differential diagnoses, esophageal stricture and megaesophagus are likelier options in Draco.

   Esophageal strictures may result from esophagitis, inflammation of the esophageal mucosa. (27, 33) Risk factors for developing esophagitis include:(13, 33)

- brachycephalic breeds*** and Shar Pei dogs:
    - these breeds are more likely to have abnormal lower esophageal sphincters
    - abnormal lower esophageal sphincters increase the risk for gastroesophageal reflux

- reflux is acidic
- acid burns the esophagus
- delayed gastric emptying
- "dry pilling" may lead to esophageal ulceration and/or stricture:
  - bisphosphonates
  - clindamycin and cats(27)
  - doxycycline and cats(27, 37, 38)
- esophageal foreign body due to abnormal ingestive behaviors***:
  - full obstruction
  - partial obstruction
- esophageal infection
- frequent vomiting
- general anesthesia
- hiatal hernia
- hypergastrinemia, e.g. as caused by a gastrinoma(27)
- radiation therapy
- trichobezoars, or hairballs.

Items that are starred (***) above are patient-specific risk factors for Draco.

Megaesophagus is a pathological condition in which the esophagus is dilated and hypomotile.(29, 30) This causes retention of food and water within the esophagus. Depending upon the severity of esophageal dilation, food and water may not make it into the lower digestive tract for processing.(29, 30) This results in regurgitation.(13) On physical examination, I might have expected to palpate an enlarged esophagus at the thoracic inlet or pain on esophageal palpation.(29, 30, 35) However, neither physical exam finding is consistent. The absence of either a palpably distended or painful esophagus cannot definitely rule out megaesophagus.

7.   Although Draco's history and clinical signs are helpful at narrowing down the list of differential diagnoses, we still need to formulate a diagnostic plan.(32) Survey images of the thoracic cavity are an appropriate first step in the work-up of a patient with esophageal disease, including megaesophagus.(29, 30, 35) Survey radiographs may require the use of contrast to highlight an esophageal foreign body (unlikely in Draco), esophageal stricture (possible in Draco), vascular ring anomaly (unlikely in Draco), or esophageal masses (rare in dogs).(28) Esophageal strictures are best highlighted by feeding barium-soaked kibble: liquid will easily pass through the stricture, but kibble will not.(28)

The patient's ability to swallow and the function of the esophagus to propel the swallowed bolus forward may also be evaluated using contrast-enhanced videofluoroscopy.(28) Although this imaging modality is not typically available in primary care companion animal practice, it is becoming increasingly common at referral (specialty) hospitals. Liquid barium is administered to the patient and boluses are tracked real-time all the way to the stomach.(28) The ability to evaluate the recording, frame by frame, facilitates diagnosis of oropharyngeal and/or esophageal dysfunction.(13, 28)

Returning to Case 24: The Dog That Can't Keep Food Down

You convince Lenny to proceed with two-view thoracic radiographs. The lateral radiograph is diagnostic (see Figure 24.2).

Round Four of Questions for Case 24: The Dog That Can't Keep Food Down

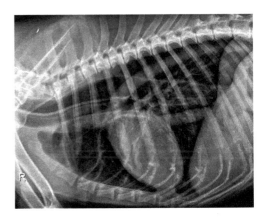

Figure 24.2 Right lateral thoracic radiograph.

1. Based upon the provided radiograph, what is Draco's diagnosis?
2. The diagnosis that you identified in Question #1 (above) may be congenital or acquired. Which canine breeds are at risk if the patient's condition is congenital? Which feline breeds are at risk?
3. If Draco has the diagnosis that you identified in Question #1, then he would have acquired it. What are causes of this condition when it is acquired?
4. What is the potential impact that Draco's diagnosis could have on his airway?
5. Draco does not have evidence of airway disease at this time. Lenny asks which clinical sign(s) he should keep an eye out for that might indicate Draco's condition has resulted in airway disease.
6. What is the best approach to managing Draco's condition?
7. Which, if any, additional tests might you pursue in any dog with megaesophagus?
8. Which, if any, additional tests might you be inclined to pursue in Draco and why?
9. How do you propose to manage idiopathic megaesophagus?

Answers to Round Four of Questions for Case 24: The Dog That Can't Keep Food Down

1. Based upon the provided radiograph, Draco's diagnosis is megaesophagus (see **Plate 11**).

2. Megaesophagus may be congenital(39–41) or acquired.(39, 42–44) The following canine breeds are at increased risk of developing congenital megaesophagus:(24, 32, 39–41)

   - Fox terriers
   - German shepherd
   - Great Dane
   - Irish Setter
   - Labrador retriever
   - Newfoundland
   - Shar Pei.

   The Siamese breed of cat is also predisposed to congenital megaesophagus.(24, 29)

3. Owing to Draco's signalment and history, this condition was acquired. Acquired megaesophagus may result from:(32, 39, 42–45)

   - botulism
   - dysautonomia
   - esophageal obstruction
   - hypoadrenocorticism
   - hypothyroidism
   - lead poisoning

- myasthenia gravis
- polymyositis
- polyneuritis
- systemic lupus erythematosus (SLE)
- thallium toxicosis.

Idiopathic acquired megaesophagus is also common.(29, 30, 32)

4. Regurgitation may cause aspiration pneumonia.(24, 27)

5. Signs of aspiration pneumonia include:(24, 27, 33)

- adventitious lung sounds – crackles
- anorexia or reduced appetite
- cough
- depression
- dyspnea
- fever
- increased respiratory effort
- increased respiratory rate
- lethargy
- mucopurulent nasal discharge
- respiratory distress.

6. In order to treat megaesophagus most effectively, you need to do your best to establish the underlying etiology.(32) When you have diagnosed the underlying etiology, you can address it and in this way hopefully reduce, if not resolve, megaesophagus. Note that resolution does not always occur. Clients should be warned that, for instance, only about half of patients with megaesophagus secondary to myasthenia gravis experience resolution of megaesophagus when the primary condition is treated.(46)

7. To establish the underlying etiology, you may wish to consider one or more of the following tests:(30, 31, 46)

- complete blood count (CBC), chemistry panel – findings may be supportive of hypoadreno-corticism and/or hypothyroidism
- ACTH stimulation test – findings will confirm or refute hypoadrenocorticism
- acetylcholine (Ach) receptor antibody test
- atropine response test – which may rule out dysautonomia
- esophagoscopy – which may confirm the presence of a stricture, mass, and/or esophagitis
- muscle biopsy – rules out polymyositis
- Tensilon test – rules out myasthenia gravis
- thyroid panel – rules out hypothyroidism.

8. Draco has a history of weight loss and slowing down. He also has caudal thigh muscle atrophy on physical exam.

Hypothyroidism is unlikely based upon his history of weight loss. However, myasthenia gravis is a condition that I would want to investigate further because it does cause focal or generalized paresis that is worsened by activity.

At rest, a patient with myasthenia gravis is typically clinically normal.(13, 30, 31) However, with exercise, the patient is easily fatigued.(13, 30, 31) Weakness is progressive until the patient is rendered non-ambulatory. The patient may be mistaken for being lame when in fact the patient is simply weak.

Weakness results from immune-mediated disease in which antibodies attack the acetylcholine receptors at neuromuscular junctions.(13, 30, 31) This interferes with acetylcholine delivering the message that it intended to transmit.(13, 30, 31) Unbound acetylcholine is destroyed by acetylcholinesterase, resulting in muted muscle stimulation that diminishes rapidly. (13, 30, 31) Clinically, this translates into a progressively weak patient.(13, 30, 31)

Based upon the history, it would behoove us to explore the possibility of this diagnosis further. The easiest in-clinic test to perform is called the Tensilon test.(13, 30, 31) A dose of a short-acting anticholinesterase, edrophonium chloride, is administered to the patient intravenously.(13, 30, 31) This allows acetylcholine to accumulate at the neuromuscular junction.(13, 30, 31) Because there is more acetylcholine available for longer periods of time, the neurochemical messages are more easily received by the affected muscle(s).(13, 30, 31) Thus, the patient with myasthenia gravis regains strength.(13, 30, 31) The effect is short-lived. If the patient has a positive Tensilon test and serology is confirmatory for acetylcholine autoantibodies, then a longer-acting, commercially available anticholinesterase, such as pyridostigmine or neostigmine bromide, can be prescribed.

9. Many cases of megaesophagus are also idiopathic, meaning that there is no known cause. In these cases, a multimodal approach to management is indicated. Management of idiopathic megaesophagus may include the following.(30, 31, 46, 47)

    • Nutritional support

        • Feed small amounts of a high-calorie diet, frequently.
        • Feed a slurry of gruel or canned food meatballs to facilitate bolus propulsion through the hypomotile esophagus.
        • Feed the patient in an elevated position, meaning that his front half is raised higher than his lower half such that gravity facilitates bolus propulsion through the hypomotile esophagus:

            • using a Bailey chair may help
            • maintain this elevated position for up to 30 minutes after eating.

        • In severe cases, a gastric tube may be placed to bypass the esophagus.

    • Reduce activity for at least 30 minutes following each meal.
    • Administer a prokinetic at least 30 minutes prior to meals to enhance motility of the smooth muscle of the gastrointestinal tract (e.g. cisapride, metoclopramide).
    • Manage esophagitis with a slurry of oral sucralfate to coat esophageal lesions and facilitate healing.
    • Prescribe an antacid to reduce gastric pH if reflux is contributing to esophagitis.

CLINICAL PEARLS

• Patients are often presented for vomiting when in fact they are regurgitating.

• When a patient presents for "vomiting," it is important to confirm if the patient truly is in fact "vomiting."

• Distinguishing between vomiting and regurgitating requires thoughtful history-taking.

    • Vomiting is an active process: it takes effort to evacuate the contents of the stomach. For this reason, a client will witness abdominal contractions. S/he will see the patient heaving before stomach contents are brought up.
    • Regurgitation is passive. The patient opens its mouth and food falls out without effort.
    • Vomiting often is associated with bile; regurgitation is not.
    • Vomiting often is preceded by nausea; regurgitation is not.
    • Regurgitated contents are often tubular in shape because food was retained in the tubular esophagus.

• Regurgitation is the hallmark of esophageal disease. Patients with esophageal disease have difficulty transporting food from the esophagus to the stomach. This may result from:

- • esophageal mass or stricture
- • esophageal dilation and/or hypomotility (megaesophagus).
- • Megaesophagus may be congenital or acquired.
- • Megaesophagus is diagnosed by radiographs. Contrast may be administered to facilitate diagnosis. Contrast also facilitates diagnosis of strictures.
- • Management of megaesophagus is improved when the underlying etiology is identified. Management of idiopathic cases requires a multimodal approach that typically includes nutritional support and prokinetic therapy.
- • Megaesophagus is difficult to treat and increases the patient's risk of presenting in respiratory distress for aspiration pneumonia.

References

1. Englar R. Writing skills for veterinarians. Sheffield: 5M Publishing; 2019.
2. King LG, Donaldson MT. Acute vomiting. Vet Clin North Am Small Anim Pract 1994;24(6):1189–206.
3. Twedt DC. Differential diagnosis and therapy of vomiting. Vet Clin North Am Small Anim Pract 1983;13(3):503–20.
4. Elwood C, Devauchelle P, Elliott J, Freiche V, German AJ, Gualtieri M, et al. Emesis in dogs: a review. J Small Anim Pract 2010;51(1):4–22.
5. Encarnacion HJ, Parra J, Mears E, Sadler V. Vomiting. Compendium 2009;31(3):E8.
6. Batchelor DJ, Devauchelle P, Elliott J, Elwood CM, Freiche V, Gualtieri M, et al. Mechanisms, causes, investigation and management of vomiting disorders in cats: a literature review. J Feline Med Surg 2013;15(4):237–65.
7. Feldman M. Nausea and vomiting. In: Sleizenger MH, Fordtran JS, editors. Gastrointestinal disease: pathophysiology, diagnosis, and management. 4th ed. Philadelphia, PA: W.B. Saunders; 1989. p. 222–38.
8. Fuchs S, Jaffe D. Vomiting. Pediatr Emerg Care. 1990;6(2):164–70.
9. Argenzio RA. Gastrointestinal motility. In: Dukes HH, Reece WO, editors. Dukes' physiology of domestic animals. 12th ed. Ithaca, NY: Comstock Pub. Associates; 2004. p. 391–404.
10. McGrotty Y. Medical management of acute and chronic vomiting in dogs and cats. Pract 2010;32(10):478–83.
11. Armstrong PJ. GI intervention: approach to diagnosis and therapy of the vomiting patient. Today's. Vet Pract 2013 (March/April):18–27.
12. Englar R. A guide to. Oral Communication in Veterinary Medicine. Sheffield: 5M Publishing; 2020.
13. Englar RE. Common clinical presentations in dogs and cats. Hoboken, NJ: Wiley/Blackwell; 2019.
14. Rossmeisl JH, Jr. Vestibular disease in dogs and cats. Vet Clin North Am Small Anim Pract 2010;40(1):81–100.
15. DeLahunta A, Glass E, Kent M. Veterinary neuroanatomy and clinical neurology. 4th ed. St. Louis, MO: Elsevier; 2015.
16. Angelaki DE, Cullen KE. Vestibular system: the many facets of a multimodal sense. Annu Rev Neurosci 2008;31:125–50.
17. Brandt T, Strupp M. General vestibular testing. Clin Neurophysiol 2005;116(2):406–26.
18. Thomas WB. Vestibular dysfunction. Vet Clin North Am Small Anim Pract 2000;30(1):227–49.
19. Troxel MT, Drobatz KJ, Vite CH. Signs of neurologic dysfunction in dogs with central versus peripheral vestibular disease. J Am Vet Med Assoc 2005;227(4):570–4.
20. Evans HE, DeLahunta A. Guide to the dissection of the dog. 6th ed. St Louis, MO: Saunders; 2004.
21. Evans HE, Miller ME. Miller's anatomy of the dog. 4th ed. St. Louis, MO: Elsevier; 2013.
22. Rylander H. Vestibular syndrome: what's causing the head tilt and other neurologic signs? DVM360 [Internet]; 2012. Available from: http://veterinarymedicine.dvm360.com/vestibular-syndrome-whats-causing-head-tilt-and-other-neurologic-signs.

23. Tams TR. Diagnosing of acute and chronic vomiting in dogs and cats. 2017. Available from: https://vvma.org/resources/2017%20VVC%20Notes/Tams-Vomiting%20in%20Dogs%20and%20Cats%20-%20Diagnosis.pdf.
24. Sherding RG. Regurgitation, dysphagia, and esophageal dysmotility. DVM; 2011. Available from: http://veterinarycalendar.dvm360.com/regurgitation-dysphagia-and-esophageal-dysmotility-proceedings. 360 [Internet].
25. Gallagher A. Regurgitation or vomiting? NAVC Clin's Brief 2012 (June):33–5.
26. Sherding RG. Regurgitation, dysphagia, and esophageal dysmotility (Proceedings). DVM360 [Internet]; 2011. Available from: https://www.dvm360.com/view/regurgitation-dysphagia-and-esophageal-dysmotility-proceedings.
27. Sherding RG. Esophagitis and esophageal stricture. DVM; 2011. 360 [Internet]. Available from: Esophagitis and esophageal stricture.
28. Pollard RE. Imaging evaluation of dogs and cats with Dysphagia. ISRN Vet Sci 2012;2012:238505.
29. Tilley LP, Smith FWK. The 5-minute veterinary consult: canine and feline. 3rd ed. Baltimore, MD: Lippincott Williams & Wilkins; 2004.
30. Côté E. Clinical veterinary advisor. Dogs and cats. 3rd ed. St. Louis, MO: Elsevier Mosby; 2015.
31. Ettinger SJ, Feldman EC, Côté E. Textbook of veterinary internal medicine: diseases of the dog and the cat. 8th ed. St. Louis, MO: Elsevier; 2017.
32. Marks SL, editor. Dysphagia and regurgitation in dogs – more common than you think! Canine Medicine Symposium; 2008.
33. Bissett S. Esophagitis. NAVC Clin's Brief 2012 (June):23–6.
34. Buchanan JW. Tracheal signs and associated vascular anomalies in dogs with persistent right aortic arch. J Vet Intern Med 2004;18(4):510–4.
35. Carlisle WT, Egger EL. Differential diagnosis of persistent dysphagia and regurgitation in the young. Iowa State Univ Vet 1980;42(1):[14–8]. Available from: https://lib.dr.iastate.edu/cgi/viewcontent.cgi?article=2975andcontext=iowastate_veterinarian.
36. Ridgway RL, Suter PF. Clinical and radiographic signs in primary and metastatic esophageal neoplasms of the dog. J Am Vet Med Assoc 1979;174(7):700–4.
37. Leib MS, editor. Doxycyline esophagitis/stricture in cats. Orlando: NAVC, Floria; 2005.
38. McGrotty YL, Knottenbelt CM. Oesophageal stricture in a cat due to oral administration of tetracyclines. J Small Anim Pract 2002;43(5):221–3.
39. Washabau RJ. Gastrointestinal motility disorders and gastrointestinal prokinetic therapy. Vet Clin North Am Small Anim Pract 2003;33(5):1007–28.
40. Holland CT, Satchell PM, Farrow BR. Vagal esophagomotor nerve function and esophageal motor performance in dogs with congenital idiopathic megaesophagus. Am J Vet Res 1996;57(6):906–13.
41. Holland CT, Satchell PM, Farrow BR. Selective vagal afferent dysfunction in dogs with congenital idiopathic megaoesophagus. Auton Neurosci Basic Clin 2002;99(1):18–23.
42. Gaynor AR, Shofer FS, Washabau RJ. Risk factors for acquired megaesophagus in dogs. J Am Vet Med Assoc 1997;211(11):1406–12.
43. Shelton GD, Willard MD, Cardinet GH, 3rd, Lindstrom J. Acquired myasthenia gravis. Selective involvement of esophageal, pharyngeal, and facial muscles. J Vet Intern Med 1990;4(6):281–4.
44. Shelton GD, Schule A, Kass PH. Risk factors for acquired myasthenia gravis in dogs: 1,154 cases (1991–1995). J Am Vet Med Assoc 1997;211(11):1428–31.
45. Fracassi F, Tamborini A. Reversible megaoesophagus associated with primary hypothyroidism in a dog. Vet Rec 2011;168(12):329b.
46. Ridgway MD. Megaesophagus. DVM360 [Internet]; 2010. Available from: https://www.cliniciansbrief.com/article/megaesophagus#.
47. Plumb DC. Plumb's veterinary drug handbook. 9th ed. Hoboken, NJ: Pharma Vet Inc.; 2018.

Case 25

The Vomiting Dog

You have known Soli since he was 12 weeks old. Much to the dismay of his owner, Xander Beasley, Soli has been a repeat customer. Xander often joked that he had paid for the new wing of the clinic with Soli's medical bills!

Soli had always been a mouthy pup, sampling everything that he could wrap his muzzle around. It didn't matter if it was food or not. If it were accessible, then he would try it. At three months old, he presented for electrical burns after chewing on computer cords. At 4 months old, you removed a crayon from his pharynx. At 5 months old, he ate a slipper, and at 6 months old, a golf ball. To his credit, everything had passed (or had been removed by you before it could cause an obstruction!).

Xander had hoped that Soli would grow out of it, but it was becoming apparent that Soli was a lost cause. At age 3, he hadn't slowed down his enthusiasm for eating items that were not legitimately his. **Plates 12–18** show the items that have been retrieved (non-surgically) from Soli's digestive tract after at-home or in-clinic induction of emesis.

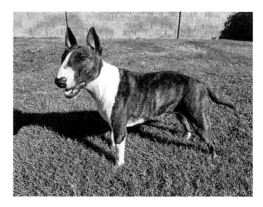

Figure 25.1 Meet your new patient, Soli, a 3-year-old castrated male Bull Terrier dog. Courtesy of Danielle Nicole.

Round One of Questions for Case 25: The Vomiting Dog

1. **Plates 12–14** demonstrate examples of foreign bodies that Soli ingested. Had these items not been vomited up, what is a potential complication of foreign body ingestion?
2. When foreign body ingestion leads to the complication that you identified in Question #1 (above), patients often present with so-called acute abdomen. What does this refer to?
3. Which clinical signs are suggestive of acute abdomen?
4. **Plates 15–18** demonstrate examples of ingested items that, if allowed to remain in the digestive tract, could lead to toxicosis. Link each item to the clinical signs and underlying pathology that might be expected if toxicosis developed.
5. The vignette does not describe how vomiting was induced. If Xander had telephoned from home to report ingestion of a toxin that you felt was safe to vomit up, what would you instruct him to administer to Soli?
6. If Soli were at your clinic right now and required induction of emesis, what would you administer?
7. If Soli were a cat, instead of a dog, and he was at your clinic right now, needing you to induce emesis, what would you administer?
8. What are contraindications to inducing vomiting?
9. If induction of emesis is successful, Soli will throw up. Describe the vomiting process.

Answers to Round One of Questions for Case 25: The Vomiting Dog

1. Foreign body ingestion may lead to foreign body obstruction at any point within the digestive tract.(1)

2. Acute abdomen refers to sudden onset of severe abdominal pain.(1–10) Such pain can result from a spectrum of medical and/or surgical presentations, some of which are life-threatening.(1–10)

3. The clinical signs may be supportive of acute abdomen:(1–4, 8–22)

    * abnormal posturing:

        * hunched, with either an arched back or the so-called "prayer posture," which resembles a play bow:

            * extended forelimbs
            * lowered chest
            * elevated rump

        * abdominal distension
        * depressed mentation
        * inability to settle
        * ptyalism
        * retching, particularly if non-productive
        * tenseness on abdominal palpation
        * abdominal splinting.

4. Chocolate contains methylxanthines, theobromine and caffeine.(1) The amount of each that is contained in chocolate varies depending upon brand and type. However, in general, the darker the chocolate, the less it takes to be toxic.(1) Dry cocoa powder is most concentrated, followed by unsweetened (baker's) chocolate, semi-sweet, and dark.(23) Milk chocolate can still create toxicosis, but more of it must be consumed to cause toxicosis.(23) White chocolate is insignificant: it mostly contains fat.(23) Clinical signs of chocolate toxicosis depend upon the severity of ingestion. Mild toxicosis occurs at 20 mg/kg of methyxanthines(23). At this dose, the gastrointestinal tract is adversely affected. Patients typically present for vomiting or diarrhea. At 40–50 mg/kg, tachycardia and hypertension may develop.(23) At doses that exceed 60 mg/kg, seizure activity is likely.(23) Toxicity calculators are available online to guide clients that telephone in on emergency as to the relative risk based upon what specifically was consumed and how much.

    Sugar-free snacks often contain xylitol.(24, 25) Xylitol is relatively safe for people to consume. People who overindulge in it may develop diarrhea.(24) However, dogs interpret xylitol ingestion as if glucose itself had been consumed.(24, 26, 27) Insulin is released, causing a hypoglycemic crisis.(24, 27, 28) Affected patients often exhibit generalized weakness and ataxia.(24, 25, 29, 30) They may also seize.(24, 25, 29, 30) Patients can survive these fits without sustaining damage to the nervous system.(24) However, weeks to months following xylitol ingestion, dogs may develop hepatopathy.(24, 25, 30–32)

    Snail bait typically contains metaldehyde.(23) This is metabolized to acetaldehyde within the stomach.(23) Both enter circulation after being absorbed from the gastrointestinal tract, and impact neurotransmission.(23) Metaldehyde reduces concentrations of the inhibitory neurotransmitter, γ-aminobutyric acid.(23) This causes neuroexcitation.(23) Metaldehyde also reduces circulating concentrations of serotonin and norepinephrine, which precipitates convulsions.(23) Patients initially may present for evaluation of muscle tremors and hyperesthesia.(23) As toxicosis progresses, patients may present in opisthotonos with full-blown seizure activity.(1, 23)

    Raisins (and grapes) cause acute kidney injury (AKI) in some, but not all dogs. The mechanism by which this occurs is poorly understood. AKI results in pathologic oliguria.(1)

5. The vignette does not describe how vomiting was induced. If Xander had telephoned from home to report ingestion of a toxin that I felt was safe to vomit up, then I would have instructed him to administer either of the following drugs:(23)

- hydrogen peroxide

  - 2 mL/kg PO
  - Maximum of 45 mL
  - Okay to repeat once if vomiting is not induced with one dose within 10 to 15 minutes of administration

- syrup of ipecac

  - 10–20 mL PO.

6. If Soli is at your clinic right now and requires induction of emesis, then I would administer apomorphine parenterally: 0.05–0.1 mg/kg.(23) An alternate route is to crush a 6.25 mg tablet, mix it with sterile 0.9% saline, and instill it within the conjunctival sac.(33)

7. If Soli were a cat instead of a dog, then I would be inclined to administer xylazine to induce emesis.(34) Xylazine is thought to be more efficacious in cats than either hydrogen peroxide or apomorphine.(34)

8. You would not want to induce vomiting if:(23)

- the patient is non-responsive
- the patient is seizing
- the patient is at increased risk for aspiration pneumonia, i.e. a patient with megaesophagus
- the patient has no swallowing reflex
- the swallowed item is corrosive or erosive, i.e. petroleum distillates or volatile hydrocarbons.

9. The vomiting center, located within the medulla oblongata, receives input from the periphery to make a decision about whether to proceed with emesis.(35–39) Once this decision has been made, the vomiting center coordinates a sequence of events aimed at evacuating the stomach. (35–37)

- Nausea typically precedes vomiting.(35, 36)
- Stomach tone decreases.(36)
- Proximal small bowel contractions increase.(36)
- Bile and pancreatic juices flow retrograde into the stomach.(36, 40)
- Retching is initiated:

  - the patient reflexively closes the glottis while moving the chest wall and diaphragm as they would during inspiration(36, 37)
  - simultaneously, the antral and pyloric parts of the stomach contract to trigger emesis(36)
  - stomach contents forced into the esophagus and out through the mouth.(36, 37) This requires the cardia of the stomach to relax.(36)

Returning to Case 25: The Vomiting Dog

Soli and Xander had visited a neighbor's home earlier today to help with a garage sale. Xander had turned his back for a minute. The next thing he knew, he was wrestling a box of rodenticide out of Soli's mouth.

Xander is not sure if Soli ate any of it. The neighbor says that the box was empty, but Xander is not taking any chances. He rushes Soli in to be evaluated by you on an emergency basis.

Your technician takes Soli's vital signs before paging you that your next patient is here.

Weight: 65.2 lb (29.6 kg)
BCS: 4/9
Mentation: BAR

Round Two of Questions for Case 25: The Vomiting Dog

TPR

T: 101.8°F (38.8°C)
P: 92 beats per minute
R: 28 breaths per minute

1. Xander is concerned that Soli is going to "bleed out" if he did in fact ingest rodenticide. Which category of rodenticide would Soli have had to ingest for development of clinical or subclinical hemorrhage to occur?
2. What is/are the active ingredient(s) in the category of rodenticide that you identified in Question #1 (above)?
3. How do(es) the active ingredient(s) cause bleeding?
4. When does hemorrhage occur relative to ingestion if there is no medical intervention? Is it immediate or is it delayed?
5. How is this kind of rodenticide medically managed?
6. If ingestion of this kind of rodenticide is not medically managed – or if medical management is discontinued too soon – which clinical signs would you expect to see in your patient?
7. Identify other major categories of rodenticides that dogs and cats may inadvertently ingest, outline their mechanisms of action, and identify commonly associated clinical signs.

Answers to Round Two of Questions for Case 25: The Vomiting Dog

1. Anticoagulant rodenticides cause clinical or subclinical hemorrhage to occur.(23, 41, 42)

2. Active ingredients in anticoagulant rodenticides include:(23, 41, 42)

   - brodifacoum
   - bromadiolone
   - difethialone
   - warfarin.

3. Activation of the coagulation cascade is how hemorrhage is stopped.(23, 41, 42) Hemorrhage consumes coagulation factors, which are required for clotting.(23, 41, 42) These coagulation factors must be regenerated. Vitamin K is an ingredient of coagulation factors 2, 7, 9, and 10.(23, 41, 42)

   In health, Vitamin K is recycled so that these factors can be regenerated. This process is catalyzed by the enzyme, Vitamin K epoxide reductase. Anticoagulant rodenticides inhibit this enzyme, which means that these coagulation factors are not recycled.(23, 41, 42) Once coagulation factors are consumed, they are not regenerated.(23, 41, 42) Thus, the patient bleeds out internally, externally, or both.

4. Hemorrhage is not immediate; it is delayed.(23) It usually occurs within 72 hours after ingestion. (23) However, there is variation in the onset of clinical presentation following anticoagulant rodenticide ingestion. Why such variation? How long it takes for patients to develop clinical signs depends upon how long it takes for the supply of clotting factors in circulation to be depleted.(23) This is contingent upon:(23)

   - the species of the patient
   - the dose of the rodenticide

- whether the rodenticide is so-called "first-generation," "second-generation," etc.:

  - as a "first-generation" anticoagulant, warfarin often requires several ingestions to develop toxicosis
  - "second-generation" anticoagulants, such as brodifacoum, bromadiolone, and diethiolone, can create clinical signs after a single ingestion.

5. Medical management of anticoagulant rodenticide includes the following.(23, 41, 42)

   - Induction of vomiting, if recently ingested.
   - Monitoring prothrombin time (PT) and only administering oral Vitamin K1 (phytonadione) if clinical signs of hemorrhage develop.

     - The PT test measures how quickly Soli's blood clots.
     - Factor VII is the first clotting factor affected by anticoagulant rodenticides because it has the shortest half-life.
     - When factor VII is depleted, PT elevates.
     - PT elevates within 36–72 hours of ingesting a toxic dose of anticoagulant rodenticide.

   Many clients (and clinicians!) feel uncomfortable monitoring for signs of hemorrhage to start Vitamin K1 therapy. They would prefer to initiate treatment prophylactically to guard against potential coagulopathy. This is an appropriate choice for medical management.(33)

6. If ingestion of this kind of rodenticide is not medically managed, I would expect to see one or more of the following clinical signs:(23, 41, 42)

   - non-specific malaise, often referred to in clinical practice as "ADR" – "ain't doing right"
   - bruising:

     - petechiations
     - ecchymoses

   - epistaxis
   - dyspnea, if bleeding into chest
   - hemoptysis, coughing up blood
   - hematuria, bloody urine
   - hematemesis, bloody vomit
   - hematochezia, stool coated with fresh red blood from the lower digestive tract
   - melena, tarry black stool coated with digested blood from the upper digestive tract
   - sudden death.

7. Other major categories of rodenticides that dogs and cats may inadvertently ingest include the following.(23, 41, 42)

   - Bromethalin – mechanism of action:

     - causes uncoupling of oxidative phosphorylation
     - ATP is depleted
     - the sodium-potassium pump cannot function without ATP
     - cerebral edema results
     - patients present with neurologic signs:

       - within hours:
       - the patient is hyperexcitable
       - the patient has hyperesthesia
       - the patient has focal motor seizures
       - the patient is sensitive to light and noise

- - days later:
  - the patient is depressed
  - the patient has hindlimb weakness that may or may not progress to paralysis
  - the patient has decreased to absent conscious proprioception
  - the patient may lose deep pain response.
- Cholecalciferol-based, mechanism of action:
  - cholecalciferol is activated to calcidiol and calcitriol in the body
  - these hormones cause an increase in circulating calcium
  - sustained pathologic levels of circulating calcium cause metastatic calcification
  - when the calcium-phosphorus product (Ca × P) exceeds 60, tissue mineralization is likely to occur in these tissues:
    - blood vessels
    - cardiac muscle
    - kidneys
    - ligaments
    - gastrointestinal tract
    - skeletal muscle
  - hypercalcemia may cause the following clinical signs:
    - decreased appetite or even anorexia
    - vomiting
    - changes in thirst, excessive
    - changes in urination:
    - initially polyuric
    - progresses to oliguria or anuria
- Zinc phosphide, mechanism of action:
  - zinc phosphide combines with gastric acid and water in the stomach
  - phosphine gas is produced:
    - acts as a direct irritant to gastric mucosa
    - inhibits cytochrome C oxidase, tissue hypoxia
  - clinical signs are quick in onset (often within 20 minutes)
  - clinical signs mirror strychnine poisoning:
    - rigid limbs (all!)
    - stiff limbs (all!)
    - muscle spasms
    - opisthotonus
    - seizures
    - dyspnea
  - veterinary clients and members of the veterinary team will also be exposed to phosphine gas when patients exhale
  - veterinary team members can be exposed to phosphine gas during necropsy
    - by the time you smell it, it's too late: you've been exposed!

Returning to Case 25: The Vomiting Dog

You ask Xander if he has the ingredient label handy for the product that Soli got into within the past 90 minutes. Xander provides you with the package. The active ingredient is brodifacoum. Even though you aren't certain if Soli ate any, you explain your concern about the potential for toxicosis and recommend inducing vomiting right away. Xander agrees. You crush a 6.25 mg tablet of apomorphine, mix it in sterile 0.9% sterile saline, and instill it into his conjunctival sac. Within minutes, he produces green-colored vomit (see **Plate 19**).

Despite successful induction of vomiting, you advise prophylactically starting Soli on oral Vitamin K to protect against the possibility that some rodenticide was absorbed into his circulation before he was able to receive medical attention. Xander agrees that it is better to be safe than sorry. Xander waits for the prescription to be filled in-house before checking out at the discharge office. He is just about to depart from the clinic with Soli in tow when Soli heaves all over the waiting room.

Round Three of Questions for Case 25: The Vomiting Dog

1. What is the most likely explanation for Soli vomiting a second time?
2. Xander was not expecting to see Soli vomit again. This unexpected turn of events rattled him. After you explain to him why Soli vomited and that he is truly okay to be discharged, Xander asks you to repeat the discharge instructions. How long do you instruct Xander to give Soli Vitamin K1?
3. Xander asks why you didn't give Soli an injection of Vitamin K1 to jumpstart treatment?
4. Xander asks if he ought to give Vitamin K1 on any empty stomach?
5. Which diagnostic test should you check after the last dose of Vitamin K has been given?
6. How long after the last dose of Vitamin K should the test you identified in Question #3 (above) be performed?
7. What if the test is abnormal at Soli's recheck?

Answers to Round Three of Questions for Case 25: The Vomiting Dog

1. You did not rinse the conjunctival sac following successful induction of emesis with apomorphine.(34) This means that residual apomorphine is still being absorbed into Soli's circulation and can trigger protracted vomiting.(34)

2. You need to treat with Vitamin K for an extended period based upon the active ingredient in the rodenticide.(43) Many clinicians prescribe a 30-day supply to cover all their bases, particularly if the active ingredient is unclear.

   In this case, we know that the active ingredient is bromadialone, so Soli only needs to receive treatment for 21 days.(43) Treatment for all other second-generation anticoagulant rodenticides is typically rounded up to one month.(43) On the other hand, if Soli had ingested warfarin, then treatment could be shortened to two weeks.(43)

3. Vitamin K1 is not typically administered intravenously because it can cause an anaphylactic reaction in some, but not all, patients.(33) Anaphylaxis is also possible if Vitamin K1 is administered as an injectable through intramuscular and subcutaneous routes.(43) Oral therapy is the best approach to treatment because it delivers Vitamin K1 to the liver, which is the site of clotting factor activation.(43)

4. It is not ideal to administer Vitamin K1 on an empty stomach. Giving Vitamin K1 with fatty food enhances its absorption.(43)

5. You should check Soli's PT after the last dose of Vitamin K has been given.

6. You should perform the PT test 48–72 hours after Soli receives his last dose of Vitamin K.

7. If Soli's PT is elevated at his recheck appointment, then he would need to resume treatment with oral Vitamin K1 for another 14–21 days. PT should be retested 48–72 hours after the last dose.

Returning to Case 25: The Vomiting Dog

Soli is discharged with instructions to administer Vitamin K1 for 21 days to guard against coagulopathy. You instruct Soli to return in 23–24 days to assess his PT to evaluate efficacy of treatment. Ten days later, Soli presents to the overnight emergency service for acute onset of unproductive retching. Triage examination identifies a swollen abdomen and increased respiratory effort.

Round Four of Questions for Case 25: The Vomiting Dog

1. What are broad causes of abdominal distension in a canine patient?
2. Which cause did you identify in Question #1 (above) that is also consistent with non-productive retching?
3. What is the colloquial (common) name for this condition?
4. What is the appropriate medical name for this condition?
5. If your presumptive diagnosis is correct, which organ do you expect to feel on abdominal palpation?
6. Should you be able to feel that organ in a normal (healthy) patient on routine physical examination?
7. Which diagnostic test must you perform immediately to confirm your suspicion?

Answers to Round Four of Questions for Case 25: The Vomiting Dog

1. Abdominal distension in a canine patient can result from:(1)

   • organomegaly
   • gaseous distension of abdominal viscera
   • peritoneal effusion.

2. Gaseous distension of the stomach is most concerning. This can explain both abdominal distension and non-productive retching if there is accompanying volvulus that essentially cuts off the inflow tract to the stomach.(1, 44, 45) This prevents the stomach from evacuating its contents through the esophagus and out the oral cavity.

3. The condition that is described in Question #2 (above) is commonly referred to as "bloat."(1)

4. The appropriate medical term for "bloat" is gastric dilatation and volvulus (GDV).(1)

5. If I am correct and Soli is presenting with GDV, then I would expect to be able to feel his distended, taut, and painful stomach on abdominal palpation.(1, 2, 44, 46)

6. No, you should not be able to feel the stomach in a normal (healthy) patient on routine physical examination.(1, 47)

7. A right lateral abdominal radiograph is essential to confirm GDV.(3, 12, 19, 22, 48)

Returning to Case 25: The Vomiting Dog

Xander authorizes you to take a right lateral abdominal radiograph (see Figure 25.2).

Round Five of Questions for Case 25: The Vomiting Dog

1. What is Soli's diagnosis?
2. Which breeds are predisposed to this diagnosis?
3. Xander asks what could have caused this condition. What is your response?
4. Why is it impossible for Xander to throw up in this condition?
5. Xander's BP is steadily decreasing. Why is this so?
6. What do you expect his HR to be doing in response to his tanking BP?
7. True or false: It is likely that you will see cardiac arrhythmias in patients with this condition.
8. True or false: Soli needs to go to surgery immediately.

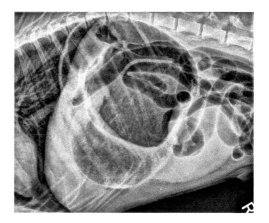

Figure 25.2 Right lateral abdominal radiograph.

Answers to Round Five of Questions for Case 25: The Vomiting Dog

1. Soli has GDV.

2. GDV most commonly occurs in deep-chested, large-breed dogs.(1, 47, 49–51) These include:(1)

   - Alaskan malamutes
   - German Shepherds
   - Great Danes
   - Irish Wolfhounds
   - Labrador retrievers
   - Saint Bernard.

3. An exact etiology is unknown; however, the following links have been suggested in the current veterinary medical literature:(44, 49, 50, 52–55)

   - type of diet – commercial cereal and/or soy-based diets may increase risk
   - amount fed at one sitting – eating large meals may encourage repeated stretch of the hepatogastric and hepatoduodenal ligaments, increasing the risk of volvulus
   - delayed gastric emptying
   - rigorous activity after meals
   - post-prandial stress
   - body condition – underweight dogs are thought to be at increased risk
   - age – older animals are thought to be at increased risk
   - prior splenectomy.

4. When volvulus occurs, the stomach migrates from its normal anatomical position.(47) The right-sided pylorus becomes cranioventral relative to the body of the stomach.(47) The pylorus then moves to the left of midline.(47) Eventually, the pylorus is positioned dorsal to the esophagus and the fundus, still to the left of midline.(44) This cuts off the inflow tract to the stomach.(1, 44, 45) This prevents the stomach from evacuating its contents through the esophagus and out

the oral cavity.(47) Because there is nowhere for the build-up of gas to go, the stomach progressively inflates.(47)

5. Dogs with GDV have compromised venous return to the heart because the portal vein and vena cava are compressed.(47) The result is a sharp decline in cardiac output along with systemic arterial pressure.(47)

6. I would expect the patient to become tachycardic in response to its tanking BP in an attempt to raise cardiac output and systolic BP. Tachycardia is a physiologic response to hypovolemic shock.(44, 56–59)

7. True. It is likely to see cardiac arrhythmias in patients with this condition.(41, 42, 47)

8. True. Soli needs to go to surgery immediately. If untreated, the stomach will rupture.(1, 47)

CLINICAL PEARLS

- Foreign bodies and toxic substances are frequently ingested by dogs.

- Induction of vomiting is often indicated in a clinical setting to evacuate gastric contents.

- Hydrogen peroxide can be administered at-home by the client to induce emesis.

- If hydrogen peroxide is not effective at inducing vomiting, the dose can be repeated once.

- At the clinic, apomorphine can be administered to induce vomiting in dogs.

- Apomorphine can be administered in injectable form or as a solution (crushed tablet, mixed with sterile saline) applied to the conjunctival sac.

- If applied to the conjunctival sac, the sac must be rinsed free of residual apomorphine to prevent protracted vomiting.

- At the clinic, xylazine is typically the preferred choice for emesis induction in cats because it tends to be more efficacious.

- Induction of vomiting is contraindicated if the ingested item is caustic or if the patient is depressed, non-responsive, unable to swallow, or at risk of aspiration.

- Supportive care and medical management after induction of emesis may be required in cases of toxicosis in the event that some of the toxin was absorbed into circulation.

- Treatment of toxicosis requires an understanding of the mechanism of action so that an appropriate course of action can be taken. For instance, anticoagulant rodenticide toxicosis is medically managed by administration of Vitamin K1.

- In addition to patients presenting for induction of vomiting, some patients present to the clinic for vomiting.

- When large-breed, deep-chested dogs present for non-productive retching, abdominal distension, and increased respiratory effort, GDV is a primary concern.

- GDV is a surgical emergency. A right lateral abdominal radiograph is diagnostic.

References

1. Englar RE. Common clinical presentations in dogs and cats. Hoboken, NJ: Wiley/Blackwell; 2019.
2. Tilley LP, Smith FWK. The 5-minute veterinary consult: canine and feline. 3rd ed.Baltimore, MD: Lippincott Williams & Wilkins; 2004.
3. Heeren V, Edwards L, Mazzaferro EM. Acute abdomen: Diagnosis. Comp Cont. Educ Pract. 2004;26(5): 350.
4. Pachtinger G. Acute abdomen in dogs and cats: step-by-step approach to patient care. Today's. Veterinary Practice. 2013 (September/October):14–9.
5. Durkan S. Approach to the acute abdomen. DVM. 360 [Internet]; 2008. Available from: http://veterinarycalendar. dvm360.com/approach-acute-abdomen-proceedings?id=andsk=anddate=andpageID=2.
6. Boag A, Hughes D. Emergency management of the acute abdomen in dogs and cats 1. Investigation and initial stabilization. In Practice 2004;26(9):476–83.
7. Swinney G. The acute abdomen and septic peritonitis. Available from: http://www.ava.com.au/sites/ default/files/AVA_website/pdfs/NSW_Division/THE%20ACUTE%20ABDOMEN%20AND%20SEPTIC%20 PERITONITIS_GSwinney.pdf.
8. Mazzaferro EM. Triage and approach to the acute abdomen. Clin Tech Small Anim Pract 2003;18(1):1–6.
9. Tello LH, editor. Dealing with the acute abdomen patient. World Small Animal Veterinary Association World Congress 2011.
10. Burrows CF, editor. The acute abdomen. World Small Animal Veterinary Association World Congress; 2002.
11. Walters PC. Approach to the acute abdomen. Clin Tech Small Anim Pract 2000;15(2):63–9.
12. Franks JN, Howe LM. Evaluating and managing acute abdomen. Vetmed-US 2000;95(1):56.
13. Kleine LJ. Radiology and acute abdominal disorders in the dog and cat: Part 1. The Compendium Collection. Yardley, PA: Veterinary Learning Systems; 1997. p. 336–41.
14. Davenport DJ, Martin RA. Acute abdomen. In: Murtaugh RJ, Kaplan PM, editors. Veterinary emergency and critical care medicine. St. Louis: Mosby; 1992. p. 153–62.
15. Leveille CR. The acute abdomen. In: Bonagura JD, Kirk RW, editors. Current veterinary therapy. XI. Philadelphia, PA: W.B. Saunders; 1992. p. 125–31.
16. Mann FA. Acute abdomen: evaluation and emergency treatment. In: Bonagura JD, editor. Kirk's current veterinary therapy. Philadelphia, PA: W.B. Saunders; 2002. p. 160–4.
17. Brady CA, Otto CM, Van Winkle TJ, King LG. Severe sepsis in cats: 29 cases (1986–1998). J Am Vet Med Assoc 2000;217(4):531–5.
18. Macintire DK. The acute abdomen – differential diagnosis and management. Semin Vet Med Surg (Small Anim) 1988;3(4):302–10.
19. Dye T. The acute abdomen: a surgeon's approach to diagnosis and treatment. Clin Tech Small Anim Pract 2003;18(1):53–65.
20. Crowe D Symposium on the Acute Abdomen – Introduction – Responding to a Life-Threatening Condition. Vet Med-Us; 1988. p. 652.
21. Crowe DT. The 1st Steps in Handling the acute abdomen Patient. Vetmed-US 1988;83(7):654-and.
22. Saxon WD. The acute abdomen. Vet Clin North Am. Small Anim Pract 1994;24(6):1207–24.
23. The Merck Veterinary Manual. Whitehouse Station, NJ: Merck & Co., Inc.; 2016.
24. Murphy LA, Coleman AE. Xylitol toxicosis in dogs. Vet Clin North Am Small Anim Pract 2012;42(2): 307–12.
25. Peterson ME. Xylitol. Top Companion Anim Med 2013;28(1):18–20.
26. Hirata Y, Fujisawa M, Sato H, Asano T, Katsuki S. Blood glucose and plasma insulin responses to xylitol administrated intravenously in dogs. Biochem Biophys Res Commun 1966;24(3):471–5.
27. Kuzuya T, Kanazawa Y, Kosaka K. Plasma insulin response to intravenously administered xylitol in dogs. Metabolism 1966;15(12):1149–52.
28. Kruth SA, Feldman EC, Kennedy PC. Insulin-secreting islet cell tumors: establishing a diagnosis and the clinical course for 25 dogs. J Am Vet Med Assoc 1982;181(1):54–8.
29. Dunayer EK. Hypoglycemia following canine ingestion of xylitol-containing gum. Vet Hum Toxicol 2004;46(2):87–8.

30. Dunayer EK. New findings on the effects of xylitol ingestion in dogs. Veterinary Medicine. 2006 (December): [791–7]. Available from: https://www.aspcapro.org/sites/pro/files/xylitol.pdf.

31. Todd JM, Powell LL. Xylitol intoxication associated with fulminant hepatic failure in a dog. J Vet Emerg Crit Car 2007;17(3):286–9.

32. Dunayer EK, Gwaltney-Brant SM. Acute hepatic failure and coagulopathy associated with xylitol ingestion in eight dogs. J Am Vet Med Assoc 2006;229(7):1113–7.

33. Plumb DC. Plumb's veterinary drug handbook. 9th ed. Hoboken NJ: Pharma Vet, Inc; 2018.

34. Martini-Johnson L. Applied pharmacology for veterinary technicians. 6 ed. Philadelphia, PA: Elsevier; 2020.

35. King LG, Donaldson MT. Acute vomiting. Vet Clin North Am Small Anim Pract 1994;24(6):1189–206.

36. Twedt DC. Differential diagnosis and therapy of vomiting. Vet Clin North Am Small Anim Pract 1983;13(3):503–20.

37. Elwood C, Devauchelle P, Elliott J, Freiche V, German AJ, Gualtieri M, et al. Emesis in dogs: a review. J Small Anim Pract 2010;51(1):4–22.

38. Encarnacion HJ, Parra J, Mears E, Sadler V. Vomiting. Compendium 2009;31(3):E8+.

39. Batchelor DJ, Devauchelle P, Elliott J, Elwood CM, Freiche V, Gualtieri M, et al. Mechanisms, causes, investigation and management of vomiting disorders in cats: a literature review. J Feline Med Surg 2013;15(4):237–65.

40. McGrotty Y. Medical management of acute and chronic vomiting in dogs and cats. In Practice 2010;32(10):478–83.

41. Côté E. Clinical veterinary advisor. Dogs and cats. 3rd ed. St. Louis, MO: Elsevier Mosby; 2015.

42. Ettinger SJ, Feldman EC, Côté E. Textbook of veterinary internal medicine: diseases of the dog and the cat. 8th ed. St. Louis, MO: Elsevier; 2017.

43. DeClementi C. Rodenticide poisoning: what to do after exposure. Today's Veterinary Practitioner. 2012. Available from: https://todaysveterinarypractice.com/rodenticide-poisoning-what-to-do-after-exposure/#.

44. Monnet E.. Gastric dilatation-volvulus syndrome in dogs. The Veterinary Clinics of North America. Small Animal Practice. 2003, 33(5):987–1005.

45. Brourman JD, Schertel ER, Allen DA, Birchard SJ, DeHoff WD. Factors associated with perioperative mortality in dogs with surgically managed gastric dilatation-volvulus: 137 cases (1988–1993). Journal of the American Veterinary Medical Association 1996;208(11):1855–8.

46. Englar RE. Performing the small animal physical examination. Hoboken, NJ: Wiley; 2017.

47. Englar RE. Performing the small animal physical examination. Hoboken, NJ: Wiley/Blackwell; 2017.

48. Aronson LR, Brockman DJ, Brown DC. Gastrointestinal emergencies. Vet Clin North Am Small Anim Pract 2000;30(3):555–79.

49. Sullivan M, Yool DA. Gastric disease in the dog and cat. Veterinary Journal 1998;156(2):91–106.

50. Glickman LT, Glickman NW, Pérez CM, Schellenberg DB, Lantz GC. Analysis of risk factors for gastric dilatation and dilatation-volvulus in dogs. Journal of the American Veterinary Medical Association. 1994;204(9):1465–71.

51. Schaible RH, Ziech J, Glickman NW, Schellenberg D, Yi Q, Glickman LT. Predisposition to gastric dilatation-volvulus in relation to genetics of thoracic conformation in Irish setters. J Am Anim Hosp Assoc 1997;33(5):379–83.

52. Hosgood G. Gastric dilatation-volvulus in dogs. Journal of the American Veterinary Medical Association 1994;204(11):1742–7.

53. Glickman LT, Glickman NW, Schellenberg DB, Raghavan M, Lee T. Non-dietary risk factors for gastric dilatation-volvulus in large and giant breed dogs. Journal of the American Veterinary Medical Association 2000;217(10):1492–9.

54. Glickman LT, Glickman NW, Schellenberg DB, Raghavan M, Lee TL. Incidence of and breed-related risk factors for gastric dilatation-volvulus in dogs. Journal of the American Veterinary Medical Association 2000;216(1):40–5.

55. Millis DL, Nemzek J, Riggs C, Walshaw R. Gastric dilatation-volvulus after splenic torsion in two dogs. Journal of the American Veterinary Medical Association 1995;207(3):314–5.

56. Hall JA. Canine gastric dilatation – volvulus update. Seminars in Veterinary Medicine and Surgery 1989;4(3):188–93.

57. Wingfield WE, Cornelius LM, Deyoung DW. Pathophysiology of the gastric dilation-torsion complex in the dog. J Small Anim Pract 1974;15(12):735–9.

58. Orton EC, Muir WW, 3rd. Hemodynamics during experimental gastric dilatation-volvulus in dogs. American Journal of Veterinary Research 1983;44(8):1512–5.

59. Muir WW. Gastric dilatation-volvulus in the dog, with emphasis on cardiac arrhythmias. Journal of the American Veterinary Medical Association 1982;180(7):739–42.

Case 26

The Scooting Cat

Kitty Perry is the on-site, live-in mascot for a ten-acre equestrian riding academy. Although Clive Burton adopted her with the intent that she would be an avid mouser, Kitty Perry has other plans. She prefers to watch the world go by as opposed to policing the rodent population. Clive has yet to witness her initiating a successful hunt. These days, Clive would be content if she initiated anything.

Kitty Perry is popular among guests and employees alike. She's learned how to work the system and frequently convinces everyone who crosses her path that Clive has forgotten to feed her. She sneaks extra meals whenever she can, and readily accepts snacks, even those that most cats would turn their nose up at.

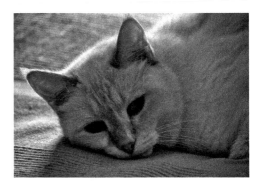

Figure 26.1 Meet your new patient, Kitty Perry, a 5-year-old spayed female Siamese mix. Courtesy of Heather Cornell.

When she's not eating, she's sleeping, which is why it was so unusual for Clive to arrive at work this morning to find her absent from her usual perch in the middle tier of the foyer cat tree.

Clive called to her and she materialized from the back-storage room, where her litter boxes were stowed. She set off in his direction, but halfway to Clive, she halted, sat on her rump, hiked up a hind leg, and cried out. She seemed intent on reaching her perineum, but could not seem to reach the mark, so she took to grooming her distal leg instead.

When Clive popped the lid off a can of food, the sound caught her attention and she resumed her journey to her breakfast dish. But twice more she eyed her flank suspiciously as if something were bothering her at her hindquarters. Clive snuck a look under her tail when she was eating and was alarmed by what he saw (see **Plate 20**).

The skin on either side of her anus is erythematous and swollen. Surrounding the swelling was what appeared to be a hole, from which a bloody discharge oozed. Clive felt faint. He wasn't sure what could have happened to her. A spat with another cat, perhaps? She certainly wasn't the one to pick a fight.

The apparent hole in her rear was all Clive needed to see to dial you up and request a home visit. Although you have only tended to his horses in the past, you are familiar with Kitty Perry and feel comfortable that, as a mixed animal practitioner, you can assist.

When you arrive, Kitty Perry is still trying to groom herself. She's reluctant to let anyone approach her rear, but you don't give her much of a choice. She vocalizes her resentment as you take her vital signs.

Weight: 14.6 lb (6.6 kg)
BCS: 7/9
Mentation: QAR

TPR

T: *** not performed ***
P: 198 beats per minute
R: 24 breaths per minute

Round One of Questions for Case 26: The Scooting Cat

1. What is the normal reference range for rectal temperature in a cat?
2. What is the appropriate medical term for depressed core body temperature?
3. What could cause a depressed rectal temperature?
4. What is/are the appropriate medical term(s) for elevated core body temperature?
5. What could cause an elevated rectal temperature?
6. Why did you not take Kitty Perry's temperature rectally?
7. Some states in the US require TPR to be documented at each physical examination. How do you get around the fact that you did not assess her rectal temperature?
8. Other than the rectum, where else can you take a cat's temperature?
9. How do readings from these sites compare, in terms of accuracy, to the rectal temperature?
10. If you had to venture a guess, do you think that Kitty Perry's temperature will be normal, low, or high?
11. Let's turn our attention now to perineal anatomy. Kitty Perry has a swollen perineum. Which structures are present in and around the vicinity of the feline perineum that could be involved?
12. Based upon what you see in **Plate 20**, which structure(s) is/are most likely implicated?
13. What is a common clinical condition that involves the structure(s) that you identified in Question #12 (above)? [Hint: it is more commonly thought of as a problem in dogs, but can occur in cats, too]
14. Kitty Perry presented for scooting. What does scooting mean?
15. What is the purpose of scooting?
16. Is scooting considered normal behavior in dogs or cats?
17. Other than the issue that you identified in Question #13 (above), what else can cause scooting?

Answers to Round One of Questions for Case 26: The Scooting Cat

1. The normal reference range for feline rectal temperature is 100.5–102.5°F, although this range varies somewhat depending upon your choice of reference text.(1, 2)

2. Hypothermia is the appropriate medical term for depressed core body temperature.(3)

3. A depressed rectal temperature may result from:(3)

   - anesthesia (4–7)
   - cardiac disease
   - cold climate
   - hypoadrenocorticism
   - hypotension
   - hypothyroidism
   - immersion in ice water (i.e. falling through the ice into a semi-frozen lake)
   - renal disease
   - shock.

   A rectal temperature may also be artificially low if the rectal canal is full of feces.(8) In this case, you are essentially taking the temperature of the feces rather than having the thermometer tip seated snuggly against the rectal mucosa. The reading is likely to come back as being low, when in fact the patient is not truly hypothermic.

4. Hyperthermia and fever are two appropriate medical terms for elevated core body temperature.(9)
   Hyperthermia refers to a condition in which the patient is unable to dissipate heat sufficiently.(9) The patient's core body temperature has exceeded the hypothalamic thermal set point

for what is considered to be normal rectal temperature.(9) This may be due to ambient conditions, such as environmental heat.(9) Think of Phoenix, Arisona in July or August. Alternatively, heat production by the patient itself, as from exertion, may raise core body temperature above what constitutes normal.(9)

Fever also refers to a condition in which the patient's core body temperature is higher than anticipated; however, in cases of fever, the patient's thermal set point within the hypothalamus is raised.(9)

5. Fever may be caused by:(9)

    - infection
    - inflammation
    - pharmaceutical agent
    - neoplasia.

6. I chose not to take Kitty Perry's temperature rectally because based upon my clinical experience (and **Plate 20!**), she is likely to be exquisitely painful and sensitive in that region of her body.

    Based upon this clinical presentation, I am going to have to work on her rear end to perform the following procedures:

    - a rectal examination:

        - to evaluate the right-sided anal sac that has ruptured
        - to evaluate and/or express her intact left anal sac, which looks ready to rupture

    - a thorough flushing out of the right anal sac.

    To perform these procedures, I would like to administer sedation and analgesia. After both medications kick in, at that point, I might circle back to check a rectal temperature. However, prior to administering such medications, the discomfort to her would be too great.

    Taking her temperature at this point is not going to change my presumptive diagnosis and/or plan of attack.

7. Some states in the US require TPR to be documented at each physical examination. You get around the fact that you did not assess her rectal temperature by being transparent in your medical documentation. You record why you chose not to perform this component of TPR in her case files.

    If you omit Kitty Perry's rectal temperature without explanation, then potentially you could be cited by a state licensing board for not providing standard of care.(10) An error of omission can lead to a successful claim against you.(10) It is often said in veterinary medicine that "if it isn't charted, it didn't happen."(11–16)

    In this case, the temperature component of TPR didn't happen for a reason. It's not that you forgot. You made a conscious decision against taking a rectal temperature because doing so would cause unnecessary distress to the patient at this time. Recording that statement in your record protects you and demonstrates that you made an executive decision in favor of what was best for the patient.(10)

8. An aural (auricular) or axillary temperature may be taken in lieu of a rectal one.(8, 17)

9. Rectal temperature remains the most accurate clinical measurement of core body temperature. (8, 17) Temperatures at other sites are correlated with rectal temperature in dogs and cats; however, these temperatures are not interchangeable.(8, 17) According to a study by Goic et al.:

    "Sensitivity and specificity for detection of hyperthermia with axillary temperature were 57% and 100%, respectively, in dogs and 33% and 100%, respectively in cats; sensitivity and specificity for detection of hypothermia were 86% and 87%, respectively, in dogs and 80% and 96%, respectively, in cats."

This means that 57% of dogs and 33% of cats with hyperthermia will be identified correctly when taking an axillary temperature.(17) In other words, 43% of dogs and 67% of cats with hyperthermia will be missed.(17)

Axillary temperatures are much better at identifying which patients do not have hypothermia. Eighty-seven percent of dogs and 96% of cats that do not have hypothermia are correctly identified.(17)

10. Based upon what I am visually observing in the photograph, inflammation is present at Kitty Perry's perineum. Infection is also likely based upon my top differential diagnosis (anal sacculitis with right-sided anal-sac rupture).

     Both inflammation and infection cause fever. So, if I were to guess, Kitty Perry's rectal temperature would be elevated.

11. Kitty Perry has a swollen perineum. The following structures are present in and around the vicinity of the feline perineum and could therefore be involved:(2, 18, 19)
    - digestive tract:

        - anus
        - anal glands
        - rectum

    - urogenital tract:

        - urethra
        - vulva

    - perineum:

        - fur
        - skin
        - soft tissue
        - underlying musculature
        - nerves.

12. Based upon the photograph, Kitty Perry's anal sacs are most likely to be involved.(2, 18)

13. Anal sacculitis with right-sided anal sac rupture is the top differential diagnosis.(2, 18–23)

14. Kitty Perry presented for scooting. Scooting refers to the patient positioning himself in a sit or squat, to facilitate rubbing his rear end on the ground, floor, or carpet. It is a source of embarrassment for many owners.

15. Scooting is thought to relieve perineal itch.

16. Scooting is not normal behavior. Its presence suggests there is an underlying medical problem that needs to be addressed.

17. Other than anal sacculitis, anal sac impaction, and anal sac rupture, scooting may reflect allergic skin disease, perianal tumors, or endoparasitism (see **Plates 21 and 22**).(2, 18, 20, 24)

     Tapeworm proglottids are particularly mobile and crawl across the perineum. This causes mild perineal itch and is sufficient to cause scooting.(18)

Returning to Case 26: The Scooting Cat

After examining your patient externally, you share with Clive that Kitty Perry has anal sacculitis, which has culminated in a ruptured anal sac. Based upon the degree of swelling and redness, you suspect that the contralateral sac is about to follow suit.

Round Two of Questions for Case 26: The Scooting Cat

1. What are anal sacs?
2. Looking at the photograph, which side has ruptured, the left or the right?
3. What is the function of the anal sacs?
4. Differentiate anal sac impaction from anal sacculitis.
5. Is anal sac impaction and/or sacculitis more likely to occur in cats or dogs?
6. In addition to scooting, what are common clinical signs of feline anal sac disease?
7. What causes anal sac impactions and/or sacculitis in cats?
8. If you were to grossly examine normal (healthy) anal sac contents, what is their typical color?
9. If you were to grossly examine normal (healthy) anal sac contents, what is their typical consistency?
10. Which color(s) of anal sac secretions would make you concerned?
11. If you were to examine anal sac contents of a normal (healthy) patient under light microscopy, what would you expect to see?
12. If you were to examine anal sac contents of a normal (healthy) patient under light microscopy, what would you NOT expect to see?
13. Are there differences in cytology between normal and diseased anal sacs?
14. Is it typical to culture anal sac secretions? Why or why not?
15. How will you medically manage the ruptured anal sac?
16. How will you medically manage the contralateral sac?
17. If anal sacculitis and/or rupture of one or both anal sacs recurs, which surgical procedure might you advise?
18. What are potential risks that are associated with the surgical recommendation that you provided in Question #17 (above)?
19. Clive is concerned that Kitty Perry does not just have an anal sac rupture. He worries about anal sac cancer. How common is anal-sac neoplasia in cats?
20. If anal sac neoplasia occurs, what is the most likely type in cats?
21. Can the tumor type that you identified in Question #20 also occur in dogs?
22. What is the most common malignant rectal tumor type in dogs?
23. Benign rectal tumors can occur in dogs. Which is the most common type?
24. Can benign rectal tumors undergo malignant transformation as is seen in people?
25. Peri-anal tumors may also arise. What is the most common type of perianal tumor in the dog?
26. The tumor type that you identified in Question #25 can also be found at locations other than perianal in the dog. What are common sites of occurrence?
27. What are the risk factors for the tumor type that you identified in Question #25 as occurring in dogs?
28. How would you propose to treat the tumor type that you identified in Question #25 in a canine patient?

Answers to Round Two of Questions for Case 26: The Scooting Cat

1. The anal sacs are two small pouches located on either side of the anus, internally, at approximately the 4 o'clock and 8 o'clock positions when you are looking at the patient's perineum from

behind.(2, 18, 19, 22, 25) The anal sacs are commonly referred to as "anal glands;" however, this terminology is inaccurate: the anal glands are housed within the anal sacs.

2.   Looking at the photograph, Kitty Perry's right anal sac has ruptured.

3.   The walls of each sac are lined with many sebaceous (sweat) glands that produce a foul-smelling secretion. This secretion is released with each bowel movement.(22) It is thought to contribute to the mucous layer that coats feces and facilitates marking behavior.(19, 26–28) Fecal marking is more common in males than females.(29) Anal-sac secretions coat every bowel movement of every dog with a unique identifier (30, 31).

     Anal gland secretions in the dog also contain sialic acids and antimicrobial substances.(27) It has been suggested that the presence of these ingredients contribute to self-defense by creating a barrier to invasion of the anal mucosa by microbes.(27)

     The release of anal sac contents may also be triggered by extreme states of excitement, including fear, anxiety, and stress.(2, 23, 30) Anal secretions contain ingredients that are capable of communicating messages of danger to conspecifics as well as other species.(2, 32–34)

4.   An anal-sac impaction refers to the condition in which secretions continue to accumulate without being able to be expressed.(23) The affected anal sac will distend and if untreated, is at risk of rupture. Anal-sac impaction may result from inflammation of the anal sac, that is, anal sacculitis. (23) Anal-sac impaction may also result from an obstructed duct.(23)

5.   Anal sac impaction and anal sacculitis are relatively uncommon events in the cat as compared to the dog.(21)

6.   In addition to scooting, clinical signs of sac disease include:(19, 35)

- biting at the tail
- bouts of constipation
- dyschezia
- externally palpable anal sacs during perineal examination
- holding the tail in an unusual position
- licking the tail excessively
- perineal swelling
- perineal erythema
- perineal ulceration, with or without draining tracts
- tenesmus
- visibly swollen anal sacs when the perineum is examined.

7.   In cats, anal-sac impactions and associated sacculitis may be due to:(2, 18, 20, 21, 24, 36)

- allergic skin disease
- change in anal muscle tone
- chronic constipation
- chronic diarrhea
- dysfunction of the anal sphincter
- genetics
- hypersecretion by anal glands
- hypoplastic anal sacs
- infectious skin disease
- lack of roughage in the diet
- megacolon
- occluded anal sac duct.

8. If you were to grossly examine normal (healthy) anal-sac contents, you would find that secretions vary immensely in color from creamy white-yellow-grey to tan-yellow-orange and brown. (19, 35)

9. If you were to grossly examine normal (healthy) anal sac contents, you would find that secretions vary immensely in consistency from watery to thick like toothpaste.(19, 35) Younger cats are more likely to exhibit the former consistency.(37)

10. Red anal-sac secretions would concern me because the presence of the pigment red suggests that hemorrhage is present. In this region of the body, hemorrhage may be due to inflammatory disease, such as anal sacculitis, or anal-sac neoplasia.

11. If you were to examine anal-sac contents of a normal (healthy) patient under light microscopy, you might expect to see:(35, 37)

    - amorphous, basophilic background
    - leukocytes:

        - neutrophils
        - monocytes

    - mixed bacterial population:

        - gram positive cocci predominate

    - yeast.

12. If you were to examine anal-sac contents of a normal (healthy) patient under light microscopy, you would NOT expect to see erythrocytes or intracellular bacteria.(35, 37)

13. Differences in cytology between normal and diseased anal sacs in dogs are not statistically significant.(38) To my knowledge, no similar studies have been reported in cats. However, reports in the canine literature suggest that cytology is not an effective tool to diagnose anal-sac disease.(38)

    It is, however, still important to perform cytology to rule out other causes of anal-sac disease, such as neoplasia.

14. Anal sac secretions are not typically cultured because bacterial and yeast populations are similar in normal and diseased anal sacs.(37, 39, 40) Commonly cultured bacteria include:(37, 39, 40)

    - *Bacillus* spp.
    - *Clostridium* spp.
    - *Escherichia coli*
    - *micrococci*
    - *Proteus* spp.
    - *staphylococci*
    - *streptococci*.

15. The right ruptured anal sac is a source of infection to surrounding tissue given the abundant mixed bacterial population that resides in the anal sac, in health as well as in diseased states. (19) Cellulitis that is associated with the rupture site is a common occurrence.(19) The ruptured sac should be cannulated and lavaged with warm saline or dilute chlorhexidine.(19) Topical antibiotic ointment can be applied to the site.(19) Such ointments may or may not contain corticosteroids. Those that do will reduce local inflammation. Systemic antibiotics are indicated if the patient is febrile.(19)

    The site of rupture is left open to heal.(19) The cat should be prevented from reaching the site by means of an Elizabethan collar until the skin seals over the defect.

    Warm compresses applied to the site for 15–20 minutes, two to three times a day, may reduce swelling and discomfort.(23) If cats are tolerant, then lowering their rear into a warm basin of water may achieve the same effect. Not all cats are amenable to this approach, so you must tailor your treatment plan to the patient. If a treatment is going to incite a fight, then it is probably not worth doing.

16. The contralateral anal sac (the left one) appears to be impacted. Impaction can be managed by expressing the sac, if possible.(19, 21) This requires rectal examination, which, in a cat, calls for sedation.(21) Kitty Perry will need analgesia in addition to sedation because anal-sac ruptures are extraordinarily tender to the touch.

    If anal-sac secretions are thick, they may need to be loosened first.(19, 23) You can achieve this by cannulating the sac and infusing warm saline.(19, 23) After expressing sac contents, it is beneficial to irrigate the sac with an antiseptic solution to guard against infection.(21, 23) Acceptable choices for flushing include 0.5% chlorhexidine or 10% povidone iodine.(23)

    Anti-inflammatory medications can be infused through the anal-sac duct to reduce local swelling.(19)

    A diet change may be discussed with the client with the hopes that increased fiber content may add to fecal bulk and therefore facilitate sac emptying with bowel movements.(21, 23) Psyllium, pumpkin, or bran can be added to the patient's current diet or the patient can be switched to a prescription food.(23) Prescription foods are often of the weight loss variety to provide the fiber content that is required to stretch the anus during defecation due to added fecal bulk.(23) Fecal bulk compresses and empties the anal sacs.(23)

17. If anal sacculitis and/or rupture of one or both anal sacs recurs, then you may recommend an anal sacculectomy.(19, 21–24, 35, 36) This procedure involves surgical excision of both anal sacs so that impaction and rupture can no longer occur.(19, 21–24, 35, 36)

18. Surgical complications are uncommon, but possible and include:(19, 23)

    - fecal incontinence, which occurs if there is damage to the caudal rectal nerve during surgical excision of one or both anal sacs
        - fecal incontinence may be transient or permanent:
            - if only one side is damaged, then the anal sphincter should reinnervate within 4 to 6 weeks because the other nerve is intact(22)
            - damage to both nerves is likely to result in permanent fecal incontinence
            - if fecal incontinence persists for 3 or more months following anal sacculectomy, then nerve damage is considered permanent
    - fistula development due to persistent drainage occurs if there is incomplete excision of the anal sac or its mucosal lining
    - rectal prolapse
    - seroma formation in the immediate postoperative period
    - stricture formation.

19. You can reassure Clive that anal-sac neoplasia in cats is rare.(19, 21)

20. If anal sac neoplasia occurs in the cat, it is typically anal-sac gland adenocarcinoma.(19, 21) Sometimes this is referred to as apocrine gland adenocarcinoma of the anal sac because this tumor type arises from the apocrine glands.(21) It is ulcerative and locally aggressive.(19) It carries a poor prognosis.(19)

21. Yes, anal-sac gland adenocarcinoma can also occur in dogs.(19) It is uncommon, but possible.(19)

22. The most common malignant rectal tumor in the dog is adenocarcinoma.(19)

23. Benign rectal tumors can occur in dogs. The most common among these is the adenomatous rectal polyp.(19)

24. Yes, benign rectal tumors can undergo malignant transformation as is seen in people.(19)

25. The most common type of perianal tumor in the dog is perianal gland adenoma.(19)

26. In addition to arising at or around the rim of the anus, perianal gland adenomas in the dog may arise on the tail, scrotum, prepuce, groin, or thighs.(19)

27. Growth of perianal gland adenomas is fueled by androgen, such that intact male dogs are at increased risk of developing this condition.(19)

28. Castration of intact male dogs will cause the perianal gland adenoma to regress.(19) Alternatively, perianal gland adenomas can be removed by surgical excision.(19) Radiation therapy is also effective.(19)

CLINICAL PEARLS

- Scooting is a common sign of anal-sac disease in dogs and cats. It may also result from allergic skin disease, perianal tumors, or endoparasitism.

- Other clinical signs of anal sac disease include:
    - changes in bowel habits or frequency; painful defecation
    - externally palpable anal sacs
    - unusual or excessive grooming at the perineum or tail
    - visible perineal swelling, redness, or ulceration +/− draining tracts

- Scooting is thought to alleviate perineal itch.

- Anal-sac impaction may lead to anal sacculitis. Anal sacculitis may lead to anal-sac rupture.

- When an anal sac is impacted, it needs to be expressed. This often requires cannulation of the anal sac to infuse warm saline to loosen up the thick secretions.

- Anal sacculitis also often requires cannulation to infuse anti-inflammatory ointment to reduce swelling and ease discomfort.

- Anal-sac rupture often leads to cellulitis. Because anal sacs naturally contain mixed bacterial and yeast populations, local infection is common. Systemic infection may also develop. Fever is a sign of systemic infection.

- Anal-sac ruptures are medically managed by flushing with antiseptic, administering topical and/or systemic antibiotics as indicated, warm compresses, and preventing the patient from accessing the site. Wounds are left open to drain and heal.

- Repeat occurrences may require surgical excision of the anal sacs, anal sacculectomy.

References

1. Rijnberk A, Stokhof AA. General examination. In: Rijnberk A, van Sluijs FJ, editors. Medical history and physical examination in companion animals. New York: Elsevier Limited; 2009.
2. Englar RE. Performing the small animal physical examination. Hoboken, NJ: Wiley/Blackwell; 2017.
3. Reuss-Lamky H. Hypothermia overview. Clinician's. Brief 2015(Nov(ember):12–6.
4. Zeltzman P, editor. Hypothermia in surgical patients. ACVS; 2009.
5. Harvey R, editor. Crisis management: what to worry about. AAHA; 2009.
6. McKelvey D, Hollingshead K. Small animal anesthesia: canine and feline practice. St. Louis, MO: Mosby; 1994.
7. Kaizer-Klinger S, editor. Troubleshooting emergency anesthesia. Phoenix, AZ: IVECC; 2008.
8. Sousa MG, Carareto R, Pereira-Junior VA, Aquino MC. Comparison between auricular and standard rectal thermometers for the measurement of body temperature in dogs. Can Vet J 2011;52(4):403–6.
9. Pachtinger G, King LG. Fever of unknown origin. Clinician's. Brief 2010 (March):29–32.
10. Englar R. Writing skills for veterinarians. Sheffield: 5M Publishing; 2019.
11. Trossman S. The documentation dilemma: Nurses poised to address paperwork burden. Am Nurse 2001;33(5):1–18.
12. Page A, editor. Keeping patients safe: Transforming the work environment of nurses. Washington, DC; 2004.
13. Nguyen AVT, Nguyen DA. Learning from medical errors: Legal issues. Abingdon: Radcliffe Publishing; 2005.
14. Andrews A, St. Aubyn B. 'It it's not written down; it didn't happen.' J Commun Nurs 2015;29(5):20–2.
15. Catalano J. Nursing now! Today's Issues, Tomorrow's Trends. 7th ed. Philadelphia, PA: F. A. Davis Company; 2015.
16. David G, Vinkhuyzen E. Medical records' dynamic nature. If it isn't written down, it didn't happen. And if it is written down, it might not be what it seems. J AHIMA 2013;84(11):32–5.
17. Goic JB, Reineke EL, Drobatz KJ. Comparison of rectal and axillary temperatures in dogs and cats. J Am Vet Med Assoc 2014;244(10):1170–5.
18. Englar RE. Common clinical presentations in dogs and cats. Hoboken, NJ: Wiley/Blackwell; 2019. pages cm p.
19. Aronson LR. Rectum, anus, and perineum. In: Tobias KM, Johnston SA, editors. Veterinary surgery: small animal. St. Louis, MO: Saunders; 2012.
20. Ettinger SJ, Feldman EC, Côté E. Textbook of veterinary internal medicine: Diseases of the dog and the cat. 8th ed. St. Louis, MO: Elsevier; 2017.
21. White RN. Large intestine, rectum, and anus. In: Langley-Hobbs SJ, Demetriou J, Ladlow JF, editors. Feline soft tissue and general surgery. New York: Saunders/Elsevier; 2014.
22. Tobias KM. Anal sacculectomy. In: Tobias KM, editor. Manual of small animal soft tissue surgery. Ames, IA: Wiley/Blackwell; 2010.
23. Surgery of the digestive system. In: Fossum TW, Duprey LP, O'Connor D, editors. Small animal surgery. 3rd ed. Boston, MA: Elsevier; 2007.
24. Côté E. Clinical veterinary advisor. Dogs and cats. 3rd ed. St. Louis, MO: Elsevier Mosby; 2015.
25. Singh B, Dyce KM. Dyce, Sack, and Wensing's textbook of veterinary anatomy. St. Louis, MO: Saunders; 2018.
26. Tsukise A, Meyer W, Nagaoka D, Kikuchi K, Kimura J, Fujimori O. Lectin histochemistry of the canine anal glands. Ann Anat 2000;182(2):151–9.
27. Nara T, Yasui T, Fujimori O, Meyer W, Tsukise A. Histochemical properties of sialic acids and antimicrobial substances in canine anal glands. Eur J Histochem 2011;55(3):e29.
28. Bradshaw JWS, Brown SL. Behavioral adaptations of dogs to domestication. In: Berger IH, editor. Pets, benefits, and practice. London: British Veterinary Association Publications; 1990. p. 18–24.
29. Sprague RH, Anisko JJ. Elimination patterns in the laboratory beagle. Behaviour 1973;47(3):257–67.
30. Overall KL. Normal canine behavior. In: Overall KL, editor. Clinical behavioral medicine for small animals. St. Louis: Mosby; 1997. p. 10–44.
31. Fox MW, Bekoff M. The behaviour of dogs. In: Hafez EEE, editor. The behaviour of domestic animals. 3rd ed. Baltimore, MD: Williams & Wilkins; 1975. p. 370–409.
32. Rosen JB, Asok A, Chakraborty T. The smell of fear: Innate threat of 2,5-dihydro-2,4,5-trimethylthiazoline, a single molecule component of a predator odor. Front Neurosci 2015;9:292.

33. Samuel L, Arnesen C, Zedrosser A, Rosell F. Fears from the past? The innate ability of dogs to detect predator scents. Anim Cogn 2020;23(4):721–9.
34. Takahashi LK, Nakashima BR, Hong H, Watanabe K. The smell of danger: a behavioral and neural analysis of predator odor-induced fear. Neurosci Biobehav Rev 2005;29(8):1157–67.
35. Ruffner E, Fancher MD, Sherman C, Owens L, Tobias KM. Anal Sacculectomy in cats. Clinician's Brief 2014:31–5.
36. Bright RM. Anal sacculectomy Anal. Clinicians Brief 2003 (June):36–8.
37. Frankel JL, Scott DW, Erb HN. Gross and cytological characteristics of normal feline anal-sac secretions. J Feline Med Surg 2008;10(4):319–23.
38. James DJ, Griffin CE, Polissar NL, Neradilek MB. Comparison of anal sac cytological findings and behaviour in clinically normal dogs and those affected with anal sac disease. Vet Dermatol 2011;22(1):80–7.
39. Scarff DH. An approach to anal sac diseases. In: Foster AP, Foil CS, editors. British Small Animal Veterinary Association manual of small animal dermatology. Gloucester: British Small Animal Veterinary Association; 2003. p. 121–4.
40. Miller WH, Griffin CE, Campbell KL, Muller GH, Scott DW. Muller and Kirk's small animal dermatology. 7th ed. St. Louis, MO: Elsevier; 2013.

Case 27

The Dog with a "Swollen Eye"

Curly Fry is new to your clinic. His owner, Rana Thurman, recently moved from the UK to New York City, and it has been quite the adjustment. Both Curly Fry and Rana had been used to the rolling hillside. Now, it's a thirty-minute walk just to find their way to Central Park to feel grass beneath their feet.

Curly Fry has never been sick to Rana's knowledge and he is the "only child" in this family of two. Rana is an entrepreneur who logs long hours at the office, but she is above all attentive to details, which is why she panicked when she came home to find that Curly Fry had a swollen mass protruding from his eye (see Figure 27.1).

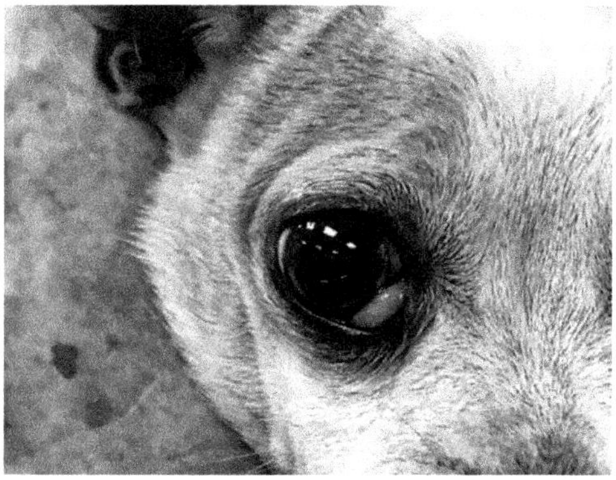

Curly Fry did not seem to be exceedingly bothered by this change in his appearance. He was at the door like always, waiting for Rana to come home, and when she opened the front door, he leaped into her arms dramatically, with a chorus of whines, as if she were the only person on earth who he'd seen in an eternity. He covered her face with wet kisses and greeted her like royalty. It wasn't until she'd returned him to the ground that she'd gotten a good glimpse of his face.

Figure 27.1 Meet your new patient, Curly Fry, a 4-year-old male castrated Chihuahua mix. Courtesy of Samantha Thurman, DVM.

At first, she thought for sure she'd made it up. But, no, on second glance, there it was – a red, bulging growth next to his eye. From time to time, he'd paw at his eye or give an unusually pronounced blink as if the growth might be interfering with his line of vision. Rana googled clinics in the area and found that yours had evening office hours. That was all she needed to know before scooping up Curly Fry and hailing a cab.

Within a half-hour, she and Curly Fry are in your waiting room, appreciative that you were able to fit them in. Your veterinary assistant-in-training logs Curly Fry's vital signs while they wait.

Your veterinary assistant-in-training briefs you on the case. This is her first day and she has never seen a clinical presentation like Curly Fry's. When you ask her to summarize the case in a sentence, she shares Curly Fry's signalment and that he is presenting today for a "swollen left eye."

Consider the following questions as you prepare for the case.

Weight: 9.9 lb (4.5 kg)
BCS: 4/9
Muscle condition score: Moderate muscle loss
Mentation: BAR
Systolic BP: 271 mmHg

TPR

T: 100.4°F (38.0°C)
P: 164 beats per minute
R: Panting

Round One of Questions for Case 27: The Dog with a "Swollen Eye"

1. The patient's photograph (Figure 27.1) was taken at check-in and is now a part of Curly Fry's medical record, which you can access. Is your veterinary assistant-in-training correct: does Curly Fry's condition involve his left eye or surrounding structures?
2. How would you document this unilateral presentation in the medical record? Which Latin abbreviation would you use to denote the laterality of the eye?
3. A swollen eye could refer to the eye itself or to its adnexa. What is the appropriate medical term for an enlarged globe?
4. What causes the condition that you identified in Question #3 (above)?
5. Based upon the patient's photograph (Figure 27.1) does it appear that Curly Fry has this condition?
6. If you wanted to be certain of your answer in Question #5 (above), which diagnostic test would you perform?
7. A swollen eye could refer to corneal edema, that is, swelling associated with the transparent outer coat of the eye. What does corneal edema look like?
8. What could cause corneal edema?
9. Based upon the patient's photograph (Figure 27.1), does it appear that Curly Fry has this condition?
10. Based upon the patient's photograph, does any aspect of Curly Fry's eye itself look swollen?
11. What does adnexa mean relative to the eye?
12. Which structures are adnexa of the eye?
13. Which of the structures that you identified in Question #12 (above) could be swollen?
14. Based upon the patient's photograph (Figure 27.1), which of these structures is most likely to be involved?
15. What is the colloquial term for the condition that Curly Fry has?
16. What is the appropriate medical term for the condition that Curly Fry has?

Answers to Round One of Questions for Case 27: The Dog with a "Swollen Eye"

1. The veterinary assistant-in-training made a rookie mistake. When she is looking at Curly Fry's face, head-on, his eye on her left is associated with the nictitans prolapse. However, that eye is Curly Fry's right rather than his left.

2. I would document this unilateral presentation as prolapsed nictitans OD. OD is Latin for oculus dexter, which means "right eye."[1]

3. The appropriate medical term for an enlarged globe is buphthalmos.[2–7]

4. Buphthalmos is caused by an increase in intraocular pressure (IOP) [2, 3, 5–7], as from glaucoma.[8]

5. No, it does not appear that Curly Fry has this condition. Although dogs with glaucoma may have a prominent nictitans, they are more likely to present with the following features on physical exam:[7–10]

   - absent menace response
     - clinically blind
   - blepharospasm
   - epiphora

- episcleral congestion
- conjunctival hyperemia
- corneal edema
- mydriasis
- "red eye" (see **Plate 23**).

6. If you wanted to be certain that Curly Fry does not have glaucoma, then you would need to assess his IOP through tonometry.(7, 8, 11)

7. Corneal edema changes the appearance of the affected eye such that its surface appears hazy-grey to blue-grey to blue.(7, 12)

8. Corneal edema may result from:(6)

- age-related endothelial degeneration(12, 13)
- glaucoma(12, 14, 15)
- traumatic injury to the globe(7)
- uveitis.(12, 14, 15)

9. No, it does not appear that Curly Fry has this condition.

10. No, based upon the photograph, it does not appear that any part of Curly Fry's right eye is swollen.

11. Adnexa of the eye refers to the surrounding structures that support the globe.(6, 7)

12. The following structures are considered adnexa of the eye:(6, 7, 16–18)

- conjunctiva
- eyelids
- lacrimal apparatus
- nictitating membrane.

13. Any of the structures that were identified in Question #12 (above) could be swollen.(6, 7)

- Conjunctivitis refers to inflammation of the conjunctiva (see **Plate 24**).
- Blepharitis refers to inflammation of the eyelids (see **Plate 25**).
- Dacryoadenitis refers to inflammation of the lacrimal gland.
- The nictitans becomes swollen when it prolapses.

14. Based upon the patient's photograph (Figure 27.1), the nictitans is most likely to be involved.

15. Cherry eye is the colloquial term for the condition that Curly Fry has.(6, 7, 19–22)

16. The appropriate medical term for cherry eye is a prolapsed nictitans. Sometimes this is referred to as a prolapsed nictitating membrane or a prolapsed third eyelid.(7)

Returning to Case 27: The Dog with a "Swollen Eye"

You take a comprehensive patient history and perform a physical exam. Your exam confirms your suspicion that Curly Fry does indeed have a prolapsed nictitans.

Round Two of Questions for Case 27: The Dog with a "Swollen Eye"

1. Where specifically within the orbit, relative to the eye, is the nictitans?
2. What maintains the position of the nictitans within the orbit?
3. What is/are the purpose(s) of the nictitans?
4. Is the nictitans typically visible in a normal (healthy) dog?
5. What does the nictitans look like in health in terms of color and appearance?
6. When the nictitans becomes prolapsed, how might its appearance change?
7. Other than a prolapse of the nictitans, what can cause the nictitans to be more prominent?
8. Rana asks if Curly Fry's condition is likely to spontaneously resolve. What do you tell her?
9. Rana asks if Curly Fry's breed has predisposed him to this condition. How will you answer her?
10. Are dogs more likely to be affected by this condition or are cats?
11. If Curly Fry were a cat instead of a dog, which breeds would be most likely to develop this condition?

Answers to Round Two of Questions for Case 27: The Dog with a "Swollen Eye"

1. The nictitans typically rests in the ventro-medial orbit.(6, 7)

2. The position of the nictitans in the orbit is maintained by the sympathetic tone of the orbital smooth muscles.(20)

3. The nictitans contains a T-shaped wedge of hyaline cartilage that acts like a windshield wiper. (7, 23) Every time the patient blinks, the nictitans glides across the cornea.(7, 23) This spreads tear film across the surface of the eye.(7, 23) In addition, the nictitans is a significant contributor to tear film.(6, 7, 20, 23, 24)

4. No, the nictitans is typically not visible in a normal (healthy) dog.(6, 7) In order to evaluate this structure during the veterinary consult, you need to learn how to bring it into view. You do this by pushing down gently, but firmly, over the upper palpebra. This will elevate the nictitans for visual inspection.(4, 6, 7)

5. The nictitans is typically pink and shiny because its surfaces are lined with moist conjunctiva. (6, 7) Its leading edge may be pigmented black.

6. When the nictitans becomes prolapsed, it no longer retains its moisture and tends to dry out.(19–21) This may cause it to appear dull, rather than shiny.(6, 7) It may also become erythematous.

7. Other than a prolapse of the nictitans, the following conditions may cause this structure to be more prominent:

    - foreign body, such as a grass awn, lodged within the orbit(4)
    - Horner's syndrome:(25–28)

        - sympathetic denervation to the eye, characterized by:(6, 7, 25, 28–30)

            - miosis
            - ptosis
            - enopthalmos
            - prominent nictitans

- neoplasia of the nictitans:(31–35)

    - uncommon in companion animal patients(31, 36)
    - more often malignant(31, 36–40)
    - most often adenocarcinoma(31, 39, 40)
    - the nictitans takes on a bulbous appearance(7)

- ocular pain or irritation, as from corneal ulceration(41)
- systemic illness, as from a heavy burden with gastrointestinal parasites:(4, 6, 7)

    - typically leads to bilateral involvement of the nictitans
    - historically this was referred to as Haws syndrome.(7)

8. Prolapse of the nictitans is often transient in the early stages.(7) However, I would expect that Curly Fry's affected nictitans will become permanently prolapsed.(7)

9. Certain breeds do appear predisposed to cherry eye; however, I have not seen Chihuahuas or Chihuahua mixes appear in any of these lists. Most common canine breeds to be affected are small to medium breeds including:(21, 22, 36, 42, 43)

- Bassett hounds
- Beagles
- Boston terriers
- Cocker Spaniels

- English Bulldogs
- Lhasa apsos
- Pekingese
- Shih tzus

Great Danes, German shepherds, Weimaraners, German shorthaired pointers, Irish setters, and Newfoundland dogs are among the larger breeds to be overrepresented.(44–49)

10. Dogs more often develop cherry eye than cats do.(36, 50–54)

11. If Curly Fry were a cat instead of a dog, he would be at greater risk of contracting this condition if he were a Burmese (51, 53, 55), Siamese(56), or Persian.(56)

Returning to Case 27: The Dog with a "Swollen Eye"

You excuse yourself from the examination room for a moment to check on an inpatient at the request of one of your colleagues. When you return to the consultation, you find Rana researching cherry eye on her smart phone. She has prepared a list of questions for you concerning treatment recommendations.

Round Three of Questions for Case 27: The Dog with a "Swollen Eye"

1. Rana has read that the preferred treatment for cherry eye is surgical excision of the nictitans. Although this procedure is still performed by some clinicians, you share with her your concerns about a potentially serious surgical outcome. What is the risk associated with removing the entire nictitans?
2. To prevent the complication that you identified in Question #1 (above), how do you recommend proceeding with this case?
3. Can recurrence of cherry eye occur after surgical correction?
4. Rana asks if the other eye could become affected. What do you say?
5. Rana is very concerned that she did something to cause this problem. She says that the apartment

is a mess and she has hardly unpacked. Dust is everywhere. Is it possible that the dust irritated his eye and caused this problem? She feels responsible for Curly Fry and is beside herself that her actions (or inactions) may have precipitated this. How do you respond to her?

Answers to Round Three of Questions for Case 27: The Dog with a "Swollen Eye"

1. Because the nictitans is a significant contributor to tear film, surgical excision of the nictitans predisposes the patient to keratoconjunctivitis sicca (KCS), otherwise known as "dry eye." (6, 7)

2. To prevent this complication, it is no longer advisable to remove the nictitans surgically as a means of correcting cherry eye. Instead, newer techniques aim to replace the nictitans within the orbit.(36) The conjunctival pocket technique is just one of many methods of restoring the nictitans to its anatomic position.(36, 43, 50, 57–60)

3. Yes, recurrence can occur after surgical correction of cherry eye. However, when the conjunctival pocket technique is used, the rate of recurrence is low.(43)

4. Unilateral presentations may progress to bilateral ones.(19, 20, 22) It is likely, though not guaranteed, that Curly Fry will develop cherry eye in his contralateral orbit.

5. Although dust can contribute to allergic conjunctivitis, Rana's lack of unpacking did not cause Curly Fry's current condition. I would normalize her feelings ("I understand why you might worry that . . ."). I would then explain that there is no link between particulate matter and nictitans prolapse. She did not cause this to occur.

CLINICAL PEARLS

- Companion animal patients often have clinical presentations that involve the eye. A "swollen eye" is a common clinical complaint. It may or may not involve the eye.

- It is important to consider the anatomy of the region of the body that is being presented for evaluation. When a patient presents for a "swollen eye", it is important to consider the surrounding structures as well as the globe itself.

- The structures that surround and support the globe include:
  - the eyelids
  - the conjunctiva
  - the nictitans / the nictitating membrane / the third eyelid
  - the lacrimal apparatus.

- Any of these structures can become swollen. Each has its own classic appearance.

- A prolapsed nictitans is readily apparent in the consultation room. It can be diagnosed based on appearance alone.

- In health, the nictitans is typically tucked into the ventro-medial pocket of the orbit.

- Its purpose is to protect the eye's surface, produce tears, and spread tear film across the cornea every time that the patient blinks.

- When the nictitans prolapses, it bulges out from the orbit and looks like a fleshy pink mass. For this reason, nictitans prolapse is often referred to as "cherry eye."

- A prolapsed nictitans may initially come and go, but over time, the prolapse is likely to become permanent.

- As the prolapse persists, the tissue may become erythematous. It also desiccates.

- Prolapse may be unilateral or bilateral. Prolapse may progress to a bilateral state.

- Surgical excision of a prolapsed nictitans was historically the treatment of choice. However, because the nictitans contributes to tear film, surgical excision of this structure is likely to result in keratoconjunctivitis (dry eye).

- A preferred approach to cherry eye is to perform a "tucking" procedure to surgically replace the gland within its anatomic location in the orbit.

References

1. Englar R. Writing skills for veterinarians. Sheffield: 5M Publishing; 2019.
2. Aiello SE, Moses MC. Merck Veterinary Manual. Whitehouse Station, NJ: Merck Sharp and Dohme, Corp. 2016.
3. Côté E. Clinical veterinary advisor. Dogs and cats. 3rd ed. St. Louis, MO: Elsevier Mosby; 2015.
4. Englar RE. Performing the small animal physical examination. Hoboken, NJ: Wiley; 2017.
5. Tilley LP, Smith FWK, Tilley LP. Blackwell's five-minute veterinary consult: canine and feline. 4th ed. Ames, IA: Blackwell; 2007.
6. Englar RE. Performing the small animal physical examination. Hoboken, NJ: Wiley/Blackwell; 2017.
7. Englar RE. Common clinical presentations in dogs and cats. Hoboken, NJ: Wiley/Blackwell; 2019. pages cm p.
8. Maggio F. Glaucomas. Top Companion Anim Med 2015;30(3):86–96.
9. Reinstein S. Under pressure: canine and feline Glaucoma. 2017. Available from: https://michvma.org/resources/Documents/MVC/2017%20Proceedings/reinstein%2005.pdf.
10. Reinstein S, Rankin A, Allbaugh R. Canine glaucoma: pathophysiology and diagnosis. Compend Contin Educ Vet 2009;31(10):450–2; quiz 2–3.
11. Wilkie DA. Determining intraocular pressure. NAVC Clin's Brief 2013;February:77–9.
12. Strom AR, Maggs DJ. Corneal opacities in dogs and cats. Today's. Vet Pract 2015;May/June:105–13.
13. Gelatt KN, Gilger BC, Kern TJMacKay EO, Gelatt KN. Veterinary Ophthalmology. Hoboken, NJ:. Wiley-Blackwell; 2013.
14. Gelatt KN. Essentials of veterinary ophthalmology. Ames, IA: John Wiley & Sons, Inc.; 2014.
15. Townsend WM. Canine and feline uveitis. Vet Clin North Am Small Anim Pract 2008;38(2):323–46.
16. Eyelids MC. In: Martin C, editor. Ophthalmic disease in veterinary medicine. London: Manson Publishing, Inc.; 2005. p. 145–82.
17. Martin CL. Conjunctiva and third eyelild. In: Martin CL, editor. Ophthalmic diseases in veterinary medicine. London: Manson Publishing, Inc.; 2005. p. 205–9.
18. Martin C. Lacrimal system. In: Martin C, editor. Ophthalmic disease in veterinary medicine. London: Manson Publishing, Inc.; 2005. p. 219–40.
19. Mazzucchelli S, Vaillant MD, Wéverberg F, Arnold-Tavernier H, Honegger N, Payen G, et al. Retrospective study of 155 cases of prolapse of the nictitating membrane gland in dogs. Vet Rec 2012;170(17):443.
20. Maggs DJ. Third eyelid. In: Maggs DJ, Miller PE, Ofri R, Slatter DH, editors. Slatter's fundamentals of veterinary ophthalmology. 5th ed. St. Louis, MO: Elsevier; 2013. p. 151–6.

21. Hendrix DVH. Canine conjunctiva and nictitating membrane. In: Gelatt KS, editor. Veterinary ophthalmology. Oxford: Blackwell Publishing; 2007. p. 662–89.
22. Plummer CE, Källberg ME, Gelatt KN, Gelatt JP, Barrie KP, Brooks DE. Intranictitans tacking for replacement of prolapsed gland of the third eyelid in dogs. Vet Ophthalmol 2008;11(4):228–33.
23. Brooks DE. Removal of the third eyelid. NAVC Clin's Brief 2005(January):47–9.
24. Gómez JB. Repairing nictitans gland prolapse in dogs. Vet Rec 2012;171(10):244–5.
25. Penderis J. Diagnosis of Horner's syndrome in dogs and cats. Pract 2015;37(3):107–19.
26. Boydell P. Horner's syndrome following cervical spinal surgery in the dog. J Small Anim Pract 1995;36(11): 510–2.
27. Garosi LS, Dennis R, Penderis J, Lamb CR, Targett MP, Cappello R, Delauche AJ. Results of magnetic resonance imaging in dogs with vestibular disorders: 85 cases (1996–1999). J Am Vet Med Assoc 2001;218(3):385–91.
28. Heller HB, Bentley E. The practitioner's guide to neurologic causes of canine anisocoria. Today's. Vet Pract 2016 (January/February):[77–83]. Available from: http://todaysveterinarypractice.navc.com/wp-content/uploads/2016/05/TVP_2016–0102_OO-Anisocoria.pdf.
29. Troxel M. Horner syndrome at a glance. Clinician's. Brief 2014 (May);25.
30. Bagley RS. The cat with anisocoria or abnormally dilated or contricted pupils. In: Rand J, editor. Problem-based feline medicine. New York: Saunders; 2006. p. 870–89.
31. Aquino SM. Management of eyelid neoplasms in the dog and cat. Clin Tech Small Anim Pract 2007;22(2):46–54.
32. Dees DD, Schobert CS, Dubielzig RR, Stein TJ. Third eyelid gland neoplasms of dogs and cats: a retrospective histopathologic study of 145 cases. Vet Ophthalmol 2016;19(2):138–43.
33. Rodriguez Galarza RMR, Shrader SM, Koehler JW, Abarca E. A case of basal cell carcinoma of the nictitating membrane in a dog. Clin Case Rep 2016;4(12):1161–7.
34. Liapis IK, Genovese L. Hemangiosarcoma of the third eyelid in a dog. Vet Ophthalmol 2004;7(4):279–82.
35. Wang AL, Kern T. Melanocytic ophthalmic neoplasms of the domestic veterinary species: a review. Top Companion Anim Med 2015;30(4):148–57.
36. Aquino SM. Surgery of the eyelids. Top Companion Anim Med 2008;23(1):10–22.
37. Gelatt KN. Surgery of the eyelids. In: Gelatt KN, Gelatt JP, editors. Small animal ophthalmic surgery. Tarrytown, NY: Pergamon; 1994. p. 60.
38. Krohne S. Ocular tumors of the dog and cat. In: Morrison WB, editor. Cancer in dogs and cats: medical and surgical management. Jackson, WY: Teton New Media; 2002. p. 701–26.
39. Wilcock B, Peiffer R, Jr. Adenocarcinoma of the gland of the third eyelid in seven dogs. J Am Vet Med Assoc 1988;193(12):1549–50.
40. Komaromy AM, Ramsey DT, Render JA, Clark P. Primary adenocarcinoma of the gland of the nictitating membrane in a cat. J Am Anim Hosp Assoc 1997;33(4):333–6.
41. Lim CC. Small animal ophthalmic atlas and guide. Oxford: Wiley; 2013.
42. Dugan SJ, Severin GA, Hungerford LL, Whiteley HE, Roberts SM. Clinical and histologic evaluation of the prolapsed third eyelid gland in dogs. J Am Vet Med Assoc 1992;201(12):1861–7.
43. Morgan RV, Duddy JM, Mcclurg K. Prolapse of the Gland of the 3rd-Eyelid in Dogs – a Retrospective Study of 89 Cases (1980 to 1990). J Am Anim Hosp Assoc 1993;29(1):56–60.
44. Allbaugh RA, Stuhr CM. Thermal cautery of the canine third eyelid for treatment of cartilage eversion. Vet Ophthalmol 2013;16(5):392–5.
45. Martin CL. Everted membrana nictitans in German Shorthaired Pointers. J Am Vet Med Assoc 1970;157(9):1229–32.
46. Moore CP, Constantinescu GM. Surgery of the adnexa. Vet Clin North Am Small Anim Pract 1997;27(5):1011–66.
47. Crispin S. Treating the everted membrana nictitans in the dog. Pract 1986;8(2):66–7.
48. Gelatt KN. Surgical correction of everted nictitating membrane in the dog. Vet Med Small Anim Clin 1972;67(3):291–2.
49. Jensen HE. Stereoscopic atlas of clinical ophthalmology of domestic animals. St. Louis, MO: Mosby; 1971.
50. Albert RA, Garrett PD, Whitley RD, Thomas KL. Surgical correction of everted third eyelid in two cats. J Am Vet Med Assoc 1982;180(7):763–6.
51. Chahory S, Crasta M, Trio S, Clerc B. Three cases of prolapse of the nictitans gland in cats. Vet Ophthalmol 2004;7(6):417–9.

52. Christmas R. Surgical correction of congenital ocular and nasal dermoids and third eyelid gland prolapse in related Burmese kittens. Can Vet J 1992;33(4):265–6.
53. Koch SA. Congenital ophthalmic abnormalities in the Burmese cat. J Am Vet Med Assoc 1979;174(1):90–1.
54. Schoofs SH. Prolapse of the gland of the third eyelid in a cat: a case report and literature review. J Am Anim Hosp Assoc 1999;35(3):240–2.
55. Williams D, Middleton S, Caldwell A. Everted third eyelid cartilage in a cat: a case report and literature review. Vet Ophthalmol 2012;15(2):123–7.
56. Cherry Eye AK. Clinician's. Brief 2004 (November):19–21.
57. Moore CP. Alternate technique for prolapsed gland of the third eyelid (replacement technique). In: Bojrab MJ, editor. Current techniques in small animal surgery. Philadelphia, PA: Lea & Febiger; 1983. p. 52–3.
58. Stanley RG, Kaswan RL. Modification of the orbital rim anchorage method for surgical replacement of the gland of the 3rd eyelid in dogs. Journal of the American Veterinary Medical Association 1994;205(10):1412–4.
59. Twitchell MJ. Surgical repair of a prolapsed gland of the 3rd eyelid in the dog. Mod Vet Pract 1984;65(3):223–.
60. Kaswan RL, Martin CL. Surgical-correction of 3rd eyelid prolapse in dogs. J Am Vet Med Assoc 1985;186(1):83.

Case 28

The Cat with Questionable Vision

Pico de Gato is new to your practice. He was adopted two years ago from a local humane organization and has not required veterinary care since then.

Pico de Gato is presenting to the weekend emergency service for evaluation of acute onset of disorientation. He seems reluctant to move. When he does, he steps hesitantly. His owner, Jacqueline Mahoney, became concerned when she saw Pico de Gato "bumping into things" tonight.

Jacqueline does not believe that he could have gotten into "anything" within the home. He is Jacqueline's only housemate and she insists that no chemicals or prescription medications are within his reach. However, Pico de Gato does lead an indoor/outdoor lifestyle, so Jacqueline cannot rule out exposure to an environmental toxin. At intake, Jacqueline mentions that she and her neighbor are in an ongoing spat about Pico de Gato hunting the songbirds next door. This raises his suspicion that foul play is involved.

"Could my neighbor have poisoned Pico de Gato?" Jacqueline asks the technician as he records the cat's vital signs in his chart below.

Your technician does not agree with or refute Jacqueline's claims. He simply acknowledges she was right to bring Pico de Gato into the clinic straight away.

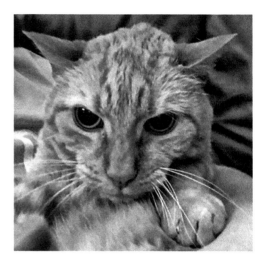

Figure 28.1 Meet your new patient, Pico de Gato, a 9-year-old, castrated male domestic shorthaired cat. Courtesy of Rachel Karner.

Weight: 11.6 lb (5.3 kg)
BCS: 3/9
Muscle condition score: Moderate muscle loss
Mentation: QAR

TPR

T: 100.6°F (38.1°C)
P: 172 beats per minute
R: 26 breaths per minute

Round One of Questions for Case 28: The Cat with Questionable Vision

1. When your technician summarizes the case for you, he shares his concern that Pico de Gato can't see. What clues might he have seen on gross inspection of Pico de Gato that would support this concern?
2. Other than blindness, what else could cause the physical exam feature(s) that you identified in Question #1 (above)?

3. How would you evaluate the patient for the condition(s) that you identified in Question #2 (above)?
4. If the patient is truly blind, will you expect to see a menace response in the affected eye(s)?
5. Describe the menace response.
6. Which two cranial nerves (CNs) does the menace response assess?
7. What are some other ways to assess vision in companion animal patients?
8. Why might it be difficult to assess cats for vision using some of the methods that you outlined in Question #7 (above)?
9. Vision is a complicated pathway that involves more than just the eye. What are other parts of the pathway that are required to be functional for the patient to be visual?
10. Deficits can occur anywhere along the visual pathway. (1, 2) Where in the pathway are lesions most likely to arise?
11. Assessment of which reflex will assist with lesion localization?
12. Describe how to assess for the reflex that you identified in Question #11 (above).
13. Which CNs does this reflex assess?
14. Before you perform any sort of physical examination on this patient, including the neurologic exam, which diagnostic test do you want to perform?
15. Why do you want to perform this test?

Answers to Round One of Questions for Case 28: The Cat with Questionable Vision

1. Patients that are blind have mydriatic pupils.(3, 4) The affected pupils will be large and saucer-like.(4)

2. Fear, anxiety, and stress (FAS) can also cause mydriatic pupils.(3–7)

3. If Pico de Gato were experiencing signs of FAS, then, in addition to mydriatic pupils, I would expect to see one or more of the following behavioral, postural, and/or physiologic changes on physical exam: (3, 5–7)

   • arching of the back
   • tachycardia
   • tachypnea
   • tense face
   • tense jaw
   • lowering of the head
   • "airplane ears," i.e., ears that swivel such that the inner pinna face sideways, in opposite directions, or are completely back and flattened against the skull
   • open mouth, associated with growling, hissing, or spitting
   • the body is tucked up to appear smaller and feet are hidden underneath of the body
   • the cat may be exhibiting piloerection of fur along the topline
   • the tail is curled around the body; the tail may or may not be piloerect
   • the tail may be thwacking rhythmically against the exam room table.

4. If Pico de Gato is blind bilaterally, then I would not expect to see a menace response in either eye.(4)

5. To perform the menace response, the clinician uses his/her hand to make a startling, threatening gesture towards each eye.(3, 4) Each eye is tested separately.(8, 9)
   Visual patients will observe the threat and blink to protect the eye, provided that both CNs II and VII are intact, and their pathways to the brain and brainstem are functional.(8, 9)

Avisual patients will not observe the threat.(3, 4) Therefore, they will not blink in response to the threat.(3, 4, 8, 9)

6. The optic (II) and facial (VII) CNs are tested by the menace response.(8, 9)

7. One can also assess vision using "tracking" and/or maze tests.(4, 10)

To "track" a patient's vision, you drop a cotton ball directly in front of the patient, and also to either side to each visual field.(4) Patients that are visual will see the falling object and follow it to the ground.(4) Patients must be paying attention for this test to be an accurate assessment of their visual status.(4) You may need to repeat the test multiple times to be sure that the patient is attentive.(4) Patients that consistently do not track the cotton ball may have diminished vision. (4, 10) If a cotton ball isn't handy, you can also make use of a laser pointer.(4) This is particularly of value during feline examinations.(4, 10)

Another way to assess the patient's vision is to create a maze of stationary objects around the room.(4) You then observe how the patient navigates through this makeshift obstacle course.(4) Obstacles do not need to be fancy.(4) Chairs or any other object within the practice will serve the function well.(4) Patients that can see will avoid the obstacles.(4) Patients that have visual deficits may stumble into objects or hesitate when walking around them.(4, 10) Mazes should be tested in a lit environment as well as in the dark to test photopic and scotopic vision.(4, 10) The maze itself should be altered between daylight and "night-time" simulated tests so that a patient does not simply memorize the course.(4, 10)

8. Cats are not always cooperative in the consultation room when we ask them to ambulate. Many freeze, hunch, or hide.(4) Refusal to move through the maze does not tell us anything about the patient's visual status.(4, 10)

9. Vision is a complicated pathway that involves more than just the eye. In order for patients to see, they also need functioning optic nerves, optic tracts, and a visual cortex.(1, 2)

10. Deficits can occur anywhere along the visual pathway.(1, 2) Common sites for lesions that result in blindness include the:(1, 2)

- retina
- optic nerve
- visual cortex.

11. Assessing the patient's pupillary light reflexes (PLRs), in addition to the patient's menace response, can facilitate lesion localization.(1, 11, 12) This is because the PLR and vision share the same neuroanatomical pathway until they reach the lateral geniculate nucleus.(1)

When lesions occur at or rostral to the lateral geniculate nucleus, meaning that they occur at one or both optic tracts, the optic chiasm, optic nerve, or retina, the patient will lack both menace responses and PLRs.(1)

When lesions that cause blindness occur beyond the lateral geniculate nucleus, PLRs will remain intact, but menace responses will be absent.(1) These patients are considered cortically blind.(11, 12) They cannot see, but they still have PLRs.

12. To test for intact PLRs, a bright light is directed at each eye. The pupil at which the light is directed should become miotic.(3, 4) That is, it should constrict and remain small for as long as the light source is present.(3, 4) This procedure assesses the patient's so-called direct PLR.(3, 4)

The indirect or consensual PLR evaluates the contralateral eye.(3, 4) If bright light is directed at the patient's right eye, then the patient's left pupil should also constrict.(3, 4)

13. The optic (II) and oculomotor (III) nerves are tested by the PLR.(11, 12)

14. Before you perform any sort of physical examination on this patient, including the neurologic exam, I would ask the technician to measure Pico de Gato's systolic blood pressure (BP).

15. Hypertension can cause retinopathy that leads to blindness.(3, 4) It is therefore essential that I check Pico de Gato's BP.

   I would want to assess Pico de Gato's BP prior to handling because some, but not all patients, get spooked at the veterinary clinic.(3, 4) These patients develop so-called "white coat syndrome" or "white coat hypertension."(3, 4) The clinic setting and how these patients are handled and examined in the consultation activates their sympathetic nervous system, resulting in situational hypertension.(3, 4)

   I want to minimize stress to the best of my ability so that the patient's resultant BP is more likely to be accurate (and not stress-induced). Therefore, BP should be measured first, particularly in feline patients. In this case, BP should have even been measured prior to taking Pico de Gato's temperature.

Returning to Case 28: The Cat with Questionable Vision

You ask your technician to take Pico de Gato's systolic BP before you examine him. Pico de Gato tolerates the procedure well. Three readings are taken and averaged. The mean is 280 mmHg.

Round Two of Questions for Case 28: The Cat with Questionable Vision

1. What value should systolic BP fall below in the cat for it not to be considered elevated?
2. Would you classify Pico de Gato's systolic BP as low, normal, or high?
3. What is the appropriate medical term for low BP?
4. What is the appropriate medical term for high BP?
5. BP may become elevated due to physiologic and pathologic changes. Discuss how physiologic changes may lead to situational hypertension.
6. Hypertension may also be pathologic. What are common causes of pathologic hypertension?
7. When systolic hypertension persists, which so-called target organs are at risk of sustaining damage?
8. Could Pico de Gato's clinical presentation have resulted from hypertension?
9. What kind of exam do you need to perform on a cat to gather evidence of hypertensive retinopathy?
10. What will you be looking for on this exam to evaluate the patient for hypertensive retinopathy?
11. Can anything else other than hypertension cause these lesions?
12. Blindness can also be caused by retinal degeneration. What causes retinal degeneration to occur?

Answers to Round Two of Questions for Case 28: The Cat with Questionable Vision

1. Systolic BP in the cat should fall below 150–160 mmHg to be considered "normal." In cats, systolic BP that is persistently greater than 160–170 mmHg is considered elevated.(4, 13–18)

2. Pico de Gato's systolic BP is considered high.

3. Hypotension is the appropriate medical term for low BP.(4)

4. Hypertension is the appropriate medical term for high BP.(4)

5. Stress causes situational hypertension and tachycardia by activating the sympathetic nervous system.(4) This fuels the fight-or-flight response, which is protective.

6. Hypertension can also be persistent and pathologic. Pathologic hypertension may be:(13, 15, 16, 19–21)

   - primary:

     - occurs more frequently in dogs than cats, but may be more common in cats than was once believed.(15, 22–26)

   - secondary:

     - often due to renal disease(13, 15–19, 27–30)
     - other causes include:(13, 15–17, 21, 28, 31–34)

       - acromegaly
       - chronic anemia
       - diabetes mellitus
       - erythropoietin treatments
       - high-salt diets
       - hyperthyroidism
       - hyperadrenocorticism
       - pheochromocytomas
       - primary hyperaldosteronism.

7. When systolic hypertension persists, the eyes, kidneys, heart, and brain are at increased risk of sustaining organ damage.(3, 4, 13)

8. Yes, Pico de Gato's clinical presentation could have resulted from hypertension. Blindness can result from hypertensive retinopathy.(4)

9. To evaluate a cat for evidence of hypertensive retinopathy, you need to perform a fundic exam. (3, 4, 13)

10. In the early stages of persistent hypertension, the retina will appear swollen during fundic exam. (13) If hypertension persists, then retinal hemorrhages may also be observed.(13, 16, 17, 21, 23, 30) Hemorrhages may be focal or extensive.(35) In severe cases, hypertensive retinopathy progresses to detachment of one or both retinas.(4)

11. Although hypertension is a common cause of retinal detachments, it is not the only etiology. Other causes of retinal detachments include:(4)

    - adverse drug reaction, e.g. overdose of phenylpropanolamine (PPA):(36, 37)

      - PPA is a synthetic, sympathomimetic drug that is prescribed to manage urinary incontinence in dogs to improve control of the urinary sphincter(36, 38–41)
      - at concentrations that are higher than prescribed, PPA potentiates the activity of catecholamines such as epinephrine by preventing them from being metabolized(36, 42, 43)
      - this may result in severe tachycardia and systemic hypertension that can induce target organ damage(36)

    - infectious chorioretinitis:(1, 44–54)

      - bacterial
      - fungal:(55–58)

        - blastomycosis
        - coccidioidomycosis
        - cryptococcosis
        - histoplasmosis

- protozoal:

    - toxoplasmosis (55)

- viral:(55, 59)

    - feline immunodeficiency virus (FIV)
    - feline infectious peritonitis (FIP)
    - feline leukemia virus (FeLV)

- lens instability, as from cataracts(60–65)
- retinal dysplasia (1)
- traumatic injury to the globe, as occurs in people.(66, 67)

12. Blindness can also be caused by retinal degeneration. This may result from the following.(4)

- A combination of ketamine with methylnitrosurea in an isolated research study.(68)
- Fluoroquinolone antibiotic administration:

    - when prescribed to dogs and cats at the original, oral dosage of 2.5 mg/kg, every 12 hours, enrofloxacin did not appear to induce retinopathy(69)
    - when the dosing range is increased from 5 to 20 mg/kg per day, either administered as a split or a single dose, adverse effects in cats began to appear in the veterinary literature(69)
    - a small percentage of cats developed blindness(69, 70)
    - blindness was partial or complete, and tended to occur within 2 to 14 days after treatment with enrofloxacin(69)
    - in most cases, blindness was permanent(69)
    - today, the incidence is estimated to be 1 out of 122,414 cats.(69)

- Sudden acquired retinal degeneration syndrome (SARDS) in middle-aged to older dogs. (1, 71, 72)
- Taurine deficiency.(73–77)

Returning to Case 28: The Cat with Questionable Vision

Given Pico de Gato's acute onset of "bumping into things" and his documented hypertension despite appearing to be relatively calm and collected, you agree with the technician that blindness is a very real possibility. The first organs that you examine are his eyes. Both eyes are mydriatic. He lacks menace responses bilaterally. When you look at both eyes, this is what you observe grossly (see **Plate 26**). Fundoscopic examination of both eyes is performed (see **Plate 27**).

Round Three of Questions for Case 28: The Cat with Questionable Vision

1. Based upon the photographs in **Plates 26 and 27**, what is Pico de Gato's diagnosis?
2. Because the diagnosis that you identified in Question #1 (above) is often associated with and results from renal disease, you would like to ask Jacqueline some clarifying questions before performing bloodwork and/or urinalysis. Which questions would you like to ask Jacqueline to gain some additional answers about Pico de Gato's urinary health?
3. If Pico de Gato has renal disease, what do you expect Jacqueline's answers to your questions in Question #2 (above) to be?
4. How will you screen for renal disease?

5.   Jacqueline shares that she feels overwhelmed. She brought Pico de Gato in today for evaluation of his vision. Now, you're telling her that not only does he have a problem with his eyes, he also may have a problem with his kidneys. Which communication skills might you make use of to address her emotions?

6.   Jacqueline asks if Pico de Gato's vision can be restored. What do you tell her?

7.   Jacqueline blames herself for not bringing him in sooner. Which communication skills might you make use of to address her guilt?

Answers to Round Three of Questions for Case 28: The Cat with Questionable Vision

1.   Based upon the photographs in **Plates 26 and 27**, Pico de Gato has bilateral retinal detachments.(4)

2.   Because the diagnosis that you identified in Question #1 (above) is often associated with and results from renal disease, I would like to ask Jacqueline the following clarifying questions before performing bloodwork and/or urinalysis.

   - Does Pico de Gato seem to be drinking more water than normal?

     - How much water is the patient offered per day?
     - How much water does the patient drink per day?
     - Does the patient seek out unusual sources of water (bathtub, toilet bowl, pool, other)?

   - Does Pico de Gato seem to be urinating more often?
   - Does Pico de Gato seem to be voiding larger volumes of urine?

   I would also want to ask about Pico de Gato's appetite and if he is vomiting. If he is vomiting, I would want to clarify the frequency of vomiting and whether the client considers this to be increased as compared to his norm.

3.   If Pico de Gato has renal disease, then I expect Jacqueline to share that:

   - he is drinking more water
   - he may be seeking out water in unusual places
   - he is urinating more often
   - he is voiding larger volumes of urine, as noted by sizeable clumps in the litter box.

   These signs are supportive of chronic kidney disease (CKD), a condition that is common in older cats.(3, 4, 78, 79)

   I might also expect Jacqueline to share that Pico de Gato's appetite is decreased and he may be vomiting more often. Both of these signs are non-specific, but supportive of CKD.(4) They occur due to the build-up of uremic toxins in the bloodstream.(4, 78, 80, 81)

4.   I will recommend screening for renal disease by gathering a minimum database:(4, 82, 83)

   - CBC
   - serum biochemistry profile
   - urinalysis.

   Refer to Case #21 to explore what clinicopathologic changes you might expect to see on the screening tests that I've outlined above.

5.   Jacqueline shares that she feels overwhelmed. To address her emotions, I might lean on the following communication skills.

- Eliciting the client's perspective:(84)

  - invites the client to share(85)
  - helps us to hear our client's expectations and concerns(86)
  - often takes the form of open-ended statements:

    - Tell me . . .
    - Share with me . . .
    - Explain to me . . .
    - Show me . . .

  - Examples:

    - Tell me what concerns you most.
    - Tell me what's on your mind.
    - Tell me what is most overwhelming for you.
    - Share with me what's going through your mind.

- Empathy:(84, 87–90)

  - is defined as identifying with another individual or imagining yourself in someone else's shoes
  - demonstrates that you are sensitive to the client's situation
  - while you may not personally understand what it is like to be your client, your use of empathetic actions or statements conveys that you are developing awareness as to how s/he is experiencing the present situation.
  - Examples of empathetic actions:(84)

    - Making eye contact.(89, 91)
    - Maintaining eye contact when a client is expressing an emotion.(89, 91)
    - Mirroring the client's posture, that is, if the client is seated, seat yourself.(89, 91–93)
    - Angling your body at a 5–10 degree angle from the horizontal line between you and the client.(92)
    - Avoiding towering above the client, if you are standing.
    - Decreasing the distance between you and the client, i.e. bringing one's chair nearer to the client or sitting beside the client on an examination room bench.
    - Talking slowly to allow the client to process details.(89)
    - Using a moment of silence.(89)
    - Using touch appropriately at one of the following locations: the client's shoulder, upper arm, forearm, or top of the hand to console.(94)
    - Touching the patient, particularly if the clinician is uncomfortable with touching the client.(95)

  - Examples of empathetic statements:(84)

    - I see that you care very deeply about Pico de Gato.
    - I can see that this wasn't the news you were expecting to hear.
    - I can tell that today's visit is really weighing on your mind.
    - I know that you would do anything in your power to fix this.

  - Sometimes empathetic statements mirror reflective listening:(84, 91)

    - It sounds like you're overwhelmed.
    - It sounds like this is a lot to absorb right now.
    - What I'm hearing you say is that you are overwhelmed about the possibility that Pico de Gato may have more than one medical condition to manage at home.

6. It is unlikely that Pico de Gato's vision can be restored. However, it is still essential to initiate treatment for his hypertension as soon as possible to protect against additional target organ damage.

7. Jacqueline blames herself for not bringing him in sooner. To address her guilt, I would first and foremost listen. I would encourage her to share what is on her mind through the use of open-ended statements ("Share with me . . .," "Tell me more . . .")

    Although I do not agree that Pico de Gato's condition is her fault, I need to hear her out. I need to listen to what is on her mind. It will not help me to negate how Jacqueline feels. Invalidating her feelings is not going to make her feel the way I want her to.

    Instead of negating her feelings about the current situation, I would focus on delivering unconditional positive regard.

    Unconditional positive regard is a concept that was initially coined by Carl Rogers, a leader in the field of human mental health.(84, 96) Although it is most typically used to describe the work of clinicians in psychiatry, social work, counseling, and psychology, unconditional positive regard can be ascribed to all human health professionals.(84) The practice of unconditional positive regard suggests that the clinician approaches each (human) patient as an individual.(84, 85) People are valued and accepted for who they are rather than held to standards that they are incapable of meeting.(84, 85)

    Many (human) patients fear being judged.(84) When patients fear judgment, they are less likely to open up to the medical team.(84) This is prohibitive to relationship-building. It also prevents the appropriate transfer of information between doctor and patient. The patient who is afraid to open up is more likely to withhold key facts and pieces of information that are essential for the physician to be aware of if s/he is to make the correct diagnosis.(84)

    The intent behind unconditional positive regard is to transform the examination room into a safe zone, where (human) patients can feel free to be themselves, ask questions, and air concerns.(84)

    Veterinary clients also fear being judged by the veterinary team.(84) They may not always do what is right, or they may delay seeking treatment for their pet because they didn't recognize that there was a problem sooner.(84) Clients still need to be encouraged and rewarded for their good intentions rather than to be beaten down for their faults.(84) This is particularly important to cat owners.(85)

    In response to Jacqueline's guilt, I might make use of one or more of the following unconditional positive regard statements.(84)

    • You're here now, that's what matters most.
    • You did the best you could.
    • Of course you didn't mean for this to happen.
    • How would you have known that he was going blind?
    • I could have missed the signs that he was going blind, too.

    I would then emphasize partnership statements. Partnership statements suggest that the veterinarian and client are coming together as one team for the benefit of common ground, the patient. (84, 97, 98) Although the veterinarian may counsel and advise, s/he is expected to be, first and foremost, a collaborator.(84, 97–102) In this role, the veterinarian is tasked with providing information and resources that are necessary for the client to make informed decisions.(84, 99) This requires the veterinarian to consider the client's needs, preferences, and desires.(84, 99)

    There are many ways that veterinarians can demonstrate partnership. Above all, remember the old adage, "There is no I in team."(84) This means that we replace "I" statements with "we" statements and actually mean them.(84)

    • We will work through this together.
    • We will get through this.
    • We are in this together – you, me, and Pico de Gato.
    • We are invested in finding the answers to manage Pico de Gato's underlying condition.

Partnership statements might also make use of the phrase, let us, or the contraction, let's.(84)

- Let's get to the bottom of what's causing Pico de Gato's high BP.
- Let's decide how best to help Pico de Gato get around the house now that he can't see.
- Let's figure out the best solution to the main problem at hand – his high BP.
- Let's establish what's going on behind the scenes – let's run some bloodwork and get some answers so that we know how to move forward with treatment.

Sometimes, the additional word, together, is tacked onto the statement to further emphasize partnership.(84)

- Let's work together to come up with a plan that will be best for you two.
- Let's put our heads together to figure out what is causing Pico de Gato's high BP.
- Let's determine together which test is most likely to provide the answer we are looking for.

CLINICAL PEARLS

- Acute onset of blindness in cats may present as subtle complaints:

    - the cat is not getting around like s/he used to
    - the cat hesitates when walking around the home
    - the cat is bumping into objects that are new to the home.

- Cats that are bilaterally blind often present with mydriatic pupils.

- Mydriasis can also result from stress. Stress activates the sympathetic nervous system to initiate "fight-or-flight" mode.

- Stress can often be ruled out as a cause of mydriasis by evaluating the patient's body language, HR, and RR. Cats that are stressed will be tachycardic and tachypneic. Cats that are not will have normal resting heart and RRs.

- Blind cats lack menace responses.

- Blind cats may or may not lack PLRs. It depends upon where in the visual pathway the lesion is located.

- BP should be assessed in any cat that becomes blind acutely.

- Hypertensive retinopathy is common in practice and often results from renal disease.

- Vision is unlikely to be restored after retinal detachments.

- A diagnostic work-up is essential to establish the underlying cause of hypertension.

- Addressing the cause of hypertension is essential in reducing target organ damage.

References

1. Meekins JM. Acute blindness. Top Companion Anim Med 2015;30(3):118–25.
2. Cook C. What do they See and How Do We Know? Clean Run 2009:[61–6]. Available from: http://veterinary-vision.com/wp-content/uploads/2012/06/VisionInDogsPart1.pdf.
3. Englar RE. Performing the small animal physical examination. Hoboken, NJ: Wiley/Blackwell; 2017.
4. Englar RE. Common clinical presentations in dogs and cats. Hoboken, NJ: Wiley/Blackwell; 2019. pages cm p.

5. Fear free L. Module 1: fear free behavior modification basics. Denver, CO, 2018.

6. Rodan I, Sundahl E, Carney H, Gagnon AC, Heath S, Landsberg G, et al. AAFP and ISFM feline-friendly handling guidelines. J Feline Med Surg 2011;13(5):364–75.

7. Moody CM, Picketts VA, Mason GJ, Dewey CE, Niel L. Can you handle it? Validating negative responses to restraint in cats. Appl Anim Behav Sci 2018;204:94–100.

8. Englar RE. Performing the small animal physical examination. Hoboken, NJ: Wiley; 2017.

9. Chrisman CL. The Neurologic Examination2006; (January): [11–6 pp.]. Available from: https://www.clinicians-brief.com/sites/default/files/sites/cliniciansbrief.com/files/7.pdf.

10. Maggs DJ, Miller PE, Ofri R. Slatter's fundamentals of veterinary ophthalmology. St. Louis, MO: Saunders; 2013.

11. Rijnberk A, van Sluijs FS. Medical history and physical examination in companion animals. Amsterdam: Elsevier; 2009.

12. DeLahunta A, Glass E, Kent M. Veterinary neuroanatomy and clinical neurology. 4th ed. Amsterdam: Elsevier; 2014.

13. Maggio F, DeFrancesco TC, Atkins CE, Pizzirani S, Gilger BC, Davidson MG. Ocular lesions associated with systemic hypertension in cats: 69 cases (1985–1998). J Am Vet Med Assoc 2000;217(5):695–702.

14. Sansom J, Rogers K, Wood JL. Blood pressure assessment in healthy cats and cats with hypertensive retinopathy. Am J Vet Res 2004;65(2):245–52.

15. Henik RA. Systemic hypertension and its management. Vet Clin North Am Small Anim Pract 1997;27(6):1355–72.

16. Littman MP. Spontaneous systemic hypertension in 24 cats. J Vet Intern Med 1994;8(2):79–86.

17. Morgan RV. Systemic hypertension in four cats: ocular and medical findings. J Am Anim Hosp Assoc 1986;22:615–21.

18. Stiles J, Polzin DJ, Bistner SI. The prevalence of retinopathy in cats with systemic hypertension and chronic-renal-failure or hyperthyroidism. J Am Anim Hosp Assoc 1994;30(6):564–72.

19. Henik RA, Snyder PS, Volk LM. Treatment of systemic hypertension in cats with amlodipine besylate. J Am Anim Hosp Assoc 1997;33(3):226–34.

20. Komáromy AM, Andrew SE, Denis HM, Brooks DE, Gelatt KN. Hypertensive retinopathy and choroidopathy in a cat. Vet Ophthalmol 2004;7(1):3–9.

21. Turner JL, Brogdon JD, Lees GE, Greco DS. Idiopathic hypertension in a cat with secondary hypertensive retinopathy associated with a high-salt diet. J Am Anim Hosp Assoc 1990;26(6):647–51.

22. Brown SA, Henik RA. Diagnosis and treatment of systemic hypertension. Vet Clin North Am Small Anim Pract 1998;28(6):1481–94.

23. Sansom J, Barnett KC, Dunn KA, Smith KC, Dennis R. Ocular disease associated with hypertension in 16 cats. J Small Anim Pract 1994;35(12):604–11.

24. Bovée KC, Littman MP, Saleh F, Beeuwkes R, r Pn W, Kinter LB. Essential hereditary hypertension in dogs: a new animal model. J Hypertens Suppl 1986;4(5):S172–1.

25. Tippett FE, Padgett GA, Eyster G, Blanchard G, Bell T. Primary hypertension in a colony of dogs. Hypertension 1987;9(1):49–58.

26. Littman MP, Robertson JL, Bovée KC. Spontaneous systemic hypertension in dogs: five cases (1981–1983). J Am Vet Med Assoc 1988;193(4):486–94.

27. Ross LA. Hypertension and chronic renal failure. Semin Vet Med Surg Small Anim 1992;7(3):221–6.

28. Kobayashi DL, Peterson ME, Graves TK, Lesser M, Nichols CE. Hypertension in cats with chronic renal failure or hyperthyroidism. J Vet Intern Med 1990;4(2):58–62.

29. Jensen J, Henik RA, Brownfield M, Armstrong J. Plasma renin activity and angiotensin I and aldosterone concentrations in cats with hypertension associated with chronic renal disease. Am J Vet Res 1997;58(5):535–40.

30. Snyder PS. Amlodipine: a randomized, blinded clinical trial in 9 cats with systemic hypertension. J Vet Intern Med 1998;12(3):157–62.

31. Peterson ME, Taylor RS, Greco DS, Nelson RW, Randolph JF, Foodman MS, et al. Acromegaly in 14 cats. J Vet Intern Med 1990;4(4):192–201.

32. Cowgill LD, James KM, Levy JK, Browne JK, Miller A, Lobingier RT, Egrie JC. Use of recombinant human erythropoietin for management of anemia in dogs and cats with renal failure. J Am Vet Med Assoc 1998;212(4):521–8.

33. Chun R, Jakovljevic S, Morrison WB, DeNicola DB, Cornell KK. Apocrine gland adenocarcinoma and pheochromocytoma in a cat. J Am Anim Hosp Assoc 1997;33(1):33–6.

34. Flood SM, Randolph JF, Gelzer AR, Refsal K. Primary hyperaldosteronism in two cats. J Am Anim Hosp Assoc 1999;35(5):411–6.

35. Crispin SM, Mould JR. Systemic hypertensive disease and the feline fundus. Vet Ophthalmol 2001;4(2):131–40.

36. Ginn JA, Bentley E, Stepien RL. Systemic hypertension and hypertensive retinopathy following PPA overdose in a dog. J Am Anim Hosp Assoc 2013;49(1):46–53.

37. Crandell JM, Ware WA. Cardiac toxicity from phenylpropanolamine overdose in a dog. J Am Anim Hosp Assoc 2005;41(6):413–20.

38. Bacon NJ, Oni O, White RA. Treatment of urethral sphincter mechanism incompetence in 11 bitches with a sustained-release formulation of phenylpropanolamine hydrochloride. Vet Rec 2002;151(13):373–6.

39. Byron JK, March PA, Chew DJ, DiBartola SP. Effect of phenylpropanolamine and pseudoephedrine on the urethral pressure profile and continence scores of incontinent female dogs. J Vet Intern Med 2007;21(1):47–53.

40. Hamaide AJ, Grand JG, Farnir F, Le Couls G, Snaps FR, Balligand MH, Verstegen JP. Urodynamic and morphologic changes in the lower portion of the urogenital tract after administration of estriol alone and in combination with phenylpropanolamine in sexually intact and spayed female dogs. Am J Vet Res 2006;67(5):901–8.

41. Scott L, Leddy M, Bernay F, Davot JL. Evaluation of phenylpropanolamine in the treatment of urethral sphincter mechanism incompetence in the bitch. J Small Anim Pract 2002;43(11):493–6.

42. Kanfer I, Dowse R, Vuma V. Pharmacokinetics of oral decongestants. Pharmacotherapy 1993;13(6 Pt 2):116S–128S.

43. Yu PH. Inhibition of monoamine oxidase activity by phenylpropanolamine, an anorectic agent. Res Commun Chem Pathol Pharmacol 1986;51(2):163–71.

44. Stiles J. Canine rickettsial infections. Vet Clin North Am Small Anim Pract 2000;30(5):1135–49.

45. Townsend WM, Stiles J, Krohne SG. Leptospirosis and panuveitis in a dog. Vet Ophthalmol 2006;9(3):169–73.

46. Wilkinson GT. Feline cryptococcosis: a review and seven case reports. J Small Anim Pract 1979;20(12):749–68.

47. Rodenbiker HT, Ganley JP. Ocular coccidioidomycosis. Surv Ophthalmol 1980;24(5):263–90.

48. Nasisse MP, van Ee RT, Wright B. Ocular changes in a cat with disseminated blastomycosis. J Am Vet Med Assoc 1985;187(6):629–31.

49. Krohne SG. Canine systemic fungal infections. Vet Clin N Am. Small 2000;30(5):1063–+.

50. Greene RT. Coccidioidomycosis in 48 cats – a retrospective study (1984–1993). J Vet Intern Med 1995;9(3):226–.

51. Gwin RM, Makley TA, Wyman M, Werling K. Multifocal ocular histoplasmosis in a dog and cat. J Am Vet Med Assoc 1980;176(7):638–42.

52. Gionfriddo JR. Feline systemic fungal infections. Vet Clin N Am. Small 2000;30(5):1029–+.

53. Davidson MG. Toxoplasmosis. Vet Clin N Am. Small 2000;30(5):1051–+.

54. Bloom JD, Hamor RE, Gerding PA, Jr. Ocular blastomycosis in dogs: 73 cases, 108 eyes (1985–1993). J Am Vet Med Assoc 1996;209(7):1271–4.

55. Stiles J. Ocular manifestations of systemic disease. Part 2: the cat. In: Gelatt KN, editor. Veterinary ophthalmology. Philadelphia, PA: Lippincott Williams & Wilkins; 1999. p. 1448–73.

56. Graves TK, Barger AM, Adams B, Krockenberger MB. Diagnosis of systemic cryptococcosis by fecal cytology in a dog. Vet Clin Pathol 2005;34(4):409–12.

57. Angell JA, Merideth RE, Shively JN, Sigler RL. Ocular lesions associated with coccidioidomycosis in dogs: 35 cases (1980–1985). J Am Vet Med Assoc 1987;190(10):1319–22.

58. Shively JN, Whiteman CE. Ocular lesions in disseminated coccidioidomycosis in 2 dogs. Pathol Vet 1970;7(1):1–6.

59. Glaze MB, Gelatt KN. Feline ophthalmology. In: Gelatt KN, editor. Veterinary ophthalmology. Philadelphia: Lippincott Williams & Wilkins; 1999. p. 997–1052.

60. Nasisse MP, Glover TL. Clinical signs, concurrent diseases, and risk factors associated with retinal detachment in dogs. Prog Vet Comp. Ophthalmologe 1997;3:87–91.

61. Glover TL, Davidson MG, Nasisse MP, Olivero DK. The intracapsular extraction of displaced lenses in dogs: a retrospective study of 57 cases (1984–1990). J Am Anim Hosp Assoc 1995;31(1):77–81.

62. Sigle KJ, Nasisse MP. Long-term complications after phacoemulsification for cataract removal in dogs: 172 cases (1995–2002). J Am Vet Med Assoc 2006;228(1):74–9.

63. Davidson MG, Nasisse MP, Jamieson VE, English RV, Olivero DK. Phacoemulsification and intraocular lens implantatioon: a study of surgical results in 182 dogs. Prog Vet Comp. Ophthalmologe 1991;1:233–8.

64. Klein HE, Krohne SG, Moore GE, Stiles J. Postoperative complications and visual outcomes of phacoemulsification in 103 dogs (179 eyes): 2006–2008. Vet Ophthalmol 2011;14(2):114–20.

65. Miller TR, Whitley RD, Meek LA, Garcia GA, Wilson MC, Rawls BH, Jr. Phacofragmentation and aspiration for cataract extraction in dogs: 56 cases (1980–1984). J Am Vet Med Assoc 1987;190(12):1577–80.

66. Ruiz RS. Traumatic retinal detachments. Br J Ophthalmol 1969;53(1):59–61.

67. Johnston PB. Traumatic retinal detachment. Br J Ophthalmol 1991;75(1):18–21.

68. Schaller JP, Wyman M, Weisbrode SE, Olsen RG. Induction of retinal degeneration in cats by methylnitrosourea and ketamine hydrochloride. Vet Pathol 1981;18(2):239–47.

69. Wiebe V, Hamilton P. Fluoroquinolone-induced retinal degeneration in cats. J Am Vet Med Assoc 2002;221(11):1568–71.

70. Gelatt KN, van der Woerdt A, Ketring KL, Andrew SE, Brooks DE, Biros DJ, et al. Enrofloxacin-associated retinal degeneration in cats. Vet Ophthalmol 2001;4(2):99–106.

71. Vainisi SJ, Schmidt GM, West CS. Metabolic toxic retinopathy preliminary report. Vet ophthalmol Coll A, Trans: 14. p. 76–81; 1983.

72. Montgomery KW, van der Woerdt A, Cottrill NB. Acute blindness in dogs: sudden acquired retinal degeneration syndrome versus neurological disease (140 cases, 2000–2006). Vet Ophthalmol 2008;11(5):314–20.

73. Aguirre GD. Retinal degeneration associated with the feeding of dog foods to cats. J Am Vet Med Assoc 1978;172(7):791–6.

74. Schmidt SY, Berson EL, Hayes KC. Retinal degeneration in cats fed casein. I. Taurine deficiency. Invest Ophthalmol 1976;15(1):47–52.

75. Schmidt SY, Berson EL, Watson G, Huang C. Retinal degeneration in cats fed casein. III. Taurine deficiency and ERG amplitudes. Invest Ophthalmol Vis Sci 1977;16(7):673–8.

76. Berson EL, Hayes KC, Rabin AR, Schmidt SY, Watson G. Retinal degeneration in cats fed casein. II. Supplementation with methionine, cysteine, or taurine. Invest Ophthalmol 1976;15(1):52–8.

77. Hayes KC. A review on the biological function of taurine. Nutr Rev 1976;34(6):161–5.

78. Bartges JW. Chronic kidney disease in dogs and cats. Vet Clin North Am Small Anim Pract 2012;42(4):669–92.

79. Langston CE, Eatroff AE. Chronic kidney disease. In: Silverstein DC, Hopper K, editors. Small animal critical care medicine. St. Louis, MO: Saunders/Elsevier; 2015. p. 661–6.

80. Polzin DJ. Chronic kidney disease in small animals. Vet Clin North Am Small Anim Pract 2011;41(1):15–30.

81. Tilley LP, Smith FWK. The 5-minute veterinary consult: canine and feline. 3rd ed. Baltimore, MD: Lippincott Williams & Wilkins; 2004.

82. Nichols R. Polyuria and polydipsia – diagnostic approach and problems associated with patient evaluation. Vet Clin N Am. Small 2001;31(5):833–+.

83. Schoeman JP, editor. Approach to polyuria and polydipsia in the dog. Proceedings of the 33rd world small animal veterinary congress; 2008; Dublin, Ireland. World Small Animal Veterinary Association (WSAVA).

84. Englar R. A guide to oral communication in veterinary medicine. Sheffield: 5M Publishing; 2020.

85. Englar RE, Williams M, Weingand K. Applicability of the Calgary-Cambridge guide to dog and cat owners for teaching veterinary clinical communications. J Vet Med Educ 2016;43(2):143–69.

86. Hunter LJ, Shaw JR. How to exceed – not merely meet – client expectations. March: Veterinary Team Brief. p. 19–22; 2018.

87. Adams CL, Kurtz SM. Skills for communicating in veterinary medicine. Oxford: Otmoor Press and Dewpoint Publishing; 2017.

88. Shaw JR. Four core communication skills of highly effective practitioners. Vet Clin North Am Small Anim Pract 2006;36(2):385–96, vii, vii.

89. Silverman J, Kurtz S, Draper J. Skills for communicating with patients. Oxford: Radcliffe Medical Press; 2008.

90. Kurtz SM, Silverman JD, Draper J. Teaching and learning communication skills in medicine. Grand Rapids, FL: Radcliffe; 2004.

91. McMurray J, Boysen S. Communicating empathy in veterinary practice. Vet Irel J 2017;7(4):199–205.

92. Shea SC. Psychiatric interviewing: the art of understanding. 2nd ed. Philadelphia, PA: W.B. Saunders Company; 1998.

93. Carson CA. Nonverbal communication in veterinary practice. Vet Clin North Am Small Anim Pract 2007;37(1):49–63; abstract viii:abstract viii.

94. Bateman SW. Communication in the veterinary emergency setting. Vet Clin North Am Small Anim Pract 2007;37(1):109–21.

95. Morrisey JK, Voiland B. Difficult interactions with veterinary clients: working in the challenge zone. Vet Clin North Am Small Anim Pract 2007;37(1):65–77.

96. Amadi C. Clinician, society and suicide mountain: reading Rogerian doctrine of unconditional positive regard (UPR). Psychol Thought 2013;6(1):75–89.

97. Shaw JR, Bonnett BN, Adams CL, Roter DL. Veterinarian-client-patient communication patterns used during clinical appointments in companion animal practice. J Am Vet Med Assoc 2006;228(5):714–21.

98. Küper AM, Merle R. Being nice is not enough-exploring relationship-centered veterinary care with structural equation modeling. A quantitative study on German pet owners' perception. Front Vet Sci 2019;6:56.

99. Cornell KK, Kopcha M. Client-veterinarian communication: skills for client centered dialogue and shared decision making. Vet Clin North Am Small Anim Pract 2007;37(1):37–47.

100. Show A, Englar RE. Evaluating Dog- and Cat-Owner Preferences for Calgary-Cambridge Communication Skills: Results of a Questionnaire. J Vet Med Educ 2018;45(4):534–43.

101. McArthur ML, Fitzgerald JR. Companion animal veterinarians' use of clinical communication skills. Aust Vet J 2013;91(9):374–80.

102. Shaw JR, Adams CL, Bonnett BN. What can veterinarians learn from studies of physician–patient communication about veterinarian-client-patient communication? J Am Vet Med Assoc 2004;224(5):676–84.

Case 29

The Dog with the Cloudy Eye

Colonel Mustard hasn't had the easiest of lives. He's been rehomed twice by families who were moving out of state and couldn't take him along for the ride. After being relinquished to the shelter for the second time, he was attacked by another boarder, who lunged at his face. His right eye proptosed and was unable to be replaced within the orbit, so he underwent enucleation surgery. He's been one-eyed now for six months.

Just when he had given up hope of finding his forever home, Mariah Parkay stopped by the shelter. She was there on business rather than to adopt. Her work had asked her to drop off donated supplies from an office fundraiser the previous weekend. She lived just around the corner from the shelter, so it was an easy commute.

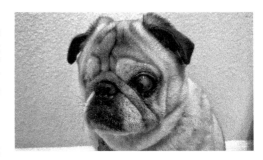

Figure 29.1 Meet your new patient, Colonel Mustard, a 10-year-old castrated male pug. Courtesy of Ashley Parker.

As Mariah was leaving the facility, Colonel Mustard, in the far cage in the left corner of the room, by the exit, caught her attention. In fact, she did a doubletake because he was the spitting image of Sir Pugsly, her childhood pet. They were the same color and same size (round!). The same quizzical brow completed the picture. Mariah's heart and mind overflowed with memories and when she asked about his backstory, she knew that she could gift him a better final chapter.

Colonel Mustard left the shelter with her that day, even though she was hardly prepared for his homecoming. It was a transition for them both. Mariah had been single for the past decade, so she'd had to relearn what it was like to share a home and tend to someone who didn't always fit her schedule. The Colonel, for instance, loved food. He had an internal timer. He knew precisely when it was time for meals, right to the exact minute. If something delayed Mariah from keeping on track, he was right there at her side, begging, like her own personal alarm clock.

Colonel Mustard was a good fit for Mariah. He completed her in a way that she hadn't expected. Before he'd come along, she wouldn't have said that anything (or anyone!) was missing from her life. Now that he's been a part of her world for the past 6 weeks, she can't imagine him not being by her side. He had a big dog's heart inside of that "little" body, and his presence had fully reshaped the house into a home.

All was well until this morning. Mariah awoke with the alarm on the nightstand blasting rock music into her right ear, as always, but when she bounced out of bed to get started on the day, she noticed that Colonel Mustard did not follow. He usually leaped off the bed in a single bound, even though she had purchased a set of pet stairs for him to facilitate his exit from such a height. Today, he was strikingly absent from her side as she put her make-up on in the bathroom. An alarm bell went off in her head. That was uncharacteristic of him.

When Mariah went to investigate, she found Colonel Mustard perched at the edge of the bed, looking hesitant. She called out to him and he lifted his head in her direction, but instead of focusing in on her, he glanced around nervously. That's when she saw his left eye. In the center, there was a haze of cloudy white. The Colonel seemed unbothered by it – he wasn't blinking or squinting or pawing at his eye – but he clearly couldn't see her, and this alarmed Mariah. Mariah contacted her work to say that she would be late, then rushed Colonel Mustard to the nearest clinic.

She is standing in your waiting room now, with the Colonel tucked in her arms, awaiting consultation. The technician has already been by to check his vital signs. They have been documented in the record as such.

The technician briefs you on the case and offers his own diagnosis. Before you enter the examination room to see for yourself, you consider the following questions.

Weight: 26 lb (11.8 kg)
BCS: 8/9
Mentation: BAR

TPR

T: 101.9°F (38.8°C)
P: 156 beats per minute
R: panting

Round One of Questions for Case 29: The Dog with the Cloudy Eye

1. Colonel Mustard is presenting for evaluation of cloudy eyes. Which anatomical structure(s) in the outer coat of the eye can cause the eye to appear cloudy?
2. What is the purpose of the anatomical structure(s) that you identified in Question #1 (above)?
3. What color should the structure that you identified in Question #1 (above) be in a healthy (normal) eye?
4. What could cause this structure to develop opacity?
5. Each etiology that you identified in Question #4 has a distinct characteristic appearance. Explain each appearance.
6. Based upon the Colonel's photograph, which was added to his patient profile at intake, does he appear to have any of these opacities?
7. Which anatomical structure(s) within the eye can cause the eye to appear cloudy?
8. What color should the structure that you identified in Question #7 (above) be in a healthy (normal) eye?
9. What shape should the structure that you identified in Question #7 (above) be in a healthy (normal) eye?
10. How is the structure that you identified in Question #7 (above) suspended in space?
11. Can the shape of the structure that you identified in Question #7 change?
12. What is the purpose of the structure that you identified in Question #7?
13. Which two conditions can cause this structure to develop opacity?
14. Describe each condition that you mentioned in Question #13 in detail, explaining what it is and how or why it develops.
15. Are any of these etiologies able to cause opacity to appear suddenly, overnight?
16. Based upon the Colonel's photograph, which is his most likely diagnosis?

Answers to Round One of Questions for Case 29: The Dog with the Cloudy Eye

1. The cornea is a structure in the outer coat of the eye.(1–5) Abnormalities within the cornea can cause the eye to appear cloudy.(6, 7)

2. The cornea helps the globe to maintain its shape and it refracts incoming light.(3, 8) This is essential to the special sense of vision.(8)

3. The healthy (normal) cornea is transparent.(6, 7) Transparency is essential in order for the cornea to perform its function as a refractive surface.(7)

    Transparency of the cornea is achieved by maintaining the stromal layer in a dehydrated state.(8) Deturgescence requires endothelial cells to actively pump fluid out of the cornea.(8)

Transparency is also achieved by not having a direct blood supply to the cornea.(5, 8, 9) Instead, the cornea is nourished by vessels at the limbus, and other nutrients are delivered to the cornea through lacrimal fluid and aqueous humor.(5)

4. Corneal opacities may result from:(8, 10)

- edema
- infiltration of inflammatory cells
- lipid deposits

- fibrosis
- melanosis
- neovascularization.

5. Each of the aforementioned etiologies has a distinct appearance:(8)

- "blue eye" results from corneal edema
- the stroma takes on a yellow-green or creamy-tan appearance when it is infiltrated with inflammatory cells
- lipid causes the cornea to take on a sparkly silver or white appearance at the site of deposition
- gray-white scarring of the cornea is seen with fibrosis
- black-brown pigment is seen in cases of corneal melanosis
- red vessels are seen in cases of neovascularization.

(See **Plates 28–31** and Figure 29.2.)

6. Based upon the Colonel's photograph, he appears to have corneal melanosis. This is a common clinical finding in pugs and other brachycephalic breeds due to their facial conformation.(7)

- The "bug-eyed" appearance is created by eyes seated in shallow sockets, causing the eyes to bulge forward.(6, 7) Depending upon how severe this conformation is, the eyelids may not be able to close completely.(6, 7) This hinders the blink reflex.(6, 7) The cornea dries

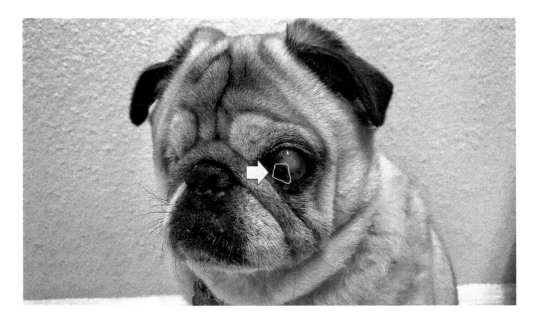

Figure 29.2 Corneal opacity with melanosis outlined. Note that the same patient also has a lens opacity, which is beyond the scope of this question. Courtesy of Ashley Parker.

out. Chronic irritation causes pigment to be laid down along the corneal surface.(7) This pigment is consistent with melanosis.(7) Sometimes, melanosis is referred to as pigmentary keratitis to reflect the inflammatory component of this process.(7)

- These patients also typically have nasal folds.(6, 7) Fur that lines the nasal folds may chronically rub against the cornea, causing the same outcome.(6, 7)

7. The lens is a structure within the eye.(6, 7) Abnormalities within the lens can cause the eye to appear cloudy.(6, 7)

8. The healthy (normal) lens is transparent.(1, 5–7, 11–13)

9. Like the cornea, the lens is transparent because it is avascular.(12–14) The hyaloid artery nourishes the lens in embryonic life, but it degenerates shortly after birth.(5, 13) After birth, the lens receives nutrients from the aqueous humor by diffusion.(5, 13–15) The healthy (normal) lens is biconvex, with anterior and posterior poles.(1, 5, 11–13)

10. The lens is suspended in space by zonular fibers that attach the equator of the lens, where the anterior and posterior poles meet, to the ciliary processes of the ciliary body.(5–7, 12)

11. Yes, the lens can change shape.(6, 7) This process is called accommodation.(13) Accommodation allows for objects in the visual field to come into focus, regardless of whether they are near or far.

How does this work?

The lens capsule is under tension.(5, 7) Without opposition, the lens will take on a spherical shape.(5, 7) This is not the case in health. The zonular fibers counter this by exerting their own pull on the equator.(13) This creates the normal biconvex resting shape of the lens.(1, 5, 11, 12) This is how the lens is able to bring distant objects into focus.(5)

When near objects need to come into focus, the ciliary body muscle contracts.(5) This brings the ciliary processes of the ciliary body closer to the lens, relaxing the zonular fibers.(5) This allows to lens to round out.(5) This trend toward a spherical shape brings near objects into focus.(5)

12. The purpose of the lens is to refract light so that it falls upon the retina for visual processing. (1, 5, 11, 12, 14) To achieve this end, the lens adjusts its shape, as was described in the question above.(5, 13)

13. Lens opacities result from:

- nuclear sclerosis(6, 7)
- cataracts.(1, 5–7, 12–14)

14. Nuclear sclerosis is a normal process that reflects aging of the lens.(12, 13, 16) As the patient ages, new cells are produced within the cortical lens, forcing the older cells inward.(17) This makes the nucleus more compact.(13, 14, 16, 17) This denseness scatters light, creating a haze that is visible to the observer(17) (see **Plate 32**).

Unlike nuclear sclerosis, cataracts are pathologic opacities of the lens or lens capsule.(1, 5, 12–14) Cataracts are often characterized by their position within the lens:(7)

- nuclear – arise from the core of the lens(18)
- cortical – arise from the periphery of the lens(18)
- capsular – arise within the lens capsule(18)
- subcapsular – arise just beneath the lens capsule
- equatorial – arise near attachment sites of the zonular fibers, which bridge the lens to the ciliary body.(5, 12)

Cataracts are also frequently characterized by their stage of development:(7)

- incipient:
    - small(14, 18)
    - do not typically obstruct the patient's vision(14)
    - do not interfere with the ability of the clinician to perform fundoscopy(14, 18)
    - immature:
    - larger than incipient cataracts, but do not take up the entire lens(14, 18)
    - does not interfere with the tapetal reflection(14, 18)
    - may compromise vision, depending upon location(14, 18)
    - may cause the lens to become edematous:(18)

        - swelling of the lens is called intumescence(14)
        - this may cause leakage of cystallins, which could incite uveitis(14, 19)
        - swelling may also obstruct the flow of aqueous humor through the pupil, causing glaucoma(14, 20)

- mature:
    - take up the entire lens
    - the clinician will be unable to appreciate a tapetal reflex(14)
    - patients will be blind(18)
    - pupillary light reflexes (PLRs) will be present if the retina is still functional, even though the patient is avisual(18)

- hypermature:
    - the lens itself is undergoing resorption(18)
    - lens fibers break apart and release crystallins(14)
    - uveitis results.(14)

(See **Plates 33–35**.)

15. Nuclear sclerosis is a gradual process. On the other hand, cataracts may well appear overnight. Clients of affected patients often report sudden onset of cloudy eye(s) and acute blindness.(18, 21)

16. Based upon the Colonel's photograph, he likely has a cataract in his left eye.

Returning to Case 29: The Dog with the Cloudy Eye

After performing a comprehensive physical exam and ophthalmoscopy, you agree with your technician's diagnosis. You share with Mariah that Colonel Mustard has developed a cataract in his left eye. Mariah is taken back. She has heard of cataracts in people but didn't know that they could occur in dogs and isn't sure what that means for the Colonel.

Walk her through the following list of typical questions that you might get asked by a client who has just heard an unfamiliar diagnosis for the first time.

Round Two of Questions for Case 29: The Dog with the Cloudy Eye

1. Mariah says, "I've heard that dogs' eyes get hazy when they get older. Couldn't that just be what this is?"

    Which condition is Mariah most likely referring to?

2. This condition is sometimes mistaken for cataracts by veterinarians and clients alike. How might these two conditions look different from one another on physical exam?

3. Gross observation during the physical exam is not the best way to differentiate these two conditions. What is?
4. Does the condition that Mariah is referring to cause blindness?
5. It is hard for Mariah to accept that the Colonel has yet another health issue. He's been through so much already. She asks, "How could this have happened? Did I cause this?"
6. Are cataracts inherited in dogs?
7. Are cataracts inherited in cats?
8. Outline etiologies for cataracts.
9. Based upon your list of etiologies in Question #5 (above), what additional clarifying questions do you want to ask about Colonel Mustard to help you to determine if one or more of these could be likely?

Answers to Round Two of Questions for Case 29: The Dog with the Cloudy Eye

1. Mariah is likely referring to nuclear sclerosis, a normal aging process within the lens.(6, 7) Sometimes this condition is called lenticular sclerosis.(7, 12, 13, 16)

2. Nuclear sclerosis is sometimes mistaken for cataracts by veterinarians and clients alike.(6, 7, 13, 17) Physical exam is not the best way to differentiate the two conditions. However, certain appearances may be more characteristic of one than the other. Nuclear sclerosis often appears as an even, pearly haze.(7) By contrast, advanced cataracts tend to take on a crushed ice appearance.(7, 17)

3. Slit lamp evaluation, also called retroillumination, is the best approach to characterize lens-associated changes.

4. No, nuclear sclerosis does not cause blindness. (13, 17)

5. You can say with certainty that Mariah is not responsible for the Colonel's current eye condition.

6. Yes, cataracts can be inherited in dogs.(22–24) Over 90 canine breeds have heritable cataracts, including, but not limited to:(23–47)

- Afghan hound
- Australian shepherd
- Bearded collie
- Bichon frise
- Boston terrier
- Brussels griffon
- Chesapeake Bay retriever
- Chow chow
- Cocker spaniel
- French Bulldog
- German shepherd
- Golden retriever
- Havanese
- Japanese chin
- Labrador retriever
- Miniature poodle
- Miniature Schnauzer
- Old English Sheepdog
- Silky terrier
- Springer spaniel
- Staffordshire bull terrier
- Standard poodle
- Toy poodle
- West Highland white terrier.

7. Cats are less likely than dogs to present with inherited cataracts.(13, 22–24, 48) However, the following breeds appear to be overrepresented in the current literature:(13, 22, 43, 49–54)

- Bengal
- Birman

- Himalayan
- Russian blue
- British shorthair
- Persian, particularly blue-smoke Persian cats.

8. Other than being inherited, cataracts may result from:

- aging, as is true in people(18)
- electrocution, as from chewing on wires(18)
- excessive exposure to ultraviolet (UV) radiation(14, 55)
- inadvertent exposure of the eye during radiation therapy(18, 56)
- nutritional deficiencies in some, but not all commercial milk replacers(18, 57)
- ocular trauma(18)
- underlying disease:(7, 58, 59)

    - diabetes mellitus(14, 46, 60–62)
    - retinal degeneration
    - uveitis.

9. Of the etiologies that are listed in Question #7 (above), I am most concerned about diabetes mellitus. Diabetic cataracts often have a history of arising overnight. Based upon my suspicion, I would like to ask Mariah the following clarifying questions to help me to determine if diabetes is or is not likely.

- Does Colonel Mustard seem to be drinking more water than normal?

    - How much water is the patient offered per day?
    - How much water does the patient drink per day?
    - Does the patient seek out unusual sources of water (e.g. bathtub, toilet bowl, pool, other)?

- Does Colonel Mustard seem to be urinating more often?
- Does Colonel Mustard seem to be voiding larger volumes of urine?
- Describe Colonel Mustard's appetite.

    - In the initial phase of diabetes mellitus, it is not uncommon for patients to exhibit polyphagia because the cells are starved of glucose and eating more is the body's natural reaction to try to provide fuel.(63) The body doesn't understand that the fuel is not able to be utilized.
    - As the disease progresses, patients may exhibit reduced appetites or they may go off feed altogether.(63)

- Have you noticed any change in weight?

    - As diabetes mellitus progresses, patients often lose weight and muscle mass.(63)

Returning to Case 29: The Dog with the Cloudy Eye

You explain to Mariah that, no, there is nothing she could have done to have prevented this. However, you are concerned that when cataracts arise suddenly like this, they may be indicative of diabetes mellitus. You ask several clarifying questions to round out the patient profile. When prompted, Mariah shares that, in retrospect, Colonel Mustard drinks a "ton" of water and "pees like a race-horse." Since Mariah has only recently adopted him, she assumed that was "normal" for him, and because he wasn't having any accidents in the house, his thirst and urination habits did not concern her.

Round Three of Questions for Case 29: The Dog with the Cloudy Eye

1. How does diabetes mellitus lead to cataract formation?
2. Which screening test(s) should you perform today to rule out diabetes mellitus?
3. Which results would you expect to see if Colonel Mustard is diabetic?
4. If Colonel Mustard is diabetic, what additional tests might you want to run to expand his minimum database?
5. Mariah is afraid of losing the Colonel. He's become an essential member of her family. She asks, "Is diabetes treatable in dogs?"
6. Mariah also googles "diabetes in pets" while you are performing your screening test(s) and sees that cats can go into remission from diabetes. She asks you, "Is that true of dogs, too? Can they be cured of diabetes?"
7. Mariah asks if you treat the diabetes, will the cataract go away? How do you respond to her?
8. Is there a surgical option to expedite cataract resolution?
9. What is a potential concern if the Colonel's lens is not operated on with expedience?

Answers to Round Three of Questions for Case 29: The Dog with the Cloudy Eye

1. The lens uses glucose as fuel. Within the lens itself, glucose is primarily acted upon by the enzyme, hexokinase.(64)

   Diabetic patients have an excess of glucose in circulation. Hexokinase converts glucose into glucose 6-phosphate and adenosine diphosphate (ADP).(64) However, the lens does not have a lot of hexokinase, so the enzyme becomes easily saturated.(14, 64)

   As a result, glucose has to be metabolized by an alternate pathway: Another enzyme within the lens, aldose reductase, converts excess glucose into sorbitol.(14, 62) Sorbitol dehydrogenase then catalyzes the transformation of sorbitol into fructose.(14, 62)

   Neither sorbitol nor fructose can cross the lens capsule.(14) Within the lens, both of these act as osmotic agents, thus drawing water into the lens from the aqueous humor.(14, 62) The lens becomes edematous, so much so that its Y-shaped sutures often become visible to the observer.(18)

   As the lens continues to swell, fibers rupture.(14, 60, 62) This promotes cataract formation. (60)

2. You should assess, at minimum, Colonel Mustard's blood glucose (BG) as a screening test to assess him for diabetes mellitus.(7, 58, 59)

3. If Colonel Mustard is diabetic, then I would expect to see hyperglycemia.(7, 58, 59)

4. If Colonel Mustard is diabetic, I would want to expand his minimum database to include:(7, 58, 59)

   - complete blood count (CBC)
   - chemistry profile
   - urinalysis.(UA)

5. You reassure Mariah that, yes, diabetes mellitus is a treatable condition in dogs, but requires parenteral administration of exogenous insulin.(58, 59)

6. You clarify that up to 30% of cats, but not dogs, may go into diabetic remission.(59) It is not a reasonable expectation to hope for remission for Colonel Mustard.

7. It is essential that the client and veterinary team work together to medically manage diabetes. However, despite treatment for diabetes, the cataract will persist.

8. Yes, there is a surgical option to expedite cataract resolution. This is called phacoemulsification. (7) The cataract is essentially blenderized using an ultrasonic headpiece into a solution that can be aspirated from the eye during surgery. An artificial lens can then be implanted.(14, 65) This can restore the patient's vision.

9. If the Colonel's lens is not operated on with expedience and it continues to swell, then the lens itself is at risk of rupturing.(7) If rupture of the lens occurs, then intense inflammation within the eye will ensue. This could lead to permanent blindness.

CLINICAL PEARLS

- It is important to understand basic eye anatomy because ocular complaints are common in clinical practice and clients often report vague signs that can mean several different things.

- The chief complaint, "cloudy eyes," may refer to corneal haze or lens-associated opacity.

- Both the cornea and the lens are transparent structures in health. Transparency is essential for both structures to serve their respective purposes.

- The cornea is a refractive surface and a protective barrier for the globe.

- The lens refracts light so that it falls upon the retina for visual processing. The lens is also able to change shape in a process called accommodation to allow objects within the visual field to come into focus, whether they are near or far.

- Corneal opacity may result from edema, inflammatory infiltrate, lipid deposits, fibrosis, melanosis, or neovascularization. Each opacity has a characteristic appearance on physical exam.

- Opacity within the lens may be due to nuclear sclerosis, a normal aging process, or cataract formation, a pathologic process.

- Nuclear sclerosis and cataracts may resemble one another on gross observations during the physical exam. Slit lamp evaluation (retroillumination) is the best way to evaluate lens-related changes.

- Cataracts may occur anywhere throughout the lens. They may even be associated with the lens capsule.

- Cataracts progress. As they do, they may cause damage to the globe. Hypermature cataracts, for example, are in the process of resorption and incite uveitis.

- Diabetic cataracts may arise overnight. Clients report acute onset of cloudiness and blindness. Treating diabetes is essential but will not reverse the cataract. Phacoemulsification surgery is the only treatment that can restore the patient's vision.

References

1. Englar RE. Performing the small animal physical examination. Hoboken, NJ: Wiley; 2017.
2. Gelatt KN. Essentials of veterinary ophthalmology. Ames, IA: John Wiley & Sons, Inc.; 2014.
3. Gelatt KN. Cornea. Merck Vet Man 2018. Available from: https://www.merckvetmanual.com/eye-and-ear/ophthalmology/cornea.
4. Evans HE, Miller ME. Miller's anatomy of the dog. 3rd ed. Philadelphia, PA: W. B. Saunders; 1993.
5. Singh B, Dyce KM. Dyce, Sack, and Wensing's textbook of veterinary anatomy. 5th ed. St. Louis, NO: Saunders; 2018.
6. Englar RE. Performing the small animal physical examination. Hoboken, NJ: Wiley/Blackwell; 2017.
7. Englar RE. Common clinical presentations in dogs and cats. Hoboken, NJ: Wiley/Blackwell; 2019. pages cm p.
8. Strom AR, Maggs DJ. Corneal opacities in dogs and cats. Today's. Vet Pract 2015; May/June:105–13.
9. Ollivier FJ. Bacterial corneal diseases in dogs and cats. Clin Tech Small Anim Pract 2003;18(3):193–8.
10. MacKay EO, Gelatt KN. Vet Ophthalmol. Wiley-Blackwell 2013;16(3):198–203.
11. Evans HE, Miller ME. Miller's anatomy of the dog. 4th ed. St. Louis, MO: Elsevier; 2013.
12. Boeve MH. Stades FC, Djajadningrat-Laanen. Eyes. In: Rijnberk A, van Sluijs FJ, editors. Medical history and physical examination in companion animals. Amsterdam: Elsevier; 2009. p. 175–201.
13. Sapienza JS. Feline lens disorders. Clin Tech Small Anim Pract 2005;20(2):102–7.
14. La Croix NL. Cataracts: when to refer. Top Companion Anim Med 2008;23(1):46–50.
15. Dziezyc J, Brooks DE. Canine Cataracts. Comp cont. Educ Pract 1983;5(2):81-and.
16. Tobias G, Tobias TA, Abood SK. Estimating age in dogs and cats using ocular lens examination. Comp Cont Educ Pract 2000;22(12):1085–91.
17. Giresi JC. Cataracts: how to uncover the imposter lenticular sclerosis. DVM. 360 [Internet]; 2005. Available from: http://veterinarynews.dvm360.com/cataracts-how-uncover-imposter-lenticular-sclerosis.
18. Mancuso L, Hendrix D. Cataracts in dogs. NAVC Clin's Brief 2016 (August):79–91.
19. Ramsey DT, editor. Cataracts: which and when to refer. Proc North Am Vet Conference; 2002.
20. Wilkie DA, Gemensky-Metzler AJ, Colitz CM, Bras ID, Kuonen VJ, Norris KN, Basham CR. Canine cataracts, diabetes mellitus and spontaneous lens capsule rupture: a retrospective study of 18 dogs. Vet Ophthalmol 2006;9(5):328–34.
21. Huang A. Canine diabetes mellitus. NAVC Clin's Brief 2012 (November):47–50.
22. Nygren K, Jalomäki S, Karlstam L, Narfström K. Hereditary cataracts in Russian Blue cats. J Feline Med Surg 2018;20(12):1105–9.
23. Davidson MG, Nelms SR. Diseases of the lens and cataract formation. In: Gelatt KN, Gilger BC, Kern TJ, editors. Veterinary ophthalmology. Ames, IA: Wiley/Blackwell; 2013. p. 1199–233.
24. Kristiansen E, Revold T, Lingaas F, Narfström K, Pedersen PB, Kielland C, et al. Cataracts in the Norwegian Buhund-current prevalence and characteristics. Vet Ophthalmol 2017;20(5):460–7.
25. Gelatt KN, Mackay EO. Prevalence of primary breed-related cataracts in the dog in North America. Vet Ophthalmol 2005;8(2):101–11.
26. Slatter D. Fundamentals of veterinary ophthalmology. Philadelphia, PA: W. B. Saunders; 2001.
27. Rubin LF. Inherited eye diseases in purebred dogs. Baltimore, MD: Williams & Wilkins; 1989.
28. Ocular disorders presumed to be inherited in purebred dogs. (CERF) CERF West Lafayette, IN: Purdue University; 1996.
29. Mellersh CS, Graves KT, McLaughlin B, Ennis RB, Pettitt L, Vaudin M, Barnett KC. Mutation in HSF4 associated with early but not late-onset hereditary cataract in the Boston Terrier. J Hered 2007;98(5):531–3.
30. Mellersh CS, Pettitt L, Forman OP, Vaudin M, Barnett KC. Identification of mutations in HSF4 in dogs of three different breeds with hereditary cataracts. Vet Ophthalmol 2006;9(5):369–78.
31. Barnett KC. Hereditary cataract in the Welsh Springer Spaniel. J Small Anim Pract 1980;21(11):621–5.
32. Barnett KC. Hereditary cataract in the Miniature Schnauzer. J Small Anim Pract 1985;26(11):635–44.
33. Barnett KC. Hereditary cataract in the German-shepherd dog. J Small Anim Pract 1986;27(6):387–95.
34. Barnett KC, Startup FG. Hereditary cataract in the Standard Poodle. Vet Rec 1985;117(1):15–6.
35. Curtis R. Late-onset cataract in the Boston Terrier. Vet Rec 1984;115(22):577–8.

36. Curtis R, Barnett KC. A survey of cataracts in golden and Labrador retrievers. J Small Anim Pract 1989;30(5):277–86.
37. Gelatt KN. Cataracts in Golden Retriever dog. Vet Med Sm Anim Clin 1972;67(10):1113-and.
38. Gelatt KN, Samuelson DA, Barrie KP, Das ND, Wolf ED, Bauer JE, Andresen TL. Biometry and clinical characteristics of congenital cataracts and microphthalmia in the Miniature Schnauzer. J Am Vet Med Assoc 1983;183(1):99–102.
39. Gelatt KN, Samuelson DA, Bauer JE, Das ND, Wolf ED, Barrie KP, Andresen TL. Inheritance of congenital cataracts and microphthalmia in the Miniature Schnauzer. Am J Vet Res 1983;44(6):1130–2.
40. Gelatt KN, Whitley RD, Lavach JD, Barrie KP, Williams LW. Cataracts in Chesapeake Bay retrievers. J Am Vet Med Assoc 1979;175(11):1176–8.
41. Koch SA. Cataracts in interrelated Old English Sheepdogs. J Am Vet Med Assoc 1972;160(3):299–301.
42. Narfström K. Cataract in the West Highland White Terrier. J Small Anim Pract 1981;22(7):467–71.
43. Narfström K. Hereditary and congenital ocular disease in the cat. J Feline Med Surg 1999;1(3):135–41.
44. Roberts SR, Helper LC. Cataracts in Afghan hounds. J Am Vet Med Assoc 1972;160(4):427–32.
45. Rubin LF. Cataract in golden retrievers. J Am Vet Med Assoc 1974;165(5):457–8.
46. Adkins EA, Hendrix DV. Outcomes of dogs presented for cataract evaluation: a retrospective study. J Am Anim Hosp Assoc 2005;41(4):235–40.
47. Collins BK, Collier LL, Johnson GS, Shibuya H, Moore CP, da Silva Curiel JM. Familial cataracts and concurrent ocular anomalies in chow chows. J Am Vet Med Assoc 1992;200(10):1485–91.
48. Williams DL, Heath MF. Prevalence of feline cataract: results of a cross-sectional study of 2000 normal animals, 50 cats with diabetes and one hundred cats following dehydrational crises. Vet Ophthalmol 2006;9(5):341–9.
49. Peiffer RL, Gelatt KN. Congenital cataracts in a Persian kitten (a case report). Vet Med Small Anim Clin 1975;70(11):1334–5.
50. Schwink K. Posterior nuclear cataracts in 2 Birman kittens. Feline Pract 1986;16(4):31–3.
51. Rubin LF. Hereditary cataract in Himalayan cats. Feline Pract 1986;16(1):14–5.
52. Collier LL, Bryan GM, Prieur DJ. Ocular manifestations of the Chédiak-Higashi syndrome in four species of animals. J Am Vet Med Assoc 1979;175(6):587–90.
53. Irby NI, editor. Hereditary cataracts in the British Shorthair cat. American College of Veterinary ophthalmology Genetics Workshop; 1983.
54. Bourguet A, Chaudieu G, Briatta A, Guyonnet A, Abitbol M, Chahory S. Cataracts in a population of Bengal cats in France. Vet Ophthalmol 2018;21(1):10–8.
55. Williams DL. Oxidation, antioxidants and cataract formation: a literature review. Vet Ophthalmol 2006;9(5):292–8.
56. Roberts SM, Lavach JD, Severin GA, Withrow SJ, Gillette EL. Ophthalmic complications following megavoltage irradiation of the nasal and paranasal cavities in dogs. J Am Vet Med Assoc 1987;190(1):43–7.
57. Ranz D, Gutbrod F, Eule C, Kienzle E. Nutritional lens opacities in two litters of Newfoundland dogs. J Nutr 2002;132(6)(Suppl 2):1688 SS-9 SS.
58. Ettinger SJ, Feldman EC, Côté E. Textbook of veterinary internal medicine: diseases of the dog and the cat. 8th ed. St. Louis, MO: Elsevier; 2017.
59. Côté E. Clinical veterinary advisor. Dogs and cats. 3rd ed. St. Louis, MO: Elsevier Mosby; 2015.
60. Basher AW, Roberts SM. Ocular manifestations of diabetes mellitus: diabetic cataracts in dogs. Vet Clin North Am Small Anim Pract 1995;25(3):661–76.
61. Beam S, Correa MT, Davidson MG. A retrospective-cohort study on the development of cataracts in dogs with diabetes mellitus: 200 cases. Vet Ophthalmol 1999;2(3):169–72.
62. Schermerhorn T. Treatment of diabetes mellitus in dogs and cats. NAVC Clin's Brief 2008 (January):35–7.
63. Tilley LP, Smith FWK. The 5-minute veterinary consult: canine and feline. 3rd ed. Baltimore, MD: Lippincott Williams & Wilkins; 2004.
64. Pottinger PK. A study of three enzymes acting on glucose in the lens of different species. Biochem J 1967;104(2):663–8.
65. Lim CC, Bakker SC, Waldner CL, Sandmeyer LS, Grahn BH. Cataracts in 44 dogs (77 eyes): A comparison of outcomes for no treatment, topical medical management, or phacoemulsification with intraocular lens implantation. Can Vet J 2011;52(3):283–8.

Case 30

The Dog with "Blue" and "Red" Eyes

Lieutenant Horatio Caine is new to your practice. He was recently taken in by Dorian Gray, the son of his original owner, who passed away from pancreatic cancer 3 months ago.

Dorian is new to pet ownership. As a traveling businessman, he was used to jet-setting. He spent more time on planes and in hotels than in his own home. However, Dorian had made a promise at his father's deathbed that the Beagle would be well cared for, and so far, he was doing everything in his power to prove his words true. Dorian now works remotely when he can. When that is an impossibility, he hires a house sitter,

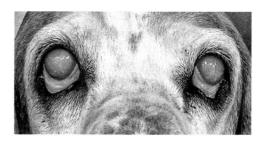

Figure 30.1 Meet 10-year-old intact male Beagle, Lieutenant Horatio Caine.

Jaycee, to stay with the Lieutenant. Jaycee has successfully gotten the Lieutenant through five trips thus far with no concerns, and she is attentive to his every need. Thanks to Jaycee, the Lieutenant has come out of his shell of depression and is starting to reinvest in life.

For the past 10 days, Dorian has been overseas. The Lieutenant has been in good spirits, but halfway through Dorian's trip, both of his eyes take on a "red" appearance. Jaycee tried to text Dorian a photograph, but his cellular phone's reception is poor, and he did not receive it. Jaycee asked Dorian what to do.

Dorian's gut reaction was that it was probably pollen related. This was the worst time of year for seasonal allergies, and from what his friends had shared, this season seemed particularly brutal. Dorian asked if the beagle's eyes seemed to irritate him. Jaycee didn't think so. Other than increased tearing, Lieutenant Horatio Caine did not seem phased. Jaycee did not observe him pawing at his face or eyes. Jaycee did not report photophobia or blepharospasm. So, Dorian asked her just to keep an eye on it.

The Lieutenant's "red eyes" persist throughout the remainder of Dorian's trip. On the evening before Dorian's homecoming, the dog's eyes looked "bloodshot." Jaycee again texted Dorian, but he was in-flight and never received the message.

When Dorian returned home this morning, he panicked when he saw Lieutenant's eyes. "They're not red!" he exclaimed! "They're blue! I don't know what that is, but that isn't allergies!"

Dorian dialed the nearest clinic and was appreciative when your customer service representative told him that the Lieutenant could be fit in.

Dorian arrives at your clinic 30 minutes later with Lieutenant Horatio Caine in tow. The technician checks them in and documents his vital signs in the medical record.

Use the questions below to help you work through this consultation.

Weight: 32.5 lb (14.8 kg)
BCS: 7/9
Mentation: BAR

TPR

T: 100.3°F (37.9°C)
P: 112 beats per minute
R: panting

Round One of Questions for Case 30: The Dog with "Blue" and "Red" Eyes

1. When Jaycee told Dorian that the Lieutenant's eyes were "red," which structure was she referring to?
2. What is the purpose of the structure that you identified in Question #1 (above)?
3. Is the structure that you identified in Question #1 (above) typically visible in a patient that is staring straight ahead?
4. In which breeds might the structure that you identified in Question #1 (above) become more prominent?
5. In what situations might the structure that you identified in Question #1 (above) become more prominent?
6. What color should the structure in Question #1 (above) be in a healthy (normal) eye?
7. Are there variations of the normal color of this structure?
8. It would be abnormal if the structure in Question #1 (above) were which color(s)?
9. What causes the color(s) that you identified in Question #8 (above)?
10. Based on the photograph of the Lieutenant, how would you describe the structure that you identified in Question #1 (above)?
11. When Dorian returned home and exclaimed that the Lieutenant's eyes were "blue," which structure was he referring to?
12. What is the purpose of the structure that you identified in Question #11 (above)?
13. What color should the structure in Question #11 (above) be in a healthy (normal) eye?
14. It would be abnormal if the structure in Question #11 (above) were which color(s)?
15. What causes the color(s) that you identified in Question #14 (above)?
16. Based on the photograph of the Lieutenant, how would you describe the structure that you identified in Question #11?

Answers to Round One of Questions for Case 30: The Dog with "Blue" and "Red" Eyes

1. When Jaycee told Dorian that the Lieutenant's eyes were "red," she was likely referring to the sclera.

2. The sclera is part of the outermost layer of the globe.(1, 2)

3. When the patient is staring straight ahead, the sclera is not typically seen.(3, 4) If the sclera does come into view, then it is usually just a sliver.(5)

4. The sclera is particularly prominent in brachycephalic patients because of their facial conformation.(3, 4) Their shallow orbits and oversized palpebral fissures cause the eyes to appear bulgy. (6) More of each eye is seen, including the sclera.

5. The sclera is also prominent in patients that are experiencing fear, anxiety, or stress (FAS).(3–5, 7) These patients are said to demonstrate "whale eye" or "crescent moon eye," meaning that the sliver of white has morphed into a sea of white.(5) This is a sign that we should exert caution when handling and restraining these patients.(3, 4) These patients are likely to react defensively or aggressively; therefore, their actions may be unpredictable. The cardinal rule in these patients is to go slow.

6. The healthy (normal) eye typically has a white sclera.(1–4)

7. Some, but not all dogs, have pigment at the limbus, the site at which the sclera and the cornea meet.(1, 8) This pigment is melanin, which may be focal or more widespread, and typically appears dark brown or black.(8) If melanin is lightly sprinkled at the limbus, then the sclera may appear to be gray.(3, 4) These are all considered variations of normal.(4)

8. It would be abnormal if the sclera were yellow or red.(3, 4)

9. If the sclera is yellow, then it is said to be icteric and the patient is jaundiced.(1, 3–5) The yellow pigment develops when bile pigments pathologically accumulate in the body.(9) It is easier to appreciate the yellow discoloration at certain sites of the body, including the sclera.(5) Other commonly assessed sites include the patient's mucous membranes and the skin, once the fur is parted.(3, 4) In cats, peri-aural (peri-auricular) alopecia is common, so the skin is easiest to examine just in front of the ears.(3, 4)

    When it occurs, icterus may be pre-hepatic, hepatic, or post-hepatic.(5, 9–12)

   - Extensive hemolysis results in pre-hepatic icterus:(4, 10, 11, 13)

     - an immune-mediated disease, drug, or toxin triggers widespread hemolysis:(4, 10–19)

       - acetaminophen
       - infectious disease:
       - hemobartonellosis, as caused by *Mycoplasma haemofelis*
       - cytauxzoonosis, as caused by *Cytauxzoon felis*
       - feline immunodeficiency virus (FIV)
       - feline leukemia virus (FeLV)
       - immune-mediated hemolytic anemia (IMHA)
       - transfusion reactions
       - neonatal isoerythrolysis (NI)
       - new methylene blue
       - onion toxicity

     - too many erythrocytes line up to be broken down at once
     - the body is overwhelmed: it can only metabolize and excrete so much bilirubin(19)
     - unconjugated bilirubin builds up within the bloodstream.(19)

   - Liver disease results in hepatic icterus.(4, 11) Hepatopathy may be primary or secondary. (4, 11) Examples include:(10–12, 19–21)

     - cholangiohepatitis
     - drugs and toxins:(10–12, 19, 20)

       - acetaminophen
       - diazepam
       - ketoconazole
       - methimazole
       - phenols
       - aflatoxins

     - hepatic lipidosis
     - hepatitis
     - infectious disease:

       - toxoplasmosis, as caused by toxoplasma gondii
       - feline infectious peritonitis (FIP)
       - leptospirosis

     - portosystemic shunts

- neoplasia:
  - lymphoma
  - biliary cystadenoma or cystadenocarcinoma
  - hepatocellular or biliary carcinoma
  - metastatic disease
- sepsis
- bile duct obstruction causes post-hepatic icterus.(11)

The sclera can also appear red. Redness can result from:(3, 4)

- scleral hemorrhage, as from trauma:(22–24)
  - ocular surgery
  - penetrating foreign bodies
- inflammation of the outermost layer of the sclera, episcleritis:(23, 25, 26)
  - episcleritis can be caused by:(23, 26, 27)
    - immune-mediated disease,(26–30) American Cocker spaniels and Golden retrievers may be predisposed(26–29, 31)
    - infectious disease, such as *Ehrlichia canis*
    - inflammatory disease (e.g. glaucoma, keratitis, uveitis)
    - parasitic infestations, including *Onchocerca* spp.
    - neoplasia
  - when episcleritis is focal, pink-tan elevations appear in the affected tissue,(23, 26) such lesions are more likely to occur in Collies(27)
  - when episcleritis is diffuse, there is generalized redness because the superficial episcleral vessels are congested,(26) the sclera may appear bloodshot, and owners are likely to complain about "red eye."

10. The Lieutenant appears to have diffuse episcleritis, which has caused a bloodshot appearance in both of his eyes. His sclera both appear significantly pinker than they ought to be, which likely accounts for Jaycee's description of "red eye."

11. When Dorian returned home and exclaimed that the Lieutenant's eyes were "blue," he was likely referring to the cornea.

12. The primary purpose of the cornea is to refract incoming light.(32, 33) In addition, the cornea and the sclera combined form the outermost layer of the globe and therefore contribute to globe shape and structural integrity.(3, 4)

13. The healthy (normal) cornea is transparent.(3, 4) For more information on how this transparency is established and maintained, refer to Case #29.

14. It would be abnormal if the cornea were any of the following colors:(4, 32, 34)
    - black-brown
    - blue
    - creamy-tan
    - red
    - silvery-white
    - yellow-green.

15. Each abnormal corneal color can be linked to a specific etiology:(4, 32, 34)

- black-brown: melanosis
- blue: corneal edema
- creamy-tan: infiltration of the cornea with inflammatory cells
- gray-white: corneal scarring, as from fibrosis
- red: neovascularization of the cornea
- silvery-white: deposition of lipid within the cornea
- yellow-green: infiltration of the cornea with inflammatory cells.

16. The Lieutenant appears to have corneal edema, which has given the appearance that both of his globes are blue-gray. This likely accounts for Dorian's description of "blue eye."

Returning to Case 30: The Dog with "Blue" and "Red" Eyes

After examining Lieutenant Horatio Caine, you validate Dorian's concerns. He is right to be alarmed. Dorian appears to have episcleritis and corneal edema, and both are bilateral. In addition, you are concerned that both of his eyes seem to be enlarged.

Use the questions below to guide your diagnostic work-up of the Lieutenant.

Round Two of Questions for Case 30: The Dog with "Blue" and "Red" Eyes

1. The shape of the globe is largely dependent upon intraocular pressure (IOP). What is the name of the fluid that is the primary determinant of IOP?
2. Where is the fluid that you identified in Question #1 produced?
3. Describe how the fluid that you identified in Question #1 flows through the eye.
4. What are lesser determinants of IOP?
5. Which procedure assesses our patient's IOP in clinical practice?
6. There are two approaches to the procedure that you identified in Question #5 (above). Name these methods and associate at least one diagnostic tool with each.
7. Which approach that you named in Question #6 (above) requires you to apply topical anesthetic to each eye before you measure IOP?
8. Which approach that you named in Question #6 (above) requires your patient's head to be positioned in a specific way?
9. What is normal IOP in a dog?
10. What is normal IOP in a cat?
11. When IOP is persistently elevated, the globe enlarges. What is the appropriate medical term for an enlarged globe?
12. Which clinical disease causes an enlarged globe?
13. Is the condition that you named in Question #12 (above) more likely to be congenital or acquired?
14. When the condition that you named in Question #12 (above) is acquired, disease may be primary or secondary. Which occurs more often in dogs?
15. When considering the condition that you named in Question #12 (above), what causes acquired primary disease in dogs?
16. Are there breed predispositions for acquired primary disease in dogs?
17. Are there breed predispositions for acquired primary disease in cats?
18. When considering the condition that you named in Question #12 (above), what causes acquired secondary disease in dogs?

19. Is acquired secondary disease typically bilateral?
20. In addition to buphthalmos, what are additional clinical signs that dogs and cats present with when they are affected by the condition that you named in Question #12 (above)?

Answers to Round Two of Questions for Case 30: The Dog with "Blue" and "Red" Eyes

1. IOP is determined primarily by the production and flow of aqueous humor.(35, 36)

2. Aqueous humor is produced by the ciliary body of the eye, and fills the globe's anterior and posterior chambers.(35–37)

3. Aqueous humor reaches the anterior chamber from the posterior chamber by flowing through the pupil of the eye.(35, 38–40) After reaching the anterior chamber, aqueous humor exits the eye through one of two pathways.(35)

   • The conventional pathway

     • This is the primary pathway.(35)
     • Aqueous humor flows from the base of the iris to the cornea, through the pectinate ligaments.(41)
     • Aqueous humor then travels from the trabecular meshwork through angular plexus, and ultimately into the episcleral veins.(41)
     • The efficient passage of aqueous humor via this route is dependent upon the iridocorneal angle (ICA).(35)

   • The uveoscleral or nonconventional pathway

     • This is the secondary route by which aqueous humor exits the eye.(35)
     • It relies upon hydrostatic pressure differences between the anterior chamber and suprachoroidal spaces to force aqueous humor into the adjacent sclera.(35, 42)

4. Other lesser determinants of IOP include:(35, 43–52)

   • age (in the cat):(53–56)

     • adult cats have IOP that is greater than kittens
     • adult cats have IOP that is greater than seniors

   • corneal health
   • diurnal variation
   • exercise
   • how the patient is restrained:

     • IOP readings will be falsely elevated if excessive restraint that compresses the jugular vein is required(35, 51, 52)

   • pharmaceutical agents:

     • the mydriatic agent, tropicamide, elevates IOP(57–59)
     • corticosteroids also elevate IOP(54)

   • the patient's species
   • the patient's temperature.

5. Tonometry is the procedure by which IOP is assessed.(35, 60)

6. In veterinary medicine, two techniques are appropriate for assessing IOP.(60, 61)

   - Applanation tonometry

     - Requires a portable device, such as the Tono-Pen.(60)
     - The Tono-Pen is tapped against the numbed cornea.(60)
     - As the device comes into contact with the cornea, the cornea is flattened.(60)
     - Force is required to achieve applanation. The Tono-Pen measures this force by averaging several readings, and offers a percent error.(60)

   - Rebound tonometry

     - Requires a portable device such as the Tono-Vet.(60)
     - This device has a lightweight probe that only requires momentary contact with the cornea to obtain a reading.
     - The probe is magnetized via an induction coil.(60)
     - The rebound of the probe upon corneal contact creates an induction current.(60)
     - This allows the device to calculate the IOP.(60)

7. Applanation tonometry, using the Tono-Pen, requires you to apply topical anesthetic to each eye before you measure IOP.(4) Rebound tonometry does not.

8. Rebound tonometry, using the Tono-Vet, requires your patient's head to be positioned so that the probe is directed horizontally.(60) Applanation tonometry does not.(60)

9. Values of IOP in healthy (normal) dogs vary depending upon which study is referenced. However, normal IOP readings in the dog via applanation tonometry have been reported as:(35, 62–64)

   - 12.9 mmHg +/– 2.7 mmHg
   - 19.2 mmHg +/– 5.5 mmHg.

   Normal IOP readings in the dog via rebound tonometry have been reported as:(35, 62, 63)

   - 10.8 mmHg +/– 3.1 mmHg
   - 9.1 mmHg +/– 3.4 mmHg.

10. What is normal IOP in a cat?
    Values of IOP in healthy (normal) cats, when determined by applanation tonometry, have been reported as 18.4 mmHg +/– 0.67 mmHg.(65)
    Values of IOP in healthy (normal) cats, when determined by rebound tonometry, have been reported as 20 mmHg +/– 0.48 mmHg.(65)

11. The appropriate medical term for an enlarged globe is buphthalmos.(5, 24, 48, 66)

12. Glaucoma is the clinical condition that causes an enlarged globe.(35)

13. Acquired glaucoma is much more likely to occur in companion animal patients than congenital glaucoma.(35, 36, 61)

14. Acquired primary glaucoma is much more likely to occur in dogs than acquired secondary glaucoma.(35, 51, 61)

15. Acquired primary glaucoma is an inherited condition in which there is either a narrowed ICA (primary closed angle glaucoma) or the fibers at the ICA, the pectinate ligaments, are misshapen, causing drainage through the conventional pathway to be impaired.(61, 67) The latter scenario is termed primary open angle glaucoma.(35)

16. American Cocker spaniels, Basset hounds, Boston terriers, and Shar Pei dogs are predisposed to primary closed angle glaucoma.(35, 36, 61, 68) Beagles and Norwegian Elkhounds are overrepresented when it comes to developing primary open angle glaucoma.(35)

17. Cats are less likely to develop primary glaucoma.(35) However, Siamese, Burmese, Persian, and domestic short-haired (DSH) are overrepresented.(54, 61)

18. Acquired secondary glaucoma occurs when the flow of aqueous humor through the eye is physically obstructed, as occurs when:(4, 61)

    - posterior synechiae attach the iris to the lens through the pupil(69)
    - the lens luxates
    - there is hyphema
    - there is hypopyon
    - there is intraocular neoplasia:(53, 54, 70–72)

        - more common in cats than dogs
        - typically involves either anterior uveal melanoma or lymphoma(53, 54, 70–72)
        - intraocular sarcomas have also been reported in cats months to years after globe-related trauma.(54, 73, 74)

19. Acquired secondary glaucoma is typically bilateral. However, the patient may present initially with unilateral involvement that later progresses to bilateral.(35, 61)

20. In addition to buphthalmos, patients with glaucoma may present with one or more of the following clinical signs:(35, 36, 61)

    - absent menace response
    - blepharospasm
    - blindness
    - conjunctival hyperemia
    - corneal edema ("blue eye")
    - epiphora
    - episcleral congestion
    - mydriasis
    - prominent nictitans
    - "red eye."

Returning to Case 30: The Dog with "Blue" and "Red" Eyes

Dorian agrees to proceed with measuring the Lieutenant's IOP via applanation tonometry. You take three values per eye. The mean IOP in each is recorded as:

- 30 mmHg OS
- 32 mmHg OD.

Round Three of Questions for Case 30: The Dog with "Blue" and "Red" Eyes

1. What is your interpretation of the Lieutenant's IOPs? Are they normal, too low, or too high?
2. Does the Lieutenant have glaucoma?
3. Dorian is concerned that the Lieutenant is in pain despite being stoic. How likely is it that the Beagle is painful?
4. What is your proposed approach to treatment?

Answers to Round Three of Questions for Case 30:
The Dog with "Blue" and "Red" Eyes

1. Lieutenant's IOP in each eye is elevated.

2. Yes, the Lieutenant has glaucoma.

3. Glaucoma is considered painful.(35, 61, 67) The pain is thought to be due to the elevation in IOP.(67) Pain lessens as IOP is reduced.(67)

4. The goal of treatment for glaucoma is to reduce IOP sufficiently to halt retinal damage and pre-serve whatever vision remains.(35) Ideally, IOP should not exceed 19–20 mmHg in dogs with glaucoma.(35) Keeping IOP at this level will alleviate pain.

    IOP is lowered by prescribing medications that either reduce aqueous humor production or improve its flow.(4)

    Topical drugs such as carbonic anhydrase inhibitors (CAIs) reduce aqueous humor produc-tion.(35) These include topical dorzolamide and brinzolamide.(35, 61, 75)

    On the other hand, prostaglandin analogs (PGAs), such as latanoprost, bimatoprost, and travoprost, act on ciliary body muscles to increase aqueous humor outflow.(4)

    Medical management stabilizes disease in the short-term, but glaucoma typically progresses.(35)

    Advanced surgical techniques can selectively target the ciliary body to reduce aqueous humor production and improve outflow.(35) Patients that are avisual, for instance, may undergo chemical ablation of the ciliary body with an intravitreal injection of gentamicin or cidofovir.(35, 61) However, these techniques are not typically available in general practice. More fre-quently, enucleation is pursued as a reasonable course of action.(35, 37) By eliminating ocular discomfort, patient quality of life is maximized despite the patient's loss of vision.(35) In truth, the patient had probably already had significantly compromised vision, if he had any at all. Dogs do surprisingly well, even if both eyes are removed.

CLINICAL PEARLS

- Dogs frequently present on emergency for "red eye."

- Note that "red eye" is not pathognomonic for glaucoma.

- "Red eye" is a generic descriptor that may result from anterior uveitis, blepharitis, conjunc-tivitis, keratitis, scleritis, and episcleritis.(29, 30)

- It is essential to understand basic eye anatomy because what clients report may be vague or may be a clinical sign, such as "red eye," that can mean several different things.

- This patient had both "red eye" from episcleritis and "blue eye" from corneal edema. This highlights a key point about clinical practice. Clinical signs rarely occur in isolation. It is up to the practitioner to establish links between signs that may be related and to read between the lines.

- Patients with glaucoma often present for "red eye", "blue eye", and/or buphthalmos.

- Buphthalmos is the appropriate medical term for an enlarged globe. It occurs with elevations in IOP, which is painful.

- Treatment of glaucoma is aimed at reducing aqueous humor production or increasing flow. Both mechanisms effectively reduce IOP and pain in the short-term. However, glaucoma progresses. Therefore, enucleation may be indicated to improve quality of life.

References

1. Boeve MH. Stades FC, Djajadiningrat-Laanen. Eyes. In: Rijnberk A, van Sluijs FJ, editors. Medical history and physical examination in companion animals. Amsterdam: Elsevier; 2009.
2. Gelatt KN. Eye structure and function in cats. In: Aiello SE, Moses MA, editors. The Merck Veterinary Manual 2016.
3. Englar RE. Performing the small animal physical examination. Hoboken, NJ: Wiley/Blackwell; 2017.
4. Englar RE. Common clinical presentations in dogs and cats. Hoboken, NJ: Wiley/Blackwell; 2019.
5. Englar RE. Performing the small animal physical examination. Hoboken, NJ: Wiley; 2017.
6. Packer RM, Hendricks A, Burn CC. Impact of facial conformation on canine health: corneal ulceration. PLloS one 2015;10(5):e0123827.
7. Fear free L. Module 1: fear free behavior modification basics. Denver, CO, 2018.
8. Gionfriddo JR. Just ask the expert: can a smoky sclera be normal? DVM. 360 [Internet]; 2011. Available from: http://veterinarymedicine.dvm360.com/just-ask-expert-can-smoky-sclera-be-normal.
9. Schaer M. Icterus NAVC Clinician's. Brief. 2008 (September):8.
10. Wray J. Canine internal medicine: what's your diagnosis? Hoboken, NJ: John Wiley & Sons, Ltd.; 2017.
11. Schaer M. The icteric dog and cat. Available from: http://www.delawarevalleyacademyvm.org/pdfs/may10/Icteric.pdf.
12. Lappin M. Feline internal medicine secrets. Philadelphia, PA: Hanley & Belfus, Inc.; 2001.
13. Schaer M. Immune-mediated hemolytic anemia. NAVC Clin's Brief 2010 (March);78.
14. Caruso K. Feline erythroparasites NAVC Clin's. Brief 2004 (June):36–8.
15. Fry JK, Burney DP. Feline cytauxzoonosis. NAVC Clin's Brief 2012 (July):85–9.
16. Haber M. Icterus and pancytopenia in a cat. NAVC Clin's Brief 2005 (July):21–3.
17. Bowles M. Identifying and treating 3 tick-borne diseases in dogs. DVM. 360 [Internet]; 2017. Available from: http://veterinarymedicine.dvm360.com/identifying-and-treating-3-tick-borne-diseases-dogs.
18. Colleran E. Tick-borne disease in cats: two to watch for. DVM. 360 [Internet]; 2017. Available from: http://veterinarynews.dvm360.com/tick-borne-disease-cats-two-watch.
19. Gordon J. Clinical approach to icterus in the cat (Proceedings). DVM. 360 [Internet]; 2011. Available from: http://veterinarycalendar.dvm360.com/clinical-approach-icterus-cat-proceedings.
20. Norsworthy GD. The icteric cat: a case study. DVM. 360 [Internet]; 2011. Available from: http://veterinarycalendar.dvm360.com/icteric-cat-case-study-proceedings.
21. Webb C. Liver conditions in dogs. NAVC Clin's Brief 2013 (May):85–7.
22. Rampazzo A, Eule C, Speier S, Grest P, Spiess B. Scleral rupture in dogs, cats, and horses. Vet Ophthalmol 2006;9(3):149–55.
23. Tilley LP, Smith FWK. The 5-minute veterinary consult: canine and feline. 3rd ed. Baltimore, MD: Lippincott Williams & Wilkins; 2004.
24. Côté E. Clinical veterinary advisor. Dogs and cats. 3rd ed. St. Louis, MO: Elsevier Mosby; 2015.
25. Laminack EB, Myrna K, Moore PA. Clinical approach to the canine red eye. Today's. Vet Pract 2013 (May/June):12–41.
26. Grahn BH, Sandmeyer LS. Canine episcleritis, nodular episclerokeratitis, scleritis, and necrotic scleritis. Vet Clin North Am Small Anim Pract 2008;38(2):291–308.
27. Sandmeyer LS, Grahn BH. Diagnostic ophthalmology. Can Vet J Rev Vet Canadienne 2008;49(11):1141–2.
28. Deykin AR, Guandalini A, Ratto A. A retrospective histopathologic study of primary episcleral and scleral inflammatory disease in dogs. Prog Vet Comp Ophthalmol 1997;7:245–58.
29. Paulsen ME, Lavach JD, Snyder SP, Severin GA, Eichenbaum JD. Nodular granulomatous episclerokeratitis in dogs: 19 cases (1973-1985). J Am Vet Med Assoc 1987;190(12):1581–7.
30. Breaux CB, Sandmeyer LS, Grahn BH. Immunohistochemical investigation of canine episcleritis. Vet Ophthalmol 2007;10(3):168–72.
31. Grahn BH, Peiffer RL. Fundamentals of veterinary ophthalmic pathology. In: Gelatt KN, editor. Veterinary ophthalmology. Ames, IA: Blackwell Publishing; 2007. p. 355–437.
32. Strom AR, Maggs DJ. Corneal opacities in dogs and cats. Today's. Vet Pract 2015; May/June:105–13.
33. Gelatt KN. Cornea. Merck Veterinary Man [Internet] 2018. Available from: https://www.merckvetmanual.com/eye-and-ear/ophthalmology/cornea.

34. MacKay EO, Gelatt KN. Veterinary ophthalmology, Oxford: Wiley-Blackwell; 2013.
35. Maggio F. Glaucomas. Top Companion Anim Med 2015;30(3):86–96.
36. Reinstein S, Rankin A, Allbaugh R. Canine glaucoma: pathophysiology and diagnosis. Compend Contin Educ Vet 2009;31(10):450–2.
37. Dietrich U. Feline glaucomas. Clin Tech Small Anim Pract 2005;20(2):108–16.
38. Evans HE, DeLahunta A. Guide to the dissection of the dog. 6th ed. St. Louis, MO: Saunders; 2004.
39. Evans HE, Miller ME. Miller's anatomy of the dog. 4th ed. St. Louis, MO: Elsevier; 2013.
40. Dyce KM, Sack WO, Wensing CJG. Textbook of veterinary anatomy. 4th ed. St. Louis, MO: Saunders/Elsevier; 2010.
41. Samuelson DA. Ophthalmic anatomy. In: Gelatt KN, Gilger BC, Kern TJ, editors. Veterinary ophthalmology. Ames, IA: Wiley/Blackwell; 2013.
42. Gum GG, MacKay EO. Physiology of the eye. In: Gelatt KN, Gilger BC, Kern TJ, editors. Veterinary ophthalmol. Ames, IA: Wiley/Blackwell; 2013.
43. Brubaker RF. Flow of aqueous humor in humans [the Friedenwald Lecture]. Invest Ophthalmol Vis Sci 1991;32(13):3145–66.
44. Koskela T, Brubaker RF. The nocturnal suppression of aqueous humor flow in humans is not blocked by bright light. Invest Ophthalmol Vis Sci 1991;32(9):2504–6.
45. Liu JH, Weinreb RN. Monitoring intraocular pressure for 24 h. Br J Ophthalmol 2011;95(5):599–600.
46. Drance SM. Effect of oral glycerol of intraocular pressure in normal and glaucomatous eyes. Arch Ophthalmol 1964;72:491–3.
47. Qureshi IA. Effects of mild, moderate and severe exercise on intraocular pressure of sedentary subjects. Ann Hum Biol 1995;22(6):545–53.
48. Aiello SE, Moses MC. Merck Veterinary Manual. Whitehouse Station, NJ: Merck Sharp and Dohme, Corp. 2016.
49. Brunton L, Chabner BA, Knollman B. General anesthetics and therapeutic gases. Goodman and Gilman's: the pharmacological basis of therapeutics. New York: McGraw-Hill Companies, Inc.; 2011.
50. Plumb DC. Plumb's veterinary drug handbook. 7th ed. Ames, IA: PharmaVet; 2011.
51. Plummer CE, Regnier A, Gelatt KN. The canine glaucomas. In: Gelatt KN, Gilger BC, Kern TJ, editors. Veterinary ophthalmology II. Ames, IA: Wiley/Blackwell; 2013. p. 1050–145.
52. von Spiessen L, Karck J, Rohn K, Meyer-Lindenberg A. Clinical comparison of the TonoVet(®) rebound tonometer and the Tono-Pen Vet(®) applanation tonometer in dogs and cats with ocular disease: glaucoma or corneal pathology. Vet Ophthalmol 2015;18(1):20–7.
53. McLellan GJ, Miller PE. Feline glaucoma--a comprehensive review. Vet Ophthalmol 2011;14;Suppl 1:15–29.
54. McLellan GJ, Teixeira LB. Feline glaucoma. Vet Clin North Am Small Anim Pract 2015;45(6):1307–33, vii, vii.
55. Adelman S, McLellan GJ, Ellinwood NM, editors. Early life intraocular pressures in normal cats and cats with primary congenital glaucoma. American College of Veterinary Ophthalmologists. Puerto Rico; 2013.
56. Kroll MM, Miller PE, Rodan I. Intraocular pressure measurements obtained as part of a comprehensive geriatric health examination from cats seven years of age or older. J Am Vet Med Assoc 2001;219(10):1406–10.
57. Stadtbäumer K, Frommlet F, Nell B. Effects of mydriatics on intraocular pressure and pupil size in the normal feline eye. Vet Ophthalmol 2006;9(4):233–7.
58. Stadtbäumer K, Köstlin RG, Zahn KJ. Effects of topical 0.5% tropicamide on intraocular pressure in normal cats. Vet Ophthalmol 2002;5(2):107–12.
59. Gomes FE, Bentley E, Lin TL, McLellan GJ. Effects of unilateral topical administration of 0.5% tropicamide on anterior segment morphology and intraocular pressure in normal cats and cats with primary congenital glaucoma. Vet Ophthalmol 2011;14;Suppl 1:75–83.
60. Wilkie DA. Determining intraocular pressure. NAVC Clin's Brief 2013 (February):77–9.
61. Reinstein S. Under pressure: canine and feline Glaucoma2017. Available from: https://michvma.org/resources/Documents/MVC/2017%20Proceedings/reinstein%2005.pdf.
62. Knollinger AM, La Croix NC, Barrett PM, Miller PE. Evaluation of a rebound tonometer for measuring intraocular pressure in dogs and horses. J Am Vet Med Assoc 2005;227(2):244–8.
63. Leiva M, Naranjo C, Peña MT. Comparison of the rebound tonometer (ICare) to the applanation tonometer (Tono-pen XL) in normotensive dogs. Vet Ophthalmol 2006;9(1):17–21.

64. Gelatt KN, MacKay EO. Distribution of intraocular pressure in dogs. Vet Ophthalmol 1998;1(2–3):109–14.
65. Rusanen E, Florin M, Hässig M, Spiess BM. Evaluation of a rebound tonometer (Tonovet) in clinically normal cat eyes. Vet Ophthalmol 2010;13(1):31–6.
66. Tilley LP, Smith FWK, Tilley LP. Blackwell's five-minute veterinary consult: canine and feline. 4th ed. Ames, IA: Blackwell; 2007.
67. Colitz CMH. Canine glaucoma. NAVC Clin's Brief 2010 (March):24–6.
68. Gelatt KN, MacKay EO. Prevalence of the breed-related glaucomas in pure-bred dogs in North America. Vet Ophthalmol 2004;7(2):97–111.
69. Heller HB, Bentley E. The practitioner's guide to neurologic causes of canine anisocoria. Today's Vet Pract 2016 (January/February):[77–83]. Available from: http://todaysveterinarypractice.navc.com/wp-content/uploads/2016/05/TVP_2016–0102_OO-Anisocoria.pdf.
70. Blocker T, Van Der Woerdt A. The feline glaucomas: 82 cases (1995–1999). Vet Ophthalmol 2001;4(2):81–5.
71. Walde I, Rapp E. Feline glaucoma: clinical and morphological aspects (a retrospective study of 38 cases). Eur J Compan Anim Pract 1993;4:87–105.
72. Wilcock BP, Peiffer RL, Jr., Davidson MG. The causes of glaucoma in cats. Vet Pathol 1990;27(1):35–40.
73. Dubielzig RR, Everitt J, Shadduck JA, Albert DM. Clinical and morphologic features of post-traumatic ocular sarcomas in cats. Vet Pathol 1990;27(1):62–5.
74. Dubielzig RR, Zeiss C. Feline Post-traumatic ocular sarcoma: three morphologic variants and evidence that some are derived from lens epithelial cells. Investig Ophth Vis Sci 2004;45:U170-U.
75. Maślanka T. A review of the pharmacology of carbonic anhydrase inhibitors for the treatment of glaucoma in dogs and cats. Vet J 2015;203(3):278–84.

Case 31

The Head-Shaking Dog

Tarragon is new to the practice. His owner, Eugene Wilkinson, recently moved from the city to the countryside. Tarragon has been a city dog for his whole life. He has never known the freedom of the rolling hills and the other amenities that rural life has to offer. One of his favorite discoveries has been the lake. For a dog that has never known how to swim, Tarragon certainly did take to water! Every morning finds him semi-submerged in the lake, paddling around like a spring chicken. Eugene is excited to see this second wind in him. Tarragon had been steadily slowing down over the past 2 years and it was hard for

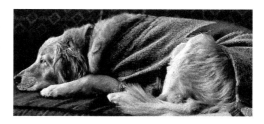

Figure 31.1 Meet your new patient, Tarragon, a 10-year-old castrated male Golden Retriever. Courtesy of Desiree Pearsall.

Eugene to think of him as getting old. Introducing the lake to Tarragon at this stage of life had awakened him, and it was as if the clock hit rewind. The pup that Eugene had fallen in love with years ago was back.

Weight: 86.8 lb (39.5 kg)
BCS: 6/9
Muscle condition score:
Moderate muscle loss
Mentation: BAR

TPR

T: 101.1°F (38.4°C)
P: 96 beats per minute
R: Panting

Life was about as good as it got, with one exception. Since discovering the lake 10 days ago, Tarragon's ears have gotten a bit pungent. His ears were never particularly appealing to smell, but they were tolerable. Lately, Tarragon has been smelling much more "doglike" than suits Eugene's tastes. Tarragon had always seemed clean before. Now, Eugene feels like he must wash his hands after handling the dog, just so that he doesn't end up carrying around the scent for the rest of the day.

What started as just an odor has morphed into a copious amount of aural debris. Eugene cleaned Tarragon's ears to the best of his ability, hoping that would help, but the discharge just came back. Eugene is presenting Tarragon to you today for evaluation. He is hoping for a speedy resolution and that you will not tell him the cure is to keep Tarragon away from the lake.

Tarragon's vital signs have been recorded below.

Use the questions below to prepare for your consultation.

Round One of Questions for Case 31: The Head-Shaking Dog

1. The entrance to the external ear canal has little to no fur in cats and most dog breeds. Which dog breeds are the exceptions to this rule?
2. Why might excessive fur at the entrance to the external ear canal be problematic?
3. The external ear canal is composed of two parts. Outline its anatomy, including its shape.
4. Where is the ear drum located relative to the canal?
5. What is the appropriate medical term for the ear drum?

6. What color is the normal ear drum?
7. How might the ear drum's appearance change in cases of otitis media?
8. How might the appearance of the ear drum change if there is fluid build-up in the middle ear?
9. What will a ruptured ear drum look like?
10. What color is ear wax in a healthy (normal) dog or cat?
11. What consistency is ear wax in a healthy (normal) dog or cat?
12. Which structure(s) produce ear wax?
13. What is the appropriate medical term for ear wax?
14. Which breeds of dog are known for producing excessive ear wax?
15. Which breeds of cat are known for producing excessive ear wax?
16. Excessive ear wax in a patient that typically does not have an appreciable amount can signify a problem with the ear itself. What other clinical signs might cause you to evaluate one or both ears?
17. Aural discharge may be described by color. Which colors are considered abnormal?
18. Aural discharge may be described by consistency or texture. What constitutes abnormal?
19. Historically, clinicians have made diagnoses based upon observation and aural odor. What might you expect to see grossly if Tarragon had ear mites?
20. Is it appropriate to make a diagnosis based upon gross appearance?
21. Which procedure will you need to perform as part of Tarragon's complete physical exam? Why is this procedure essential?
22. Which diagnostic test(s) might you need as part of Tarragon's work-up?
23. Describe what each diagnostic test that you identified in Question #22 is assessing.
24. Before you jump to any conclusions, it is essential that you complete the patient profile. What additional clarifying questions do you want to ask Eugene based upon the limited history that you received in the vignette?

Answers to Round One of Questions for Case 31: The Head-Shaking Dog

1. The entrance to the external ear canal has little to no fur in cats and most dog breeds. Dog breeds that are exceptions to this rule include Bichon Frise, Poodles, Schnauzers, Shih tzus, Lhasa Apso, and certain types of terriers.(1–3)

2. Excessive fur at the entrance to the external ear canal can occlude its opening.(2, 3) This may create favorable conditions for opportunistic pathogens and/or overgrowth of resident flora.(2–6)

3. The external ear canal includes a vertical canal, which forms the natural bridge between the ear flap (the pinna) and the horizontal canal.(1–3, 7, 8)

    The external ear canal is curvilinear.(1–3, 7, 8) It begins as cartilage and ends as osseous tissue.(1, 7, 8) The vertical canal tracks ventro-rostally before making a turn medially into the horizontal canal.(8) This junction between vertical and horizontal ear canals is angled at approximately 75 degrees.(9) When I describe this characteristic bend to clients, I often share that the ear canal is "L-shaped" to create a visual picture. This is in stark contrast to the human ear canal, which has a direct (linear) path to the ear drum.

4. The ear drum forms the anatomic barrier between the external ear and the middle ear.(1, 7, 8) The vertical ear canal feeds into the horizontal ear canal, which abuts the ear drum.(1, 7, 8)

5. The appropriate medical term for the ear drum is the tympanum or the tympanic membrane. (2, 3, 7)

6. The healthy (normal) tympanum should be transparent and intact. It consists of a greyish-blue pars tensa and a more dorsal, pinkish, elastic pars flaccida.(2, 10, 11)

7. In cases of otitis media, the tympanic membrane may take on an opaque, cloudy white appearance.(2)

8. If there is fluid build-up in the middle ear, then the tympanic membrane may bulge forward, into the horizontal canal.(2)

9. A ruptured tympanic membrane will be torn. (2, 5, 10)

10. Ear wax is typically light tan-yellow in the healthy (normal) dog or cat.(7, 9) However, the brown undertones may vary from one individual to another. For some healthy (normal) patients, ear wax may take on an amber color or even a richer brown.

11. Ear wax in a healthy (normal) dog or cat is typically ceruminous as opposed to gritty.(2, 3, 7, 9)

12. Ear wax is produced by sebaceous and ceruminous glands that line the external ear canal. (2, 3, 7)

13. Cerumen is the appropriate medical term for ear wax.(7)

14. Dogs with floppy ears, such as Bassett hounds, may overproduce ear wax. Cocker spaniels are notorious for excessive cerumen. Many develop hyperplastic ceruminous glands.(12)

    Poodles do not necessarily produce excessive cerumen; however, wax may become trapped within the external ear canal because of the excessive fur that plugs up the entrance in these dogs as well as other furry breeds.

15. The Sphynx cat overproduces cerumen.(13) This is considered normal for the breed.(2, 3) As they age, many Siamese and Persians cats also develop excessively waxy ears.(14)

16. In addition to excessive cerumen, the following clinical signs might prompt you to evaluate one or both ears:(2–4, 14)

    - malodor
    - aural pain
    - head-shaking
    - pawing at ears
    - reluctance to allow others to touch the affected ear(s)
    - scratching at ears.

17. The following colors of aural debris are reasons to investigate a patient's ear(s) further:(2, 3)

    - white or cream
    - yellow
    - yellow-green
    - green
    - dark brown to black.

18. The following consistencies or textures of aural debris are reasons to investigate a patient's ear(s) further:(2, 3)

    - dry and flaky
    - greasy
    - gritty "coffee grounds"
    - goopy or gelatinous.

19. Cats and dogs with ear mite infestations often are said to have dark brown-black, dry, crumbly, and/or gritty "coffee ground" aural debris.(9, 13)

20. Although gross appearance provides clues to examine the affected ear(s) further, it should not be used to make a definitive diagnosis because characteristics involving color are not as consistent or as reliable as they were once thought.(3, 9, 15–20)

21. Otoscopy should be performed to evaluate the entire external ear canal.(2, 3) One is limited by what one can see grossly at the entrance to the external ear canal. One cannot, for instance, examine the horizontal ear canal without an otoscope.(2)

   If you only examine the entrance to the external ear canal, then you may also miss:(2)

   • discharge that is only evident within the horizontal ear canal
   • erythema at the level of the horizontal ear canal
   • polyps or other growths within the external ear canal(8)
   • stenotic ear canals.

22. Aural debris should be evaluated by cytology.(2, 3, 5, 6, 9, 16, 17, 20–22) Samples for cytology should be taken from within the horizontal canal or, at least, the junction between the vertical and horizontal canals.(3, 9, 15, 23) Even if the patient is presenting with unilateral disease, both ears should be swabbed and evaluated microscopically.(9)

23. Aural cytology evaluates the ear canal for:(2, 3, 9)

   • bacterial populations and any associated overgrowth
   • cerumen
   • cornified squamous epithelial cells
   • erythrocytes
   • leukocytes
   • yeast populations and any associated overgrowth.

   Magnification 400×, using the high-dry, 40× objective, is sufficient for evaluation of large bacteria, yeast, erythrocytes, leukocytes, and cornified epithelium.(9) Magnification 1000×, using the oil immersion, 100× objective, is necessary for identification of smaller bacteria.(9)

   The clinician should examine an average of 5 to 10 high-powered fields, and document a rough estimate of the number of bacteria and yeast in each.(9)

24. I would want to ask Eugene the following clarifying questions.

   • When did Tarragon start swimming in the lake?
   • Eugene mentioned that the odor began 10 days ago. Did he notice anything before this?
   • Do both ears seem to be involved?
   • Has Eugene noticed any of the following changes?

      • bleeding ears
      • ears becoming exceptionally warm to the touch
      • ears becoming tender
      • excessive scratching and/or pawing at either ear
      • excoriations along the pinnae due to self-trauma (i.e. scratching)
      • head-shaking
      • red ears
      • swollen pinnae.

   • Describe the discharge in the ear(s) in terms of color and consistency, pre-cleaning.
   • How, if at all, has the discharge appeared after cleaning the ear(s)?
   • Describe the odor in the ear(s).
   • How, if at all, has the odor changed since cleaning both ear(s)?
   • Has Eugene ever had to clean Tarragon's ears before?

- How did Eugene clean Tarragon's ears?

  - Did he use cotton swabs?
  - Did he use cotton tipped applicators (i.e. Q-tips)?

- What product did Eugene use to clean the ears?

  - Is it a commercially marketed product?
  - Is it a homemade concoction?
  - What ingredients does the cleaner contain?

Returning to Case 31: The Head-Shaking Dog

You asked Eugene to describe the aural discharge. He clarifies that both ears appear to be involved and pulls out his smart phone to share two photographs with you: before and after he cleaned the ears. (See **Plates 36 and 37**.)

Eugene describes the odor as nutty, yet somewhat nauseating. There is an acridness to it that makes Eugene want to keep Tarragon an arm's length away.

You ask what Eugene used to clean the ears. He shares that he poured hydrogen peroxide into both canals, enough so that he heard a squishing sound when he massaged each. He then used cotton balls to scoop up any debris. Eugene says that Tarragon tolerated this – then again, his personality is such that he would put up with anything. According to Eugene, Tarragon did not seem particularly fond of having his ears cleaned. He's been pawing at them more since then.

Round Two of Questions for Case 31: The Head-Shaking Dog

1. What is a primary anatomical concern about cleaning the ears before they have been examined?
2. What is a primary diagnostic concern about cleaning the ears before they have been examined?
3. Which products should never be used for ear cleaning and why?

Answers to Round Two of Questions for Case 31: The Head-Shaking Dog

1. If you do not examine the ears before you clean them, then you are not certain if one or both tympanic membranes are intact.(2, 3)

2. If you clean the ears before they have been examined, then you greatly reduce and/or otherwise alter the sample that you will be taking for cytology. If the ears were cleaned just before exam, for instance, then your sample may be negative for bacterial and/or yeast overgrowth, when in fact the patient may have true infectious otitis. You also may adversely impact any sample that you intended to submit for culture.

3. Abrasive, caustic, or otherwise irritating products, such as alcohol and hydrogen peroxide, should never be used for ear cleaning because they will inflame the ear and/or potentially damage the tissue. In addition, if the client is cleaning the ear prior to ear exam, as often occurs in the home environment, then the client is not sure if the ear drum is intact. If the ear drum is not intact, then any caustic solution that is applied to the external ear will enter into and subsequently damage the middle ear.

If the ear itself is not examined or the ear drum cannot be visualized prior to cleaning, sterile saline should be used as a cleaning agent because it is safe to encounter the middle ear in the event that the tympanic membrane has ruptured.(2)

Returning to Case 31: The Head-Shaking Dog

You perform a comprehensive exam on Tarragon, including otoscopy. Both ear canals are erythematous and stenotic, but you can visualize both ear drums and they are intact. Eugene consents to aural diagnostics. You swab both ears and evaluate their contents via light microscopy. (See **Plates 38 and 39**.)

Round Three of Questions for Case 31: The Head-Shaking Dog

1. What are you likely to see on cytology if you were to swab a healthy (normal) canine or feline ear?
2. Healthy (normal) ears have resident bacteria. Which shape of bacteria – rod or cocci – is typical of the resident populations?
3. Which bacterial species typically make up the resident populations in normal (healthy) ears?
4. Does yeast make up the normal flora of the canine or feline ear?
5. What color does a Modified Wright's stain, such as Diff-Quik, stain yeast?
6. How would you describe the classic yeast shape?
7. Do you expect to see leukocytes on aural swabs of healthy (normal) ears?
8. What is the appropriate medical term for an ear infection that involves the external ear canal?
9. Which conditions may favor an ear infection that involves the external ear canal?
10. Which, if any, of the conditions that you identified in Question #9 above is/are likely in this clinical scenario?
11. When you examine Tarragon's cytology (**Plates 38 and 39**), what do you see?
12. How much bacteria is "too much?"
13. How much yeast is "too much?"
14. What is the most appropriate recommendation for how to proceed?
15. In what situations might you elect to culture the ear(s)?

Answers to Round Three of Questions for Case 31: The Head-Shaking Dog

1. If you were to swab a healthy (normal) canine or feline ear and examine the contents of the swab under light microscopy, then you would expect to see:(4, 9, 19, 24, 25)

   - cerumen – does not take up stain
   - cornified squamous epithelial cells – stain blue due to keratin when a Modified Wright's stain, such as Diff-Quik, is used
   - resident bacteria
   - resident yeast.

2. Healthy (normal) ears have resident bacteria. These bacterial populations are typically made up of cocci-shaped organisms.(3, 4, 9, 16, 24) Rod-shaped bacteria are not typically part of the normal flora of the canine or feline ear, with the exception of *Corynebacterium* spp.(3, 9, 16, 24, 26)

3. The resident bacterial populations in normal (healthy) ears include:(3, 4, 9, 16, 24)

   - coagulase-positive and coagulase-negative *Staphylococcus* spp.
   - β-hemolytic *Streptococcus*.

4. Yes, yeast make up the normal flora of the canine or feline ear.(3, 9, 19, 25, 27)

5. Yeast become purple with application of a Modified Wright's stain, such as Diff-Quik.(3, 9, 19, 25, 27)

6. When yeast reproduce, they exhibit unipolar budding.(9) This creates the classic "footprint," "peanut," or "snowman" shape.(9)

7. No, you should not expect to see leukocytes on aural swabs of healthy (normal) ears.(9, 15, 16, 23, 28)

8. Otitis externa is the appropriate medical term for an ear infection that involves the external ear canal.(2, 3)

9. The following conditions may precipitate otitis externa:(2–6)

   - excessive fur at the entrance to the external ear canal, which may occlude the entrance and help to retain humidity/moisture
   - excessive moisture within the external ear canal, as from swimming or bathing
   - floppy ears, this conformation prevents aeration of the external ear canal
   - obstructive ear canal disease, such as polyps
   - plucking hair from the external ear canal, inciting inflammation
   - the use of irritating ear rinses, such as those containing high concentrations of alcohol.

10. Tarragon has floppy ears. In addition, he has a history of swimming. Eugene also cleaned his ears with hydrogen peroxide.

11. When I examine Tarragon's cytology, I see a mixed bacterial population that includes cocci, diplococci, individual rods, and rods that are linked to one another like a necklace (**Plate 38**). I also see a cluster of yeast (**Plate 39**).

12. It has been suggested that greater than 14 bacteria per high-powered field, in cats, and 25, in dogs, indicates an abnormally increased bacterial population.(9)

13. It has been suggested by Ginel et al. that more than 5 and less than 12 yeast per high-powered field in dogs and cats respectively is abnormal.(9, 29) However, these numbers are not set in stone and they have not been validated. Only use as a guideline.(9)

14. Because of the mixed bacterial population – and especially due to the presence of rods – I would be inclined to culture Tarragon's ears.

    When cocci are observed on cytology, they are most likely to be either *Staphylococcus* ssp. or *Streptococcus* spp.(9) Cytology alone cannot differentiate between the two.(9) Cytology also cannot determine whether pre-existing bacteria are susceptible to certain classes of antibiotics. (9) The additive value of bacterial culture is that it provides this additional information. This information, in combination with cytological findings, collectively guides the therapeutic plan for the patient.(9)

    Cultures are particularly essential when cytological findings include rod-shaped bacteria because they are more likely to be multi-drug resistant.(12, 30) Therefore, it is critical to determine the susceptibility profile of the pathogenic organism(s), as through culture.(12, 30)

15. In addition to the presence of rods on aural cytology, reasons to culture include:(16, 17, 20, 31–33)

- chronic otitis
- recurrent otitis
- involvement of the middle ear
- lack of response to current treatment.

CLINICAL PEARLS

- Otitis externa is a common complaint in companion animal practice.

- Clients may complain about aural odor. In addition, they may report redness, tenderness, and scratching at the affected ear(s).

- Predisposing factors include:

  - breed
  - aural conformation, i.e. floppy ears retain moisture and humidity
  - presence/absence of excessive aural hair
  - excessive moisture within the ear canal, as from swimming
  - high humidity environments
  - obstructive growths within the external ear canal, including polyps
  - using an irritating, abrasive, or caustic agent to clean the ear(s).

- Otoscopic exam is essential at the time of the consultation so that you can evaluate the entire external ear canal, not just its entrance.

- It is important to recall the anatomy of the external ear canal. Understanding that it has a curvilinear shape facilitates how you introduce your otoscope into the horizontal canal during otoscopic exam. It is equally important to assess the integrity of the tympanum.

- Samples for cytology should be taken at the junction between the vertical and horizontal canals or within the horizontal canal itself. Recall that resident bacterial and yeast populations are present. The presence of rods is an indication for culture.

References

1. Venker-van Haagen AJ. Ears. In: Rijnberk A, van Sluijs FJ, editors. Medical history and physical examination in companion animals. St. Louis, MO: Saunders Elsevier; 2009. p. 202–6.
2. Englar RE. Performing the small animal physical examination. Hoboken, NJ: Wiley/Blackwell; 2017.
3. Englar RE. Common clinical presentations in dogs and cats. Hoboken, NJ: Wiley/Blackwell; 2019.
4. Rosser EJ, Jr. Causes of otitis externa. Vet Clin North Am Small Anim Pract 2004;34(2):459–68.
5. Gotthelf LN. Diagnosis and treatment of otitis media in dogs and cats. Vet Clin North Am Small Anim Pract 2004;34(2):469–87.
6. Thomas JS. Otitis externa. NAVC Clin's Brief 2004 (July):33–5.
7. Singh B, Dyce KM. Dyce, Sack, and Wensing's textbook of veterinary anatomy. 5th ed. St. Louis, NO: Saunders; 2018.
8. Lanz OI, Wood BC. Surgery of the ear and pinna. Vet Clin North Am Small Anim Pract 2004;34(2):567–99.
9. Angus JC. Otic cytology in health and disease. Vet Clin North Am Small Anim Pract 2004;34(2):411–24.
10. Cole LK. Otoscopic evaluation of the ear canal. Vet Clin North Am Small Anim Pract 2004;34(2):397–410.

11. Allyn W. Direct and indirect veterinary eye and ear examination instructions. Available from: https://www.welchallyn.com/content/dam/welchallyn/documents/sap-documents/LIT/80020/80020547LITPDF.pdf.

12. Paterson S. Pseudomonas otitis. NAVC Clin's Brief 2010 (June):35–9.

13. Englar RE. Performing the small animal physical examination. Hoboken, NJ: Wiley; 2017.

14. Kennis RA. Feline otitis: diagnosis and treatment. Vet Clin North Am Small Anim Pract 2013;43(1):51–6.

15. Harvey RG, Harari J, Delauche AJ. Diagnostic procedures. Ear diseases of the dog and cat. Ames, IA: Iowa State University Press; 2001. p. 43–80.

16. Scott DW, Miller WH, Griffin CE. Diseases of eyelids, claws, anal sacs, and ears. Muller and Kirk's Small animal dermatology. Philadelphia, PA: W.B. Saunders; 2000. p. 1185–235.

17. Jacobson LS. Diagnosis and medical treatment of otitis externa in the dog and cat. J S Afr Vet Assoc 2002;73(4):162–70.

18. Little C. A clinician's approach to the investigation of otitis externa. Pract 1996;18(1):9–16.

19. Morris DO. Malassezia dermatitis and otitis. Vet Clin North Am Small Anim Pract 1999;29(6):1303–10.

20. Rosychuk RA. Management of otitis externa. Vet Clin North Am Small Anim Pract 1994;24(5):921–52.

21. Little C. Medical treatment of otitis externa in the dog and cat. Pract 1996;18(2):66–71.

22. Rosser EJ, Jr. Evaluation of the patient with otitis externa. Vet Clin North Am Small Anim Pract 1988;18(4):765–72.

23. Chickering WR. Cytologic evaluation of otic exudates. Vet Clin North Am Small Anim Pract 1988;18(4):773–82.

24. Harvey RG, Harari J, Delauche AJ. The normal ear. Ear diseases of the dog and cat. Ames, IA: Iowa State University Press; 2001. p. 9–42.

25. Guillot J, Bond R. Malassezia pachydermatis: a review. Med Mycol 1999;37(5):295–306.

26. Kowalski JJ. The microbial environment of the ear canal in health and disease. Vet Clin North Am Small Anim Pract 1988;18(4):743–54.

27. Scott DW, Miller WH, Griffin CE. Fungal skin diseases. Muller and Kirk's Small animal dermatology. Philadelphia, PA: W.B BSaunders; 2000. p. 336–422.

28. Cole LK, Schwassmann M. Antibiotic use in chronic otitis externa. In: Thoday KL, Foil CS, Bond R, editors. Advances in veterinary dermatology. Oxford: Blackwell Science; 2002. p. 212–23.

29. Ginel PJ, Lucena R, Rodriguez JC, Ortega J. A semiquantitative cytological evaluation of normal and pathological samples from the external ear canal of dogs and cats. Vet Dermatol 2002;13(3):151–6.

30. Hariharan H, Coles M, Poole D, Lund L, Page R. Update on antimicrobial susceptibilities of bacterial isolates from canine and feline otitis externa. Can Vet J 2006;47(3):253–5.

31. Chester DK. Medical management of otitis externa. Vet Clin North Am Small Anim Pract 1988;18(4):799–812.

32. Greene CE. Otitis externa. In: Greene CE, editor. Infectious diseases of the dog and cat. Philadelphia, PA: W.B. Saunders; 1998. p. 549–54.

33. Griffin CE. Pseudomonas otitis therapy. In: Bonagura JD, editor. Kirk's current veterinary therapy. Philadelphia, PA: W.B. Saunders; 2000. p. 586–8.

Case 32

The Cat with the Puffy Ear

Professor Starfish is new to your practice. He joined Dottie Brinks' household at 12 weeks of age, when he was rescued from a hoarding situation. For the past six years, he has been Dottie's sole housemate. However, his world was turned upside down two weeks ago when Dottie spontaneously decided to adopt a kitten. The kitten, Mocha Latte, was one of three semi-feral "additions" to an unsuspecting neighbor's barn. Although the neighbor did not have any desire to raise kittens, Mocha Latte's mom decided that it was the perfect spot to deliver her first litter.

Shortly after birth, the queen was spooked by ongoing construction in the barn. She bolted, leaving the kittens behind. Dottie's neighbor had taken the kittens to the shelter, where they had been fostered to the appropriate age. Now, all three were in search of their forever homes.

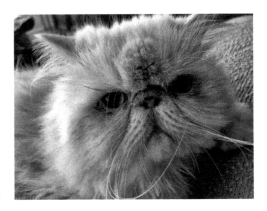

Figure 32.1 Meet your new patient, Professor Starfish. A 6-year-old castrated male Himalayan cat. Courtesy of Martha Alice MahoneyHuss.

Within a week of being advertised online, two of the three were spoken for, but no one had laid claim to Mocha Latte. When Dottie saw a photograph of the kitten, her eyes lit up. Mocha Latte was the spitting image of her childhood cat. Although Dottie doubted that the Professor would be pleased, she told herself that the company might be good for him. If anything, she hoped it would make him more sociable.

The past 2 weeks have been a bit of an uphill battle. Although Professor Starfish had accepted that Mocha Latte was a household fixture, he didn't like it one bit. At around the same time as the kitten arrived, he also started to itch at his ears. At first it was just one ear, but then the itch "spread." Dottie didn't notice initially, because the itch was sporadic. But now it's unmistakable. He's even beginning to lose some fur along the aural margins from where he's scratching with his hind paws.

Dottie had looked at both ears when she'd first noticed the itch. At that time, they hadn't seemed particularly dirty. Not 48 hours later, they were looking a bit gritty. What concerned her most, how-

Weight: 8.8 lb (4.0 kg)
BCS: 4/9
Mentation: BAR

TPR

T: 102.2°F (39°C)
P: 191 beats per minute
R: 22 breaths per minute

ever, was that the Professor's left ear seemed to puff up acutely. When Dottie awoke this morning and went to stroke his head, she discovered the ear straight away. The Professor resented any further attempt at an in-depth investigation, so she didn't get to take a closer peek, but it seemed to her that the ear was swollen and warm to the touch.

Dottie has arrived at your clinic for you to evaluate this sudden change in the Professor's health. She assumes that he and Mocha Latte got into a scuffle overnight. Could Mocha Latte have bitten him? Would that have caused such a big lesion? It seems like a bit much for a little kitten bite. Then again, the Professor had always been delicate, and it didn't take much to ruffle his fur.

As Dottie awaits your consultation, the technician documents the Professor's vital signs in his chart.

When the technician briefs you on the case, his eyes light up because he thinks he knows exactly what the problem is. He pulls out his smartphone and shows you a photograph that he retrieved from a google search (see Figure 32.2).

Use the following questions to help you prepare for your consultation.

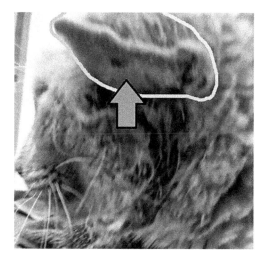

Figure 32.2 Swelling of the left pinna in a feline patient. Courtesy of Patricia Bennett, DVM.

Round One of Questions for Case 32: The Cat with the Puffy Ear

1. Assuming that the photograph is an accurate representation of Professor Starfish's presenting complaint, what is his diagnosis?
2. If you were to tap the swelling that is associated with the Professor's left ear, what color do you expect the fluid that the swelling contains to be? Which cell would predominate if you then looked at a sample of the fluid under the microscope?
3. What causes this swelling to occur?
4. If this swelling is not tended to, what is likely to happen and how might this impact the patient's appearance?
5. Dottie is particularly fond of Professor Starfish's face and does not want him to appear any differently. To prevent the change in appearance that you noted in Question #4 (above), what needs to happen?
6. After medical intervention that you outlined in Question #5, is recurrence likely?
7. In the event that the patient's aural hematoma continues to refill, what might you do to facilitate drainage?
8. What else could you do, surgically, to resolve an aural hematoma? (Hint: this is done more routinely in dogs with floppy ears)
9. In addition to treating the swelling itself, what else do you need to consider about case management moving forward?

Answers to Round One of Questions for Case 32: The Cat with the Puffy Ear

1. Assuming that the photograph is an accurate representation of Professor Starfish's presenting complaint, he has an aural hematoma. An aural hematoma is a condition in which blood accumulates between the skin and the two flaps of auricular cartilage, forming a visible and palpable pocket of fluid.(1–3)

2. If you were to tap the swelling that is associated with the Professor's left ear, the resultant fluid would be serosanguinous. Its color would be red. The predominant cell would be an erythrocyte.

453

3. An aural hematoma develops when blood vessels that supply the ear burst.(2, 3) This occurs when the patient vigorously shakes its head and/or traumatizes the ear, as through incessant scratching.(2, 3)

   Vessels are easily damaged in floppy-eared dogs. (2, 3) The force of the pinnae flapping against the head, over and over again, damages the auricular cartilage.(2, 3) Internal hemorrhage causes blood to pool between the skin and auricular cartilage.(1–3) This creates the aural hematoma.(2, 3)

   It is harder to appreciate how vessels become damaged in a cat's ear because whether the ears are erect or folded, as in the Scottish Fold, they are not flappable. However, cats can do a significant amount of damage with their claws and hind paws. Punctures to the ear, as from fight wounds, can also precipitate an aural hematoma.

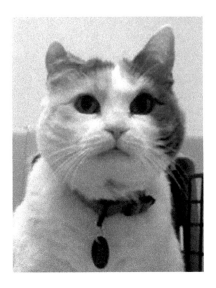

Figure 32.3 Classic "crinkle" shape or "cauliflower ear" in a cat that did not receive treatment for its aural hematoma. The hematoma resolved on its own. Courtesy of Patricia Bennett, DVM.

4. If this swelling is not tended to, the fluid will eventually reabsorb, over time. However, in the process, granulation tissue forms, causing the affected pinna to undergo fibrosis.(1–3) Fibrosis causes the ear to shrivel up.(1–3) The ear takes on a crinkled, deformed appearance.(2–4) In general practice, the patient is sometimes said to have a "cauliflower ear."(2–4) (See Figure 32.3.)

5. To prevent a change in Professor Starfish's appearance, you need to drain the aural hematoma before fibrosis has started to occur.(1, 5)

6. When presentations are acute, drainage alone can be effective.(1) However, it is not uncommon for aural hematomas to recur.(1) The fluid is more likely to refill within the pocket between the aural cartilage if the patients continue head-shaking and/or scratching at their ears.(1)

7. You can place a temporary drain or teat cannula to facilitate drainage so that fluid is not allowed to continuously build up in cartilaginous flaps of the affected pinna.(1, 6–10)

8. You could place the patient under general anesthesia and cut through the auricular cartilage into the aural hematoma to achieve incisional drainage.(3) You then could place mattress sutures parallel to aural vasculature.(1, 3, 5) These sutures are placed close together so as to bring the skin and both flaps of cartilage together, without any gaps between them for fluid to accumulate. (3) As long as the pinna is immobilized to guard against further trauma, the ear is forced to heal. (1, 3) This technique works well in floppy-eared dogs. Immobilization is typically achieved by bandaging the ear over the top of the head.(1, 3) Scarring of the pinna may occur. I have not performed this technique on cats.

9. In addition to treating the aural hematoma, you need to address the primary problem that caused it to form.(2, 3) Otherwise, the aural hematoma is likely to recur.

Returning to Case 32: The Cat with the Puffy Ear

After greeting the client, taking history, and examining the patient, you share with Dottie that Professor Starfish has an aural hematoma. You explain the diagnosis and how to medically manage it. However, you emphasize the importance of looking deeper. If the primary problem is not addressed, then the aural hematoma is likely to recur. Your otoscopic exam revealed an abundance of dark brown-black debris that looks like coffee grounds. You tell Dottie that you need to investigate this further to get to the bottom of the Professor's troubles.

Round Two of Questions for Case 32: The Cat with the Puffy Ear

1. What is your presumptive diagnosis?

Answers to Round Two of Questions for Case 32: The Cat with the Puffy Ear

1. I suspect that Professor Starfish has ear mites based upon the description of the aural debris (dark black-brown coffee ground debris) and the fact that this has all developed since bringing the new kitten in the household.(2, 3)

Returning to Case 32: The Cat with the Puffy Ear

Based upon the appearance of color and consistency of the aural debris, you suspect that ear mites may have triggered the itchiness that caused incessant scratching, which led to the aural hematoma.
    Use the following questions to guide how you plan on addressing your suspicions in your diagnostic work-up of the Professor.

Round Three of Questions for Case 32: The Cat with the Puffy Ear

1. What is the Latin name for the ear mite that is seen in cats?
2. Ear mites are often associated with cats. Can the same species also infest dogs? What about ferrets?
3. What causes the "coffee ground" aural debris in ear mite infestations?
4. Would an ear mite infestation be consistent with the Professor's history of pruritus?
5. What is the best way to diagnose ear mites?
6. If you were interested in evaluating the Professor for bacterial and/or yeast otitis, would that change your approach to the diagnostic test that you identified in Question #5 above?
7. If the Professor has ear mites, where did they likely come from?

Answers to Round Three of Questions for Case 32: The Cat with the Puffy Ear

1. The Latin name for the ear mite that is seen in cats is *Otodectes cynotis*.(2–4, 11–15)

2. Although *Otodectes cynotis* prefers cats, the mite is not species-specific.(2, 3, 11, 12, 16–21) Therefore, it will also infest dogs(2, 3) and ferrets.(22)

3. The aural debris that resembles coffee grounds in pets with ear mite infestation is a mixture of cerumen, dried blood, and mite feces.(23)

4. Ear mite infestations are exceptionally pruritic, particularly for those patients that develop a hypersensitivity reaction to mite antigen.(4, 12, 23)

5. Ear mites can be diagnosed by otic cytology.(2, 3) Ear debris can be sampled using a cotton tip applicator. The tip of the applicator is then rolled through a droplet of mineral oil that has been placed on a clean slide.(2–4, 12) This action dislodges the sample onto the slide and mineral oil provides an appropriate medium for you to visualize the mites by way of light microscopy.

   Low magnification using a 4× objective will reveal adult, eight-legged mites; six-legged larva; and eggs.(12) Finding one or more of these stages is diagnostic for ear mite infestation.(12)

6. If you wanted to also evaluate the Professor for bacterial and/or yeast otitis, then you would need to make use of a different slide prep.

   As before, a sample of each ear would be obtained using a cotton tip applicator.(3) The slide may be heat-fixed to adhere the sample to the slide.(12) There is ongoing debate as to whether heat-fixing is preferred.(3) It is thought to be of benefit in helping to remove the cerumen from the slide because it is largely lipid. Heating it will loosen it up and allow it to wash away during the staining process.(3)

   Each slide is then stained using a Modified Wright's stain, such as Diff-Quik.(12, 24) Gram staining is rarely performed as an add-on procedure because most aural cocci will be Gram positive (+) and most aural rods will be Gram negative.(12)

   After staining, each slide is air dried, then examined by light microscopy. Low magnification is used initially to find an area of interest.(12) Once this is in view, magnification is increased. Magnification 400×, using the high-dry, 40× objective, is sufficient for evaluation of large bacteria, yeast, erythrocytes, leukocytes, and cornified epithelium.(12) Magnification 1000×, using the oil immersion, 100× objective, is necessary for identification of smaller bacteria.(12)

Returning to Case 32: The Cat with the Puffy Ear

You swab the Professor's ears using both preps. A photomicrograph of the slide that you prepared with mineral oil is provided in Figure 32.4 for your review.

   Use the photomicrograph to answer the following questions.

Round Four of Questions for Case 32: The Cat with the Puffy Ear

1. What is the Professor's diagnosis?
2. How will you treat this condition?
3. What else must you consider when you formulate a treatment plan?

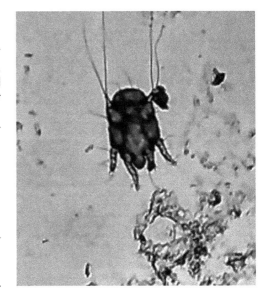

Figure 32.4 Otic prep using cytology prepared with mineral oil.

Answers to Round Four of Questions for Case 32:
The Cat with the Puffy Ear

1. The Professor does have at least one ear mite. Because ear mites should not be seen in healthy (normal) ears, just seeing one alone is indicative of an ear mite infestation.

    The presence of an ear mite does not rule out bacterial or fungal otitis. These conditions may be concurrent with ear mite infestation, so it is still important that you examine the other slide, the one that was stained with Diff-Quik.(11)

2. There are lots of options for managing Professor Starfish's ear mites, including the following: (22, 25)

    * otic preparations that contain ivermectin:

        * Acarexx®, which is a 0.01% ivermectin otic suspension
        * MilbeMyte, which contains milbemycin
        * Tresaderm, which contains thiabendazole

    * topical preparations:

        * Revolution, which contains selamectin
        * Frontline, which contains fipronil
        * Advantage Multi, which contains moxidectin

    * oral preparations:

        * off-label use of Bravecto, which contains fluralaner

    * systemic prescriptions:

        * injectable or oral ivermectin.

    Please note that the Professor's ears will need to be thoroughly cleaned in order to remove debris and all lifestages of the mites, including mite eggs.

    Ears may be cleaned with mineral oil for the added purpose of smothering mites at the same time as cleansing them from the ear.

3. Ear mites have a three-week life cycle – it takes three weeks for them to mature into an adult from an egg – and as adults, they can live for an average of two months.(22, 26) They also can live quite well in the environment, which means that you rarely only need to treat once. You need to prolong treatment to reach all life stages, and you need to pair treatment with environmental clean-up to rid the environment of the mites. This also means that every dog and cat (and ferret!) in the household should be treated, even if they are not demonstrating clinical signs.(22) Ear mites are highly infectious dog-to-dog, cat-to-cat, cat-to-dog, and dog-to-cat so if only one pet in the household is treated, ear mite infestation is simply going to "jump" into the untreated pets, creating a vicious cycle that is difficult for owners to stay on top of. In Dottie's case, this means that she is also going to need to treat Mocha Latte. Unfortunately, you have not yourself met Mocha Latte, so you are unable to prescribe anything to manage the ear mites in the kitten. You need to first establish a veterinarian-client-patient relationship before you are legally able to write or fill a prescription. Therefore, Professor Starfish is the only one who will receive treatment today. Dottie will need to schedule an appointment for the kitten to be examined and evaluated.

CLINICAL PEARLS

- Otitis externa is a common complaint in companion animal practice.

- Infectious (bacterial/viral/fungal) and parasitic (*Otodectes cynotis*) causes of otitis externa are routinely diagnosed.

- Both can case focal pruritus at the affected ear(s) that triggers headshaking and/or scratching.

- Headshaking in floppy-eared dogs and pawing or scratching at the ear in cats can cause damage to the auricular cartilage. Repetitive damage causes auricular vessels to burst.

- When auricular vessels burst, blood pools between both auricular cartilages, causing a fluid-filled pocket to form.

- This pocket is both visible and palpable. It is called an aural hematoma.

- If left untreated, the fluid will eventually reabsorb, but the affected ear(s) will undergo fibrosis. This leads to a "crinkling" effect or the so-called "cauliflower ear." This appears as a cosmetic defect. While it does not hurt the cat, it may be aesthetically displeasing to some owners.

- Acute presentations of aural hematoma are easily treated with draining the ear through a needle and syringe.

- Placement of a teat canula may facilitate drainage in cases in which the aural hematoma recurs.

- Surgical management is more commonly performed in dogs and involves the placement of very close sutures parallel to the vasculature in the affected pinna to stitch the cartilages together. Without spaces in between the sutures, there is little to no room for fluid to accumulate.

- It is not enough to treat the aural hematoma. It is critical that you investigate further to discover the primary cause.

- If the primary cause is not addressed, then the issue is likely to return.

References

1. Lanz OI, Wood BC. Surgery of the ear and pinna. Vet Clin North Am Small Anim Pract 2004;34(2):567–99.
2. Englar RE. Performing the small animal physical examination. Hoboken, NJ: Wiley/Blackwell; 2017.
3. Englar RE. Common clinical presentations in dogs and cats. Hoboken, NJ: Wiley/Blackwell; 2019.
4. Englar RE. Performing the small animal physical examination. Hoboken, NJ: Wiley; 2017.
5. MacPhail C. Current treatment options for auricular hematomas. Vet Clin North Am Small Anim Pract 2016;46(4):635–41.
6. Swaim SF, Bradley DM. Evaluation of closed-suction drainage for treating auricular hematomas. J Am Anim Hosp Assoc 1996;32(1):36–43.
7. Romatowski J. Nonsurgical treatment of aural hematomas. J Am Vet Med Assoc 1994;204(9):1318.
8. Wilson JW. Treatment of auricular hematoma, using a teat tube. J Am Vet Med Assoc 1983;182(10):1081–3.
9. Kagan KG. Treatment of canine aural hematoma with an indwelling drain. J Am Vet Med Assoc 1983;183(9):972–4.
10. Pavletic MM. Use of laterally placed vacuum drains for management of aural hematomas in five dogs. J Am Vet Med Assoc 2015;246(1):112–7.

11. Rosser EJ, Jr. Causes of otitis externa. Vet Clin North Am Small Anim Pract 2004;34(2):459–68.
12. Angus JC. Otic cytology in health and disease. Vet Clin North Am Small Anim Pract 2004;34(2):411–24.
13. August JR. Otitis externa. A disease of multifactorial etiology. Vet Clin North Am Small Anim Pract 1988;18(4):731–42.
14. Scott DW, Miller WH, Griffin CE. Diseases of eyelids, claws, anal sacs, and ears. Muller and Kirk's Small Animal dermatology. Philadelphia, PA: W.B. Saunders; 2000.
15. Chickering WR. Cytologic evaluation of otic exudates. Vet Clin North Am Small Anim Pract 1988;18(4):773–82.
16. Kennis RA. Feline otitis: diagnosis and treatment. Vet Clin North Am Small Anim Pract 2013;43(1):51–6.
17. Becskei C, Reinemeyer C, King VL, Lin D, Myers MR, Vatta AF. Efficacy of a new spot-on formulation of selamectin plus sarolaner in the treatment of Otodectes cynotis in cats. Vet Parasitol 2017;238;Suppl 1:S27–S30.
18. Perego R, Proverbio D, Bagnagatti De Giorgi GB, Della Pepa A, Spada E. Prevalence of otitis externa in stray cats in northern Italy. J Feline Med Surg 2014;16(6):483–90.
19. Nardoni S, Ebani VV, Fratini F, Mannella R, Pinferi G, Mancianti F, et al. Malassezia, Mites and Bacteria in the External Ear Canal of Dogs and Cats with otitis Externa. Slov Vet Res 2014;51(3):113–8.
20. Taenzler J, de Vos C, Roepke RK, Frénais R, Heckeroth AR. Efficacy of fluralaner against Otodectes cynotis infestations in dogs and cats. Parasit Vectors 2017;10(1):30.
21. Roy J, Bédard C, Moreau M. Treatment of feline otitis externa due to Otodectes cynotis and complicated by secondary bacterial and fungal infections with Oridermyl auricular ointment. Can Vet J 2011;52(3):277–82.
22. Côté E. Clinical veterinary advisor. Dogs and cats. 3rd ed. St. Louis, MO: Elsevier Mosby; 2015.
23. Arther RG. Mites and lice: biology and control. Vet Clin North Am Small Anim Pract 2009;39(6):1159–71.
24. Cole LK, Schwassmann M. Antibiotic use in chronic otitis externa. In: Thoday KL, Foil CS, Bond R, editors. Advances in veterinary dermatology. Oxford: Blackwell Science; 2002. p. 212–23.
25. Plumb DC. Plumb's veterinary drug handbook. 9th ed. Hoboken, NJ: Pharma Vet Inc.; 2018.
26. Bowman DD. Georgis parasitology for veterinarians. 11th ed. Philadelphia, PA: Elsevier; 2020.

Case 33

The Crusty Cat

Midge is new to your practice. She is owned by Joby and Carl Salina, who are long-term customers of yours, but Midge has never been examined because she's been the healthiest member of the three-cat household since her adoption 2 years ago. Joby and Carl have had to concentrate their efforts on their other two high-maintenance fur kids. Moss, their 9-year-old, is a diabetic that took at least 6 months to regulate. It was not an easy journey to get to this point, and the process of finding an insulin type (and dose!) that he responded to had enough ups and downs to last a lifetime. Meanwhile, Juniper, their 12-year-old, was facing an ongoing battle with alimentary lymphoma. Joby and Carl had their hands full. Midge, on the other hand, had never needed medical care. She'd always been their easy keeper. She balanced out the others' nearly constant medical needs and gave Joby and Carl a moment to catch their breath in between their daily triage.

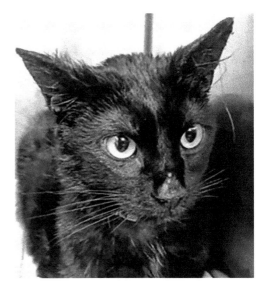

Figure 33.1 Meet Midge, a 6-year-old spayed female domestic shorthaired (DSH) cat. Courtesy of Lauren Bessert.

All three cats are indoor-only and get along well. They have never gotten into any kind of scuffle, not even when Midge joined the household. So, when Joby noticed some scabs along the backside of Midge's right ear 3 weeks ago, the very last thing on her mind was the possibility of a cat fight. At first, she thought that perhaps the scabs resulted from overzealous grooming. Midge had a tendency to be an overachiever in that department. She was fastidious, to the point that she often groomed the others if she deemed their coats unfit to be on display.

Joby ignored the scabs at first, assuming that Midge had overdone it with her hind claws. It was not uncommon for Midge to dig at her ears as if they itched, yet neither had ever contained any debris, redness, or odor. It was a habit, perhaps, like kids and thumb-sucking.

It was easy enough to overlook the scabs, until a week later, when they had multiplied. Before long, they had taken over both ears, including the edges of each pinna (see **Plates 40 and 41**).

The affected sites steadily lost fur until they were bald. Only erythematous skin remained. When the scabs flaked off, the underlying tissue appeared scalded and raw. Lesions spread down the bridge of the nose and also ventrally, encircling some, but not all of Midge's nipples.

All four paws developed crusts and thick caseous debris at and around each nailbed. For a cat who always appeared at her personal best, Midge looked increasingly unkempt. Her feet seemed dirty. They also were quite tender. Although Midge had never been fond of others touching her feet, she had never resented it as much as now. Just the other day, when Joby went to trim her claws, Midge let out a hiss the moment her paw was grasped. This reaction took Joby by surprise. Midge had never been this close to striking anyone. That she had reached this point made Joby question if something was really wrong. Joby contacted the clinic to schedule the next available appointment, confident that if anyone can get to the bottom of this, you can.

Joby has arrived at the clinic just now with Midge. The technician takes Midge's vital signs as Joby wonders aloud whether Midge could have developed ringworm. Some of the photographs that she has stumbled across during her recent online searches look just like Midge. Joby warns the technician that what Midge has may be contagious and that he might want to consider wearing gloves. He hesitates for a moment before donning a pair to gather the necessary information for Midge's chart.

While the technician jots down Midge's chief complaint, "crusty ears", Joby mentions that Midge has sore feet and at times seems lame. "Her feet also look puffy to me," Joby says, and the technician agrees that Midge's nailbeds seem inflamed.

Use the following questions to guide your preparation for this consultation.

Weight: 9.4 lb (4.3 kg)
BCS: 4/9
Mentation: QAR

TPR

T: 103.2°F (39.6°C)
P: 202 beats per minute
R: 25 breaths per minute

Round One of Questions for Case 33: The Crusty Cat

1. The skin forms an essential barrier between the patient and the outside world. How is the skin put together to perform this protective function?
2. Several types of lesions threaten the integrity of the skin. Differentiate primary from secondary skin lesions.
3. Provide examples of primary lesions and define them using appropriate dermatological terms.
4. Provide examples of secondary lesions and define them using appropriate dermatological terms.
5. Jody and the technician both reported the lesions as being "scabs." Why do scabs form?
6. How are scabs and crusts related?
7. Other than what has been described in Question #6, what are common causes of crusts in cats?
8. In the clinical vignette, you were given a description as to where the scabs are located on Midge. Why is lesion location important? Give an example to support your answer.
9. In addition to location, what other information about skin lesions may prove helpful as you craft your list of differential diagnoses?
10. When your technician briefs you on the case, he shares that Midge is losing fur. Differentiate the following dermatological terms that relate to fur loss: hypotrichosis and alopecia.
11. What are major categories of differential diagnoses for thinning and/or loss of fur? Develop a comprehensive list.
12. Of the differential diagnoses that you outlined in Question #11, which broad category is most likely in this patient given the patient's signalment and health history?
13. Joby expressed concern to the technician that Midge could have ringworm. What is the appropriate medical term for ringworm and what is/are the causative agent(s)?
14. Is ringworm contagious cat-to-cat?
15. Is ringworm zoonotic?
16. If you are concerned about ringworm, what could you do to investigate further?
17. Your technician shares that Midge's nailbeds appear to be inflamed. What is the correct medical terminology for this clinical presentation?
18. You ask the technician for clarification: is Midge's nailbed swelling asymmetrical or symmetrical? What do these terms mean?
19. What causes asymmetrical claw bed disease?
20. What causes symmetrical claw bed disease?
21. Based upon the description of Midge that your technician has relayed, is she likely to have asymmetrical or symmetrical claw bed disease?

22. Are there any additional clarifying conditions that you would like to ask Joby when you enter the consultation room to expand upon the history that your technician gathered?

23. After history-taking, what is the next appropriate step in the diagnostic work-up?

Answers to Round One of Questions for Case 33: The Crusty Cat

1. For the skin to serve as an essential barrier between the patient and the outside world, it needs to maintain a relatively tight seal.(1) This seal is provided by the epidermal layer of keratinocytes, which are tightly connected to one another.(2) Adhesion between keratinocytes is made possible by desmosomes and hemidesmosomes.(2, 3) The former connect the cells to one another and the latter connect the cells to the basement membrane.(2, 3)

2. The skin forms an essential barrier between the patient and the outside world. Several types of lesions threaten the integrity of this barrier. Primary skin lesions are those that develop at the onset of clinical disease.(1, 2, 4, 5) Secondary skin lesions develop as the disease progresses. (1, 2, 4, 5) They may reflect the evolution of primary lesions or the response of the patient to the clinical presentation.(1, 2, 4, 5) For example, excoriations are secondary lesions that result from self-trauma.

3. Examples of primary skin lesions include:(1, 2, 4, 5)

    • macule: a flat area of color change as compared to surrounding skin
    • papule: a small solid elevation of the skin
    • nodule: a large papule, typically measuring greater than 0.25 cm in diameter, but less than 1.0 cm
    • tumor: a large nodule, typically measuring greater than 1.0 cm in diameter
    • pustule: a pus-filled papule ("a pimple")
    • vesicle: a fluid-filled elevation that does not contain pus
    • bullae: a large vesicle, typically measuring greater than 0.5 cm in diameter
    • wheal: a focal allergic reaction that is characterized by an irregularly shaped solid elevated patch of cutaneous edema
    • plaque: an elevation with a flat, rather than rounded top.

4. Examples of secondary skin lesions include:(1, 2, 4, 5)

    • scale: loose flakes of skin ("dandruff")
    • collarette: what remains behind after a pustule ruptures
    • crust: a hard layer of dried exudate and keratin that forms over the skin's surface
    • scab: dried fibrin and platelet plug that caps the surface of a wound, under which a new layer of skin begins to form
    • comedone: a plug of oil and dead skin cells at the surface of a pore ("a blackhead")
    • lichenification: abnormally thick, leathery skin that typically signifies chronic skin irritation, inflammation, and/or infection
    • hyperpigmentation: dark gray to black discoloration of the skin that typically signifies chronic skin irritation, inflammation, and/or infection.

5. Scabs form to protect wounds from infection and to allow the tissue beneath to undergo repair.

6. Wounds often ooze in the early stages of healing. When this ooze dries, it forms crusts. It is likely that Midge has a combination of scabs and crusts. Crusts are evident in **Plates 40 and 41**.

7. Other than what has been described in Question #6 (above), common causes of crusts in cats include:(2, 4)

- autoimmune skin disease
- fly bite dermatitis(6)
- fungal dermatopathy
- mange
- mosquito bite hypersensitivity(6)
- pyoderma(7, 8)
- squamous cell carcinoma.(6)

8. Lesion location is important because many differential diagnoses are known for targeting certain regions of the body, but not others.(1) Understanding where lesions have developed and how they have progressed from a geographical standpoint on the patient's body provide important clues that narrow down the list of the most likely causes of clinical disease.(1) Consider, for example, papules, pustules, and comedones at the chin of a feline patient. This combination of lesions and location is most consistent with a disorder of follicular keratinization in cats that is called chin acne.(9, 10)

9. In addition to location, it is helpful to note the following information about the lesions, as identified through a combination of history-taking and the physical exam.

- How many lesions?
- What is/are the size(s) of the lesions?
- How are the lesions configured?
- Have the lesions progressed and, if so, how?

10. Hypotrichosis refers to thinning of the fur, whereas alopecia indicates that the affected skin is entirely bare.(11–14)

11. The major categories of differential diagnoses for thinning and/or loss of fur include:(1, 15)

- species-specific alopecia:

    - feline peri-aural (pre-auricular) alopecia

- tardive hypotrichosis or alopecia: patients are born with normal coats; however, the coats thin as they age:

    - pattern baldness:

        - pinnal alopecia: dogs (especially dachshunds) > cats
        - bald thigh syndrome: dogs (especially greyhounds)

    - black hair follicular dysplasia: abnormalities in hair shafts and follicles lead to loss of black fur only
    - color dilution alopecia: typically targets those with blue, red, and fawn coats

- non-color-linked, cyclical follicular dysplasias:

    - seasonal flank alopecia

- non-color-linked, non-cyclical follicular dysplasias:

    - alopecia X: typically targets Nordic breeds and others with plush coats

- non-endocrine, non-inflammatory hair loss:

    - congenital hypotrichosis and alopecia:

        - canine:(16)
        - Mexican hairless or xoloitzcuintli
        - Chinese crested
        - Inca hairless
        - Peruvian Inca orchid

- feline:
- Sphynx
- Donskoy
- the elf cat: a hybrid of the American Curl cat and the Sphynx
- the Ukranian Levkoy: a hybrid of the Scottish Fold cat and the Sphynx
- the Bambino: a hybrid of the Munchkin and the Sphynx

- endocrine, non-inflammatory hair loss:
    - hyperadrenocorticism
    - hyperestrogenism
    - hypothyroidism
    - exposure to human topical hormone replacement therapy

- non-endocrine, inflammatory hair loss:
    - bacterial pyoderma
    - dermatophytosis
    - immune-mediated
    - mange

- hepatocutaneous syndrome
- chemotherapy
- radiation therapy
- alopecia associated with topical medications
- non-medical causes of hair loss:
    - pressure alopecia

- nutritional causes of alopecia:
    - zinc deficiency
    - deficiency in linoleic acid

- environmental cause of alopecia
- compulsive and/or displacement disorders:
    - acral lick dermatitis
    - flank sucking
    - fur mowing.

12. Of the differential diagnoses that were outlined above in the answer to Question #11, the following category is MOST likely in this patient:

    - non-endocrine, inflammatory hair loss:
        - bacterial pyoderma
        - dermatophytosis
        - immune-mediated
        - mange.

13. Joby expressed concern to the technician that Midge could have ringworm. Dermatophytosis is the appropriate medical term for ringworm.(1, 2, 4, 17–19) *Microsporum canis* is the primary source of ringworm in cats.(20–23)

14. Yes, dermatophytosis is highly contagious and can be spread cat-to-cat.(24)

15. Yes, dermatophytosis is a zoonotic disease.(1, 15, 24, 25)

16. If you are concerned about ringworm, you could perform one or more of the following tests to investigate further:(1, 4)

    - Wood's lamp examination.(15, 24)
    - trichogram(23, 24, 26) with potassium hydroxide (KOH) prep(27–30) or other stains, such as lactophenol cotton blue or India Ink(27, 30–32)
    - fungal culture using special media, such as DTM.(24, 26, 27)

    Refer to Case #10 (The Alopecic Kitten) for additional details.

17. Your technician shares that Midge's nailbeds appear to be inflamed. The appropriate medical terminology for this clinical presentation is paronychia.(1, 4)

18. Asymmetrical claw bed disease implies that only one foot is affected.(4, 33) Symmetrical claw bed disease implies that multiple feet are involved.(4)

19. Asymmetrical claw bed disease is typically caused by trauma or idiopathic claw deformity.(20, 34) When trauma to the nail or nailbed occurs, it predisposes the patient to secondary bacterial infections with organisms such as *Staphylococcus intermedius*.(20, 35)
    Neoplastic disease is also possible, although it is far less common in both dogs and cats.(4) Aged large-breed dogs are more likely to develop subungual squamous cell carcinoma (SCC) or malignant melanoma.(4) When claw bed neoplasia occurs in the cat, it is typically due to metastatic disease, such as lung-digit syndrome in the cat, which is caused by primary bronchial adenocarcinoma or bronchoalveolar carcinoma.(35–41)

20. When a patient has symmetrical claw bed disease, then systemic disease is likely.(42) Many conditions have been associated with symmetrical claw bed disease including:(1, 4, 42–47)

    - endocrine:
        - hyperadrenocorticism in dogs and cats(48)
        - hypothyroidism in dogs
    - immune-mediated:
        - pemphigus foliaceus(35)
        - symmetrical lupoid onychodystrophy (SLO) in dogs(19, 20, 49)
    - infectious:
        - fungal:
            - overgrowth of the commensal skin organism, *Malassezia pachydermatis*, may cause nailbed infection(20–22)
            - claw lesions may also develop due to dermatophytosis, as from invasion of keratin by *Microsporum canis*(20)
            - deep systemic mycoses, such as blastomycosis, cryptococcosis, and sporotrichosis, can also cause claw and claw bed disease, but these occur infrequently by comparison to the others that have been listed here(20, 21)
        - parasitic:
            - hookworms, such as *Ancylostoma* spp. and *Uncinaria* spp., have been associated with nailbed disease in dogs(42)
            - dogs with demodicosis may also develop paronychia, whereas neither *Demodex cati* nor *Demodex gatoi* tends to affect the claws or claw bed in cats
            - mange mite infestation with *Sarcoptes scabiei* and *Notoedres cati* in cats may involve the nail beds

- protozoal:

  - *Leishmania* spp.(42, 50–52)

- nutritional
- vasculitis.

21. Based upon the description that your technician has relayed, Midge likely has symmetrical claw bed disease. All four feet are involved.

22. I would like to ask Joby the following clarifying questions.

    - What is Midge's attitude? Is she acting like her normal self or is she acting "off"?
    - How is Midge's appetite? Is her appetite normal or is it "off"?
    - What is Midge eating?
    - Has there been a change in Midge's diet?
    - Has Midge experienced any change in weight recently?
    - How is Midge's thirst? Has her thirst changed at all?
    - Is Midge pruritic? If so, what is the intensity of the itch?
    - Other than the scabs and fur loss, has Joby seen any other skin lesions?
    - Has the consistency of her coat changed?
    - Does Midge's skin or coat have an odor?
    - Is Midge's skin or coat dry and flaky?
    - Is Midge's skin or coat greasy?
    - Does Midge's fur epilate easily?
    - Are either Moss or Juniper exhibiting similar symptoms?
    - Have there been any new additions to the household:

      - new cats?
      - new dogs?
      - other pets?
      - visitors?
      - visitors with pets?

    - Has there been any change to the cats' indoor-only lifestyle?
    - Has any topical medication (prescription or other) been applied to Midge?
    - Have any oral medications (prescription or other) been given to Midge?
    - Is Midge exhibiting any additional symptoms unrelated to her skin (vomiting, diarrhea, other)?
    - Have either Joby or Carl developed skin lesions?

23. After history-taking, the next appropriate step in the diagnostic work-up is for you to perform a comprehensive physical examination.(1, 4)

Returning to Case 33: The Crusty Cat

You enter the consultation room. Joby shares that Midge has been unusually quiet for the past few days. She seems unwell and has taken to hiding. Midge is also lethargic. Her diet hasn't changed, but she is surprisingly less interested in eating her food. She seems more invested in scratching at her ears than in pursuing her next meal. When you ask her to clarify the intensity of the itch, she says that the scratching keeps her and Carl up at night. Midge and the other two cats usually sleep on their bed. When Midge doesn't sleep on account of incessant scratching, no one does.

  When you examine Midge, you find that she has the following combination of skin lesions:

- hypotrichosis to alopecia at the base of each ear
- hyperkeratosis of the footpads (**Plate 42**)
- crusts along the margins of each ear, face, footpads and ungual folds of all claws
- erosive lesions where crusts have flaked off
- isolated, large, coalescing pustules on the muzzle, nasal planum, and concave pinnae.

Midge's unaffected skin appears healthy.

Round Two of Questions for Case 33: The Crusty Cat

1. What is hyperkeratosis?
2. What causes hyperkeratosis of the footpads?
3. Of the possibilities that you listed in Question #2 (above), which is/are most likely in Midge?
4. If Midge's skin appeared papery or fragile, which underlying disease might you have suspected?
5. Based upon the additional information that you gleaned from the updated history and physical exam findings, which differential diagnoses will you prioritize?
6. What is/are the next appropriate step(s) in your diagnostic plan?

Answers to Round Two of Questions for Case 33: The Crusty Cat

1. Hyperkeratosis refers to thickening of the outermost layer of the epidermis, the stratum corneum, typically due to overproduction of keratin.(1, 2, 4)

2. Footpad hyperkeratosis may be caused by:(2, 53–56)

   - constant pressure, as from persistent exposure to hard surfaces, such as concrete, which results in callus formation
   - genetics, as in cases of familial hyperkeratosis
   - immune-mediated disease:(2, 53–55, 57, 58)

     - pemphigus foliaceus
     - systemic lupus erythematosus

   - infectious disease, such as canine distemper virus (CDV)(2, 51, 53–55)
   - neoplastic disease
   - zinc-responsive dermatoses.

   Hyperkeratosis may also be idiopathic, although this is more likely to occur in aged dogs.(2, 54, 55, 59)

3. Of the possibilities that I listed in the answer to Question #2 (above), immune-mediated disease is most likely.

   Midge is an indoor-only cat. She is not exposed to hard surfaces, such as concrete, or constant pressure that may result in callus formation. Familial hyperkeratosis tends to occur in dogs, typically Labrador retrievers or Labrador crosses.(54, 60)

   Although CDV is known to cause disease in wild felids, in clinical practice it is associated with causing "hard pad disease" in dogs, not cats.(1, 4)

   Neoplastic diseases that cause footpad hyperkeratosis, such as cutaneous lymphoma or hepatocutaneous syndrome, are relatively rare.(2, 53) Zinc-responsive dermatoses is often associated with young Siberian Huskies and Alaskan Malamutes.(61–64)

4. If Midge's skin appeared papery or fragile, I might have suspected hyperadrenocorticism.(48)

5. Based upon the additional information that was gleaned from the updated history and physical exam findings, I will prioritize infectious and immune-mediated diseases as the most likely causes of Midge's clinical presentation. Midge's pustules, crusts, alopecia, and claw bed involvement could all be explained by:(1, 4)

- bacterial pyoderma:
    - primary disease is possible
    - secondary disease is more likely(7, 8, 65–69)
- dermatophytosis
- mange mites
- pemphigus foliaceus.

6. I will prioritize cytology to explore potential infectious and immune-mediated diseases. These diagnostic tests may include the following.(1, 4)

- Acetate tape preps to explore the possibility of yeast overgrowth and to search for *Cheyletiella* spp., although this so-called walking dandruff would have been expected to be paired with appreciable scale.(70, 71)
- Impression smears of primary lesions and fine-needle aspirates (FNAs) of pustules to evaluate the patient for pyoderma and pemphigus foliaceus
- Skin scrapes to look for mange mites:(72–76)
    - superficial scrapes to rule out *Demodex gatoi*, *Sarcoptes scabiei*, and *Notoedres cati*
    - deep scrapes to rule out *Demodex cati*.
- Trichogram to assess the patient for evidence of dermatophytosis.(23, 24, 26–32)

This list of diagnostic tests is intentionally not exhaustive. It provides a starting point to gather data. Additional tests can then be layered as needed to fill in gaps, clarify ambiguous test results, support or establish safety of treatment.

Returning to Case 33: The Crusty Cat

Joby asks you to stage the work-up. She would prefer not to do "everything" at once. She asks you to determine the most reasonable starting point. You suggest performing cytologic exam of an intact pustule. Joby agrees. (See **Plate 43**.)

Round Three of Questions for Case 33: The Crusty Cat

1. What do you see when you examine the cytology in **Plate 43**?
2. Based upon the cytological findings, what is your suspected diagnosis?
3. Is this diagnosis definitive?
4. Which layer of the skin does this condition affect?
5. Describe the pathogenesis of this condition.
6. What are potential triggers for this condition?
7. Assuming that your diagnosis is correct, how will you proceed with treatment of the primary problem?
8. What will you need to share with the client concerning treatment of this condition?
9. What are potential side effects of therapy?
10. What can you do to reduce the chance of side effects?
11. What might you need to do to monitor for potential side effects of therapy?

Answers to Round Three of Questions for Case 33: The Crusty Cat

1. I see acantholytic keratinocytes in **Plate 43**. Acantholytic keratinocytes are free-floating rafts of cells that have lost their anchor to the epidermis.(4)

2. The presence of acantholytic keratinocytes supports a diagnosis of pemphigus foliaceus.(1, 4)

3. Acantholytic keratinocytes are not pathognomonic for pemphigus foliaceus. A definitive diagnosis of pemphigus must come from a biopsy.(77) Intact pustules are the best lesions to sample for biopsy, followed by crusts. Crusts may keep micropustules hidden from view.(77)

4. Pemphigus foliaceus targets the epidermis.(2, 4, 17, 19)

5. Pemphigus foliaceus is an immune-mediated disease.(2, 4, 17, 19) Autoantibodies are created by the patient against desmosomes.(2, 3) This disrupts the integrity of the skin's surface by forcing keratinocytes apart.(2, 3)

6. Potential triggers for pemphigus foliaceus include:

   - exposure to ultraviolet (UV) light(3)
   - reactions to drugs.(3, 4, 20)
     The development of pemphigus foliaceus is also thought to be influenced by genetics.(3)

7. Treatment of pemphigus foliaceus typically involves the administration of long-term immunosuppressive agents such as prednisolone and/or chlorambucil.(1–4, 17–19, 35, 78, 79)
     Patients with pemphigus foliaceus often demonstrate a rapid response to therapy.(3)

8. This condition is chronic, meaning that although it may go into remission, it is unlikely to ever resolve.(3) Most patients experience a waxing and waning course.(1–4, 17–19, 35, 78, 79) This can be frustrating for clients, who understandably would prefer an easy fix and a permanent solution.

9. Side effects are often linked to the administration of glucocorticoids and include:(3, 18, 19, 79)

   - polyuria and polydipsia (PU/PD)
   - polyphagia
   - ulcerations within the gastrointestinal tract.

   Long-term administration of glucocorticoids may increase the risk of developing diabetes mellitus.(3, 18, 79)
     Long-term administration of glucocorticoids also may predispose to secondary infections because these medications are intentionally administered at immunosuppressive doses.(3, 18, 79) These infections may be bacterial; however, patients that receive long-term immunosuppressive agents are also more likely to develop demodicosis or dermatophytosis.(3) This presents a diagnostic challenge because these clinical presentations may resemble a flare-up of pemphigus foliaceus.(3) Clients may become frustrated by the need to repeat diagnostic tests, such as skin scrapes, trichograms, and fungal cultures, yet they are essential to evaluate the patient for opportunistic invaders.(3)

10. To reduce the frequency and severity of side effects, it is customary to taper the immunosuppressive agent to the lowest effective dose.(3)

11. It is wise to monitor any patient that is receiving long-term immunosuppressive therapy for secondary infections. For example, routinely culturing the urine is an effective strategy to monitor for subclinical urinary tract infections.(3)

CLINICAL PEARLS

- The skin serves many functions, not the least of which is to be a protective barrier.

- Presentations that disrupt the integrity of the skin are common in clinical practice.

- Skin lesions may be primary or secondary. Secondary lesions appear as the condition evolves and/or may be self-induced, such as excoriations.

- Many dermatologic presentations look alike. There are many diseases that cause papules, fur loss, crusts, and claw bed disease.

- History-taking is an essential part of the diagnostic process. It is critical to clarify the following:

    - Onset of disease – when did clinical signs start?
    - Where are skin lesions concentrated? Are they focal or generalized?
    - Is the patient pruritic?
    - Progression of disease – how have clinical signs changed?

- The physical exam is also an essential tool because you may identify lesions that the client missed and/or you may identify subtle changes that influence how you choose to proceed with your diagnostic work-up. For example, isolated intact pustules can be sampled to assess the patient for bacterial pyoderma and/or immune-mediated disease.

- Pemphigus foliaceus is one of several types of immune-mediated disease that is associated with facial dermatitis and paronychia.

- The presence of acantholytic keratinocytes within an aspirated pustule are supportive of a diagnosis of pemphigus foliaceus.

- A definitive diagnosis of pemphigus foliaceus requires a biopsy.

- Treatment of pemphigus foliaceus is aimed at suppressing the immune system. Glucocorticoids are frequently prescribed at high doses to turn off autoantibody production.

- Glucocorticoid therapy is not curative and is not without adverse effects. Clients need to be informed that treatment is long-term and requires dose adjustments as needed to achieve clinical effects while minimizing drug reactions or drug-associated sequelae.

References

1. Englar RE. Performing the small animal physical examination. Hoboken, NJ: Wiley/Blackwell; 2017.
2. Miller WH, Griffin CE, Campbell KL, Muller GH, Scott DW. Muller and Kirk's small animal dermatology. 7th ed. St. Louis, MO: Elsevier; 2013.
3. Canine and feline pemphigus foliaceus: improving your chances of a successful outcome. DVM360 [Internet]; 2009. Available from: https://www.dvm360.com/view/canine-and-feline-pemphigus-foliaceus-improving-your-chances-successful-outcome.
4. Englar RE. Common clinical presentations in dogs and cats. Hoboken, NJ: Wiley/Blackwell; 2019.
5. Rijnberk A, Sluijs FJv. Medical history and physical examination in companion animals. 2nd ed. New York: Saunders/Elsevier; 2009.
6. Nuttall T, Harvey RG, McKeever PJ. Skin diseases of the dog and cat. Boca Raton, FL: Taylor & Francis; 2009.
7. Wildermuth BE, Griffin CE, Rosenkrantz WS. Feline pyoderma therapy. Clin Tech Small Anim Pract 2006;21(3):150–6.

8. Favrot C. Feline non-flea induced hypersensitivity dermatitis: clinical features, diagnosis and treatment. J Feline Med Surg 2013;15(9):778–84.

9. Jazic E, Coyner KS, Loeffler DG, Lewis TP. An evaluation of the clinical, cytological, infectious and histopathological features of feline acne. Vet Dermatol 2006;17(2):134–40.

10. Moriello KA. Feline skin diseases. In: Little SE, editor. The cat: clinical medicine and management. St. Louis, MO: Saunders; 2012. p. 398–9.

11. Moriello KA. Dermatology. In: Little SE, editor. The cat: clinical medicine and management. St. Louis, MO: Elsevier Saunders; 2012. p. 371–424.

12. Breathnach RMS, Shipstone M. The cat with alopecia. In: Rand J, editor. Problem-based feline medicine. Toronto: Elsevier Saunders; 2006. p. 1052–66.

13. Kennis RA. Disorders causing focal alopecia. In: Morgan RV, editor. Handbook of small animal practice. 5th ed. St. Louis, MO: Saunders/Elsevier; 2008. p. 834–40.

14. Ghubash RM. Disorders causing symmetrical alopecia. In: Morgan RV, editor. Handbook of small animal practice. 4th ed. Philadelphia, PA: Saunders; 2003. p. 841–9.

15. Englar RE. Common clinical presentations in dogs and cats. Hoboken, NJ: Wiley/Blackwell; 2019.

16. Mecklenburg L. An overview on congenital alopecia in domestic animals. Vet Dermatol 2006;17(6):393–410.

17. Ettinger SJ, Feldman EC, Côté E. Textbook of veterinary internal medicine: diseases of the dog and the cat. 8th ed. St. Louis, MO: Elsevier; 2017.

18. The Merck veterinary manual. Whitehouse Station, NJ: Merck & Co., Inc.; 2016.

19. Côté E. Clinical veterinary advisor. Dogs and cats. 3rd ed. St. Louis, MO: Elsevier Mosby; 2015.

20. Warren S. Claw disease in dogs: Part 2 – diagnosis and management of specific claw diseases. Companion Anim 2013;18(5):226–31.

21. Outerbridge CA. Mycologic disorders of the skin. Clin Tech Small Anim Pract 2006;21(3):128–34.

22. Colombo S, Nardoni S, Cornegliani L, Mancianti F. Prevalence of Malassezia spp. yeasts in feline nail folds: a cytological and mycological study. Vet Dermatol 2007;18(4):278–83.

23. DeBoer DJ, Moriello KA. Cutaneous fungal infections. In: Greene CE, editor. Infectious diseases of the dog and cat. 3rd ed. St. Louis, MO: Saunders/Elsevier; 2006. p. 551–69.

24. Frymus T, Gruffydd-Jones T, Pennisi MG, Addie D, Belák S, Boucraut-Baralon C, et al. Dermatophytosis in cats: ABCD guidelines on prevention and management. J Feline Med Surg 2013;15(7):598–604.

25. Moriello KA, Kunkle G, DeBoer DJ. Isolation of Dermatophytes from the Haircoats of Stray Cats from Selected Animal Shelters in two Different Geographic Regions in the United States. Vet Dermatol 1994;5(2):57–62.

26. Moriello KA. Diagnostic techniques for dermatophytosis. Clin Tech Small Anim Pract 2001;16(4):219–24.

27. Moriello KA, Coyner K, Paterson S, Mignon B. Diagnosis and treatment of dermatophytosis in dogs and cats: Clinical Consensus Guidelines of the World Association for Veterinary Dermatology. Vet Dermatol 2017;28(3):266–e68.

28. Dasgupta T, Sahu J. Origins of the KOH technique. Clin Dermatol 2012;30(2):238–41; discussion 41–2.

29. Achten G. The use of detergents for direct mycologic examination. J Invest Dermatol 1956;26(5):389–97.

30. Robert R, Pihet M. Conventional methods for the diagnosis of dermatophytosis. Mycopathologia 2008;166(5–6):295–306.

31. Georg LK. The diagnosis of ringworm in animals. Vet Med 1954;49:157–66.

32. Taschdjian CL. Fountain pen ink as an aid in mycologic technic. J Invest Dermatol 1955;24(2):77–80.

33. Boord MJ, Griffin CE, Rosenkrantz WS. Onychectomy as a therapy for symmetric claw and claw fold disease in the dog. J Am Anim Hosp Assoc 1997;33(2):131–8.

34. Foil CS. Facial, pedal, and other regional dermatoses. Vet Clin North Am Small Anim Pract 1995;25(4):923–44.

35. Scarff DH. Nail disease in the dog and cat. Small Anim Dermatol 2004;9(7):1–4.

36. Apple S. Senior cat with front paw swelling and pain. Today's Vet Pract 2015 (September/October):41–4.

37. Maritato KC, Schertel ER, Kennedy SC, Dudley R, Lamm C, Barnhart M, Kass P. Outcome and prognostic indicators in 20 cats with surgically treated primary lung tumors. J Feline Med Surg 2014;16(12):979–84.

38. Mehlhaff CJ, Mooney S. Primary pulmonary neoplasia in the dog and cat. Vet Clin North Am Small Anim Pract 1985;15(5):1061–7.

39. Gottfried SD, Popovitch CA, Goldschmidt MH, Schelling C. Metastatic digital carcinoma in the cat: a retrospective study of 36 cats (1992–1998). J Am Anim Hosp Assoc 2000;36(6):501–9.

40. Goldfinch N, Argyle DJ. Feline lung-digit syndrome: unusual metastatic patterns of primary lung tumours in cats. J Feline Med Surg 2012;14(3):202–8.

41. Wobeser BK, Kidney BA, Powers BE, Withrow SJ, Mayer MN, Spinato MT, Allen AL. Diagnoses and clinical outcomes associated with surgically amputated feline digits submitted to multiple veterinary diagnostic laboratories. Vet Pathol 2007;44(3):362–5.

42. Rouben C. Claw and claw bed diseases. Clinician's Brief 2016 (April):35–40.

43. Warren S. Claw disease in dogs: Part 1 – anatomy and diagnostic approach. Companion Anim 2013;18(4):165–70.

44. Mueller RS. Diagnosis and management of canine claw diseases. Vet Clin North Am Small Anim Pract 1999;29(6):1357–71.

45. Scott DW, Miller WH. Disorders of the claw and clawbed in Dogs. Comp cont. Educ Pract 1992;14(11):1448-and.

46. Scott DW, Miller WH. Disorders of the claw and clawbed in Cats. Comp cont. Educ Pract 1992;14(4):449-and.

47. Rosychuk RAW. Diseases of the claw and claw fold. In: Bonagura JD, editor. Kirk's current veterinary therapy. XII. Philadelphia, PA: W.B. Saunders; 1995.

48. Boland LA, Barrs VR. Peculiarities of feline hyperadrenocorticism: update on diagnosis and treatment. J Feline Med Surg 2017;19(9):933–47.

49. Verde MT, Basurco A. Symmetrical lupoid onychodystrophy in a crossbred pointer dog: long-term observations. Vet Rec 2000;146(13):376–8.

50. Koutinas AF, Carlotti DN, Koutinas C, Papadogiannakis EI, Spanakos GK, Saridomichelakis MN. Claw histopathology and parasitic load in natural cases of canine leishmaniosis associated with Leishmania infantum. Vet Dermatol 2010;21(6):572–7.

51. Ciaramella P, Oliva G, Luna RD, Gradoni L, Ambrosio R, Cortese L, et al. A retrospective clinical study of canine leishmaniasis in 150 dogs naturally infected by Leishmania infantum. Vet Rec 1997;141(21):539–43.

52. Koutinas AF, Polizopoulou ZS, Saridomichelakis MN, Argyriadis D, Fytianou A, Plevraki KG. Clinical considerations on canine visceral leishmaniasis in Greece: a retrospective study of 158 cases (1989–1996). J Am Anim Hosp Assoc 1999;35(5):376–83.

53. Catarino M, Combarros-Garcia D, Mimouni P, Pressanti C, Cadiergues MC. Control of canine idiopathic nasal hyperkeratosis with a natural skin restorative balm: a randomized double-blind placebo-controlled study. Vet Dermatol 2018;29(2):134–e53.

54. Pagé N, Paradis M, Lapointe JM, Dunstan RW. Hereditary nasal parakeratosis in Labrador Retrievers. Vet Dermatol 2003;14(2):103–10.

55. Kwochka KW. Primary keratinization disorders of dogs. In: Griffin CE, Kwochka KW, Macdonald JM, editors. Current veterinary dermatology, the science and art of therapy. St. Louis, MO: Mosby; 1993. p. 176–90.

56. Kunkle GA. Zinc-responsive dermatoses in dogs. In: Kirk RW, editor. Current veterinary therapy VII. Philadelphia, PA: W. B. Saunders Co.; 1980. p. 472–6.

57. Ihrke PJ, Stannard AA, Ardans AA, Griffin CE, Kallet AJ. Pemphigus foliaceus of the footpads in three dogs. J Am Vet Med Assoc 1985;186(1):67–9.

58. August JR, Chickering WR. Pemphigus foliaceus causing lameness in 4 Dogs. Comp cont. Educ Pract 1985;7(11):894.

59. Yager JA, Wilcock BP. Color atlas and text of surgical pathology of the dog and cat, dermatopathology and skin tumors. London: Wolfe Publishing; 1994.

60. Peters J, Scott DW, Erb HN, Miller WH. Hereditary nasal parakeratosis in Labrador retrievers: 11 new cases and a retrospective study on the presence of accumulations of serum ("serum lakes") in the epidermis of parakeratotic dermatoses and inflamed nasal plana of dogs. Vet Dermatol 2003;14(4):197–203.

61. Willemse T. Zinc-related cutaneous disorders of dogs. In: Kirk RW, Bonagura JD, editors. Kirk's current veterinary therapy. XI. Philadelphia, PA: W. B. Saunders; 1992. p. 532–4.

62. Brown RG, Hoag GN, Smart ME, Mitchell LH. Alaskan Malamute chondrodysplasia. V. Decreased gut zinc absorption. Growth 1978;42(1):1–6.

63. Colombini S. Canine zinc-responsive dermatosis. Vet Clin North Am Small Anim Pract 1999;29(6):1373–83.

64. Colombini S, Dunstan RW. Zinc-responsive dermatosis in northern-breed dogs: 17 cases (1990–1996). J Am Vet Med Assoc 1997;211(4):451–3.

65. Ravens PA, Xu BJ, Vogelnest LJ. Feline atopic dermatitis: a retrospective study of 45 cases (2001–2012). Vet Dermatol 2014;25(2):95–102.

66. Vogelnest LJ, Cheng KY. Cutaneous adverse food reactions in cats: retrospective evaluation of 17 cases in a dermatology referral population (2001–2011). Aust Vet J 2013;91(11):443–51.

67. Bloom P. Canine superficial bacterial folliculitis: current understanding of its etiology, diagnosis and treatment. Vet J 2014;199(2):217–22.

68. Bajwa J. Canine superficial pyoderma and therapeutic considerations. Can Vet J 2016;57(2):204–6.

69. Craig M. Lesion morphology in veterinary dermatology. Companion Animal 2009;14(3):54–60.

70. Schmidt V, Nuttall T. Malassezia in dogs and cats: Part 1. Small Anim Dermatol 2008;13(4):55–61.

71. Arther RG. Mites and lice: biology and control. Vet Clin North Am Small Anim Pract 2009;39(6):1159–71.

72. Hillier A, Lloyd DH, Weese JS, Blondeau JM, Boothe D, Breitschwerdt E, et al. Guidelines for the diagnosis and antimicrobial therapy of canine superficial bacterial folliculitis (antimicrobial Guidelines Working Group of the International Society for Companion Animal Infectious Diseases). Vet Dermatol 2014;25(3):163–e43.

73. Beco L, Fontaine F, Bergvall K. Comparison of skin scrapes and hair plucks for detecting demodex mites in canine demodicosis, a multicentre, prospect study. Vet Dermatol 2007;18:381.

74. Mueller RS, Bensignor E, Ferrer L, Holm B, Lemarie S, Paradis M, et al. Treatment of demodicosis in dogs: 2011 clinical practice guidelines. Vet Dermatol 2012;23(2):86–96.

75. Mueller RS, Bettenay SV. Skin scrapings and skin biopsies. In: Ettinger SJ, Feldman EC, editors. Skin scrapings and skin biopsies. Philadelphia, PA: W. B. Saunders; 2010. p. 368–71.

76. Young S. Feline demodicosis: prevalence, diagnostics, treatment. DVM360. 2010 (May).

77. Tater KC, Olivry T. Canine and feline pemphigus foliaceus: improving your chances of a successful outcome. DVM; 2010. Available from: http://veterinarymedicine.dvm360.com/canine-and-feline-pemphigus-foliaceus-improving-your-chances-successful-outcome?id=andsk=anddate=and%0AA%09%09%09andpageID=4.

78. Bizikova P, Burrows A. Feline pemphigus foliaceus: original case series and a comprehensive literature review. BMC Vet Res 2019;15(1):22.

79. Plumb DC. Plumb's veterinary drug handbook. 9th ed. Hoboken, NJ: Pharma Vet, Inc.; 2018.

Case 34

The Cat with Facial Swelling

You met Piper once, last year, shortly after she had been adopted from a local humane organization by Ricardo (Ricky) Juarez as a surprise for his wife, Shelby. Ricky had stumbled across a photograph of her on their friend Josephine's social media profile. Josephine worked as the director of the shelter, and frequently advertised cats and dogs that were in the market for their forever homes. In the past, she had never gotten Ricky to take the bait, but the instant that she posted about the buff orange tabby, she knew that Shelby would be sold. She and Shelby were best friends through grade school. From first grade through eighth, Shelby's family had owned a tabby not unlike this one. PS was his name – short for Pumpkin Spice – and he was the most docile, dog-like cat that Josephine had ever seen. He loved seeing the world from the vantage point of Shelby's shoulder. She carried him everywhere that she went, except for school. PS even came along for road trips and weekend campouts. He walked with her to the bus stop every morning and was there to greet her every afternoon. One day, he never showed up. Shelby never did find him, though she and Josephine searched high and low. His absence broke Shelby's heart and she vowed never to own another.

Then Piper came along. The moment that Josephine saw her, she knew that Shelby would approve. Piper was practically the reincarnation of Pumpkin Spice, right down to the piercing yellow-green eyes. There are some people who argue that all orange cats look alike, but Josephine disagreed. Piper was striking because she was unique, and she was unique because she was the only cat in 25 years that Josephine had come across that looked just like PS. And Josephine had seen a lot of cats!

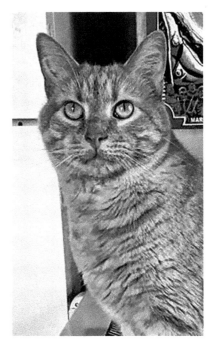

Figure 34.1 Meet your patient, Piper, a 3-year-old female spayed domestic shorthaired (DSH) cat.

When Josephine told Ricky about Piper, he questioned how Shelby would react. But ultimately, he trusted Josephine just enough to give it a try, and thankfully, she'd been right. Shelby melted with happiness the instant she saw Piper waiting on the landing when she walked through the front door. At first, she did a double take. Then she rubbed her eyes. She allowed herself to believe, just for an instant, that Pumpkin Spice had come home for good. Then she awoke to the reality that Piper was, well, Piper – a new cat with a new personality to love, who needed Shelby as much as Shelby needed her to heal.

Piper had an easy transition into the Juarez household other than her battle with fleas just two days into her adoption becoming "Facebook official." It required bombing the house, bathing Piper, and applying flea preventative. Piper took it all in stride, except for the fact that she had a severe reaction to the flea saliva. Within 24 hours of being flea-bitten, she developed a horrific itch. The itch was so intense that she dug herself raw. That was when you met Piper for the first time. You diagnosed Piper with military dermatitis, brought on by an apparent flea bite hypersensitivity. She had responded well to treatment, but you warned them that it would need to continue, particularly if she maintained her indoor-outdoor lifestyle. Piper seemed to enjoy her time outdoors, even if she was restricted to supervised visits on harness and leash. Piper complied with topical treatments for as long as they were applied. Then fall came.

At the first sign of frost, Ricky and Shelby discontinued Piper's flea preventative and they settled in for a cold, wet winter. Four months later, spring arrived. Late, but better than never. Life was busier than ever. Ricky and Shelby were now expecting their first child.

It had been a particularly hectic week. Ricky was logging long hours at the office and Shelby was feeling under the weather. Ricky was just getting home after dark for the third night in a row to find Piper waiting in the foyer for dinner. "Yes, Piper, I know, I'm late again," he fussed, preparing her food as she chirped feistily underfoot. It was only when Ricky bent down to place her food dish on the kitchen tile that he noticed Piper's face (see **Plate 44**).

Concerned, Ricky sent a screen shot of Piper's face to the emergency service. You were on call and offered to see Piper, but after speaking with you about what this could be, Ricky did not feel that Piper's pouty lip was urgent enough to warrant an emergency visit. You scheduled an appointment for Piper for today. She is here now to be evaluated.

Work through the following questions to prepare you for this consult.

Weight: 11.3 lb (5.1 kg)
BCS: 6/9
Mentation: BAR

TPR

T: 100.7°F (38.2°C)
P: 192 beats per minute
R: 24 breaths per minute

Round One of Questions for Case 34: The Cat with Facial Swelling

1. Describe the location of Piper's swelling, as is seen in **Plate 44**.
2. Describe the appearance of Piper's swelling.
3. Based upon the case history and the lesion's appearance, what is the presumptive diagnosis?
4. What is the most common location for this condition to arise?
5. Based upon the presumptive diagnosis, is this lesion likely to be pruritic?
6. Based upon the presumptive diagnosis, is this lesion likely to be unilateral or bilateral?
7. Is this presumptive diagnosis associated with any other abnormal physical exam findings?
8. If your presumptive diagnosis is correct, what is the most likely trigger of this condition?
9. Other than what you identified in Question #8 (above), what are additional triggers of this condition?
10. Based upon your understanding of potential triggers for this condition, what additional clarifying questions do you want to ask Ricky about Piper?

Answers to Round One of Questions for Case 34: The Cat with Facial Swelling

1. Piper's swelling is located at the mucocutaneous junction that is associated with the lower lip.

2. Piper's swelling is raised, nodular, and well-circumscribed. It is salmon pink in color and its surface is smooth.

3. Based upon the case history and the lesion's appearance, the presumptive diagnosis is a rodent ulcer. Sometimes this lesion is referred to as an indolent or eosinophilic ulcer.(1–6)

4. The most common location for rodent ulcers to arise is at the mucocutaneous junction that is associated with the upper lip, philtrum, or adjacent to the maxillary canine tooth.(1, 3, 5)

5. Rodent ulcers do not appear to be pruritic.(4, 5)

6. Rodent ulcers are typically unilateral.(1, 4) However, they enlarge significantly to the point that they often cross over midline.(4)

7. Rodent ulcers may be associated with regional lymphadenopathy.(1) The submandibular lymph node on the ipsilateral side may be palpably enlarged.

8. If the presumptive diagnosis is correct, then it is most likely a manifestation of an underlying allergic disease.(2, 3, 7–14) Sensitivity to arthropods, particularly fleas, has been implicated. (1, 4, 5, 11) Flea-allergic cats are prone to developing this condition in response to flea saliva. (3, 11) Other insects, such as cockroaches, may also incite sensitivity responses.(4) So, too, can *Cheyletiella* spp.(6)

9. Additional triggers for rodent ulcers include hypersensitivity to allergens contained in food or within the environment itself.(3) Both cutaneous adverse food reactions and atopic dermatitis have been known to cause these lesions.(3) It has also been proposed that autoallergens may play a role, that is, the patient develops an allergy to itself.(3, 15, 16)

   Some reports have suggested that infectious disease is also a primary cause of this condition. (3) Bacterial colonization of rodent ulcers has been documented.(17) However, these may arise secondary to the lesion as opportunistic invaders.(3)

10. Because this condition has been associated with hypersensitivity to fleas and because this patient has a history of flea bite hypersensitivity, I would want to ask Ricky if Piper is still receiving monthly topical flea preventative. Along those same lines, I would also want to ask Ricky if he or Shelby have seen any fleas or evidence of flea infestation, such as flea dirt.

    In addition, I would clarify if Piper's lifestyle has changed and if there have been any adjustments to the home environment. For instance, was a new pet brought into the home? Or has Piper recently visited someone else that has pets that might have re-exposed her to fleas?

    Because this condition is also potentially associated with adverse reactions to food, I would want to take a complete diet history.(6) What is Piper being fed?(6) Has any new diet been introduced?(6)

    Has Piper travelled anywhere recently? Has she been boarded?(6) Does she frequent a grooming salon?(6)

Returning to Case 34: The Cat with Facial Swelling

Your clarifying questions reveal that Piper's exposure to the great outdoors persists, although these days find her tethered to a leash and harness rather infrequently – at most, once per week. When Piper does go outside, she is not as invested in exploring. She would prefer to sit in the grass and watch the world go by. Ricky shares that he wouldn't be surprised if, after the baby arrives, they discontinue her outdoor adventures. They no longer seem to be high up on Piper's priority list.

Your review of the medical record reveals that Piper's prescription of topical flea preventative ran out 6 months ago. You ask if Piper is still receiving topical monthly flea preventative, hoping that Ricky had decided to price-shop and purchase it elsewhere. Ricky shares that he and Shelby discontinued the product over winter. When spring arrived, it hadn't occurred for them to restart her on preventative.

Ricky asks, "Do you really think that's what could have caused this? We haven't seen a single flea!"

Ricky adds that Shelby is "very concerned" about oral neoplasia: "Do you think there's any chance it could be cancer? Shelby was in tears last night just thinking about it."

Round Two of Questions for Case 34: The Cat with Facial Swelling

1. Are most oral tumors in cats benign or malignant?
2. What is the most common type of oral neoplasia in cats?
3. Within the oral cavity, where does this type of neoplasia prefer to reside?
4. What is the second most common type of oral neoplasia in cats?
5. Based upon lesion location, is it possible that Piper has oral neoplasia?
6. Patients with oral tumors typically present with which of the following clinical signs?
7. Do these clinical signs fit with Piper's clinical presentation?
8. How likely is oral neoplasia in Piper based upon the patient's history and physical exam?

Answers to Round Two of Questions for Case 34: The Cat with Facial Swelling

1. Most oral tumors in cats are malignant.(18–22)

2. Squamous cell carcinoma (SCC) is the most common type of oral neoplasia in cats.(19, 20, 22–25)

3. Within the oral cavity, SCC prefers the following locations:(18, 19, 22)

   - beneath the tongue
   - buccal mucosa
   - caudal pharynx
   - lip
   - mandible
   - maxilla
   - tongue.

4. The second most common oral malignancy in cats is fibrosarcoma.(26)

5. Yes, is it possible that Piper has oral neoplasia.

6. Patients with oral tumors typically present with the following signs:(18, 22)

   - blood-tinged saliva
   - decreased appetite
   - discolored coat from discolored saliva
   - dysphagia
   - halitosis
   - inability to close the mouth
   - increased mobility associated with neighboring teeth
   - oral swelling
   - pain upon opening the mouth
   - ptyalism
   - reduction in grooming behaviors
   - thick, ropy saliva
   - weight loss.

7. The only clinical sign that fits with Piper's presentation is a swelling that is associated with the oral cavity.

8. Although oral cancer cannot be ruled out based upon lesion appearance and location alone, it is less likely given the patient's history. While it is true that SCC and other oral tumors may progress rapidly,(22) it is unlikely to have cropped up overnight. If it were that aggressive of a lesion, then

I might have expected it to appear ulcerated or necrotic. Such lesions are also typically paired with bloody saliva and a distinctly rancid, rotting odor that originates from a combination of blood and decomposing tissue.

Returning to Case 34: The Cat with Facial Swelling

You share with Ricky that while SCC can target the lip in cats, Piper is not presenting with the most common clinical signs. In addition, the fact that this swelling popped up overnight in this location, with a history of flea allergy hypersensitivity and a report from the client that flea preventative was discontinued during a heavy flea season, makes another differential more probable. You suspect a rodent ulcer, otherwise known as an eosinophilic or indolent ulcer. You share that this type of lesion is one of several that is included within the umbrella term, eosinophilic granuloma complex.

Round Three of Questions for Case 34: The Cat with Facial Swelling

1. In addition to rodent ulcers, which other clinical presentations are part of the feline eosinophilic granuloma complex?
2. Describe each clinical presentation that you identified in Question #1 (above) and provide a list of differential diagnoses.
3. You share with Ricky that you are "fairly certain" that you've arrived at the correct diagnosis and that Piper's lesion is not cancerous. If Ricky wanted you to confirm your suspicions, what should you do?
4. Assuming that your diagnosis is correct, how is this condition typically managed? Identify potential adverse effects of treatment when applicable.
5. What do you need to share with your client about this condition's prognosis?

Answers to Round Three of Questions for Case 34: The Cat with Facial Swelling

1. In addition to rodent ulcers, eosinophilic plaques and eosinophilic granulomas are part of the feline eosinophilic granuloma complex.(3–5, 22, 27)

2. Eosinophilic plaques are alopecic, flat-topped, solid elevations of tissue that can appear anywhere on the body, but are most commonly found along the ventrum, at the axilla, or inguinal regions.(3, 6, 28) Affected skin is erythematous and alopecic.(2, 3) Pruritus is intense and incites patients with these lesions to overgroom.(2, 3, 6) The surfaces of lesions quickly become ulcerated. (2, 3, 6)

   Differential diagnoses for eosinophilic plaques include:(2, 3)

   - foreign body reaction
   - fungal infection:

     - dermatophytosis
     - deep mycoses

   - mycobacterial infection
   - neoplasia:

     - cutaneous lymphoma
     - mast cell tumor
     - SCC

- viral infection:

  - cowpox

Eosinophilic granulomas are typically alopecic, ulcerated, raised and nodular lesions that arise anywhere on the body, but seem to prefer the hard palate and tongue, pelvic limbs, and footpads. (1–3, 7, 28) The same list of differential diagnoses applies.

3. The diagnosis of eosinophilic granuloma complex is typically presumptive.(4) You could perform impression smears of oozing lesions. Cytology that demonstrated an abundance of eosinophils is supportive of the presumptive diagnosis.(3, 4) However, a biopsy is the only way to rule out neoplasia and other non-allergic disease.(3) Incisional biopsies are typically performed rather than excisional biopsies due to location to obtain a definitive diagnosis. Tissue can also be submitted for culture, following the biopsy procedure, if infectious disease is suspected.(3)

4. The following are treatment options for management of eosinophilic granuloma complex.(3, 6)

- Glucocorticoids:

  - Prescribed systemically as a tapered dose of either prednisolone or dexamethasone.
  - Long-term use may potentiate diabetes mellitus, gastric ulceration, demodicosis, or infections with opportunistic microorganisms.(7, 28, 29)

- Cyclosporine:

  - Can be as effective as prednisolone.(13)
  - May cause mild gastrointestinal upset.(13, 30–37)

- Chlorambucil:

  - An option to consider when patients do not respond to either of the above options.

- Interferon omega:

  - Efficacy is unknown; however, anecdotal reports suggest that subcutaneous injections may be of benefit.

- Megoestrol acetate:

  - Considered to be a last resort because chronic use has been associated with the development of diabetes mellitus, mammary hyperplasia, and pyometra.

Note that serological status for feline immunodeficiency virus (FIV), feline leukemia virus (FeLV), and toxoplasma should be evaluated prior to initiating treatment with immunomodulators and/or immunosuppressive agents.(3)

5. It is important to share with the client that this condition tends to respond well to treatment, but it is likely to recur unless the underlying issue is addressed. This may require one or more of the following diagnostic interventions and/or therapeutic trials to identify the trigger(s) for the eosinophilic granuloma complex:(3, 4)

- acetate tape impressions
- elimination diet(38)
- impression smear cytology
- intradermal skin tests
- skin scrapings
- treatment with parasiticide to address ectoparasites, including fleas
- trichograms.

Clients may become frustrated if they are not fully prepared to launch a comprehensive diagnostic investigation. Transparency is essential so that all parties are on the same page. I would share with Ricky that treating this condition is more of a marathon rather than a sprint.

CLINICAL PEARLS

- Allergic skin disease is a common presentation in clinical practice.

- Allergic skin disease may be triggered by any number of inciting factors, of which the following are repeat offenders in veterinary patients:
  - food allergens → cutaneous adverse drug reactions
  - hypersensitivity to insects → flea bite hypersensitivity, mosquito bite hypersensitivity
  - environmental allergens → atopic dermatitis.

- Other skin conditions may mimic allergic skin disease, including, but not limited to:
  - bacterial pyoderma
  - dermatophytosis
  - foreign body reaction
  - neoplasia.

- The eosinophilic granuloma complex is a manifestation of allergic skin disease in cats and includes:
  - eosinophilic granuloma
  - eosinophilic plaque
  - eosinophilic or indolent or so-called rodent ulcer.

- These lesions may appear overnight, particularly eosinophilic plaques.

- Rodent ulcers create a "pouty lip" appearance. Although they typically appear at the upper lip, at the philtrum, or adjacent to the maxillary canine tooth, they can also develop at the lower lip. Lesions are typically alopecic, well-circumscribed, nodular, and erythematous. The surface is usually smooth but can ulcerate.

- Rodent ulcers respond well to systemic treatment with immunosuppressive agents or immunomodulators. However, lesions are likely to recur if the underlying cause is not addressed.

- An extensive diagnostic investigation may be required to identify the etiological agent and address it.

- Transparency in clinical conversations with clients is essential.

References

1. Medleau L, Hnilica KA. Small animal dermatology: a color atlas and therapeutic guide. 2nd ed. St. Louis, MO: Saunders Elsevier; 2006.
2. Miller WH, Griffin CE, Campbell KL, Muller GH, Scott DW. Muller and Kirk's small animal dermatology. 7th ed. St. Louis, MO: Elsevier; 2013. ix, 938 p. p.
3. Buckley L, Nuttall T. Feline eosinophilic granuloma complex(ities): some clinical clarification. J Feline Med Surg 2012;14(7):471–81.
4. Foil CS. Facial, pedal, and other regional dermatoses. Vet Clin North Am Small Anim Pract 1995;25(4):923–44.

5. Friberg C. Feline facial dermatoses. Vet Clin North Am Small Anim Pract 2006;36(1):115–40.

6. Power HT, Ihrke PJ. Selected feline eosinophilic skin diseases. Vet Clin North Am Small Anim Pract 1995;25(4):833–50.

7. Bloom PB. Canine and feline eosinophilic skin diseases. Vet Clin North Am Small Anim Pract 2006;36(1):141–60.

8. Lee Gross T, Ihrke PJ, Walder EJ, Affolter VK. Spongiotic and vesicular diseases of the epidermis. Skin diseases of the dog and cat: clinical and histopathologic diagnosis. 1. Oxford: Blackwell Science; 2005.

9. Lee Gross T, Ihrke PJ, Walder EJ, Affolter VK. Nodular and diffuse diseases of the dermis with prominent eosinophils, neutrophils, or plasma cells. Skin diseases of the dog and cat: clinical and histopathologic diagnosis. 1. Oxford: Blackwell Science; 2005.

10. Schmidt V, Buckley LM, McEwan NA, Rème CA, Nuttall TJ. Efficacy of a 0.0584% hydrocortisone aceponate spray in presumed feline allergic dermatitis: an open label pilot study. Vet Dermatol 2012;23(1):11–6.

11. Colombini S, Hodgin EC, Foil CS, Hosgood G, Foil LD. Induction of feline flea allergy dermatitis and the incidence and histopathological characteristics of concurrent indolent lip ulcers. Vet Dermatol 2001;12(3):155–61.

12. Taglinger K, Day MJ, Foster AP. Characterization of inflammatory cell infiltration in feline allergic skin disease. J Comp Pathol 2007;137(4):211–23.

13. Wisselink MA, Willemse T. The efficacy of cyclosporine A in cats with presumed atopic dermatitis: a double blind, randomised prednisolone-controlled study. Vet J 2009;180(1):55–9.

14. Bardagí M, Fondati A, Fondevila D, Ferrer L. Ultrastructural study of cutaneous lesions in feline eosinophilic granuloma complex. Vet Dermatol 2003;14(6):297–303.

15. Wisselink MA, van Ree R, Willemse T. Evaluation of Felis domesticus allergen I as a possible autoallergen in cats with eosinophilic granuloma complex. Am J Vet Res 2002;63(3):338–41.

16. Gelberg HB, Lewis RM, Felsburg PJ, Smith CA. Antiepithelial autoantibodies associated with the feline eosinophilic granuloma complex. Am J Vet Res 1985;46(1):263–5.

17. Russell RG, Slattum MM, Abkowitz J. Filamentous bacteria in oral eosinophilic granulomas of a cat. Vet Pathol 1988;25(3):249–50.

18. Bilgic O, Duda L, Sánchez MD, Lewis JR. Feline oral squamous cell carcinoma: clinical manifestations and literature review. J Vet Dent 2015;32(1):30–40.

19. Liptak JM, Withrow SJ. Oral tumors. In: Withrow SJ, Vail DM, editors. Small animal clinical oncology. St. Louis, MO: Saunders Elsevier; 2007. p. 455–78.

20. Stebbins KE, Morse CC, Goldschmidt MH. Feline oral neoplasia: a ten-year survey. Vet Pathol 1989;26(2):121–8.

21. Harvey CE, Emily P. Oral neoplasms. In: Harvey CE, Emily P, editors. Small animal dentistry. St. Louis, MO: Mosby; 1993. p. 306.

22. Englar RE. Common clinical presentations in dogs and cats. Hoboken, NJ: Wiley/Blackwell; 2019.

23. Perrone JR. Top 5 feline Oral Health concerns. Vet Team Brief 2016 (January/February).

24. Garrett LD, Marretta SM. Feline oral squamous cell carcinoma: an overview. DVM. 360 [Internet]; 2007. Available from: http://veterinarymedicine.dvm360.com/feline-oral-squamous-cell-carcinoma-overview.

25. Pellin M, Turek M. A review of feline oral squamous cell carcinoma. Today's. Vet Pract 2016 (November/December):24–33.

26. Tilley LP, Smith FWK. The 5-minute veterinary consult: canine and feline. 3rd ed. Baltimore, MD: Lippincott Williams & Wilkins; 2004.

27. Englar RE. Performing the small animal physical examination. Hoboken, NJ: Wiley/Blackwell; 2017.

28. Foster A. Clinical approach to feline eosinophilic granuloma complex. Pract 2003;25(1):2–9.

29. Lowe AD, Graves TK, Campbell KL, Schaeffer DJ. A pilot study comparing the diabetogenic effects of dexamethasone and prednisolone in cats. J Am Anim Hosp Assoc 2009;45(5):215–24.

30. Guaguere E, Prelaud P. Efficacy of cyclosporin in the treatment of 12 cases of eosinophilic granuloma complex. Vet Dermatol 2000;11;S 31.

31. Heinrich NA, McKeever PJ, Eisenschenk MC. Adverse events in 50 cats with allergic dermatitis receiving ciclosporin. Vet Dermatol 2011;22(6):511–20.

32. Latimer KS, Rakich PM, Purswell BJ, Kircher IM. Effects of cyclosporin A administration in cats. Vet Immunol Immunopathol 1986;11(2):161–73.

33. Noli C, Scarampella F. Prospective open pilot study on the use of ciclosporin for feline allergic skin disease. J Small Anim Pract 2006;47(8):434–8.

34. Plumb DC. Plumb's veterinary drug handbook. 9th ed. Hoboken, NJ: Pharma Vet Inc.; 2018.
35. Robson DC, Burton GG. Cyclosporin: applications in small animal dermatology. Vet Dermatol 2003;14(1):1–9.
36. Vercelli A, Raviri G, Cornegliani L. The use of oral cyclosporin to treat feline dermatoses: a retrospective analysis of 23 cases. Vet Dermatol 2006;17(3):201–6.
37. Nuttall T, Harvey RG, McKeever PJ. Feline eosinophilic granuloma complex. A colour handbook of skin diseases of the dog and cat. 1. London: Manson Publishing; 2009. p. 102–5.
38. Bryan J, Frank LA. Food allergy in the cat: a diagnosis by elimination. J Feline Med Surg 2010;12(11):861–6.

Case 35

The Lumpy Bumpy Dog

Carly and her owner, Mariposa Pachenko, are long-term customers of yours. Mariposa is one of your favorites. She owns five champion bitches and two stud dogs. She has built a successful canine breeding operation from nothing, and has worked her way up to the top, learning the nuts and bolts of canine theriogenology with the help of mentor Paul Cinna. Now Mariposa is a leader in her field, yet she remembers her roots and is never too busy to show the ropes to those new to the discipline.

Mariposa is wholly committed to her dogs and rarely leaves their sides, particularly at and around whelping times. Unfortunately, her out of state mother has taken ill, forcing Mariposa to leave the kennel in the hands of her wife, Radina. Radina is an accomplished financial analyst and avid dog-lover, but she isn't particularly savvy when it comes to triaging medical predicaments. Radina has always leaned on Mariposa to tend to the health and welfare of their dogs. Like most couples, they balance their responsibilities and play to their strengths. Mariposa takes charge of anything and everything veterinary-related, while Radina oversees their finances and balances the books. This system has worked well for them, and Radina has never had to consult with your clinic on her own until today.

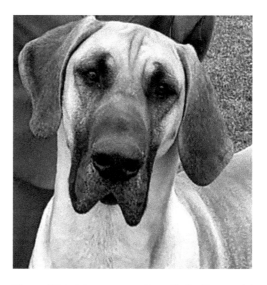

Figure 35.1 Meet your patient, Carly, 5-year-old intact female Great Dane. Courtesy of Georgia Hymmen.

It had been a typical Monday at the office, with phones ringing off the hook. You were just packing up to call it a night, three hours after your shift had officially ended, when you spot a car speed into the parking lot in front of the clinic. Radina pops out of the driver's side of the vehicle and runs through the front door.

"Doc, come quick!" She exclaims, "It's Carly! Something's happened and she's all puffed up!"

You grab your stethoscope and race out to the car to investigate. (See **Plates 45 and 46.**)

Consider the following questions as a guide to assist the progression of this consult.

Round One of Questions for Case 35: The Lumpy Bumpy Dog

1. Describe the appearance of the lesions that you see in **Plate 45**.
2. Using appropriate medical jargon, how would you define these lesions?
3. What is the colloquial name for these lesions?
4. What, in broad terms, causes these lesions to appear?
5. Which circulating cell mediates this response via degranulation?

6. Which substance(s) are released by the cell that you named in Question #5 (above) during degranulation that causes these lesions to develop?
7. What do(es) the substance(s) that you identified in Question #6 (above) do to the body?
8. How would you describe Carly's muzzle, shown in **Plate 46**, using appropriate medical jargon?
9. What conditions can mimic the condition that you identified in Question #8 (above)?
10. If you were to palpate Carly's muzzle, what do you suspect it would feel like?
11. What concerns do you have regarding Carly's wellbeing if no treatment is initiated?
12. Based upon what you observe in Carly (refer to **Plates 45 and 46**), which type of shock are you concerned that she is experiencing?
13. When the condition that you identified in Question #12 (above) is triggered by insect stings or bites, which immunoglobulin is involved?
14. When the immunoglobulin that you named in Question #13 (above) is involved, which type of hypersensitivity reaction is the patient experiencing?
15. Can other immunoglobulins cause the condition that you identified in Question #12 (above)?
16. If your presumptive diagnosis is correct, as identified in your answer to Question #12 (above), which additional clinical signs might you expect to see in Carly?
17. What does "shock organ" refer to?
18. Why does it matter where a patient's "shock organ" is?
19. What is/are the shock organ(s) in the dog and how might this relate to clinical signs?
20. What is/are the shock organ(s) in the cat and how might this relate to clinical signs?
21. Could Carly's lesions in theory resolve on their own?
22. Is this a medical emergency? Why or why not?
23. Which clarifying question(s) will you need to ask Radina to successfully manage this case?

Answers to Round One of Questions for Case 35: The Lumpy Bumpy Dog

1. The lesions that Carly has developed, as captured in **Plate 45**, are located along the left caudoventral flank and abdomen as well as the left caudolateral rump and thigh. There are dozens of raised, dome-shaped nodules, most of which are isolated and well-circumscribed. Some of the lesions are coalescing. They range in size. Some appear to be just a few millimeters in diameter while others appear to be nickel or even quarter sized. There is no evidence of hypotrichosis or alopecia. Because the lesions are covered with fur, I cannot assess the skin.

2. These lesions are characteristic of urticaria.(1–7)

3. The colloquial name for these lesions is hives.(1–3, 6, 7)

4. The development of urticaria is suggestive of an acute immune response, specifically an allergic hypersensitivity reaction.(1, 6–8)

5. Mast cells mediate the patient's response to antigen via degranulation.(1, 4, 6–8)

6. Histamine is released by mast cells during degranulation, in addition to cytokines, prostaglandins, leukotrienes, heparin, tryptase, and platelet activating factor (PAF).(8–13) These substances promote the development of urticaria.(8, 9)

7. These substances, primarily histamine and PAF, increase vascular permeability.(8) This causes vessels to become leaky. Leaky vessels allow leukocytes and other lines of defense to break out of the circulation at the affected site(s), where they can hopefully fight off any invaders.

The problem is that in an allergic reaction, the body is not responding to harmful invaders. The body is overresponding to a false alarm, that is, a harmless substance. If the increase in vascular permeability is widespread, then the patient is at risk for developing cardiovascular collapse. (8) This is because during a hypersensitivity reaction, approximately one-third of the intravascular volume can shift into the interstitial space.(8, 11, 14) This dramatic shift in volume causes significant hypotension.(8) Hypotension is intensified through peripheral vasodilation, which is triggered by prostaglandins.(11)

In addition, PAF incites bronchoconstriction.(8) This may result in respiratory distress.

8. I would describe Carly's muzzle, shown in **Plate 46**, as being edematous and erythematous. (2, 3) The abrupt changes in the appearance of her muzzle are consistent with angioedema.

9. Cellulitis and contact dermatitis may mimic angioedema.(15)

10. If I were to palpate Carly's muzzle, it would likely feel thickened and firm like cooked steak. This change in texture and consistency of the tissue is due to dermal edema.(8)

11. If no treatment is initiated, then I am concerned about the potential for Carly to experience cardiovascular collapse and acute respiratory distress.(8) Respiratory distress results from PAF-triggered bronchoconstriction. Angioedema contributes to respiratory distress when it involves tissues that surround the airway, for instance, the muzzle and throat. Swelling at and around the nares as well as laryngeal edema may essentially close off the breathing circuit, causing dyspnea, and tachypnea.

12. Based upon what is observed in Carly, I am concerned that she is experiencing anaphylactic shock. Anaphylactic shock, sometimes referred to as anaphylaxis, is a systemic reaction to a specific antigen after prior exposure and sensitization.(1, 8, 11, 16–20)

13. When anaphylaxis is triggered by insect stings or bites, then IgE is the mediator.(11, 16, 21)

14. When IgE is the mediator, anaphylaxis is triggered by a type 1 hypersensitivity reaction.(5, 7)

15. Yes, other immunoglobulins can cause anaphylaxis. For instance, IgG and IgM can mediate type II and type III hypersensitivity reactions.(5, 7, 11, 16, 17, 19)

16. If Carly is indeed experiencing anaphylaxis, then I might expect to see one or more of the following clinical signs in addition to urticaria:(8, 22)

- allergic conjunctivitis
- allergic rhinitis
- progressive erythema
- pruritus
- ptyalism, as from nausea
- wheals
- worsening facial edema.

17. A "shock organ" is defined as the location in the body where the most mast cells reside.(11, 23)

18. Different species exhibit different constellations of clinical signs based upon the location of their "shock organ(s)."(11)

19. The shock organs in the dog are the liver and the gastrointestinal tract.(5, 11, 24, 25) During anaphylaxis, histamine enters the portal vein from the digestive tract.(11)

In addition to dermal signs, dogs that present with anaphylaxis often exhibit vomiting.(8, 11, 22, 23, 25–28) Anorexia and diarrhea are also possible.(8, 22, 23, 25–28)

20. The shock organs in the cat are the lungs.(5, 11, 24, 25, 29–31)
    In addition to dermal signs, cats that present with anaphylaxis often exhibit acute respiratory distress: dyspnea, tachypnea, and open-mouth breathing.(2, 3, 5, 11, 25, 30–32) Respiratory distress is exacerbated by pharyngeal and laryngeal edema.(22)

21. In theory, yes, Carly's lesions could resolve on their own.(1) When spontaneous resolution occurs, it typically takes 1 to 2 days.(1) However, it is ill-advised to wait it out. Clinical signs progress over minutes to hours and it is difficult to know who is going to be "okay" versus who will require emergency intervention.(9, 11, 17, 25)

22. Yes, this is a medical emergency. In general, how quickly clinicals appear after exposure to the offending antigen determines how severe anaphylaxis will be.(9, 11, 25, 33–36) However, exerting caution and expedient intervention are keys to successful patient outcomes. Your client does not want to risk a situation in which the potential for badness progresses to worst case scenario as would be true if suddenly the patient's airway were compromised, and s/he cannot breathe.

23. To successfully manage this case, you will need to ask Radina the following questions.

    - Is this Carly's first health crisis of this nature? Has this ever happened before?
    - Does she know what Carly may have been exposed to?(1, 8, 11, 26, 37–46) Disclosure of the following would be significant:

        - food
        - insects that sting or bite:

            - ants
            - bees
            - black flies
            - caterpillars
            - hornets
            - mosquitoes
            - spiders
            - wasps

        - medications:

            - antimicrobial drugs
            - non-steroidal anti-inflammatory drugs
            - opioids
            - radiographic contrast material
            - other

        - transfusion-associated blood products
        - venomous animals

            - rattlesnakes.

Returning to Case 35: The Lumpy Bumpy Dog

You commend Radina for seeking veterinary care because this is a true medical emergency. You share that Carly appears to be experiencing an anaphylactic reaction that, if untreated, could potentially be fatal.

You ask your technician to take Carly's vital signs urgently so that you can initiate treatment right away.

Weight: 112 lb (50.9 kg)
BCS: 4/9
Mentation: BAR

TPR

T: 104.6°F (40.3°C)
P: 165 beats per minute
R: Panting

Round Two of Questions for Case 35: The Lumpy Bumpy Dog

1. How do Carly's vital signs compare to the normal reference ranges for large-breed dogs?
2. How can you explain the changes that you see in her vital signs? Are her vital signs consistent with what you would expect to see?
3. Although Carly is panting, she does not appear to be in respiratory distress. If she were in respiratory distress, what must you do to intervene?
4. Which categories of medications might you need to administer to Carly?
5. Name a drug that belongs in each category that you identified in Question #4 (above). List the route(s) of administration and your proposed dose(s) in milligrams per kilogram (for injectable drugs).
6. Using Carly's body weight and the proposed doses (milligrams per kilogram) for injectable drugs that you provided in your answer to Question #5 (above), calculate how much of each drug (in milligrams) you plan to administer to Carly.
7. Based upon Carly's history, presentation, and vital parameters, you suspect hypotension secondary to anaphylaxis. In addition to the injectable drugs that you outlined in Question #5 (above), what else should you administer to prevent cardiovascular collapse?

Answers to Round Two of Questions for Case 35: The Lumpy Bumpy Dog

1. Reference ranges vary somewhat depending upon which resource(s) you drawn upon. However, in general, the normal reference range for canine rectal temperature is 99.5–102.5°F.(2, 3, 47) Carly's temperature is significantly elevated.

   The normal reference range for canine heart rate (HR) is dependent upon the size of the dog. In general, the HR ranges between:(2–5)

   - 60–100 beats per minute in large-breed dogs, such as Carly
   - 80–120 beats per minute in medium-breed dogs
   - 90–140 beats per minute in small-breed dogs.

   Carly's HR is significantly elevated. She has tachycardia.
   The normal reference range for canine respiratory rate (RR) is 10–30 breaths per minute.(2–5) Carly is panting. She is exhibiting tachypnea.

2. Tachycardia is a common clinical finding in patients that are experiencing anaphylaxis. The body responds to hypovolemia through a physiologic increase in HR.(22)

   Tachypnea is a common clinical finding in patients that are experiencing anaphylaxis. Pharyngeal and laryngeal edema, in addition to bronchoconstriction, make it challenging to move air through the respiratory tree.(22) The patient has to work harder to get air into the system, which means that RR and effort typically climb.

   Hyperthermia is a common clinical finding in patients that are experiencing anaphylaxis. It is caused by histamine as well as secondary mediators, such as prostaglandins.

3. If Carly were in respiratory distress, then you would need to assess and secure the airway.(22) The patient will benefit from delivery of high-flow, concentrated oxygen by means of a face mask, nasal cannula, or oxygen cage.(11) If laryngeal edema is narrowing the airway, then an endotracheal tube can be placed to ensure that the airway stays patent.(22) Oxygen can then be delivered directly through the endotracheal tube. If swelling is severe enough to prevent endotracheal tube placement, then you will need to perform a tracheotomy to place a temporary trach tube.(22)

4. You may need to consider administering one or more of the following categories of medications to Carly:(3–5, 22, 48)

    - antihistamine
    - bronchodilator
    - glucocorticoid
    - vasopressor.

5. Diphenhydramine is an antihistamine. When used to treat anaphylaxis, it is typically administered intramuscularly (IM) at a dose of 1–4 mg/kg.(3–5, 22, 48–50)

    Albuterol is an inhalant bronchodilator that is used to open up the airway to improve oxygen delivery to the lungs for oxygen exchange. When used to treat anaphylaxis, it is typically administered as one to two puffs of a 90 g/puff inhaler.(3–5, 22, 48, 51)

    Dexamethasone sodium phosphate (DexSP) is a glucocorticoid that is commonly used in clinical practice to treat anaphylaxis even though its use has not been supported by a Cochrane systematic review.(11, 52) When used to manage anaphylaxis, it is dosed at 0.1–4 mg/kg and administered intravenously (IV).(4, 6, 11, 22, 24, 48) This range is admittedly wide and depends largely upon which resource is referenced.

    Epinephrine is a vasopressor.(11, 48) In human healthcare and in some veterinary texts, it is the recommended drug for acute management of anaphylaxis.(11, 17, 24, 25, 53) However, its use as a first-line treatment in canine clinical practice is controversial.(8, 54) The dose is 0.01–0.02 mg/kg of a 1:1000 (1 mg/mL) solution administered IV or IM.(4, 11, 22) Dose may vary depending upon which resource is consulted and which route the drug is administered. For example, the dose is typically higher if administered via an endotracheal tube.(22)

6. Using Carly's body weight and the proposed dose (milligrams per kilogram), I can calculate how much drug (in milligrams) I may administer:

Table 35.1

Drug Name	Dose (mg/kg)	Patient's weight (kg)	Amount of drug to administer (mg)
Diphenhydramine (Benedryl)	2 mg/kg (range given in Q#5 was 1–4 mg/kg)	50.9	101.8
Dexamethasone sodium phosphate (DexSP)	0.1 mg/kg (range given in Q#5 was 0.1–4 mg/kg)	50.9	5.09
Epinephrine	0.01 mg/kg (range given in Q#5 was 0.01–0.02 mg/kg)	50.9	0.51

7. In addition to the drugs outlined in Question #5 and 6 (above), I would provide resuscitative support to the patient by means of IV fluid therapy.

Returning to Case 35: The Lumpy Bumpy Dog

You explain to Radina that you need to treat Carly immediately for anaphylaxis. Radina authorizes you to "do anything you need to, just make sure that Carly pulls through this."

You rush Carly to the treatment area and need to provide a plan for your technical staff to leap into action. Use the following questions to facilitate the next steps as you outline your treatment plan for the team.

Round Three of Questions for Case 35: The Lumpy Bumpy Dog

1. Even though the use of DexSP is not supported by a Cochrane systematic review,(11, 52) you decide to administer it IV anyway because in the past that's what you've always done and anecdotally it seems to help. The injectable DexSP that you have in stock is labeled at 4 mg/mL concentration. Calculate how many milliliters of DexSP that you will inject IV if you want to administer 0.1 mg/kg.
2. Which peripheral vessel(s) is/are typically used to administer IV injections in the dog?
3. What is/are potential risks of administering IV injections?
4. What should you consider to reduce the risk(s) that you outlined in Question #3 (above)?
5. The injectable diphenhydramine that you have in stock is labelled at 50 mg/mL concentration. Calculate how many milliliters of diphenhydramine that you will inject IM, if you want to administer 2 mg/kg.
6. At which sites in the canine patient is it appropriate to administer IM injections?
7. Administering an IM injection at one of the aforementioned sites in the canine or feline patient may result in neuropathy. Which nerve are you concerned about damaging?
8. If this nerve were damaged, what would you expect to observe clinically in the patient?
9. If you cannot avoid IM injection at the site at which nerve damage is possible, what can you do to reduce the risk?
10. In addition to administering DexSP and diphenhydramine, you would like to start IV fluid therapy. What is your clinical reasoning for administering fluids, considering that Carly is not dehydrated?
11. In response to your desire to administer IV fluid therapy to Carly, your technician selects a bag of crystalloids from the dispensary. Are most crystalloids isotonic or hypertonic?
12. What is an example of a commonly used crystalloid fluid in veterinary medicine?
13. Your technician asks if you want to administer a shock dose. How do you calculate a shock dose of crystalloids in the canine patient?
14. Based upon your calculations, what would Carly's shock dose be in milliliters and also in liters?
15. How do you calculate a shock dose of crystalloids in the feline patient?
16. How do you answer your technician: do you wish to administer a shock dose of crystalloids?
17. How will you know whether Carly is responding to treatment?
18. What are suggested parameters for optimal small animal fluid resuscitation?
19. Which clinical signs or presentation might suggest that you overdid it with IV fluid therapy, that is, Carly is now overhydrated?
20. Once Carly is stable, she will be discharged to the care of Radina. Will she require any additional medication at time of discharge?
21. Radina asks how she and Mariposa can be better prepared for this type of reaction in the future. How will you answer her?

Answers to Round Three of Questions for Case 35: The Lumpy Bumpy Dog

1. The injectable DexSP that you have in stock is labelled at 4 mg/mL concentration.

    If you want to administer 0.1 mg/kg and Carly weighs 50.9 kg, then you will need to draw up 5.09 mg.

    5.09 mg × [1 mL/4 mg] = 1.3 mL

    You will administer 1.3 mL of DexSP (4 mg/mL) IV.

2. IV injections are typically administered into either cephalic vein in a canine patient. IV injections may be also injected, via catheter, into the lateral saphenous vein in dogs.

3. Extravasation is possible if you were intending to deliver an injection IV, yet your needle inadvertently slipped outside of the vessel, thereby delivering the drug to the surrounding tissues. Certain drugs can cause extensive injury, including blistering or sloughing of tissue, if they leak outside of the IV space. Pain and inflammation are also likely sequelae of inadvertently administering an IV injectable outside of circulation.

4. Placing an IV catheter and checking its patency prior to administering an IV injectable will reduce the risk of extravasation.

5. The injectable diphenhydramine that you have in stock is labelled at 50 mg/mL concentration. If you want to administer 2.0 mg/kg IM and Carly weighs 50.9 kg, then you will need to draw up 101.8 mg.

$$101.8 \text{ mg} \times [1 \text{ mL}/50 \text{ mg}] = 2.0 \text{ mL}$$

You will administer 2.0 mL of diphenhydramine (50 mg/mL).

6. It is appropriate to administer IM injections in the dog at the following sites:(55, 56)

   - epaxial muscles in the lumbar region
   - quadriceps muscle
   - triceps muscle
   - +/– hamstrings (the semimembranosus and semitendinosus).

7. Injecting the hamstrings may result in sciatic neuropathy.(55–58)

8. If the sciatic nerve were damaged during IM injection, then you might expect to observe one or more of the following clinical signs:(57, 58)

   - acute loss of function of the affected limb:

     - paresis of the affected limb
     - pelvic limb lameness

   - decreased flexion at the hock when testing the withdrawal reflex
   - decreased motor and/or sensory innervation to the caudal thigh and gluteal muscles
   - knuckling of the affected hind paw +/– scuffing injuries (i.e. abrasions) along its dorsum
   - muscle atrophy of the affected limb within 1–3 weeks of the IM injection.

9. If you must administer an IM injection at the hamstrings, then you can reduce the risk of sciatic nerve injury by directing the needle at a 45 degree angle directed caudally.(56)

10. IV fluids prevent cardiovascular collapse by infusing the vasculature with volume.(59) Recall that histamine and PAF increase vascular permeability.(8) When this leakiness of the vasculature becomes widespread, as much as one-third of the intravascular volume can shift into the interstitial space.(8, 11, 14) This causes appreciable hypotension.(8) Administering resuscitative volumes of IV fluids combats hypotension.(11, 59)

11. Most crystalloids are isotonic to plasma.(59–61)

12. Commonly used crystalloid fluids in veterinary medicine include 0.9% sodium chloride.(59–61) Other examples are Plasmalyte-A, Normosol-R, and Lactated Ringers Solution (LRS).(59–61)

13. A shock dose of crystalloids in the canine patient is 90 mL/kg/dog.(11, 59–61)

14. Carly's shock dose of crystalloids is:

    90 mL/kg/dog × 50.9 kg = 4509 mL = 4.5 L

15. A shock dose of crystalloids in the feline patient is 60 mL/kg/cat.(11, 59–61)

16. I would ask the technician to deliver 1/4 to 1/3 of Carly's shock dose of crystalloids over 15 minutes and then reassess.(59, 60)

17. I will monitor Carly's response to treatment by evaluating trends in the following parameters:(59–61)

    - blood pressure
    - capillary refill time
    - HR
    - mentation
    - mucous membrane color
    - oxygen saturation
    - pulse strength or quality
    - respiratory effort
    - RR
    - venous or arterial blood gases.

18. Suggested parameters for optimal small animal fluid resuscitation are as follows:(11)

    - euthermia
    - normal mentation
    - systolic BP of 100–120 mmHg.

19. The following signs might indicate that I overhydrated Carly with fluid therapy:(60, 61)

    - ascites
    - chemosis
    - crackles on thoracic auscultation
    - increased respiratory effort
    - increased RR
    - peripheral edema
    - serous nasal discharge, bilaterally
    - weight gain.

20. Some, but not all, clinicians elect to discharge the patient with instructions to continue administration of diphenhydramine orally at a dose of 1–4 mg/kg every 8 to 12 hours.(11)

21. Ideally, the source that triggered Carly's episode would be avoided.(11) Unfortunately, in this circumstance, we do not know what caused her to go into anaphylactic shock. All we can do from here on out is to consider prescribing an EpiPen and training Radina and Mariposa how to use it so that if Carly exhibits signs of anaphylaxis in the future, they can administer it en route to the clinic. EpiPens are sold at human pharmacies for people with histories of anaphylaxis and contain 0.3 mg epinephrine. These devices are typically reserved for dogs that weigh over 45–50 lb. An EpiPen would be an appropriate choice for Carly.

    What if Carly were not a Great Dane and weighed significantly less? The EpiPen Jr. is sold at human pharmacies for children with histories of anaphylaxis and is appropriately prescribed to dogs that weigh between 20 and 45 lb. In patients that weigh less than 20 lb, a calculated dose of epinephrine can be drawn up into a syringe for use as needed.

CLINICAL PEARLS

- Hypersensitivity reactions in companion animal patients require urgent medical attention.

- There are many triggers for hypersensitivity reactions, including:

  - food
  - insects that sting or bite
  - medications
  - transfusions
  - venomous animals.

- In order for patients to develop a hypersensitivity today, they must have previously been exposed to the inciting agent.

- Patients that experience hypersensitivity reactions present with one or more of the following signs:

  - angioedema
  - conjunctivitis
  - erythematous skin
  - pruritus
  - rhinitis
  - urticaria.

- Additional clinical signs may develop based upon the species-specific shock organ. In dogs, the shock organ is the gut; in cats, the shock organ is the lung.

  - Vomiting and diarrhea may develop in dogs in response to anaphylaxis.
  - Dyspnea, tachypnea, open-mouth breathing, and respiratory stridor may develop in cats in response to anaphylaxis.
  - Both dogs and cats may have difficulty getting air into the respiratory tract because of pharyngeal and laryngeal edema.

- Anaphylaxis is a medical emergency. Patients in anaphylactic shock are typically tachycardic, tachypneic, hyperthermic, and hypotensive.

- Treatment is tailored to the individual patient, but may include administration of antihistamines, bronchodilators, glucocorticoids, and vasopressors.

- It is helpful to have a poster in the treatment area that outlines emergency doses based upon patient weight. This allows you to expedite treatment without having to dive knee deep into calculations, particularly if math is not your strong suit.

References

1. The Merck veterinary manual. Whitehouse Station, NJ: Merck & Co., Inc.; 2016.
2. Englar RE. Performing the small animal physical examination. Hoboken, NJ: Wiley/Blackwell; 2017.
3. Englar RE. Common clinical presentations in dogs and cats. Hoboken, NJ: Wiley/Blackwell; 2019.
4. Côté E. Clinical veterinary advisor. Dogs and cats. 3rd ed. St. Louis, MO: Elsevier Mosby; 2015.
5. Ettinger SJ, Feldman EC, Côté E. Textbook of veterinary internal medicine: diseases of the dog and the cat. 8th ed. St. Louis, MO: Elsevier; 2017.
6. Medleau L, Hnilica KA. Small animal dermatology: a color atlas and therapeutic guide. 2nd ed. St. Louis, MO: Saunders Elsevier; 2006.

7. Miller WH, Griffin CE, Campbell KL, Muller GH, Scott DW. Muller and Kirk's small animal dermatology. 7th ed. St. Louis, MO: Elsevier; 2013.

8. Hoehne SN, Hopper K. Hypersensitivity and anaphylaxis. In: Drobatz KJ, Hopper K, Rozanski E, Silverstein DC, editors. Textbook of small animal emergency medicine. Hoboken, NJ: John Wiley and Sons; 2019. p. 936–41.

9. Khan BQ, Kemp SF. Pathophysiology of anaphylaxis. Curr Opin Allergy Clin Immunol 2011;11(4):319–25.

10. Sala-Cunill A, Guilarte M. The role of mast cells mediators in angioedema without wheals. Curr Treat Options Allergy 2015;2(4):294–306.

11. Shmuel DL, Cortes Y. Anaphylaxis in dogs and cats. J Vet Emerg Crit Care (San Antonio) 2013;23(4):377–94.

12. Simons FE. Anaphylaxis: recent advances in assessment and treatment. J Allergy Clin Immunol 2009;124(4): 625–36; quiz 37–8.

13. Pushparaj PN, Tay HK. H'Ng SC, Pitman N, Xu D, McKenzie A, et al. The cytokine interleukin-33 mediates anaphylactic shock. Proc Natl Acad Sci USA 2009;106(24):9773–8.

14. Kitoh K, Watoh K, Chaya K, Kitagawa H, Sasaki Y. Clinical, hematologic, and biochemical findings in dogs after induction of shock by injection of heartworm extract. Am J Vet Res 1994;55(11):1535–41.

15. Nedelea I, Deleanu D. Isolated angioedema: an overview of clinical features and etiology. Exp Ther Med 2019;17(2):1068–72.

16. Simons FE. Anaphylaxis pathogenesis and treatment. Allergy 2011;66;Suppl 95:31–4.

17. Simons FE, Ardusso LR, Bilò MB, El-Gamal YM, Ledford DK, Ring J, et al. World Allergy Organization anaphylaxis guidelines: summary. J Allergy Clin Immunol 2011;127(3):587.

18. Simons FE, Ardusso LR, Bilò MB, El-Gamal YM, Ledford DK, Ring J, et al. World Allergy Organization guidelines for the assessment and management of anaphylaxis. World Allergy Organ J 2011;4(2):13–37.

19. Simons FE. 9. Anaphylaxis. J Allergy Clin Immunol 2008;125(2):S402–7.

20. Lucke WC, Thomas H, Jr. Anaphylaxis: pathophysiology, clinical presentations and treatment. J Emerg Med 1983;1(1):83–95.

21. Lieberman P. Definition and criteria for the diagnoses of anaphylaxis. In: Castells MC, editor. Anaphylaxis and hypersensitivity reactions. New York: Humana Press; 2011. p. 1–12.

22. Lyons JL, Scherk JR. Anaphylactic shock: how to effectively diagnose and treat. Today's veterinary practice [Internet]. Available from: https://todaysveterinarypractice.com/anaphylactic-shock-effectivelydiagnose-treat/.

23. Quantz JE, Miles MS, Reed AL, White GA. Elevation of alanine transaminase and gallbladder wall abnormalities as biomarkers of anaphylaxis in canine hypersensitivity patients. J Vet Emerg Crit Care (San Antonio) 2009;19(6):536–44.

24. Cohen RD. Systemic anaphylaxis. In: Bonagura JD, Kirk RW, editors. Kirk's current veterinary therapy. XII Small Animal Practice. Philadelphia, PA: W.B. Saunders Co; 1995. p. 150–2.

25. Dowling PM. Anaphylaxis. In: Silverstein DC, Hopper K, editors. Small animal critical care medicine. St. Louis, MO: Saunders Elsevier; 2009. p. 727–30.

26. Moore GE, HogenEsch H. Adverse vaccinal events in dogs and cats. Vet Clin North Am Small Anim Pract 2010;40(3):393–407.

27. Peters LJ, Kovacic JP. Histamine: metabolism, physiology, and pathophysiology with applications in veterinary medicine. J Vet Emerg Crit Care (San Antonio) 2009;19(4):311–28.

28. Lautt WW, Legare DJ. Effect of histamine, norepinephrine, and nerves on vascular pressures in dog liver. Am J Physiol 1987;252(4 Pt 1 Pt. 1):G472–8.

29. Greenberger PA, Rotskoff BD, Lifschultz B. Fatal anaphylaxis: postmortem findings and associated comorbid diseases. Ann Allergy Asthma Immunol 2007;98(3):252–7.

30. Litster A, Atwell R. Physiological and haematological findings and clinical observations in a model of acute systemic anaphylaxis in Dirofilaria immitis-sensitised cats. Aust Vet J 2006;84(5):151–7.

31. McCusker HB, Aitken ID. Anaphylaxis in the cat. J Pathol Bacteriol 1966;91(1):282–5.

32. Aitken ID, McCusker HB. Feline anaphylaxis: some observations. Vet Rec 1969;84(3):58–61.

33. Johnson RF, Peebles RS. Anaphylactic shock: pathophysiology, recognition, and treatment. Semin Respir Crit Care Med 2004;25(6):695–703.

34. Schaer M, Ginn PE, Hanel RM. A case of fatal anaphylaxis in a dog associated with a dexamethasone suppression test. J Vet Emerg Crit Care 2005;15(3):213–6.

35. Lieberman P. Anaphylaxis and anaphylactoid reactions. In: Adkinson NF, Yunginger JW, Busse WW, editors. Middleton's allergy: principles and practice. St. Louis, MO: Mosby; 2003. p. 1497–522.

36. Tran PT, Muelleman RL. Allergy, hypersensitivity and anaphylaxis. In: Marx JA, Hockberger RS, Walls RM, editors. Rosen's emergency medicine, concepts and clinical practice. Philadelphia, PA: Mosby Elsevier; 2006. p. 1818–38.

37. Fitzgerald KT, Flood AA. Hymenoptera stings. Clin Tech Small Anim Pract 2006;21(4):194–204.

38. Girard NM, Leece EA. Suspected anaphylactoid reaction following intravenous administration of a gadolinium-based contrast agent in three dogs undergoing magnetic resonance imaging. Vet Anaesth Analg 2010;37(4):352–6.

39. Heller J, Mellor DJ, Hodgson JL, Reid SW, Hodgson DR, Bosward KL. Elapid snake envenomation in dogs in New South Wales: a review. Aust Vet J 2007;85(11):469–79.

40. Hume-Smith KM, Groth AD, Rishniw M, Walter-Grimm LA, Plunkett SJ, Maggs DJ. Anaphylactic events observed within 4 h of ocular application of an antibiotic-containing ophthalmic preparation: 61 cats (1993–2010). J Feline Med Surg 2011;13(10):744–51.

41. Miyaji K, Suzuki A, Shimakura H, Takase Y, Kiuchi A, Fujimura M, et al. Large-scale survey of adverse reactions to canine non-rabies combined vaccines in Japan. Vet Immunol Immunopathol 2012;145(1–2):447–52.

42. Niza MM, Félix N, Vilela CL, Peleteiro MC, Ferreira AJ. Cutaneous and ocular adverse reactions in a dog following meloxicam administration. Vet Dermatol 2007;18(1):45–9.

43. Ohmori K, Masuda K, Maeda S, Kaburagi Y, Kurata K, Ohno K, et al. IgE reactivity to vaccine components in dogs that developed immediate-type allergic reactions after vaccination. Vet Immunol Immunopathol 2005;104(3–4):249–56.

44. Tocci LJ. Transfusion medicine in small animal practice. Vet Clin North Am Small Anim Pract 2010;40(3):485–94.

45. Walker T, Tidwell AS, Rozanski EA, DeLaforcade A, Hoffman AM. Imaging diagnosis: acute lung injury following massive bee envenomation in a dog. Vet Radiol Ultrasound 2005;46(4):300–3.

46. DeBoer DJ. Complications: cutaneous adverse drug reactions. NAVC Clin's Brief 2005 (August):7–10.

47. Rijnberk A, Stokhof AA. General examination. In: Rijnberk A, van Sluijs FJ, editors. Medical history and physical examination in companion animals. New York: Elsevier; 2009.

48. Plumb DC. Plumb's veterinary drug handbook. 9th ed. Hoboken, NJ: Pharma Vet Inc; 2018.

49. Sheikh A, Ten Broek V, Brown SG, Simons FE. H1-antihistamines for the treatment of anaphylaxis: cochrane systematic review. Allergy 2007;62(8):830–7.

50. Sheikh A, ten Broek Vm, Brown SG, Simons FE. H1-antihistamines for the treatment of anaphylaxis with and without shock. Cochrane Database Syst Rev 2007;1(1):CD006160.

51. Lee JK, Vadas P. Anaphylaxis: mechanisms and management. Clin Exp Allergy 2011;41(7):923–38.

52. Choo KJ, Simons E, Sheikh A. Glucocorticoids for the treatment of anaphylaxis: cochrane systematic review. Allergy 2010;65(10):1205–11.

53. Kemp SF, Lockey RF, Simons FE, World Allergy Organization ad hoc Committee on Epinephrine in Anaphylaxis. Epinephrine: the drug of choice for anaphylaxis. A statement of the World Allergy Organization. Allergy 2008;63(8):1061–70.

54. Dean HR, Webb RA. The morbid anatomy and histology of anaphylaxis in the dog. J Pathol 1924;27(1):51–64.

55. Sirois M. Principles and practice of veterinary technology. 4th ed. St. Louis, MO: Elsevier; 2017.

56. Sirois M. Elsevier's veterinary assisting textbook. 2nd ed. St. Louis, MO: Elsevier; 2017.

57. Au J. Rehabilitation therapy: sciatic nerve injury. Clinician's brief [Internet]. Available from: https://www.cliniciansbrief.com/article/rehabilitation-therapy-sciatic-nerve-injury.

58. Forterre F, Tomek A, Rytz U, Brunnberg L, Jaggy A, Spreng D. Iatrogenic sciatic nerve injury in eighteen dogs and nine cats (1997–2006). Vet Surg 2007;36(5):464–71.

59. Day TK, Bateman S. Shock syndromes. In: DiBartola SP, editor. Fluid, electrolyte, and acid–base disorders in small animal practice. 4th ed. St. Louis, MO: Saunders/Elsevier; 2012.

60. Lyons BM. Fluid therapy in hospitalized patients, Part 1: Patient Assessment and Fluid Choices. Today's Veterinary Practice [Internet]. Available from: https://todaysveterinarypractice.com/fluid-therapy-part-1fluid-therapy-hospitalized-patients-patient-assessment-fluid-choices/.

61. Davis H, Jensen T, Johnson A, Knowles P, Meyer R, Rucinsky R, et al. 2013 AAHA/AAFP fluid therapy guidelines for dogs and cats. J Am Anim Hosp Assoc 2013;49(3):149–59.

Case 36

The Wounded Dog

Pippen has had a rough week. He was relinquished, as an intact male, to a local humane organization on Saturday for inappropriate elimination. He was neutered on Monday. On Wednesday, he was attacked by another dog at the shelter when being walked outdoors by a volunteer. According to the volunteer, Pippen was minding his own business when one of the other dogs in the fenced yard managed to get loose. That dog, a Boston Terrier, made a beeline straight for Pippen and proceeded to bite him between his shoulder blades. Shelter employees managed to break up the fight, but not before Pippen's skin was torn (see **Plate 47**).

Because there was no veterinarian on site at the time that Pippen sustained the injury, the shelter director, Logan Fischer, had to seek medical attention elsewhere. Logan is one of your established clients. He brings his own pets to your clinic. Given that he has always had a positive experience with you and your team, he felt confident that you could handle Pippen.

He and Pippen have just arrived in your waiting room. Because Pippen is so visibly anxious, your technician expedites the check-in process and walks them directly to the first available consult room. The technician successfully takes Pippen's vital signs but requires two extra team members to restrain him. As soon as they release Pippen, he tucks himself into a corner of the room, beneath Logan's chair, and flattens himself against the floor, bracing himself for the next assault.

Work through the following questions as you consider an approach to wound management for this patient.

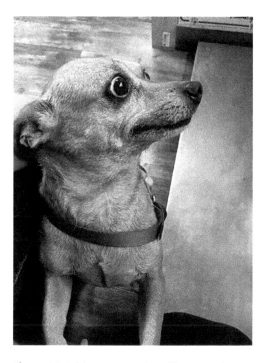

Figure 36.1 Meet your patient, Pippen, a 4-year-old castrated male mixed breed dog. Courtesy of Maki RCHS.

Weight: 14.3 lb (6.5kg)
BCS: 4/9
Mentation: QAR

TPR

T: 103.1°F (39.5°C)
P: 184 beats per minute
R: 34 breaths per minute

Round One of Questions for Case 36: The Wounded Dog

1. From a public health perspective, it is essential that you inquire about one specific aspect of the patient's history that

will impact how you will proceed with treatment. What do you need to know about Pippen and why?

2. Wound management is often staged. What constitutes immediate wound care?
3. What is the purpose of immediate wound care?
4. Define lavage.
5. Which solutions are appropriate to use for lavage from the standpoint of not causing tissue damage?
6. Which solutions are inappropriate for use for lavage?
7. What is primary wound closure?
8. What does delayed primary closure mean?
9. Why might you consider delaying primary closure?
10. What is second intention healing?
11. How do you determine whether to leave a wound open or to actively take measures to close it?
12. Which factors impact wound healing?
13. As a surgeon, what can you do to improve wound healing?
14. Which factors increase the risk that the wound will become infected?
15. Bite wounds are considered contaminated as opposed to clean. Which endogenous flora are likely to contaminate wounds?
16. What else might bite wounds contain?
17. If bite wounds of dogs and cats are cultured, which organisms are likely to predominate?
18. How might you choose to deal with surface contamination prior to wound closure?
19. How might you choose to protect the wound prior to wound closure?
20. Pippen's wound was sustained less than 6–8 hours ago. How does this timeframe impact your plan of attack?
21. What is debridement?

Answers to Round One of Questions for Case 36: The Wounded Dog

1. You need Logan to share documentation with you concerning Pippen's vaccination status, specifically whether he has been vaccinated against rabies and whether his vaccination is up to date.

   Rabies can be transmitted to the victim in the biter's saliva.(1–3) Each overseeing body of authority in veterinary medicine provides guidance concerning the appropriate management of cases that might involve transmission of this fatal zoonotic disease.(4) For instance, within the United States, the American Veterinary Medical Association (AVMA) has established recommendations about how to handle bites in vaccinated and unvaccinated dogs and cats.(4, 5) If a bite wound is sustained on US soil and the victim of the attack is current on its rabies vaccination at the time of injury, then the victim should be revaccinated immediately and observed for 45 days.(1, 4) If, on the the other hand, the victim has never been vaccinated against rabies – and the rabies status of the biter is unknown – then humane euthanasia and subsequent testing is advised by the AVMA.(4) However, clinicians should consult with local and state regulations.(4, 5) Clients that refuse to euthanize may have the option of a 6-month quarantine, during which time the bite victim is vaccinated against rabies 1 month prior to release.(1, 4)

   At the same time that you are exploring Pippen's vaccination status, you will want to confirm the vaccination status of the biter. If the biter is currently up to date on its rabies vaccination, then Pippen will not need to have his rabies immunization boostered.

2. Immediate wound care involves triaging the wound at initial presentation, irrigating the wound, and protecting it until the wound can be properly managed.(6) This may be as simple as placing an Elizabethan collar on the patient so as to prevent the patient from contacting the wound, licking it, and inciting self-trauma.(6)

3. The purpose of immediate wound care is to prevent further injury and/or environmental contamination of the wound while awaiting wound repair.(6)

4. Lavage is a fancy way of describing the process of irrigating the wound to rid the tissues of gross contaminants.(6) At this stage of wound management, it is less important what you use to irrigate, in terms of sterility, and more important that you are generous with how much you use.(6) Volume is essential to remove particulate material from the wound bed.(6)

5. The following solutions are appropriate to use for lavage from the standpoint of not causing tissue damage:

    • sterile 0.09% saline
    • dilute (0.01–0.05%) chlorhexidine diacetate
    • dilute (0.1%) povidone iodine.

    In human healthcare trials, irrigation with tap water is equally effective at reducing contamination of wounds without increasing the chance of wound infection or damaging the tissue, despite its hypotonicity.(6)

6. The following solutions are inappropriate for use for lavage because of their potential for cytotoxicity:

    • acetic acid
    • alcohol
    • hydrogen peroxide.

7. Primary wound closure is the process of apposing wound edges with bandages, tissue glue, sutures, or staples to achieve so-called first intention healing.(6) Apposing wound edges makes the defect in skin integrity minimal.(6) Healing is relatively rapid because keratinocytes do not have to migrate very far to repair the gap.(6)

8. Delayed primary closure means that you postpone wound edge-to-edge apposition for 3 to 5 days.(6)

9. Delayed primary closure is helpful when the wound would benefit from additional de-contamination and/or debridement to maximize health of the wound bed prior to healing.(6)

10. Second intention healing refers to the process by which the wound is left to heal by its own devices, through contraction and epithelialization, without you taking measures to physically bring the wound edges together.(6)

11. Whether to leave a wound open or to actively take measures to close it depends upon a variety of factors including the following.(6, 7)

    • How contaminated the wound bed is – infection impedes healing.
    • How damaged the tissue at the wound bed is – necrotic tissue is difficult to heal because it has a poor blood supply.
    • How much time has passed between the actual wounding and the present.
    • The size of wound.
    • Species differences when it comes to healing:(8)

        • open wounds in cats heal more slowly than dogs
        • sutured wounds in cats are less strong than those at the same location in dogs.

12. The following factors impact wound healing:(6, 7, 9)

- Medications

    - Antineoplastic agents reduce wound tensile strength and slow fibroblast proliferation.
    - Corticosteroids cause atrophy of the epidermis and reduce wound tensile strength.

- The patient's age.
- The patient's nutritional status, particularly protein intake.

    - Protein is required to facilitate wound healing because protein comprises collagen.
    - Diets that are deficient in protein will slow wound healing, so you need to ask yourself the following questions.

        - Is the patient malnourished?
        - Does the patient have dietary deficiencies?
        - Does the patient have hypoproteinemia? (Serum TP <1.5–2.0 g/dL may impede healing; wounds that have healed will be less strong.)

- The patient's systemic health:(8)

    - Does the patient have diabetes mellitus?

        - The inflammatory response in human diabetic patients is blunted.
        - Human diabetic patients have impaired chemotaxis.
        - Human and veterinary diabetic patients are susceptible to secondary infections, which impede healing.

    - Does the patient have hepatopathy?

        - This may cause clotting factor deficiencies

    - Does the patient have hyperadrenocorticism?

        - These patients overproduce cortisol, which slows wound healing

    - Does the patient have an infectious disease?

        - feline immunodeficiency virus (FIV) [cats only]
        - feline leukemia virus (FeLV) [cats only]

    - Does the patient have uremia?

        - Patients that have elevated blood urea nitrogen (BUN) and creatinine, as from renal disease, are said to be azotemic.
        - Azotemia impairs wound healing.

- The temperature at the site of the wound, warmer temperatures hasten healing.
- Vascular supply to wound.
- Whether the tissue is edematous.
- Whether the tissue is infected.
- Wound location:(8)

    - How likely is it that you can close the wound successfully, as through suturing?
    - Will the suture line be under significant tension?
    - Will the suture line be exposed to excessive motion? e.g. wounds at the caudal elbow or cranial stifle are difficult to heal unless the associated joint is immobilized.
    - Will there be unacceptable dead space?

13. As a surgeon, you can improve healing by:(6, 7, 9)

- achieving hemostasis
- apposing tissues well
- eliminating dead space(8)
- handling tissue gently
- using aseptic technique.

14. The following factors increase the chance that the wound will become infected:(7, 10–14)

- breach in aseptic technique
- clipping the patient well in advance of the surgical procedure
- if wounded tissue is devitalized(11)
- if wounded tissue has previously been irradiated
- lengthy general anesthesia
- obesity (in human patients)
- poor patient prep of the surgical site
- prolonged hospital stays
- protracted surgical procedures
- shaving the surgical site instead of clipping(15–17)
- the presence of particulate matter, i.e. road debris, and other contamination
- using injectable propofol as the sole injection agent.

15. Wounds may become contaminated with endogenous microbial flora. The most likely offenders are *Staphlococcus* spp. and *Streptococcus* spp.(13)

16. Bite wounds are inoculated with bacteria from the biter's teeth.(18–20)

17. Bite wound bacteria are often a mix of aerobes and anaerobes.(18) The most common bacteria that is cultured from bite wounds of dogs and cats is *Pasteurella multocida*.(19, 20)

18. As part of immediate wound care, you may elect to manage surface contamination prior to wound closure by applying a broad-spectrum topical antimicrobial agent directly to the wound. (6, 8)

19. A clean, dry bandage is an optimal way to protect a wound during immediate wound care.(6)

20. Pippen's wound was sustained less than 6–8 hours ago. This means that you are still in the so-called "golden period" of wound care in which the wound is said to be contaminated, but not infected.(7) After 6–8 hours, bacterial numbers are expected to exceed 105 organisms, at which point the wound crosses over into the infected category.(7)

    It is optimal to initiate wound management within the golden period because the wound is at its cleanest and there is greater chance that the wound will knit together well.

    Because Pippen's wound is less than 6–8 hours old, it is ideal to lavage and debride it, followed by primary closure.(7)

21. Debridement is the removal of devitalized tissue from the wound.(7) Dead tissue is trimmed back until wound margins freshly bleed.(7) This improves the chance that wound edges will knit together.(7)

Returning to Case 36: The Wounded Dog

Pippen is placed under general anesthesia late this afternoon to undergo wound closure, after base-line bloodwork establishes that he is a stable candidate for surgical repair. Consider the following questions to assist you as you plan Pippen's procedure.

Round Two of Questions for Case 36: The Wounded Dog

1. Once Pippen is placed under general anesthesia, you instruct your technicians to initiate patient prep. What does this entail?
2. You need to remove fur from around your patient's wound in order to suture it closed. Which tool should you avoid?
3. How should you hold the clippers?
4. Which size clipping blade(s) is/are appropriate for fur removal?
5. How specifically should you clip the patient relative to the direction of fur growth?
6. What are two important considerations about the clipping blade that you need to keep in mind during fur removal?
7. Logan does not want Pippen to be bald and warns against excessive shaving. "It's just a little bite," he says. "I don't want you to shave half his body." What do you tell Logan? How much fur is appropriate to clip?
8. You could not fit Pippen into surgery for four hours after his initial presentation. Should your technicians have shaved Pippen four hours ago as opposed to now, in the perioperative period? Why or why not?
9. How do you protect the wound before your technicians shave Pippen?
10. What should you use to disinfect the blades after you have finished clipping Pippen?
11. Which disinfectants are not effective when used on clippers to inhibit bacterial growth?
12. Differentiate disinfectant from antiseptic. Which should you use on living tissue?
13. Which are commonly used products that are applied to the patient's skin to cleanse it during the initial prep if tissue is intact (i.e. to cleanse the ventrum of a dog that is undergoing ovariohysterectomy)?
14. Compare and contrast the products that you identified in Question #13 (above).
15. What should you use to rinse the scrub products that you identified in Question #13 (above) in cases where the patient's tissues are intact?
16. Pippen's tissue is not intact. His wound reflects exposed tissue. In this case, which materials are appropriate to use as part of the initial prep to cleanse the wound?
17. What should you use to rinse the cleansing solution(s) that you identified in Question #16 (above)?
18. Consider what you might do if Pippen's wound were near his eye. How do you protect the eye during the initial wound prep?
19. Patient skin prep works via contact time, not scrubbing. What is the appropriate contact time for the two products that you named in answer to Question #13 (above)?
20. How does the presence of organic material impact patient prep?

Answers to Round Two of Questions for Case 36: The Wounded Dog

1. Once Pippen is placed under general anesthesia, you instruct your technicians to initiate patient prep. Patient prep is essentially preparation of the surgical site for the procedure. This involves the following steps: (13)

- fur removal
- initial skin preparation
- patient positioning in the operating room
- sterile skin preparation
- draping the patient into surgery.

2. You should avoid fur removal with a razor.(13) Razors have the potential to cause micro-abrasions that can irritate the skin and potentiate infection at the surgical site.(13) It is preferred that you use clippers instead.(13)

3. A pencil grip is the appropriate way to handle clippers.(13)

4. A No. 40 blade is an effective means of shaving most patients.(13) A No. 10 blade precedes use with a No. 40 when the patient's coat is dense.(13)

5. To clip most efficiently, remove the bulk of the hair by clipping in the same direction as fur growth.(21) The closest shave is then obtained by clipping in the opposite direction.(21)

6. The clipping blade gets overheated easily. Be sure to check the blade's heat from time to time so that the patient does not experience thermal burns at the surgical site.

    In addition, blades need to be disinfected between uses, particularly after coming into contact with wounds or orifices, such as the anus or genitalia.(21) Blades can be fomites.(21) They can easily transmit microbes from patient to patient, causing nosocomial infections.(21) In particular, clippers may transfer the following microorganisms:(21)

- *Actinomyces*
- *E. coli*
- *Pseudomonas*
- *Staphylococcus.*

7. It is essential that you clip "enough" fur – not only to rid the surgical site of fur, but also to anticipate potential complications including the following.(13)

    - Having to extend the surgical site.

        - Many bite wounds look small, but when you surgically explore them, you find extensive pockets of dead space when the skin has been avulsed from underlying musculature.
        - You will need to be able to access any and all pockets of dead space within a sterile field, which means that you need to shave much more fur than it might seem on cursory glance.

    - Having to place surgical drains.

    It is a good rule of thumb to anticipate shaving any fur within 20 cm (7.9 in) of the incision.(13) Pippen may therefore look "bald" to Logan, but it is essential. The fur will regrow.

8. No, your technicians should not have shaved Pippen well in advance of his procedure. Doing so would have increased his risk of a surgical site infection (SSI).(13, 22) To reduce this risk, you should instruct your surgical team to clip immediately prior to surgery, as they are doing now.(13)

9. It is important that you protect the wound before your technicians shave Pippen so that the wound does not become even more contaminated with particulate matter, including fur. To protect the wound, you can pack it with sterile surgical lubricant and sterile gauze.

10. You can disinfect the clipping blades with one of the following products to inhibit bacterial growth:(21, 23, 24)

   - ethanol and phenylphenol based spray
   - 70% alcohol
   - 2% percent chlorhexidine solution.

11. The following solutions are not effective means of disinfecting the clipping blades:(21, 23, 24)

   - saline
   - isopropanol and phenylphenol
   - ethanol/dimethyl benzyl ammonium chloride/o-phenylphenol spray.

12. Disinfectants and antiseptics are both applied to surfaces to slow or stop the growth of microbes. The former are applied to non-living surfaces, such as exam room tables or clipper blades, whereas antiseptics are applied to living tissue, such as the patient's skin.

13. If tissue, such as skin, is intact, then it is typical to use one of the following antiseptics in undiluted form:(13)

   - chlorhexidine gluconate 4%
   - povidone iodine (betadine).

   These concentrates are typically called scrubs to reflect that they have not been diluted.

14. Chlorhexidine gluconate 4% is a broad-spectrum antiseptic that has residual activity up to 48 hours, as compared to povidone iodine, which is effective for 4–6 hours. Povidone iodine also has some activity against mycobacteria and viruses.(13) Povidone iodine is deactivated in the presence of organic material, such as pus and other exudate, whereas chlorhexidine is more resistant. (13) Povidone iodine stains and is more likely to cause a hypersensitivity reaction. Chlorhexidine is more readily tolerated by patients; however, there are certain regions of the body where its use is contraindicated. These include periocular tissue, mucous membranes (cats exhibit some sensitivity), and external ear canals in cases where the integrity of the tympanic membrane is questionable. Chlorhexidine can cause deafness in patients if it contacts the middle or inner ear.

15. When the patient's skin is intact, you can rinse in between scrubs with 70% isopropyl alcohol.

16. Because Pippen's tissues are exposed, it is inappropriate to use concentrates, such as scrubs. Instead, you should make use of solutions. Solutions are diluted preparations of scrubs. An example of an appropriate solution is 0.05 chlorhexidine gluconate.

17. Because Pippen's tissues are exposed, it is inappropriate to use isopropyl alcohol as a rinse. Instead, you should rinse with sterile physiologic (0.9%) sodium chloride.

18. If Pippen's wound were near his eye, then you should protect his eye during wound prep by applying lubricant. You also should avoid use of chlorhexidine around the eye, in scrub or solution form. A 1:50 dilution of betadine (0.2%) is the most appropriate cleanser, followed by a sterile physiologic saline rinse. Additionally, gauze should not be used during the scrubbing process because there is too great of a risk of corneal injury. Soft cotton balls are preferred.

19. Patient skin prep works via contact time, not scrubbing.(13) Two minutes is an appropriate contact time for either chlorhexidine gluconate or povidone iodine.

20. Povidone iodine is inactivated by organic material, such as pus and other exudates, whereas chlorhexidine gluconate is not.(13)

Returning to Case 36: The Wounded Dog

After the initial patient prep, Pippen is moved into the surgical suite to undergo the sterile prep.

Round Three of Questions for Case 36: The Wounded Dog

1. You ask your technician for a drape. He says that there are disposable drapes and cloth drapes. Provide advantages and disadvantages of each.
2. When you start Pippen's wound closure, you know that you need to freshen the wound's edges. What does freshen the wound's edges mean and why is this necessary?
3. One concern about bite wounds is their resultant dead space. What does this mean?
4. Why might dead space be a concern?
5. What might you do to eliminate dead space?
6. Your technician is gathering supplies to facilitate the procedure. You ask him to remember to obtain suture to close the wound. What are the ideal properties of suture?
7. How is suture characterized?
8. How do you ask your technician for "3–0 suture?" How is "3–0" pronounced?
9. Which size of suture, 1–0 or 4–0, is larger?
10. Which size of suture, 3–0 or 3, is larger?
11. Which advantages and potential challenges are associated with braided suture?
12. Which advantages and potential challenges are associated with monofilament suture?
13. You elect to place skin sutures (see **Plate 48**). Which characteristics of suture will you select given this decision?
14. You tell Logan that Pippen's skin sutures need to stay in for how many days?

Answers to Round Three of Questions for Case 36: The Wounded Dog

1. Disposable drapes come in a variety of shapes and sizes. They are non-fenestrated so that you can custom-cut an opening to fit the patient in terms of size and shape. They are also fluid-resistant. A potential disadvantage is cost.

    Cloth drapes are pre-sized and come with a pre-cut fenestration. Cloth drapes are less expensive than paper because they are reusable and reduce waste. However, there is a high labor cost associated with them because your surgical team has to prepare them for the next patient. This involves:

    - pre-cleaning to remove gross contamination
    - laundering with stain removal
    - tracking the number of washes because fabric breaks down over time
    - re-folding
    - re-packaging
    - sterilization.

2. Freshening the wound's edges is essentially the same as debridement. Dead tissue is trimmed back until wound margins freshly bleed.(7) This improves the chance that wound edges will knit together.(7)

3. Dead space is a defect that leaves a gap between two parts of the body where no gap should be. Bite wounds often create dead space because when teeth strike at acute angles, they create tensile force.(1, 25) This essentially separates the skin from the underlying musculature, and a pocket of space forms between the two layers.(1, 25)

4. Dead space is a concern for wound management because the body doesn't like empty spaces. It tends to fill them up. Dead space represents a perfect gap to fill with fluid. Dead spaces promote the formation of seromas and hematomas. Fluid accumulation delays healing and also provides a literal sea of favorable conditions in which to harbor infection.

5. To eliminate dead space, you can provide external bandage compression. You can also suture the wound closed and aspirate as needed.(8) Alternatively, you can insert a surgical drain.

6. The ideal suture would have the following properties:

   - affordability
   - associated with low capillary action – it does not wick or draw potential contaminants
   - ease of handling – it has minimal "memory," meaning that it does not kink based upon the way that it was stored in the package
   - good shelf life
   - knot security
   - minimal drag – it can be passed through tissues easily
   - minimally reactive within tissue – it incites minimal inflammation
   - tensile strength.

7. Suture is characterized according to the following properties:(26)

   - size (suture diameter)

     - size is based upon the standardized numbering system that has been established by the United States Pharmacopeia (USP) – suture ranges in size from size 12.0 to size 7

   - whether it is absorbable

     - absorbable suture is broken down by the patient's body, examples include: chromic gut, vicryl, PDS

   - whether it is braided or monofilament

     - braided suture contains many filaments that are bound together into one strand. these strands may or may not be coated with a substance to reduce drag, examples include silk, chromic gut, braunamid, vicryl, and nylon
     - monofilament suture is composed of a single extruded strand, examples include nylon and the polyester, poly (p-dioxanone), otherwise known as PDS.

   Note that some suture can be manufactured as either braided or monofilament. Nylon is a good example.

8. If you want to ask your technician for "3–0 suture," then you pronounce 3–0 as "three-oh" or "three-ought."

9. 1–0 is larger than 4–0 suture.(26)

10. 3 is larger than 3–0 suture.(26)

11. Braided suture is easier to handle than monofilament. It is soft and pliable, with good knot strength and security. Disadvantages of braided suture are that it more readily harbors bacteria and wicks contaminants. For this reason, you should generally avoid using braided suture to close the skin. You should also avoid using it to close internal hollow organs, such as the gastro-intestinal tract. In addition to its wicking potential, braided suture causes more drag when pulled through tissue, which means that braided suture is more traumatic than monofilament suture.

12. Monofilament suture is smooth, which means that it creates less drag than braided suture. Monofilament suture is therefore less traumatic to the tissues that are being sutured. Monofilament suture does not wick and does not harbor bacteria, so it is a good choice for closing skin and internal organs. Disadvantages of monofilament suture are that it is more challenging to handle because it contains "memory." This may reduce knot security. Cut ends are also more irritating than braided suture.

13. Skin sutures should be monofilament and non-absorbable.(8) Absorbable sutures would be more appropriate for use in intradermal patterns.(8)

14. You tell Logan that Pippen's skin sutures need to stay in for approximately 10–14 days, although the exact recommendations may vary depending upon suture type, wound location, and patient status.(26) For instance, debilitated patients often taken longer to heal, which means that sutures will need to stay in longer.(26)

CLINICAL PEARLS

- Bite wounds are a common clinical occurrence in veterinary practice. When they occur, we need to triage the patient first and then consider the optimal approach to the injury site based upon:

  - degree of wound contamination
  - duration: how long has the wound been present?
  - patient stability

  - tissue viability
  - vascular supply
  - wound location
  - wound size.

- Bite wounds are classified as contaminated rather than clean. Bite wounds contain microbial flora from the victim's skin as well as microbial flora from the biter's oral cavity. These pathogens can set up shop within the wound and establish potentially serious infections. Such infections may be already present at time of surgery, or surgical conditions (i.e. inadequate irrigation of the wound and/or breach in aseptic technique) may potentiate them.

- How wounds are managed prior to surgical exploration is essential for a positive patient outcome.

- Wound management also needs to take into consideration the potential for infectious diseases that can spread from the biter to the victim.

- Some of these infections are species-specific, i.e. FeLV and FIV.

- Other infections are not species-specific and in fact may have zoonotic potential, such as rabies virus.

- It is easy to overlook patient vaccination status during triage; however, knowing the vaccination status of the victim and the biter (whenever possible) is essential to mitigate the spread of rabies to animals and people alike.

- Word of mouth that suggests the patient is current on rabies prophylaxis is insufficient confirmation. Documentation is important. Without it, you are putting you and your team's health (and lives) on the line.

- Wounds that are sustained by an otherwise healthy patient and are <6–8 hours old are typically managed by lavage, debridement, and primary closure.

- Primary closure is delayed when the wound would benefit from additional decontamination prior to healing. Healing by second intention means that the wound is left open.

References

1. Holt DE, Griffin G. Bite wounds in dogs and cats. Vet Clin North Am Small Anim Pract 2000;30(3):669–79.
2. Pavletic MM, Trout NJ. Bullet, bite, and burn wounds in dogs and cats. Vet Clin North Am Small Anim Pract 2006;36(4):873–93.
3. Englar RE. Common clinical presentations in dogs and cats. Hoboken, NJ: Wiley/Blackwell; 2019.
4. Englar RE. Common clinical presentations in dogs and cats. Hoboken, NJ: Wiley/Blackwell; 2019.
5. AVMA model rabies control ordinance. American Veterinary Medical Association. Available from: https://www.avma.org/KB/Policies/Documents/avma-model-rabies-ordinance.pdf.
6. Hosgood G. Open wounds. Veterinary surgery: small animal. In: Tobias KM, Johnston SA, editors. Veterinary surgery: small animal. St. Louis, MO: Saunders; 2012.
7. Hedlund CS. Surgery of the integumentary system. In: Fossum TW, Duprey LP, O'Connor D, editors. Small animal surgery. 3rd ed. Boston, MA: Elsevier; 2007.
8. Fahie MA. Primary wound closure. In: Tobias KM, Johnston SA, editors. Veterinary surgery. St. Louis, MO: Saunders; 2012.
9. Tobias KM. Primary wound closure. In: Tobias KM, editor. Manual of small animal soft tissue surgery. Ames, IA: Wiley/Blackwell; 2010.
10. Shales C, editor. Surgical wound infection and antibiotic prophylaxis. WSAVA/FECAVA/BSAVA World Congress; 2012.
11. Zeltzman P; 2018. How to reduce surgical site infections. Veterinary Practice News [Internet]. Available from: https://www.veterinarypracticenews.com/how-to-reduce-surgical-site-infections/.
12. Brown C. Wound infections and antimicrobial use. In: Tobias KM, Johnston SA, editors. Veterinary surgery. St. Louis, MO: Saunders; 2012.
13. Fossum TW. Preparation of the operative site. In: Fossum TW, Duprey LP, O'Connor D, editors. Small animal surgery. 3rd ed. Boston, MA: Elsevier; 2007.
14. Fossum TW. Preparation of the surgical team. In: Fossum TW, Duprey LP, O'Connor D, editors. Small animal surgery. 3rd ed. Boston, MA: Elsevier; 2007.
15. Alexander JW, Fischer JE, Boyajian M, Palmquist J, Morris MJ. The influence of hair-removal methods on wound infections. Arch Surg 1983;118(3):347–52.
16. Balthazar ER, Colt JD, Nichols RL. Preoperative hair removal: a random prospective study of shaving versus clipping. South Med J 1982;75(7):799–801.
17. Ko W, Lazenby WD, Zelano JA, Isom OW, Krieger KH. Effects of shaving methods and intraoperative irrigation on suppurative mediastinitis after bypass operations. Ann Thorac Surg 1992;53(2):301–5.
18. Brook I. Management of human and animal bite wounds: an overview. Adv Skin Wound Care 2005;18(4):197–203.
19. Goldstein EJ, Richwald GA. Human and animal bite wounds. Am Fam Phys 1987;36(1):101–9.
20. Talan DA, Citron DM, Abrahamian FM, Moran GJ, Goldstein EJ. Bacteriologic analysis of infected dog and cat bites. Emergency Medicine Animal Bite Infection Study Group. N Engl J Med 1999;340(2):85–92.
21. Zeltzman P. Tips and tricks to clip like a pro. 2017. Available from: https://www.veterinarypracticenews.com/tips-and-tricks-to-clip-like-a-pro/.
22. Mangram AJ, Horan TC, Pearson ML, Silver LC, Jarvis WR. Guideline for prevention of surgical site infection, 1999. Hospital Infection Control Practices Advisory Committee. Infect Control Hosp Epidemiol 1999;20(4):250–78.
23. Ley B, Silverman E, Peery K, Dominguez D. Evaluation of commonly used products for disinfecting clipper blades in veterinary practices: A Pilot Study. J Am Anim Hosp Assoc 2016;52(5):277–80.
24. Mount R, Schick AE, Lewis TP, Newton HM. Evaluation of bacterial contamination of clipper blades in small animal private practice. J Am Anim Hosp Assoc 2016;52(2):95–101.
25. Trott A. Mechanisms of surface soft tissue trauma. Ann Emerg Med 1988;17(12):1279–83.
26. Fossum TW. Biomaterials, Suturing, and Hemostasis. In: Fossum TW, Duprey LP, O'Connor D, editors. Small animal surgery. 3rd ed. Boston, MA: Elsevier; 2007.

Case 37

The Collapsing Dog

Cleo, short for Cleopatra, is new to your practice. Her owner, Jackson Carter, has presented her to the overnight emergency service for what he describes as "a heart attack." When the technician meets him in the waiting area to triage Cleo and asks him to clarify what specifically he saw, Jackson says that Cleo "fell over" in the middle of chasing a frisbee in the backyard. One minute she was eagerly invested in the chase and the next, she was gone to the world.

He had called out to her, but she didn't respond. At least not initially. After what seemed like "forever," she suddenly "woke up." Her tail wagged when she caught sight of Jackson kneeling beside her, but she remained sedate.

For a dog that had never been ill a day before in her life, Cleo's episode was enough to give Jackson pause. So, he scooped her up in his arms, all 65 pounds of her, and carried her to the car because she seemed too weak to stand on her own.

Jackson drove straight here. To his knowledge, she hasn't lost consciousness since the episode, but this is the quietest that she's ever been in the car, and that alarms him. The technician takes Cleo's vital signs and tells Jackson that you'll be right there.

Consider the following questions as you prepare to initiate this consultation.

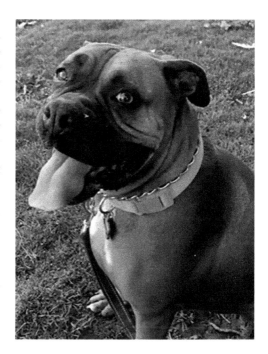

Figure 37.1 Meet your patient, Cleo, a 5-year-old female spayed Boxer dog. Courtesy of Troy Holder, DVM.

Round One of Questions for Case 37: The Collapsing Dog

1. What is the normal reference range for heart rate (HR) in an adult dog?
2. How does Cleo's HR compare to normal?
3. Where do you routinely assess mucous membrane color in the dog?
4. What color should Cleo's mucous membranes be?
5. Which colors of mucous membranes are considered abnormal?

Weight: 65.0 lb (29.5 kg)
BCS: 6/9
Mentation: Depressed

TPR

T: 101.7°F (38.7°C)
P: 265 beats per minute
R: 30 breaths per minute

Mucous membrane color: Pale pink

Capillary refill time (CRT): 3 seconds

6. What might explain the change that you see in Carly's mucous membranes?
7. What does capillary refill time (CRT) measure?
8. How do you assess CRT?
9. Which CRT is considered normal in a healthy adult dog?
10. How might you explain the change in Cleo's CRT?
11. When a patient presents with a history of collapse, one of two body systems is likely to be involved. Which two systems will you prioritize in your investigation?
12. Drawing from the two systems that you choose to prioritize in Question #11 (above), what are the top two differential diagnoses for collapse?
13. The two differential diagnoses that you identified in Question #12 are often hard to discern from one another. Which clinical signs might help you to differentiate between the two?
14. You have been provided with an abbreviated history. Which differential diagnosis are you leaning toward based upon the information that you have been given?
15. Which differential diagnosis are you leaning towards based upon the patient's signalment?
16. Which differential diagnosis are you leaning towards based upon the patient's vital signs?
17. You examine Cleo and find that her pulses are weak. There are also occasional pulse deficits. Where do you feel for a pulse in a dog?
18. What is pulse?
19. What is pulse quality?
20. What determines pulse quality?
21. What do bounding pulses mean?
22. What do weak pulses signify?
23. True or false: For every heartbeat, there should be a palpable pulse.
24. What is a pulse deficit and what does it mean?
25. Based upon this new information, what is an essential step in the diagnostic process?

Answers to Round One of Questions for Case 37: The Collapsing Dog

1. Reference ranges vary somewhat depending upon which resource(s) you drawn upon. In addition, the normal reference range for canine HR is dependent upon the size of the dog. In general, the HR ranges between:(1–4)

    • 60–100 beats per minute in large-breed dogs, such as Cleo
    • 80–120 beats per minute in medium-breed dogs
    • 90–140 beats per minute in small-breed dogs.

2. Cleo's HR is significantly elevated. She has tachycardia.

3. In clinical practice, the gingiva (the gums) are commonly used to assess mucous membrane color.(1, 2) However, when the gums are not accessible because of patient temperament, the clinician can assess the color of the conjunctival sac.(1, 2) The clinician may also evaluate a dog's mucous membrane color by assessing the color of the vulvar lips (in Cleo) or the inner lining of the prepuce (if Cleo were male).

4. Cleo's mucous should be a healthy pink.(1, 2) However, some patients have black pigment throughout their gums or mottled black and pink gums.(1, 2) This is considered to be a variation of normal.(1, 2)

5. The following colors are not considered normal if they are associated with canine or feline mucous membranes:(1, 2, 5)

    • white
    • pale pink
    • cherry red

    • cyanotic (blue-purple)
    • dark red or brick red
    • icteric (yellow).

6. Pale mucous membranes typically indicate one of two things. Either Cleo is in shock or she is anemic.(1, 2, 5)

7. CRT is one way to assess the patient's circulation.(1, 2)

8. The clinician uses his finger or the end of a tongue depressor to press down on the gingiva firmly – typically at the level of the maxillary canine.(1, 2) This action forces blood out of the capillaries where pressure has been applied.(1, 2) The site will blanch under the pressure.(1, 2) When the clinician releases pressure, blood returns to the capillaries, restoring normal mucous membrane color.(1, 2)

9. A healthy adult dog should have a CRT of 1–2 seconds.(1, 2) This means that within 1–2 seconds of releasing your fingertip from the gingiva, where you were applying pressure, the mucous membranes should pink up.(1, 2) Circulation has thus been restored.

10. The fact that Cleo's CRT is prolonged means that she is in shock or dehydrated, or both.(1, 2) In either of these circumstances, blood is slower to refill, hence the delay in CRT.(1, 2)

11. When a patient presents with a history of collapse, I prioritize my evaluation of the cardiovascular and neurological systems.(1, 2)

12. When I consider the cardiovascular and neurological systems as causing collapse, then my top two diagnoses are syncope or seizure activity.(1, 2, 6–10)
    Syncope may be:(1, 2, 7)

- cardiogenic

  - the most common cause of syncope in companion animal patients
  - results from insufficient cardiac output because there has been a structural or functional change within the heart(7)

- hypotensive:(7)

  - drug-induced vasodilation
  - hypovolemic shock:

    - blood loss
    - diarrhea
    - diuresis
    - vomiting

- neural-mediated:

  - poorly understood
  - more commonly occurs in people in response to emotional shock, such as a phobia, or a specific trigger like the sight of blood(7, 11)
  - less commonly occurs in dogs, but can, particularly if their body has been cued for "fight or flight"(11)
  - other precipitating events in dogs may include:(7, 11)

    - agitation
    - barking
    - coughing
    - defecation
    - pain
    - vomiting.

Seizures are distinct from syncopal events.(1, 2) Seizures are caused by a surge of electrical activity from the central nervous system (CNS) in which there is an imbalance between excitatory and inhibitory impulses.(1, 2, 12–14)

509

13. Collapse may be due to syncope or seizures.(1, 2, 6–10, 15) These episodes may appear to be visually similar, particularly if witnessed by a novice or someone who is not in the medical field. (1, 2, 10, 16–18)

Syncope ("fainting") occurs due to a lapse in perfusion of the brain.(7) This causes weakness and/or ataxia just before the patient passes out.(7) The episode is brief in duration.(7) Patients are most often flaccid when they collapse, only to promptly rise again as if everything is normal.(7)

Generalized seizures, on the other hand, are characterized by stiffness rather than flaccidity. (19) The limbs tend to be toned.(19) Opisthotonus and extensor rigidity are common, and, if present, tonic-clonic actions cause the limbs to appear as if they are paddling.(20, 21)

Autonomic activity during a generalized seizure is common.(19) Patients often lose bladder and bowel function.(20, 21)

Many patients will also perform one or more of the following unconscious actions during a generalized seizure:(2, 22)

- chewing actions
- grinding teeth
- licking at the air
- swallowing hard
- vocalizing.

Seizures often last longer than syncope, and seizing patients take more time to recover.(7) There is a so-called post-ictal period after a seizure, during which time the patient acts mentally "off."(21, 22) This recovery phase is variable in duration, but typically is on the order of minutes to hours.(21, 22) During this time, patients may exhibit one or more of the following clinical signs:(2, 13, 21–25)

- ataxia
- blindness
- circling or pacing
- disorientation.

14. Based upon my answer to Question #13 and the history that Jackson provided, I am leaning towards syncope rather than seizure activity. Cleo was fine immediately before the episode, and although she has acted weak following the event, her mentation has been normal. She also did not appear to exhibit autonomic activity during the short-lived episode, which would have been expected had she experienced a generalized seizure.

15. The patient is a middle-aged Boxer dog. This breed and age group is predisposed to cardiac disease.(15, 26, 27) Specifically, Boxers are at greater risk for development of arrhythmogenic right ventricular cardiomyopathy (ARVC), which is sometimes referred to as Boxer dog cardiomyopathy.(26–30) The condition is inherited in Boxer dogs as an autosomal dominant trait.(26, 27, 31)

Although I may be incorrect with my presumption, pattern recognition gives me a starting point.(32, 33) My clinical experience allows me to make associations between new patient presentations and past events to guide my diagnostic approaches.(32–34)

16. The patient is significantly tachycardic, not just borderline, with a prolonged CRT. Neither change from the normal reference range for healthy dogs can be explained by a seizure disorder, but both can be explained by shock and/or heart disease.

17. The most common site of pulse detection in the dog is the femoral artery, which runs bilaterally in the creases of the inner thighs.(1)

18. The pulse is a wave generated by ventricular contraction within the heart, during which blood forcibly passes from the left ventricle of the heart to the aorta.(1) What is felt as the pulse is the peripheral artery stretching to accommodate incoming blood.(1, 35)

19. Pulse quality refers to how strong or weak a pulse is on palpation.(1)

20. How strong or weak a pulse is depends upon the difference between systolic and diastolic BPs. (1) The greater the difference, the stronger the pulse.(1) The weaker the difference, the poorer the pulse.(1, 35)

21. "Bounding" pulses are more pronounced than is typical.(1, 5) These result from a reduction in diastolic pressure, an elevation in systolic pressure, or both.(1, 5, 35)

22. Weak pulses are caused by a reduction in systolic pressure, an elevation in diastolic pressure, or both (1, 5, 35). Sometimes these pulses may be called "thready" to reflect that they are the opposite of strong.(1)

23. True, for every heartbeat, there should be a palpable pulse.(1, 2)

24. A pulse deficit means that sometimes there is not a palpable pulse for every heartbeat.(1) In other words, the pulses are not synchronous with HR.(1) This means that there are so-called "dropped beats" of the heart as can occur with cardiac arrhythmias.(1) When contraction of the heart occurs prematurely due to the electrical activity of an ectopic focus, the ventricles may not have had a chance to fill such that ventricular output is reduced.(1) The resultant stroke volume may be insufficient to translate into a palpable pulse.(1, 36)

25. Based upon this new information, an electrocardiogram (ECG, EKG) is an essential step in the diagnostic process.(1, 15) We need to explore what is happening at the level of the heart. Why is the patient tachycardic to the degree that she is and why are the pulse deficits there?
    We may also elect to perform cardiac imaging to evaluate changes in the structure of the heart in the presence of underlying dysfunction.(15)

Returning to Case 37: The Collapsing Dog

You share your concerns with Jackson that Cleo essentially passed out from an underlying issue that you need to get to the bottom of right away. Because of Cleo's history of acute collapse, depression, pale mucous membranes, tachycardia, weak pulses, pulse deficits, and prolonged CRT, you are particularly concerned about Cleo's cardiovascular system. You recommend that an electrocardiogram (ECG) be performed on Cleo to explore possible etiologies that involve her heart. Jackson consents to this diagnostic test. Two still images of Cleo's ECG are provided in Figures 37.2 and 37.3 for you to review.

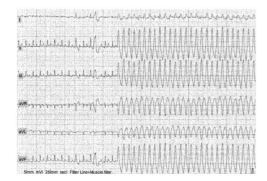

Figure 37.2 Jackson's ECG – Part 1. Courtesy of Jennifer Mulz, DVM, DACVIM (Cardiology).

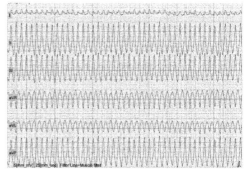

Figure 37.3 Jackson's ECG – Part 2. Courtesy of Jennifer Mulz, DVM, DACVIM (Cardiology).

Round Two of Questions for Case 37: The Collapsing Dog

1. What, in broad terms, does an ECG measure?
2. Which measurements can you take from an ECG that can facilitate diagnosis making?
3. Sometimes you need to pair an ECG with an echocardiogram. What is this diagnostic tool?
4. What kind of information does an echocardiogram give you that you cannot obtain from an ECG?
5. Prior to performing Cleo's ECG, you told Jackson that you suspected syncope. What are the pathophysiologic mechanisms that lead to cardiogenic syncope?
6. Which of the mechanisms that you identified in Question #5 (above) can an ECG screen for?
7. Of the mechanisms that you listed in Question #6 (above), what do you suspect to find on Cleo's ECG?
8. Which abnormal finding(s) do you see in Cleo's ECG?
9. What is the impact of the abnormal finding(s) on the patient?
10. Can Cleo's ECG explain her acute history of collapse?
11. What is Cleo at risk for?
12. Given that Cleo is hemodynamically unstable at this time, you initiate treatment with an anti-arrhythmic drug. Which anti-arrhythmic will you administer based upon Cleo's ECG findings?
13. What is the recommended dose of the drug that you identified in Question #12 (above)?
14. Based upon Cleo's weight, how many mg will you administer?

Answers to Round Two of Questions for Case 37: The Collapsing Dog

1. An ECG measures the electrical activity of the heart.(37–39) This allows you to evaluate a patient's heart rhythm and to characterize it as being normal or abnormal.(37–39)

2. An ECG allows you to track the cardiac cycle by featuring the following aspects on paper:(37–41)

    - the patient's P wave – atrial depolarization
    - the patient's PR interval – how long it takes for the impulse to be conducted to the ventricles from the sinoatrial node
    - the patient's QRS complex – ventricular depolarization
    - the patient's T wave – ventricular repolarization.

    The presence or absence of wave forms and/or complexes is readily apparent on the ECG and can shed light into potential cardiac dysfunction.(37)

    Changes in height or duration of wave forms or complexes can indicate chamber enlargement and/or abnormalities in conduction.(37, 39)

    You can also calculate the patient's HR from the ECG.(37)

3. An echocardiogram is an ultrasound of the heart.(42)

4. During an echocardiogram, high-frequency sound waves are used to image the heart in such a way that you can view the heart pumping as chambers contract and relax in real-time.(38, 42) The echocardiogram provides greater detail than the ECG in terms of the structure of the heart. The ECG can predict chamber enlargement.(39) However, the echocardiogram allows you to physically measure the degree to which the chamber is dilated or the degree to which the chamber wall is thickened, how rapid blood flow is in terms of velocity per second, and whether blood flow is moving in the right direction.(42)

5. Prior to performing Cleo's ECG, we suspected syncope. The pathophysiologic mechanisms that lead to cardiogenic syncope include:(2, 43)

- bradyarrhythmias:
    - associated with bradycardia, that is, a low HR(44)
    - the patient's HR may be consistently slow or the patient may experience pauses in the normal heart rhythm(44, 45)
    - examples include:(7, 45–49)
        - atrial standstill
        - atrioventricular (A-V) heart block
        - sick sinus syndrome
- outflow obstructions, i.e. pulmonary hypertension, stenotic valves
- reduced ability of the myocardium to contract, i.e. dilated cardiomyopathy (DCM)
- reduced filling of the heart with blood – conditions that reduce pre-load, i.e. pericardial effusion
- tachyarrhythmias:
    - associated with tachycardia, that is, an elevated HR(44)
    - the patient's HR may be consistently fast or the patient may experience bursts of tachycardia interposed between periods of normal heart rhythm(44, 45)
    - examples include:(3, 44, 45, 50–54)
        - atrial fibrillation
        - atrial flutter
        - supraventricular tachycardia
        - ventricular fibrillation
        - ventricular tachycardia.

6. An ECG can detect bradyarrhythmias and tachyarrhythmias.(38–41, 43, 55–57)

7. Of the mechanisms that I listed in my answer to Question #6 (above), I would expect to find that Cleo has a tachyarrhythmia.

8. I see a ventricular premature complex (VPC) in Figure 37.2 followed by a run of ventricular tachycardia ("v tach") that continues throughout Figure 37.3. This configuration of v tach is referred to as torsades de points (see Figure 37.4).

    VPCs have a characteristic wave form on the ECG that makes them relatively easy to spot:(39–41, 55, 56)

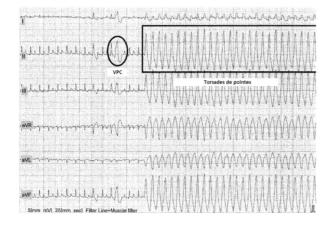

Figure 37.4 Jackson's ECG – Part 1 – with abnormalities circled and defined. Original photograph is courtesy of Jennifer Mulz, DVM, DACVIM (Cardiology). I amended the photograph to highlight the problem areas.

- QRS complexes are not associated with P waves
- QRS complexes are considered "wide and bizarre"
- polarity of the T wave may be reversed.

Isolated VPCs may or may not be associated with heart disease. In people, they have been associated with increased stress, increased caffeine consumption, and the use of certain medications.

When the patient's HR exceeds 100 beats per minutes and VPCs occur in runs, the patient is said to experience ventricular tachycardia.(39–41, 55, 56) Ventricular tachycardia is characterized as having an abnormally rapid HR that originates within the ventricles.(2) Ventricular contractions occur independently of atrial contractions.(2) Patients with v tach do have appreciable cardiac disease and are at risk for developing ventricular fibrillation.(39)

9. Tissue perfusion is markedly reduced during bouts of ventricular tachycardia.(2, 43)

10. Yes, Cleo's ECG explain her acute history of collapse. Syncope results from diminished perfusion of the brain.(29–31, 58)

11. Cleo is at risk for sudden death.(43, 55)

12. I will administer lidocaine as an intravenous (IV) bolus.(43, 55)

13. The recommended dose of lidocaine, when administered as an IV bolus, is 2 mg/kg.

14. Based upon Cleo's weight, I will administer:

$$29.5 \text{ kg} \times (2 \text{ mg/kg lidocaine}) = 59 \text{ mg}$$

Returning to Case 37: The Collapsing Dog

After administering a lidocaine bolus, Cleo's ventricular tachycardia resolved. Cleo was started on a continuous rate infusion (CRI) of lidocaine for the next 24 hours. An echocardiogram was performed the next morning and was negative for structural abnormalities. Systolic function was deemed normal.

Cleo was weaned off the CRI that evening while undergoing continuous ECG monitoring in-hospital. Ventricular tachycardia did not recur.

Cleo was discharged to the care of her owner with a prescription for sotalol and instructions to return for a recheck examination in two to three weeks following Holter monitoring.

Round Three of Questions for Case 37: The Collapsing Dog

1. Why was a CRI necessary if the lidocaine bolus was effective?
2. Why was sotalol prescribed to Cleo? What is it and what will it do?
3. What is Holter monitoring and why is it advantageous?
4. What will you be looking for when you evaluate the results from Cleo's Holter monitoring?
5. Jackson is concerned that Cleo could have another episode. What do you tell him?
6. If sotalol alone is ineffective, what could you prescribe as an add-on therapy?
7. Jackson read online that dogs with syncope are at risk of sudden death. What do you say?
8. Jackson wants to know what caused Cleo's condition. What is your top differential diagnosis?
9. Describe the condition that you identified in Question #8 (above)?
10. Are Boxers the only dogs to develop the condition that you identified in Question #8?

Answers to Round Three of Questions for Case 37: The Collapsing Dog

1. The half-life of lidocaine is short (just a few hours) so if you want the patient to benefit from this drug for an extended period of time, then you need to administer a CRI after the IV bolus has resolved v tach.(43, 59)

2. Sotalol is an anti-arrhythmic drug that exerts effects on the heart by blocking potassium channels.(43, 59) In addition, the drug has beta-adrenergic blocking potential.(43, 59)

    Although sotalol has not been proven to prevent sudden death in Boxers with heart disease, sotalol reduces the frequencies of VPCs.(43, 55) The hope is that if you reduce their occurrence, then the patient is less likely to launch into runs of VPCs that could potentiate ventricular fibrillation.

3. Holter monitoring is continuous ambulatory electrocardiography.(2, 60) It allows the patient to be hooked up to an ECG monitor for extended periods of times, which overcomes the limitations of the standard in-house ECG, which is more of a spot-check.(2, 60) On average, the in-clinic ECG records three minutes of cardiac activity. This represents a mere 0.2% of cardiac depolarizations within a 24 hour period.(61) It is not uncommon for this spot-check to be normal.(62) This is concerning because many arrhythmias are transient.(60, 61) They may go undetected if only in-clinic ECG is used as a diagnostic tool.(60, 62) This diagnostic delay puts the patient at increased risk, particularly for dogs with syncope that are at risk for sudden death, such as dogs with arrhythmogenic right ventricular cardiomyopathy (ARVC).(26–28, 63–66)

    Unlike in-clinic ECGs, Holter monitors provide continuous recordings so that clinicians can track electrical activity of the heart over the course of one or more days. Cardiac arrhythmias are more likely to be identified or excluded as the cause for the patient's clinical signs.(67) In addition, the patient's response to treatment is better assessed.

    Holter monitoring of both dogs and cats has been described.(60, 61, 67–76)

4. I will quantify VPCs and runs of VPCs when evaluating the results from Cleo's Holter monitoring. As monitoring persists over the course of several months, I will assess her response to treatment. The goal of treatment with oral medications, such as sotalol, is to reduce how often ventricular ectopy occurs by 85%.(43)

5. I would tell Jackson that, yes, unfortunately Cleo could have another episode of syncope at any time. Therapy is not curative. The hope is that therapy will reduce the episodes, rather than eliminate them.

6. If sotalol alone is ineffective, I could prescribe mexiletine an add-on therapy. Mexiletine is a sodium-channel blocker.(43, 55, 59) Patients that are still refractory to treatment may require additional treatment with procainamide or amiodarone.(55)

7. Unfortunately, yes, what Jackson read is true. Dogs with syncope are at risk of sudden death. (26, 27)

8. The top differential diagnosis for Cleo is ARVC, otherwise known as Boxer dog cardiomyopathy. (26–30)

9. ARVC was identified in the 1980s as a disease of Boxer dogs.(26–28) Dogs with ARVC develop cardiac muscle atrophy and fatty infiltrates within the heart.(26–30) This leads to dysfunctional cardiac tissue that is predisposed to ventricular arrhythmias.(43)

The condition is genetic in Boxer dogs and is characterized as an autosomal dominant trait. (26, 27, 31) The trait codes for a mutation in the striatin gene, which results in structurally weak connections between desmosomes in affected dogs.(27, 77) Connectivity is essential for effective communication between myocytes. Without intact connections between desmosomes, conversations between myocytes fall apart and the electrical activity of the heart decompensates.(27)

ARVC is also characterized by a mutation in the cardiac ryanodine receptor, which is involved with calcium channels activity and therefore excitation-contraction coupling in the heart.(78, 79) This has profound effect on ventricular function, in particular, the right ventricle, causing inefficiency of the heart as a pump.(79)

Affected dogs fit into one of three categories:(2, 26–28)

- asymptomatic:

    - incidental findings of occasional VPCs on ECG

- symptomatic:

    - history of exercise intolerance
    - history of syncope
    - evidence of tacchyarrhythmias, e.g. ventricular tachycardia

- symptomatic, with congestive heart failure (CHF) secondary to systolic dysfunction and ventricular dilation.

Cleo is classified as symptomatic.

10. No, Boxer dogs are not the only ones to develop ARVC. Although rare, ARVC has also been reported in a handful of case reports involving cats.(80, 81)

CLINICAL PEARLS

- A history of acute collapse in a companion animal patient should prompt you to consider syncope versus seizure activity.

- Syncope and seizure activity may be difficult for clients to distinguish. Therefore, it is essential that you take a thorough history to clarify what actions they observed to guide your diagnostic approach.

    - Patients with syncope tend to be flaccid during the event. Syncopal events tend to be brief. They are not associated with autonomic activity.
    - Patients that experience generalized seizure activity tend to be stiff during the event. Seizures may be protracted. One episode may blend immediately into another. Seizures do tend to be associated with autonomic activity. Patients may lose control over their bladder and bowels during a seizure. They may exhibit tonic-clonic actions. Following the seizure, there is a post-ictal or recovery phase, during which time the patient is disoriented. The patient may exhibit ataxia, blindness, circling, or pacing.

- It is critical to pair a thorough patient history with a comprehensive physical exam.

- Physical exam findings that are vital to the assessment of the cardiovascular system include:

    - HR
    - mucous membrane color
    - CRT

    - pulse presence/absence and synchrony
    - pulse strength or quality
    - pulse deficits.

- Tachycardia, pale mucous membranes, and prolonged CRT are suggestive of shock and/or cardiac disease.

- The presence of an arrhythmia requires further investigation. An electrocardiogram (ECG) is an important diagnostic tool for the evaluation of arrhythmias because it diagrams the electrical activity of the heart.

- An in-clinic ECG is an important starting point, but only captures a snapshot in time.

- Continuous ambulatory electrocardiography captures extended periods of time, which enhances diagnostic capabilities as well as monitoring response to treatment.

References

1. Englar RE. Performing the small animal physical examination. Hoboken, NJ: Wiley/Blackwell; 2017.
2. Englar RE. Common clinical presentations in dogs and cats. Hoboken, NJ: Wiley/Blackwell; 2019.
3. Ettinger SJ, Feldman EC, Côté E. Textbook of veterinary internal medicine: diseases of the dog and the cat. 8th ed. St. Louis, MO: Elsevier; 2017.
4. Côté E. Clinical veterinary advisor. Dogs and cats. 3rd ed. St. Louis, MO: Elsevier Mosby; 2015.
5. Hogan DF. Cardiac examination and history. Clinician's. Brief 2008 (July).
6. Kraus MS, editor. Syncope in small-breed dogs. ACVIM; 2003.
7. Schwartz DS, editor. The syncopal dog. World Small Animal Veterinary Association World Congress Proceedings; Sao Paulo, Brazil; 2009.
8. Thawley V, Silverstein D. Collapse. NAVC Clin's Brief 2012 (November):14–5.
9. Estrada A. Differentiating syncope from seizure. NAVC Clin's Brief 2017 (July):50–5.
10. Dutton E, Dukes-McEwan J, Cripps PJ. Serum cardiac troponin I in canine syncope and seizures. J Vet Cardiol 2017;19(1):1–13.
11. Kraus MS. Syncope: diagnosis and treatment. Available from: https://d12geb6i3t2qxg.cloudfront.net/webinar_resources/uploads/2017/01/Syncope_Diagnosis_and_Treatment_Marc_Kraus.pdf.
12. Tilley LP, Smith FWK. The 5-minute veterinary consult: canine and feline. 3rd ed. Baltimore, MD: Lippincott Williams & Wilkins; 2004.
13. De Risio L, Bhatti S, Muñana K, Penderis J, Stein V, Tipold A, et al. International veterinary epilepsy task force consensus proposal: diagnostic approach to epilepsy in dogs. BMC Vet Res 2015;11:148.
14. Fisher RS, van Emde Boas W, Blume W, Elger C, Genton P, Lee P, Engel J. Epileptic seizures and epilepsy: definitions proposed by the International League Against Epilepsy (ILAE) and the International Bureau for Epilepsy (IBE). Epilepsia 2005;46(4):470–2.
15. Mandese WW, Estrada AH. The clinical cardiology history and diagnostics. Clin's Brief 2017 (May).
16. Penning VA, Connolly DJ, Gajanayake I, McMahon LA, Luis Fuentes V, Chandler KE, Volk HA. Seizure-like episodes in 3 cats with intermittent high-grade atrioventricular dysfunction. J Vet Intern Med 2009;23(1):200–5.
17. Motta L, Dutton E. Suspected exercise-induced seizures in a young dog. J Small Anim Pract 2013;54(4):213–8.
18. Barnett L, Martin MW, Todd J, Smith S, Cobb M. A retrospective study of 153 cases of undiagnosed collapse, syncope or exercise intolerance: the outcomes. J Small Anim Pract 2011;52(1):26–31.
19. Englar RE. Common clinical presentations in dogs and cats. Hoboken, NJ: Wiley/Blackwell; 2019.
20. Lavely JA. Pediatric seizure disorders in dogs and cats. Vet Clin North Am Small Anim Pract 2014;44(2):275–301.
21. Thomas WB. Idiopathic epilepsy in dogs and cats. Vet Clin North Am Small Anim Pract 2010;40(1):161–79.
22. Mariani CL. Terminology and classification of seizures and epilepsy in veterinary patients. Top Companion Anim Med 2013;28(2):34–41.
23. Berendt M, Gram L. Epilepsy and seizure classification in 63 dogs: a reappraisal of veterinary epilepsy terminology. J Vet Intern Med 1999;13(1):14–20.
24. Pákozdy A, Leschnik M, Tichy AG, Thalhammer JG. Retrospective clinical comparison of idiopathic versus symptomatic epilepsy in 240 dogs with seizures. Acta Vet Hung 2008;56(4):471–83.

25. Patterson EE, Armstrong PJ, O'Brien DP, Roberts MC, Johnson GS, Mickelson JR. Clinical description and mode of inheritance of idiopathic epilepsy in English springer spaniels. J Am Vet Med Assoc 2005;226(1):54–8.

26. Meurs KM. Boxer dog cardiomyopathy: an update. Vet Clin North Am Small Anim Pract 2004;34(5):1235–44.

27. Meurs KM. Arrhythmogenic right ventricular cardiomyopathy in the Boxer dog: an update. Vet Clin North Am Small Anim Pract 2017;47(5):1103–11.

28. Palermo V, Stafford Johnson MJ, Sala E, Brambilla PG, Martin MW. Cardiomyopathy in Boxer dogs: a retrospective study of the clinical presentation, diagnostic findings and survival. J Vet Cardiol 2011;13(1):45–55.

29. Harpster N. Boxer cardiomyopathy. In: Kirk R, editor. Current veterinary therapy VIII. Philadelphia, PA: W.B. Saunders; 1983. p. 329–37.

30. Harpster NK. Boxer cardiomyopathy. A review of the long-term benefits of antiarrhythmic therapy. Vet Clin North Am Small Anim Pract 1991;21(5):989–1004.

31. Meurs KM, Spier AW, Miller MW, Lehmkuhl L, Towbin JA. Familial ventricular arrhythmias in boxers. J Vet Intern Med 1999;13(5):437–9.

32. Maddison J. Clinical reasoning skills. In: Hodgson JL, Pelzer JM, editors. Veterinary medical education: a practical guide. Hoboken, NJ: John Wiley and Sons; 2017.

33. Englar R. Writing skills for veterinarians. Sheffield: 5M Publishing; 2019.

34. May SA. Clinical reasoning and case-based decision making: the fundamental challenge to veterinary educators. J Vet Med Educ 2013;40(3):200–9.

35. Gompf RE. The history and physical examination. In: Tilley LP, Smith FWK, Oyama MA, Sleeper MM, editors. Manual of canine and feline cardiology. St. Louis: Elsevier Saunders; 2008. p. 2–23.

36. Cote E, Harpster NK. Feline cardiac arrhythmias. In: Kirk RW, editor. Kirk's current veterinary therapy XIV. St. Louis, MO: Elsevier Saunders; 2009. p. 731–9.

37. Green HW. Reading electrocardiograms. Clin's Brief 2010 (November).

38. Smith FWK, Tilley LP, Oyama MA, Sleeper MM. Manual of canine and feline cardiology. 5th ed. St. Louis, MO: Elsevier; 2016.

39. Smith FWK, Tilley LP. Manual of canine and feline cardiology. In: Smith FWK, Tilley LP, Oyama MA, Sleeper MM, editors. Manual of canine and feline cardiology. 5th ed. St. Louis, MO: Elsevier; 2016.

40. Bulmer B. Interpreting ECGs with confidence: Part 1. Clin's Brief 2012 (May).

41. Bulmer B. Interpreting ECGs with confidence: Part 2. Clin's. Brief 2012 (June).

42. Fuentes VL. Echocardiography and Doppler ultrasound. In: Smith FWK, Tilley LP, Oyama MA, Sleeper MM, editors. Manual of canine and feline cardiology. 5th ed. St. Louis, MO: Elsevier; 2016.

43. Leach S. Ventricular tachycardia. Clin's Brief 2016 (May).

44. DeFrancesco TC. Management of cardiac emergencies in small animals. Vet Clin North Am Small Anim Pract 2013;43(4):817–42.

45. Bulmer B. Interpreting ECGs with confidence: Part 2. NAVC Clin's Brief 2012 (June):102–5.

46. Scansen BA. Interventional cardiology for the criticalist. J Vet Emerg Crit Care (San Antonio) 2011;21(2):123–36.

47. Strickland KN. Congenital heart disease. In: Tilley LP, Smith FWK, Oyama MA, Sleeper MM, editors. Manual of canine and feline cardiology. 4th ed. Philadelphia, PA: W. B. Saunders; 2008. p. 215–39.

48. Bulmer BJ. The cardiovascular system. In: Peterson ME, Kutzler MA, editors. Small animal pediatrics: the first 12 months of life. St. Louis, MO: Saunders/Elsevier; 2011. p. 289–304.

49. Englar RE. Performing the small animal physical examination. Hoboken, NJ: Wiley; 2017

50. Bulmer B. Management tree: tachyarrhythmia NAVC Clin's Brief 2012 (June);107.

51. French A, editor. Arrhythmias: recognition and treatment. Dublin, Ireland: World Small Animal Veterinary Congress; 2008.

52. MacDonald K. Get with the beat! Analysis and treatment of cardiac arrhythmias. DVM 2009;360.

53. Jones A, Estrada A. Top 5 arrhythmias in dogs and cats. NAVC Clin's Brief 2014 (January):94–100.

54. Stepien RL, editor. Emergency arrhythmias. British Small Animal Veterinary Congress; 2008.

55. Jones A, Estrada AH. Top 5 arrhythmias in dogs and cats. NAVC Clin's Brief 2014 (January).

56. DeFrancesco T, Case E. Review. NAVC Clin's Brief 2012 (May).

57. Jones A, Estrada A. Top 5 arrhythmias in dogs and cats. NAVC Clin's Brief 2014 (January):94–100.

58. Thomason JD, Kraus MS, Surdyk KK, Fallaw T, Calvert CA. Bradycardia-associated syncope in 7 Boxers with ventricular tachycardia (2002–2005). J Vet Intern Med 2008;22(4):931–6.

59. Plumb DC. Plumb's veterinary drug handbook. 9th edition. ed. Stockholm, Wisconsin Hoboken. NJ: Pharma Vet Inc.; 2018.

60. Goodwin JK. Holter monitoring and cardiac event recording. Vet Clin North Am Small Anim Pract 1998;28(6):1391–407.

61. Miller RH, Lehmkuhl LB, Bonagura JD, Beall MJ. Retrospective analysis of the clinical utility of ambulatory electrocardiographic (Holter) recordings in syncopal dogs: 44 cases (1991–1995). J Vet Intern Med 1999;13(2):111–22.

62. MacKie BA, Stepien RL, Kellihan HB. Retrospective analysis of an implantable loop recorder for evaluation of syncope, collapse, or intermittent weakness in 23 dogs (2004–2008). J Vet Cardiol 2010;12(1):25–33.

63. Rasmussen CE, Falk T, Domanjko Petrič A, Schaldemose M, Zois NE, Moesgaard SG, et al. Holter monitoring of small breed dogs with advanced myxomatous mitral valve disease with and without a history of syncope. J Vet Intern Med 2014;28(2):363–70.

64. Borgarelli M, Savarino P, Crosara S, Santilli RA, Chiavegato D, Poggi M, et al. Survival characteristics and prognostic variables of dogs with mitral regurgitation attributable to myxomatous valve disease. J Vet Intern Med 2008;22(1):120–8.

65. Buchanan JW. Chronic valvular disease (endocardiosis) in dogs. Adv Vet Sci Comp Med 1977;21:75–106.

66. Detweiler DK, Patterson DF, Hubben K, Botts RP. The prevalence of spontaneously occurring cardiovascular disease in dogs. Am J Public Health Nations Health 1961;51:228–41.

67. Bright JM, Cali JV. Clinical usefulness of cardiac event recording in dogs and cats examined because of syncope, episodic collapse, or intermittent weakness: 60 cases (1997–1999). J Am Vet Med Assoc 2000;216(7):1110–4.

68. Ware WA, editor. Holter monitoring in cats. 15th Annual Forum. American College of Veterinary Internal Medicine; 1997.

69. Goodwin JK, Lombard CW, Ginex DD. Results of continuous ambulatory electrocardiography in a cat with hypertrophic cardiomyopathy. J Am Vet Med Assoc 1992;200(9):1352–4.

70. Vannoort R, Vanhemel NM, Voorhout G, Stokhof AA. Ambulatory electrocardiographic (Holter) monitoring in the dog. Tijdschr Diergeneesk 1993;118:S66–SS7.

71. Hall LW, Dunn JK, Delaney M, Shapiro LM. Ambulatory electrocardiography in dogs. Vet Rec 1991;129(10):213–6.

72. Ulloa HM, Houston BJ, Altrogge DM. Arrhythmia prevalence during ambulatory electrocardiographic monitoring of beagles. Am J Vet Res 1995;56(3):275–81.

73. Calvert CA, Jacobs GJ, Pickus CW. Bradycardia-associated episodic weakness, syncope, and aborted sudden death in cardiomyopathic Doberman Pinschers. J Vet Intern Med 1996;10(2):88–93.

74. Marino DJ, Matthiesen DT, Fox PR, Lesser MB, Stamoulis ME. Ventricular arrhythmias in dogs undergoing splenectomy: a prospective study. Vet Surg 1994;23(2):101–6.

75. Moize N, DeFrancesco TC. Twenty-four hour ambulatory electrocardiography (Holter monitoring). In: Bonagura JD, editor. Kirk's current veterinary therapy. XII. Philadelphia, PA: W.B. Saunders; 1995. p. 792–9.

76. Moïse NS, Gilmour RF, Jr., Riccio ML, Flahive WF, Jr. Diagnosis of inherited ventricular tachycardia in German shepherd dogs. J Am Vet Med Assoc 1997;210(3):403–10.

77. Meurs KM, Mauceli E, Lahmers S, Acland GM, White SN, Lindblad-Toh K. Genome-wide association identifies a deletion in the 3' untranslated region of Striatin in a canine model of arrhythmogenic right ventricular cardiomyopathy. Hum Genet 2010;128(3):315–24.

78. Oyama MA, Reiken S, Lehnart SE, Chittur SV, Meurs KM, Stern J, Marks AR. Arrhythmogenic right ventricular cardiomyopathy in Boxer dogs is associated with calstabin2 deficiency. J Vet Cardiol 2008;10(1):1–10.

79. Meurs KM, Lacombe VA, Dryburgh K, Fox PR, Reiser PR, Kittleson MD. Differential expression of the cardiac ryanodine receptor in normal and arrhythmogenic right ventricular cardiomyopathy canine hearts. Hum Genet 2006;120(1):111–8.

80. Harvey AM, Battersby IA, Faena M, Fews D, Darke PG, Ferasin L. Arrhythmogenic right ventricular cardiomyopathy in two cats. J Small Anim Pract 2005;46(3):151–6.

81. Fox PR, Maron BJ, Basso C, Liu SK, Thiene G. Spontaneously occurring arrhythmogenic right ventricular cardiomyopathy in the domestic cat: A new animal model similar to the human disease. Circulation 2000;102(15):1863–70.

Case 38

The Cat with Cold Feet

Jocelyn Engel grew up with Sphynx cats underfoot. Her parents loved the breed and passed this passion on to their daughter. They had only owned fur-less cats and never bred them, but with Jocelyn's strong background in science and her undergraduate degree in biochemistry, she was able to realize her dream of establishing the cattery, Nudes R Us. She decided to start small, with just a single stud and two queens.

Jocelyn breeds two litters per queen per year and prides herself on providing affordable companions to her community. She maintains contact with her clients and is committed to following up to be sure that her kittens thrive in their new homes. Jocelyn is well-intentioned and wants others to experience Sphynx cats for themselves the way that they forever changed her world, for the better.

Squab is Jocelyn's sole tomcat. She purchased him online as a 10-week-old kitten. He never came with any papers, but Jocelyn was told he was descended from a long list of champions. He is extroverted and personable, used to being in everyone's face and the center of attention. He is the first to greet prospective clients when they visit Jocelyn's cattery, which is operated out of her home. In fact, he greets them at the door to lead the grand tour. Because he is sociable, Squab is the posterchild of Jocelyn's growing enterprise. He is also Jocelyn's shadow. Everywhere she goes within the home, he follows.

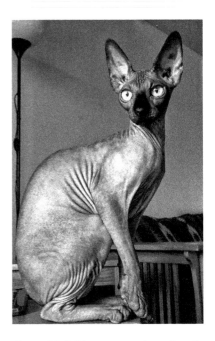

Figure 38.1 Meet your patient, Squab, a 5-year-old intact male Sphynx cat. Courtesy of Brittany Hyde.

Last night, Jocelyn left Squab home alone. She'd been out late at a friend's bachelorette party. By the time the group left the pub, it was well after midnight, so she decided to spend the night on her best friend's couch.

She returned home this morning just after 10am. The house was unusually quiet when she arrived, and Squab was not in his usual spot on the kitchen counter, waiting for her re-entry. At first, she thought he was pouting because he had never before been left alone. She grew concerned when she heard a guttural wail coming from her guest bedroom. Jocelyn found Squab laterally recumbent. He was fully aware of his surroundings, yet frantic. He tried to get up repeatedly on all four legs, but found that he was only able to drag his hind end.

Two thoughts went running through Jocelyn's mind.

1. Had he fallen off the bed and injured himself?
2. Was he blocked?

Jocelyn had heard horror stories online about cats that could not urinate. She googled urinary tract obstruction (UTO), and saw her worst nightmare materialize before her eyes. The website that she pointed her browser to said that blocked cats were an emergency and that if they were not treated, they could die! She was not ready to lose Squab, so she scooped him up and drove the 45 minutes across town to your clinic.

You're familiar with Jocelyn. She brings all three of her cats to you for routine preventative care. When she arrives, you ask your head technician to triage the case and report back to you whether Squab is blocked.

Your technician escorts Squab and Jocelyn into an empty consultation room and proceeds to take his vital signs.

During triage, your technician auscults a grade II/VI systolic parasternal murmur when he assesses Squab's heart rate (HR). This is a new finding for Squab.

During triage, your technician also palpates Squab's abdomen and reports that he doesn't think Squab is obstructed. Jocelyn breathes a sigh of relief momentarily before asking, "What could it be?"

Your technician responds that if anyone can get to the bottom of it, you can.

Use the following questions to guide your approach to this case.

Weight: 8.9 lb (4.0 kg)
BCS: 4/9
Mentation: BAR

TPR

T: 99.2°F (37.3°C)
P: 208 beats per minute
R: 44 breaths per minute

Round One of Questions for Case 38: The Cat with Cold Feet

1. Which organ did your technician palpate to assess whether Squab was blocked?
2. If Squab were blocked, which clinical signs would Jocelyn most likely have reported?
3. If Squab were blocked, what should your technician have felt upon abdominal palpation?
4. Does Squab's mildly low temperature fit the clinical picture of being blocked? In other words, are blocked cats often hypothermic?
5. What should Squab's rectal temperature be?
6. Squab also now has a heart murmur, according to your technician. What is a heart murmur?
7. What is a physiologic heart murmur?
8. What causes physiologic heart murmurs?
9. Heart murmurs may also be age-related. Squab is not a kitten, but kittens may be clinically normal, yet have non-pathologic murmurs that are systolic, low-grade, and louder at the left side of the chest.(1) What causes these innocent murmurs to occur?
10. By what age should innocent murmurs resolve in kittens?
11. Heart murmurs may also be pathologic. What are the broad types of heart disease in the cat or dog?
12. Describe major causes of each type of heart disease that you identified in Question #11 (above)
13. If Squab has heart disease, which of the two broad categories is he most likely to have?
14. Which diagnostic tool is required to identify a murmur?
15. Keeping in mind the answer that you gave for Question #14 (above), what information can you obtain when you identify a murmur?
16. Where in the cardiac cycle can a heart murmur occur?
17. How are heart murmurs graded?
18. True or false: heart murmurs can progress in terms of grade.
19. Based upon the patient history, it sounds like Squab is down in his hind end. Your technician confirms that Squab is either reluctant or unable to move his pelvic limbs. What could cause this sort of paresis or paralysis?
20. Which of the etiologies that you identified in Question #19 fits Squab's clinical picture?
21. You will need to perform a full physical exam on Squab, both to confirm your technician's findings and to pick up on any additional clues as to the cause of his presentation. Based upon your proposed differential(s) in Question #20, which features of the physical exam do you want to prioritize?

Answers to Round One of Questions for Case 38: The Cat with Cold Feet

1. Your technician palpated Squab's urinary bladder to determine if he were blocked.(1, 2)

2. If Squab were blocked, then Jocelyn most likely would have reported one or more of the following clinical signs:(1, 3–7)

   - anorexia
   - dysuria
   - emesis
   - extruded penis
   - frequent visits to the litterbox
   - hematuria
   - house-soiling
   - lack of urine produced in litterbox
   - pollakiuria
   - pulsating prepuce, due to urethral spasms
   - stranguria.

3. If Squab were blocked, then your technician should have felt a rock-hard, painful, turgid, non-compressible urinary bladder.(1, 2, 7, 8)

4. Yes, Squab's mildly low temperature is consistent with a history of being blocked. Most blocked cats are hypothermic at time of presentation.(7, 8)

5. The normal reference range for feline rectal temperature is 100.5–102.5°F, although this range varies somewhat depending upon your choice of reference text.(1, 9)

6. A heart murmur is an abnormal heart sound that results from turbulent blood flow.(1, 8)

7. A physiologic murmur is one that results from conditions outside of the heart rather than structural issues with the heart itself.(8, 10)

8. Physiologic causes of heart murmurs are:(8, 10, 11)

   - anemia
   - body condition, i.e. athletes (12–14)
   - body shape:(12–14)

     - deep-chested, large-breed dogs, such as Boxers
     - thin-chested cats and dogs, such as Greyhounds

   - hypertension
   - hyperthermia
   - hypoproteinemia
   - increased sympathetic tone, as from fear, anxiety, or stress (FAS) (cats) (12, 15)
   - pain (cats)
   - pregnancy.

9. Innocent murmurs in kittens are due to turbulence within the heart and vessels because the heart is still developing.(1, 8, 16)

10. Innocent murmurs in kittens should resolve by five months of age.(1, 8, 16)

11. Heart disease in the cat or dog may be congenital or acquired.(1, 8)

12. Congenital heart disease is relatively uncommon in companion animal practice. When it occurs, it is more likely to occur in the dog than in the cat: its incidence is 4 to 8.5 dogs out of every

1000 compared to 0.2 to 1.0 cats out of 1000 that present to university clinics annually.(10, 16, 17) Congenital defects are typically related to volume and/or pressure overload of the heart, including:(2, 16, 18–27)

- atrial septal defect (ASD):(8, 20, 28)

    - an abnormal connection between the right and left atria(28)
    - because the left side of the heart is under higher pressure than the right, oxygenated blood from the left atrium is shunted into the right atrium(28)
    - this added volume overloads the right atrium(28)

- mitral valve dysplasia (MVD)
- patent ductus arteriosus:(PDA)

    - an abnormal condition in which a fetal vascular structure, the ductus arteriosus, persists after birth(2, 16, 18, 29–33)
    - rather than closing over to form the ligamentum arteriosum, the ductus arteriosus remains patent(2, 16, 18)
    - left-to-right PDAs are more common than right-to-left(2, 29–32)
    - patients with left-to-right PDAs experience shunting of blood from the pressurized aorta into the pulmonary circulation
    - this additional volume overwhelms the pulmonary vasculature, which drains into the left atrium(2, 29–31)
    - over time, the left atrium becomes overwhelmed(2, 29–31)

- pulmonic stenosis (PS):

    - there is an outflow obstruction at the level of the pulmonic valve
    - this obstruction prevents the right ventricle from emptying completely
    - to overcome this obstruction, the right ventricle has to pump harder to force blood out through the right ventricular outflow tract(2)
    - over time, this increase in pressure causes the right ventricular wall to thicken(2)

- subaortic stenosis (SAS):

    - there is an outflow obstruction, a band of tissue, just below the aortic semilunar valves
    - this mechanical obstruction prevents the left ventricle from emptying completely(2)
    - to overcome this obstruction, the left ventricle has to pump harder to force blood out through the left ventricular outflow tract(2)
    - over time, this increase in pressure causes the left ventricular wall to thicken(2)

- tetralogy of Fallot

    - dextroposition or overriding of the aorta
    - PS
    - right ventricular hypertrophy
    - ventricular septal defect (VSD)

- tricuspid valve dysplasia (TVD)
- VSD:

    - an abnormal connection between the right and left ventricle(28)
    - moderate-to-large defects will volume overload the right side of the heart(28)
    - blood that is shunted from left to right ultimately ends up in the pulmonary circulation(28)
    - this means that more blood returns from the lungs to the left side of the heart(28)
    - in time, the left side of the heart becomes volume overloaded as well
    - the development of congestive heart failure (CHF) is likely.(28)

Murmurs are not unique to pediatric patients. In fact, they more commonly occur in adult or geriatric dogs and cat. These murmurs may be physiologic, as outlined in the answer to Question #8 (above).(8, 10, 11) Alternatively, these murmurs may be pathologic.

In the dog, acquired pathologic murmurs are most commonly due to mitral regurgitation (MR).(8, 10, 21) MR may result from:(8, 10)

- degenerative mitral valve disease (DMVD)
- dilated cardiomyopathy (DCM)
- infectious endocarditis.

DMVD is characterized by progressive changes in mitral valve morphology.(8, 34)

- Valve leaflets enlarge and become thickened.(34)
- As these changes in tissue thickness progress, valve leaflets begin to bulge.(34)
- They ultimately prolapse into the associated atrium.(34–37)
- In addition, chordae tendineae often elongate and may even rupture.(34)
- The net result is mitral regurgitation (MR).(34) Mild MR does not have any significant impact on cardiac chamber, wall thickness, heart function as a pump, or systemic circulation.(34) However, as MR worsens, the heart compensates for diminished stroke volume by increasing HR and the force of contraction.(34)
- Over time, there is pathologic remodeling of the heart.(34) Left atrial and left ventricular wall hypertrophy ensues.(34)
- If MR is severe enough, it may result in the development of CHF.(34)

Acquired pathologic murmurs also develop in cats that have:(8)

- degenerative myxomatous atrioventricular valve disease:

    - MR
    - tricuspid regurgitation
    - hyperthyroidism(10)
    - hypertrophic cardiomyopathy (HCM).(1, 8, 10, 15, 38–47)

13. Given his age at time of clinical presentation, Squab most likely has acquired heart disease.

14. Auscultation is the primary means by which murmurs are identified.(1, 8, 10, 48–53)

15. Through auscultation, you can identify the following details about the murmur.(1, 8, 10)

- Character

    - Crescendo murmurs increase in intensity toward completion.
    - Diamond-shaped or crescendo-decrescendo murmurs first increase and then decrease toward completion. These are typically associated with turbulent flow across the right or left ventricular outflow tracts, as occurs with aortic or PS.
    - Decrescendo murmurs decrease in intensity toward completion.
    - Regurgitant murmurs are harsh sounding because they are caused by blood leaking backward through circulation, as in a left-to-right shunt from left to right ventricle in a patient with a ventricular septal defect.
    - Systolic clicks are typically heard over the left apex and are high-frequency sounds that are most often associated with mitral valve disease.

- Intensity or grade
- Location
- Point of maximal intensity (PMI)

    - The location at which the murmur is the loudest:

- apical murmurs are loudest at the apex of the heart
- basilar murmurs are loudest at the heart base
- parasternal murmurs are common in cats.(54)

- The valve that the loudest part of the murmur is nearest:

  - pulmonic
  - aortic
  - mitral
  - tricuspid.

16. Heart murmurs can occur at different points throughout the cardiac cycle. They can be:(1, 8)

- systolic
- diastolic
- continuous.

Systolic murmurs are most common in companion animal practice.(10, 12, 54) These are whooshing sounds that occur between the first and second heart sound, S1 and S2:(2, 8, 55)

| S1 | WHOOSH | S2 | S1 | WHOOSH | S2 |
| "Lub" | WHOOSH | "Dub" | "Lub" | WHOOSH | "Dub" |

Diastolic murmurs are whooshing sounds that occur between S2 and S1:(2, 8, 55)

| S1 | S2 | WHOOSH | S1 | S2 | WHOOSH | S1 | S2 | WHOOSH |
| "Lub" | "Dub" | WHOOSH | "Lub" | "Dub" | WHOOSH | "Lub" | "Dub" | WHOOSH |

Continuous murmurs occur throughout both systole and diastole.(2, 8, 12) Because the whooshing sound is constant, these are sometimes referred to as machinery or "washing machine" murmurs.(8, 12)

17. Heart murmurs are graded by their intensity on a scale of 1 to 6.(1, 2, 8, 12, 55, 56)
    Grade 1 murmurs are the softest of all murmurs.(12) They are difficult to auscultate and may be present intermittently.(12) Sometimes, the only indication of their presence is an apparently prolonged S1, which occurs when the murmur blends into the first heart sound.(2)
    Grade 2 murmurs are more distinct than grade 1 murmurs, although they are not much louder.(2, 12) They tend to concentrate over one valve.(12) Because of this, Grade 2 murmurs are said to be focal.(12)
    Grade 3 murmurs are obvious murmurs of moderate intensity.(2, 12) These may be focal or they may radiate to other areas of the chest.(12)
    Grade 4 murmurs are louder than Grade 3 and more extensive in terms of their distribution patterns.(12)
    Grade 5 murmurs are loud and they radiate widely.(12) In addition, they are associated with a palpable thrill.(12) A palpable thrill is a vibration that can be felt across the chest wall.(2, 12)
    Grade 6 murmurs are the loudest type, and are routinely audible without a stethoscope, or with a stethoscope that is barely touching the body wall.(2, 12)

18. It is true that heart murmurs can progress in terms of grade.(1, 8)

19. Hind end paresis or paralysis could be caused by an abnormality within the:(1, 8)

- cardiovascular system,(57, 58), e.g. aortic thromboembolism (ATE), also known as a saddle thrombus(59–61)
- musculoskeletal system, i.e. trauma, e.g. pelvic fracture, vertebral fracture
- neurological system, i.e. trauma, e.g. femoral nerve injury, sciatic nerve injury, spinal cord compression or infectious meningomyelitis.(62)

20. There is no history of trauma. Although musculoskeletal and neurological system abnormalities cannot be definitively ruled out at this time, I would prioritize cardiovascular system differentials, particularly when considering the patient history and the new clinical finding of a heart murmur in a feline patient.

21. Although I will perform a comprehensive physical examination, I want to prioritize features of the exam that provide clues as to the patient's cardiovascular health including:

- evaluation of distal hind limbs to assess warmth
- evaluation of paw pads to assess color
- palpation of femoral pulses
- thoracic auscultation.

In addition, I will want to assess the patient's motor function and deep pain sensation in both pelvic limbs.

Returning to Case 38: The Cat with Cold Feet

You enter the consultation room. Your exam confirms the technician's findings. In addition, you identify the following abnormal physical exam findings:

- absent femoral pulses bilaterally
- muffled heart sounds ventrally
- increased bronchovesicular sounds bilaterally
- swollen gastrocnemius muscles bilaterally
- palpably cold hind paws
- cyanotic digital and metatarsal pads
- cyanotic nail beds
- negative for voluntary motor function in both pelvic limbs
- negative for deep pain sensation in both pelvic limbs.

Round Two of Questions for Case 38: The Cat with Cold Feet

1. Based upon these new physical exam findings, what most likely caused Squab's acute onset of paraparesis?
2. The cause of Squab's paraparesis that you identified in Question #1 (above) is likely secondary to underlying heart disease. What is the name of the presumptive diagnosis?
3. Describe the pathophysiology of the presumptive diagnosis that you identified in Question #2.
4. Describe how the presumptive diagnosis that you identified in Question #2 (above) could precipitate Squab's clinical presentation.
5. Why are Squab's limbs cold?
6. Squab's distal hind limbs are cooler to the touch than Squab's forelimbs. What is the appropriate medical term to describe the condition by which internal temperature varies depending upon the location where it is measured?
7. Why are Squab's paw pads and nail beds cyanotic?
8. What is the link between Squab's presumptive diagnosis and the changes in lung sounds that you auscultated during his physical exam?
9. If this patient is stable enough to take thoracic radiographs, what might you expect to see?
10. Which additional imaging study may be helpful in terms of establishing Squab's prognosis and why? Which important information will the imaging studies provide that will impact case management?

11. If you were to perform baseline bloodwork on Squab in the form of a serum chemistry profile, what might you expect to see?

12. Which additional bloodwork is helpful for case management?

Answers to Round Two of Questions for Case 38: The Cat with Cold Feet

1. Based upon these new physical exam findings, the most likely cause of Squab's acute onset of paraparesis is ATE.

2. ATE is often associated with hypertrophic cardiomyopathy (HCM).(59) This condition is characterized by excessive thickening of the muscular wall of the heart, which reduces the efficiency of this organ as a pump.

3. Patients with HCM develop progressive left ventricular hypertrophy.(63) In order to fill the left ventricle with blood , the left atrium has to raise its pressure.(63) This in turn increases the pressure of the pulmonary vein, which is tasked with the filling of the left atrium.(63)

   The pathophysiology of HCM is a vicious cycle.(63) The body attempts to compensate for reduced filling and cardiac output by increasing HR.(63) Tachycardia requires the myocardium to work harder, such that the heart's need for oxygen increases.(63) However, the heart remains inefficient.(63) Coronary perfusion time decreases.(63) This perpetuates ischemia.(63)

   In addition, the stiffness of the left ventricle impairs its ability to relax during diastole. This further hinders filling.(63)

   Additional structural changes are often present with HCM, including MR and dynamic left ventricular outflow obstruction.(63) Dynamic left ventricular outflow obstruction results from the mitral valve becoming displaced against the inner wall of the left ventricle. This causes a mechanical obstruction for blood that is attempting to pass from the left ventricle through the aortic valve and into systemic circulation.

4. HCM potentiates thrombus formation.(59, 64, 65) Dilation of the left atria exposes endocardial collagen, which may incite platelet aggregation.(60, 64, 66–69) When platelets aggregate, they activate the coagulation cascade.(60, 64, 66–69) The resultant fibrin combines with platelet clumps to form an intracardiac thrombus.(64)

   The thrombus can break off from its site of origin, within the heart, and enter the aorta, where at some point it will occlude the arterial vasculature.(60, 64)

   The distal aortic trifurcation is the most common site of obstruction in cats in that more than 90% of emboli lodge here.(64) When they do, affected patients are said to have a "saddle thrombus."(60, 64)

   Patients with a "saddle thrombus" present acutely with pelvic limb paresis or paralysis that involves one or both legs.(59–61) Bilateral involvement is most common.(60) In these cases, one limb may appear to be clinically worse than the other.(59, 60)

5. Assuming that he has HCM with ATE, Squab's limbs are cold because he is experiencing vascular occlusion. Without blood flow, the affected limbs become cold.(59)

   Infrared thermography demonstrates that temperatures of affected versus unaffected limbs may vary by up to 36.3°F (2.4°C).(62)

6. Poikilothermy is the appropriate medical term that describes how Squab's internal temperature varies depending upon the location where it is measured. This is pathological. His distal hind limbs should not be colder than his forelimbs.

7. Assuming that he has HCM with ATE, Squab's paw pads and nailbeds are cyanotic because the reduction in blood supply to the pelvic limbs has led to hypoxemic tissues.(59, 60)

8. Many patients with ATE have concurrent CHF at the time of initial presentation.(59) These patients often exhibit changes in lung sounds during thoracic auscultation. The clinician may auscult increased bronchovesicular lung sounds. Alternatively, s/he may auscult adventitious lung sounds, including crackles.(60, 70)

9. If Squab were stable enough to take thoracic radiographs, then I might expect to see one or more of the following changes, reflective of cardiomyopathy and/or CHF.(57, 58)

    - Cardiomegaly, as evident by an increased vertebral heart score:
        - left atrial enlargement
        - left ventricular enlargement.
    - Pulmonary edema, as characterized by a pulmonary interstitial pattern:
        - in dogs, this distribution tends to be caudodorsal and/or perihilar
        - in cats, this distribution may be more varied.
    - Pulmonary venous distension.

10. An echocardiogram is not necessary to make the diagnosis; however, it is a valuable tool to evaluate the severity of underlying cardiomyopathy.(59, 60, 70) An echocardiogram will confirm hypertrophy of the left ventricular wall, which is consistent with a diagnosis of HCM.(57)

    The presence of so-called "smoke," that is, spontaneous echo contrast, is common.(59, 71) It tells us that the heart chamber(s) in which it occurs is dilated and that there is appreciable blood stasis.(57)

    Some clinicians also believe that "smoke" confers increased risk that the patient will succumb to additional episodes of ATE.(59, 71)

11. If I drew blood on Squab to perform a serum chemistry profile, then I might expect to find the following changes:(59, 60)

    - azotemia due to poor systemic perfusion
    - elevation of creatine kinase (CK) due to muscle ischemia
    - elevation of aspartate aminotransferase
    - elevation of lactate dehydrogenase
    - stress hyperglycemia.

12. Coagulation profiles (PT/PTT) are essential to rule out coagulopathy.(57)

Returning to Case 38: The Cat with Cold Feet

You share with Jocelyn your concerns that Squab has appreciable HCM, which led to ATE. You are also concerned that he might have CHF. You discuss the need for diagnostic studies to confirm your suspicions and to establish a suitable treatment plan for him. Jocelyn allows you to pursue a diagnostic work-up.

Squab is not hypertensive. Baseline bloodwork is unremarkable except for a marked elevation in CK. A thyroid panel rules out hyperthyroidism. Coagulation profiles rule out coagulopathy.

Squab was stable enough to undergo thoracic radiography with the help of flow-by oxygen. This thoracic imaging study demonstrates the following abnormalities:

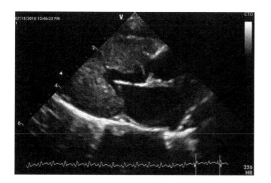

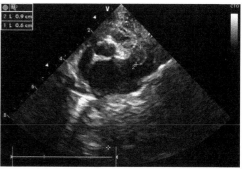

Figure 38.2 Echocardiography (right parasternal long axis view): Concentric hypertrophy of the left ventricle. Courtesy of Justin Thomason, DACVIM (Cardiology; SAIM), Wildcat Cardiology, and Christy Zimmer Coyle, RVT.

Figure 38.3 Echocardiography (right parasternal short axis basilar view): Consistent with left atrial dilation with a thrombus in the left atrium. Courtesy of Justin Thomason, DACVIM (Cardiology; SAIM), Wildcat Cardiology, and Christy Zimmer Coyle, RVT.

- an increased vertebral heart score
- left atrial enlargement
- left ventricular enlargement
- pulmonary edema.

Squab's echocardiogram confirms your presumptive diagnosis. Significant findings include:

- enlarged left atrium
- "smoke" within the left atrium
- thrombus within the left atrium
- left ventricular concentric hypertrophy.

(See Figures 38.2 and 38.3).

Round Three of Questions for Case 38: The Cat with Cold Feet

1. Which breeds of cat are predisposed to HCM?
2. Which gender is predisposed to HCM?
3. Which gender is predisposed to ATE?
4. What is the general approach to treating acute cases of ATE?
5. What are potential complications that are associated with treating ATE?
6. What is the general approach to treating CHF?
7. What is Squab's prognosis?

Answers to Round Three of Questions for Case 38: The Cat with Cold Feet

1. Certain breeds are predisposed to HCM, including Maine coons, Persians, Burmese, Siamese, American shorthairs, Ragdolls, and Norwegian Forest cats.(61)

2. Males are more likely to develop HCM.(59, 72)

3. Because males are more likely to develop HCM, male cats appear to be at greater risk for development of ATE.(59, 72)

4. The general approach to treating acute cases of ATE with underlying HCM involves:(57, 58)
   - analgesia: patients are acutely painful(59–61)
   - anticoagulant therapy:
     - aspirin
     - unfractionated heparin
     - low molecular weight heparin
   - monitoring for signs of reperfusion injury, i.e. hyperkalemia(59)
   - physiotherapy of affected limbs
   - thromboprophylaxis:
     - low-dose aspirin
     - clopidogrel (Plavix).

   It is not advisable to administer thrombolytic therapy due to the high potential for life-threatening adverse events.(58)

5. Reperfusion injury and the development of ischemic necrosis at affected sites (i.e. the limbs) are potential concerns associated with management of ATE.(57, 58)
   Reperfusion injury occurs when vascular occlusion has been removed and blood flow is reestablished.(73) Inflammatory mediators and toxic byproducts that had previously built up in tissue are now released into general circulation.(73) Some of these products combine with oxygen to form reactive oxygen species (ROS).(73) These cause damage to cells throughout the body. ROS may also trigger lipid peroxidation, which impairs cellular membranes and sets the stage for cell death.(73) In addition, hyperkalemia is a common result of reperfusion.(59)

6. The general approach to treating CHF involves:(57, 58)
   - administration of diuretics, i.e. furesemide (Lasix)
   - angiotensin-converting enzyme (ACE) inhibitors
   - oxygen therapy.

7. Historically, the majority of cats with ATE were euthanized on initial presentation.(59) However, although the average patient's prognosis is guarded, some patients do better than others.(59) Survival is most likely among those with unilateral involvement: as many as 70–80% survive to discharge.(59, 71, 72, 74)

CLINICAL PEARLS

- An acute onset of paresis and/or paralysis in a feline patient without a history of trauma should make you suspicious of ATE or "saddle thrombus."

- ATE is an extraordinarily painful condition is which a thrombus breaks off from its site of origin within the heart and enters the aorta, where it can occlude the arterial vasculature.

- The most common site is the distal aortic bifurcation.

- When thrombi lodge at this site, they occlude blood flow to the distal limbs.

- Occlusion of hind limb vasculature most often affects both legs simultaneously; however, unilateral involvement is possible.

- Without blood supply to the affected limb(s), the limb(s) become(s) cool to the touch.

- In addition, affected tissues become hypoxemic. This results in cyanotic paw pads and nail beds in the affected limb(s).

- The most common cause of ATE in the cat is underlying heart disease, specifically HCM.

- Patients with HCM develop left ventricular hypertrophy. This reduces left ventricular compliance. The left atria now must work that much harder to pump blood into the left ventricle. This results in increased left atrial pressure. Over time, the left atria dilates to accommodate the back-up of blood trying to get through the ventricle.

- The body tries to compensate for reduced cardiac output by increasing HR. However, tachycardia only makes the heart work harder. It does nothing to improve the efficiency of the heart, which has become an ineffective pump.

- Patients may or may not have signs of CHF at the time.

- Patients that present with ATE must be managed acutely through this crisis but will require lifelong management for HCM.

- Sudden death is possible.

References

1. Englar RE. Performing the small animal physical examination. Hoboken, NJ: Wiley/Blackwell; 2017.
2. Englar RE. Performing the small animal physical examination. Hoboken, NJ: Wiley/Blackwell; 2017.
3. Sabino CV. Urethral obstruction in cats. Vet Team Brief 2017 (April):37–41.
4. Segev G, Livne H, Ranen E, Lavy E. Urethral obstruction in cats: predisposing factors, clinical, clinicopathological characteristics and prognosis. J Feline Med Surg 2011;13(2):101–8.
5. Lee JA, Drobatz KJ. Characterization of the clinical characteristics, electrolytes, acid–base, and renal parameters in male cats with urethral obstruction. J Vet Emerg Crit Car 2003;13(4):227–33.
6. Thomovsky EJ; 2011. Managing the common comorbidities of feline urethral obstruction. DVM 360 [Internet]. 2011. Available from: http://veterinarymedicine.dvm360.com/managing-common-comorbidities-feline-urethral-obstruction.
7. George CM, Grauer GF. Feline urethral obstruction: diagnosis and management. Today's. Vet Pract 2016 (July/August):36–46.
8. Englar RE. Common clinical presentations in dogs and cats. Hoboken, NJ: Wiley/Blackwell; 2019.
9. Rijnberk A, Stokhof AA. General examination. In: Rijnberk A, van Sluijs FJ, editors. Medical history and physical examination in companion animals. New York: Elsevier; 2009.
10. Côté E, Edwards NJ, Ettinger SJ, Fuentes VL, MacDonald KA, Scansen BA, et al. Management of incidentally detected heart murmurs in dogs and cats. J Vet Cardiol 2015;17(4):245–61.
11. Estrada AH. Physiologic murmur. Clinician's brief [Internet]. Available from: https://www.cliniciansbrief.com/cardiac-library/heart-sound/physiologic-murmur.
12. Mandese WW, Estrada AH. The basic cardiology examination. NAVC Clin's Brief 2017 (May):91–7.
13. Garcia JL. Journal Scan: Physiological heart murmurs are more common in our veterinary patients than we may think. 2015. DVM. Available from: http://veterinarymedicine.dvm360.com/journal-scan-physiological-heart-murmurs-are-more-common-our-veterinary-patients-we-may-think.
14. Drut A, Ribas T, Floch F, Franchequin S, Freyburger L, Rannou B, et al. Prevalence of physiological heart murmurs in a population of 95 healthy young adult dogs. J Small Anim Pract 2015;56(2):112–8.

15. Wagner T, Fuentes VL, Payne JR, McDermott N, Brodbelt D. Comparison of auscultatory and echocardio-graphic findings in healthy adult cats. J Vet Cardiol 2010;12(3):171–82.

16. Strickland KN. Congenital heart disease. In: Tilley LP, Smith FWK, Oyama MA, Sleeper MM, editors. Manual of canine and feline cardiology. 4th ed. Philadelphia. PA: W. B. Saunders; 2008. p. 215–39.

17. Patterson DF. Epidemiologic and genetic studies of congenital heart disease in the dog. Circ Res 1968;23(2):171–202.

18. Bulmer BJ. The cardiovascular system. In: Peterson ME, Kutzler MA, editors. Small animal pediatrics: the first 12 months of life. St. Louis, MO: Saunders/Elsevier; 2011. p. 289–304.

19. Schrope DP. Prevalence of congenital heart disease in 76,301 mixed-breed dogs and 57,025 mixed-breed cats. J Vet Cardiol Off J Eur 2015;17(3):192–202.

20. MacDonald K; 2011. Murmurs in puppies and kittens DVM 360 [Internet]. 2011. Available from: http://veterinarycalendar.dvm360.com/murmurs-puppies-and-kittens-proceedings.

21. Rishniw M. Canine heart murmur. NAVC Clin's Brief 2011 (May):49–52.

22. Oliveira P, Domenech O, Silva J, Vannini S, Bussadori R, Bussadori C. Retrospective review of congenital heart disease in 976 dogs. J Vet Intern Med 2011;25(3):477–83.

23. Buchanan JW. Prevalence of cardiovascular disorders. In: Fox PR, Sisson DD, Moize NS, editors. Textbook of canine and feline cardiology. Philadelphia, PA: W. B. Saunders; 1998. p. 457–70.

24. Baumgartner C, Glaus TM. [Congenital cardiac diseases in dogs: a retrospective analysis]. Schweiz Arch Tierheilkd 2003;145(11):527–33.

25. Hunt GB, Church DB, Malik R, Bellenger CR. A retrospective analysis of congenital cardiac anomalies (1977–1989). Aust Vet Pract 1990;20(2):70–5.

26. Tidholm A. Retrospective study of congenital heart defects in 151 dogs. J Small Anim Pract 1997;38(3):94–8.

27. MacDonald KA. Congenital heart diseases of puppies and kittens. Vet Clin North Am Small Anim Pract 2006;36(3):503–31.

28. Tilley LP, Smith FWK. The 5-minute veterinary consult: canine and feline. 3rd ed. Baltimore, MD: Lippincott Williams & Wilkins; 2004.

29. Côté E. Clinical veterinary advisor. Dogs and cats. 3rd ed. St. Louis, MO: Elsevier; 2015.

30. Tilley LP, Smith FWK, Tilley LP. Blackwell's five-minute veterinary consult: canine and feline. 4th ed. Ames, IA: Blackwell; 2007.

31. The Merck veterinary manual. Whitehouse Station, NJ: Merck & Co., Inc. 2016.

32. Arora M. Reversed patent ductus arteriosus in a dog. Can Vet J 2001;42(6):471–2.

33. Scurtu I, Pestean C, Lacatus R, Lascu M, Mircean M, Codea R, et al. Reverse PDA – less common type of patent ductus arteriosus – case report. Bull UASVM Vet Med;2106(73 (2)):351–5.

34. Haggstrom J, Pedersen HD, Kvart C. New insights into degenerative mitral valve disease in dogs. Vet Clin N Am. Small 2004;34(5):1209.

35. Buchanan JW. Chronic valvular disease (endocardiosis) in dogs. Adv Vet Sci Comp Med 1977;21:75–106.

36. Kogure K. Pathology of chronic mitral valvular disease in the dog. Nihon Juigaku Zasshi 1980;42(3):323–35.

37. Whitney JC. Observations on the effect of age on the severity of heart valve lesions in the dog. J Small Anim Pract 1974;15(8):511–22.

38. Côté E, Manning AM, Emerson D, Laste NJ, Malakoff RL, Harpster NK. Assessment of the prevalence of heart murmurs in overtly healthy cats. J Am Vet Med Assoc 2004;225(3):384–8.

39. Paige CF, Abbott JA, Elvinger F, Pyle RL. Prevalence of cardiomyopathy in apparently healthy cats. J Am Vet Med Assoc 2009;234(11):1398–403.

40. Bonagura JD. Feline echocardiography. J Feline Med Surg 2000;2(3):147–51.

41. Dirven MJ, Cornelissen JM, Barendse MA, van Mook MC, Sterenborg JA. Cause of heart murmurs in 57 apparently healthy cats. Tijdschr Diergeneeskd 2010;135(22):840–7.

42. Nakamura RK, Rishniw M, King MK, Sammarco CD. Prevalence of echocardiographic evidence of cardiac disease in apparently healthy cats with murmurs. J Feline Med Surg 2011;13(4):266–71.

43. Fuentes VL. Cardiomyopathy: establishing a diagnosis. In: August JR, editor. Consultations in feline internal medicine. St. Louis, MO: Saunders Elsevier; 2006. p. 301–10.

44. Ferasin L, Sturgess CP, Cannon MJ, Caney SM, Gruffydd-Jones TJ, Wotton PR. Feline idiopathic cardiomyopathy: a retrospective study of 106 cats (1994–2001). J Feline Med Surg 2003;5(3):151–9.

45. Rishniw M, Pion PD. Is treatment of feline hypertrophic cardiomyopathy based in science or faith? A survey of cardiologists and a literature search. J Feline Med Surg 2011;13(7):487–97.

46. Freeman LM, Rush JE, Stern JA, Huggins GS, Maron MS. Feline hypertrophic cardiomyopathy: A spontaneous large animal model of human HCM. Cardiol Res 2017;8(4):139–42.

47. Payne JR, Brodbelt DC, Luis Fuentes V. Cardiomyopathy prevalence in 780 apparently healthy cats in rehoming centres (the CatScan study). J Vet Cardiol 2015;17;Suppl 1:S244–57.

48. Dennis S. Sound advice for heart murmurs. J Small Anim Pract 2013;54(9):443–4.

49. Szatmári V, van Leeuwen MW, Teske E. Innocent cardiac murmur in puppies: prevalence, correlation with hematocrit, and auscultation characteristics. J Vet Intern Med 2015;29(6):1524–8.

50. Marinus SM, van Engelen H, Szatmári V. N-terminal pro-B-type natriuretic peptide and phonocardiography in differentiating innocent cardiac murmurs from congenital cardiac anomalies in asymptomatic puppies. J Vet Intern Med 2017;31(3):661–7.

51. Fonfara S. Listen to the sound: what is normal? J Small Anim Pract 2015;56(2):75–6.

52. Abbott J. Auscultation: what type of practice makes perfect? J Vet Intern Med 2001;15(6):505–6.

53. Naylor JM, Yadernuk LM, Pharr JW, Ashburner JS. An assessment of the ability of diplomates, practitioners, and students to describe and interpret recordings of heart murmurs and arrhythmia. J Vet Intern Med 2001;15(6):507–15.

54. Hogan DF. Cardiac examination and history. NAVC Clin's Brief 2008 (July):49–53.

55. Gompf RE. The history and physical examination. In: Tilley LP, Smith FWK, Oyama M, Sleeper MM, editors. Manual of canine and feline cardiology. St. Louis, MO: Saunders; 2008. p. 2–23.

56. Estrada A. Cardiac physical examination. NAVC clinician's brief [Internet]. Available from: https://www.cliniciansbrief.com/article/cardiac-physical-examination.

57. Laughlin DS, Oyama MA. Acute pelvic limb paresis and respiratory effort in a cat. Clinician's. Brief 2013 (September):51–6.

58. Rishniw M. Feline aortic thromboembolism. Clin's Brief 2006 (November):17–20.

59. Luis Fuentes VL. Arterial thromboembolism. Risks, realities and a rational first-line approach. J Feline Med Surg 2012;14(7):459–70.

60. Smith SA, Tobias AH. Feline arterial thromboembolism: an update. Vet Clin North Am Small Anim Pract 2004;34(5):1245–71.

61. Rishniw M. Feline aortic thromboembolism. NAVC Clin's Brief 2006 (November):17–20.

62. Pouzot-Nevoret C, Barthélemy A, Goy-Thollot I, Boselli E, Cambournac M, Guillaumin J, et al. Infrared thermography: a rapid and accurate technique to detect feline aortic thromboembolism. J Feline Med Surg 2018;20(8):780–5.

63. Bonagura JD. Feline hypertrophic cardiomyopathy. Vet Q 1997;19(sup1):5–6.

64. Falconer L, Atwell R. Feline aortic thromboembolism. Aust Vet Pract 2003;33(1):20–+.

65. Borgeat K, Wright J, Garrod O, Payne JR, Fuentes VL. Arterial thromboembolism in 250 cats in general practice: 2004–2012. J Vet Intern Med 2014;28(1):102–8.

66. Fox PR Fox PR, Sisson D, Moize SN, editors. Textbook of canine and feline cardiology: principles and practice. Philadelphia, PA: Saunders; 1999.

67. Fox PR. In: Ettinger SJ, Feldman EC, editors. Textbook of veterinary internal medicine. Philadelphia, PA: Saunders; 2000. p. 896.

68. Rodriguez DB, Harpster N. Aortic thromboembolism associated with feline hypertrophic cardiomyopathy. Comp Cont Educ Pract 2002;24(6):478–82.

69. Rush JE. Therapy of feline hypertrophic cardiomyopathy. Vet Clin North Am Small Anim Pract 1998;28(6):1459–79.

70. Smith SA, Tobias AH, Jacob KA, Fine DM, Grumbles PL. Arterial thromboembolism in cats: acute crisis in 127 cases (1992–2001) and long-term management with low-dose aspirin in 24 cases. J Vet Intern Med 2003;17(1):73–83.

71. Schober KE, Marz I. Doppler echocardiographic assessment of left atrial appendage flow in cats with cardiomyopathy. J Vet Intern Med 2003;17(5):739.

72. Moore KE, Morris N, Dhupa N, Murtaugh RJ, Rush JE. Retrospective study of streptokinase administration in 46 cats with arterial thromboembolism. J Vet Emerg Crit Care 2000;10(4):245–57.

73. How to handle feline aortic thromboembolism. DVM360 [Internet]; 2010. Available from: https://www.dvm360.com/view/how-handle-feline-aortic-thromboembolism.

74. Laste NJ, Harpster NK. A retrospective study of 100 cases of feline distal aortic thromboembolism: 1977–1993. J Am Anim Hosp Assoc 1995;31(6):492–500.

Case 39

The Dog with Exercise Intolerance

Darby is new to your practice. He was seized from a hoarding investigation after a landlord discovered the extent to which a rental home was damaged by a tenant's collection of 12 dogs and 62 cats. The animals were found in deplorable conditions and most had to be euthanized. Darby was among those few whose gentle disposition made him a good candidate for foster care. The hope was that he could learn what normal living was like before he found his forever home.

Darby's transition from a state of squalor into his new residence was smoother than anticipated. He settled in nicely and his two new foster parents, Janice and Leeroy Billings, gave him more attention than he had known in a lifetime.

Janice and Leeroy described him as sweet,

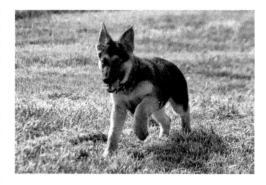

Figure 39.1 Meet your patient, Darby, a 1-year-old intact male German Shepherd Dog. Courtesy of Jayne Regan.

yet shy, and anything but young at heart. When they had agreed to take the young adult dog into their home, they had envisioned a gregarious soul, livening up the home. Janice and Leeroy hoped that Darby would be a great fit for their two grandchildren, age 12 and 14. The kids were stir crazy indoors, and the couple thought for sure that Darby would do the trick by keeping them occupied in the yard for hours on end. They pictured sitting on the back porch in the early evening, watching Darby and the grandkids play catch.

That vision had yet to materialize. For starters, Darby didn't know what to do with a ball. He'd never seen one before. The first time one was tossed into the yard, he whined like Shepherds do, tucked his tail, and tried to hide under Leeroy's chair.

Weight: 54.2 lb (24.6 kg)
BCS: 3/9
Mentation: QAR

TPR

T: 100.6°F (38.1°C)
P: 96 beats per minute
R: Panting

Okay, so he wasn't a fan of baseball, Janice thought. Maybe he'd be more of a frisbee dog? No such luck. The frisbee terrified him, too. In the days that followed, they tried everything. Even when Darby didn't react in a frightened manner, he never seemed engaged in what life had to offer. Instead, he seemed content to watch the world go by.

At first, they chalked it up to him never having learned how to play. After all, he'd been caged for most of his life. Then, after noticing that short walks to the mailbox left him winded, they began to wonder if his lack of get-up-and-go was due to a medical condition rather than apathy.

Janice and Leeroy are here today with Darby to meet you and to investigate his apparent exercise intolerance. Your technician documents his vital signs as they await your consult.

In addition to sharing these vital signs with you, your technician alerts you that Darby's heart sounds "odd."

Use the following questions to guide your approach to this case.

Round One of Questions for Case 39: The Dog with Exercise Intolerance

1. The heart is a pump. In order to deliver blood to the body effectively and efficiently, it must work through a coordinated cycle. What is this cycle called and which are its two components?
2. Describe the flow of blood through the normal canine heart, beginning with its entrance into the right atrium. Include the names of the valves through which blood passes.
3. Which valves are the so-called A-V valves of the heart?
4. Which valves are the so-called semi-lunar valves of the heart?
5. It is normal to hear the heart during thoracic auscultation. What action within the heart causes normal heart sounds to occur?
6. Which heart sounds are normal to hear in a canine (or feline) heart?
7. Describe normal heart sounds: what do they sound like?
8. If you want to focus on hearing normal heart sounds, which side of the stethoscope should you rely upon: the bell or the diaphragm? Explain your answer.
9. What if your stethoscope does not have a separate bell and diaphragm? What will you do?
10. Which additional heart sounds are unlikely to be heard in a normal canine (or feline) heart?
11. Are these additional heart sounds likely to be evident on an electrocardiogram (ECG)?
12. When these extra sounds are heard, the patient is said to have a gallop rhythm. Describe two main types of gallop rhythms in companion animal patients.
13. Which kinds of cardiomyopathy cause these gallop rhythms to occur in companion animal patients?
14. If you suspected a gallop rhythm and you needed to listen for the associated extra heart sounds, which side of the stethoscope would you need to rely upon: the bell or the diaphragm? Explain your answer.
15. What is a summation gallop?
16. Your technician clarifies that, when he said Darby's heart sounded "odd," he did not mean to imply that there were extra heart sounds. It just sounded "off." What two additional findings could he be referring to?
17. Identify potential causes of each item that you identified in Question #16 (above).
18. You will need to listen to Darby's heart yourself to be certain. However, you know that cardio-thoracic auscultation is an imperfect diagnostic tool. What are its potential limitations?
19. In addition to cardiothoracic auscultation, which other structures will you need to assess during Darby's physical exam to make conclusions about his cardiovascular health?
20. Which additional heart-specific studies might you need, after his physical exam, to round out your understanding of Darby's cardiovascular health?

Answers to Round One of Questions for Case 39: The Dog with Exercise Intolerance

1. The cardiac cycle is the process by which the heart delivers blood to the body effectively and efficiently by means of coordinated contraction (systole) followed by relaxation (diastole).(1) Diastole is as critical a component in the cardiac cycle as systole because relaxation of the cardiac muscle is necessary in order for the chambers to fill with blood for the next cycle of coordinated contraction.

2. Blood flows from the right atrium into the right ventricle through the right atrioventricular (A-V) valve, the tricuspid valve.(1–5) During systole, blood is forced from the right ventricle through the pulmonic valve to the pulmonary artery to the lungs.(2, 3, 5) Here, gas exchange takes place and the blood is re-oxygenated.(2, 3, 5) Oxygen-rich blood then returns to the heart through the pulmonary vein to fill the left atrium and left ventricle during diastole, the state of cardiac relaxation.(2, 3, 5) To fill the left ventricle, blood passes through the left A-V valve, otherwise known as the mitral valve.(1–5) When systole recurs, the cycle repeats.(2, 3, 5) Oxygenated blood is now actively pumped from the left ventricle through the aortic valve to the aorta, which disseminates it to the rest of the body.(1–6) Blood perfuses the tissues after being transported from arteries to arterioles to capillary beds.(2, 3, 5) Once deoxygenated, blood is gathered up in venules, which pool into veins, which return to the right atrium through the venae cavae.(2, 3, 5)

    For simplicity, I have traced the blood from one side of the heart to the other, but it is important to remember that both sides of the heart pump simultaneously. During systole, both the left and the right ventricles contract.(1, 7, 8) During diastole, both sides of the heart relax.(1, 7, 8)

3. The mitral and tricuspid valves are the so-called A-V valves of the heart because they bridge the corresponding atrium and ventricle.(1–6) The left A-V valve is the mitral and the right A-V valve is the tricuspid.(1–6)

    Some remember which is which by remembering the mnemonic RAT – the "R" stands for the right side of the heart and the "T" stands for tricuspid. Others remember LAM, pronounced "lamb" – the "L" stands for the left side of the heart and the "M" stands for mitral.

4. The pulmonic and aortic valves are the so-called semi-lunar valves of the heart.(1–6) The pulmonic valve bridges the right ventricle and the pulmonary artery and is important for the flow of blood out of the heart to the lungs to reoxygenate.(1–6) The aortic valve bridges the left ventricle and the aorta and is important for the flow of blood out of the heart to the body for tissue perfusion with oxygen.(1–6)

5. It is normal to hear the heart during thoracic auscultation. Normal heart sounds result from the coordinated closing of heart valves.(1, 5–8)

6. The S1 and S2 heart sounds are normally auscultated when you listen to a normal canine (or feline) heart.(1, 2, 5)

    Closure of the A-V valves to facilitate forward flow of blood during ventricular contraction is what causes S1.(1, 5–9)

    Closure of the pulmonic and aortic valves to allow the heart to fill in between ventricular contractions is what causes S2.(1, 5–9)

7. S1 and S2 combined sound like "lub-dub."(1, 5) The S1 sound is the "lub" and the S2 sound is the "dub."(1, 5) These sounds should be easy to distinguish when you auscultate the heart.(1, 5, 7, 9)

8. To focus on hearing S1 and S2, you should make use of the diaphragm of the stethoscope.(5) Both S1 and S2 are high-frequency sounds, and these are preferentially transmitted by the diaphragm, as opposed to the bell, which transmits lower frequency sounds.(5)

9. Not all stethoscopes have two sides of the chest piece, a bell and a diaphragm.(5) Many of the newer models have a single dual-sided chest piece.(5) If this is true of yours, then you will need to reference your stethoscope's instruction manual to learn how to switch between each.(5) Usually, you do so by changing the amount of pressure that you apply against the chest piece when it is against the patient's chest wall.(5)

10. S3 and S4 are additional heart sounds that are unlikely to be heard in a normal canine (or feline) heart.(1, 5) When either is audible, it typically reflects cardiac pathology.(1, 5)

11. No, S3 and S4 are not likely to appear on an electrocardiogram (ECG).(5)

12. There are two main types of gallop rhythms.

     S3 is the ventricular gallop sound.(1, 10) It occurs in early diastole, when the ventricles are filling with blood.(1, 10, 11) Ordinarily, this event does not translate into a heart sound.(1, 10) However, certain cardiac pathologies result in diastolic dysfunction.(1, 10) Affected patients require greater investment of pressure to encourage filling of the ventricles.(1, 10) This creates a third heart sound, S3.(1, 9, 10) The result is a so-called gallop rhythm:(1, 7, 9)

1	2–3	1	2–3	1	2–3	1	2–3

     As you can see, S3 arrives on the coat tails of S2 as blood flows from the atria into the now relaxed, partially filled ventricles.(1, 5)

     S4 is the atrial gallop sound.(10) It occurs during the "atrial kick," when the atria contract just before ventricular systole.(11) The purpose of the "atrial kick" is to increase preload by providing one last push of blood into the ventricles before it is pumped into systemic circulation. S4 develops in patients that have impaired ventricular relaxation.(10) Because their ventricles are inadequately relaxed, they have greater filling pressures.(10) The atria must exert more energy than is normal to force additional blood volume into the ventricles to maintain cardiac output.(10) This creates a fourth heart sound, S4.(9, 10) The result is yet another so-called gallop rhythm:(7, 9)

4–1	2	4–1	2	4–1	2	4–1	2

13. S3 is more likely to be audible when there is appreciable ventricular dilation, such as dilated cardiomyopathy (DCM). DCM is more likely to occur in dogs than cats.(1, 5) When it occurs in cats, it is most often secondary to taurine deficiency.(1, 5)

     S4 is more likely to be audible when there is appreciable atrial dilation, such as hypertrophic cardiomyopathy (HCM).(1, 5) S4 also occurs in some patients that have systemic hypertension.(1)

14. You would want to use the bell of the stethoscope to listen closely for S3 and S4 because these are low frequency sounds.(12, 13)

15. A summation gallop occurs when the patient has both S3 and S4.(10) Usually S3 and S4 occur in isolation from one another. When the patient has both, then its heart sounds translate into:(1)

4–1	2–3	4–1	2–3	4–1	2–3	4–1	2–3

16. When the technician says that Darby's heart sounded "odd", he could have meant that Darby's heart sounds were muffled. This means that they are difficult to hear. Alternatively, the technician could have meant that Darby had a heart murmur, which has a characteristic whooshing sound when the chest is auscultated.(1, 5, 7, 8, 14)

17. Muffled heart sounds typically result from abnormal tissue or fluid getting in between the heart and the stethoscope, which is firmly placed against the body wall. This creates an extra layer or obstacle through which sound must travel to be heard. Morbidly obese patients may have muffled heart sounds because the insulating layer of fat represents a sound barrier. Muffled heart sounds may also result from cardiac or respiratory pathology, including pericardial and pleural effusions.(15–22)

     Murmurs, on the other hand, reflect turbulent blood flow.(1, 5) When they occur, heart murmurs may be physiologic or pathologic, congenital or acquired.(1)

     Physiologic murmurs result from conditions outside of the heart, rather than structural issues with the heart itself:(1, 23, 24)

- anemia
- body condition, i.e. athletes(14, 25, 26)
- body shape:(14, 25, 26)

    - deep-chested, large-breed dogs, such as Boxers
    - thin-chested cats and dogs, such as Greyhounds

- hypertension
- hyperthermia
- hypoproteinemia
- increased sympathetic tone, as from FAS (cats)(14, 27)
- pain (cats)
- pregnancy

Congenital murmurs include:(7, 28–38)

- atrial septal defect (ASD) (1, 31, 39)
- mitral valve dysplasia (MVD)
- patent ductus arteriosus (PDA)
- pulmonic stenosis (PS)
- subaortic stenosis (SAS)
- tetralogy of Fallot
- tricuspid valve dysplasia (TVD)
- VSD.

Acquired pathologic murmurs most often result from degenerative myxomatous atrioventricular valve disease, which causes mitral and/or triscuspid regurgitation.(1, 24, 32)
For additional information on murmurs, refer to Case #38.

18. A potential limitation of thoracic auscultation is its accuracy in terms of localizing a murmur and providing a diagnosis. Although murmur characteristics, such as intensity, character, and PMI, can guide you to make a provisional diagnosis, that diagnosis is not always correct.(1) In fact, auscultation without follow-up cardiac imaging is error-prone.(24) In a study of murmurs in Whippet dogs, auscultation exhibited low specificity: 89% of dogs with murmurs were incorrectly diagnosed based upon the acoustics of their murmurs.(1, 24)

19. In addition to cardiothoracic auscultation, I need to assess the following structures on physical exam to obtain a more complete picture about Darby's cardiovascular health:

- capillary refill time (CRT)
- mucous membrane color
- pulse quality/pulse strength
- pulse synchrony: is there a pulse for every heartbeat?

20. I may need to perform an electrocardiogram (ECG) and/or echocardiogram to round out my understanding of Darby's cardiovascular health.

Returning to Case 39: The Dog with Exercise Intolerance

When you place your stethoscope on Darby's chest, you instantly understand what your technician was referring to in terms of the dog's heart. There is a continuous heart murmur. In addition, Darby has bilaterally symmetrical pulses that are bounding.

Round Two of Questions for Case 39: The Dog with Exercise Intolerance

1. Where in the cardiac cycle can a heart murmur occur?
2. What does it mean when you say that Darby has a continuous heart murmur?
3. What is one way to describe to Janice and Leeroy what a continuous heart murmur sounds like?
4. What causes a continuous heart murmur?
5. How will you confirm the cause of Darby's continuous heart murmur?

Answers to Round Two of Questions for Case 39: The Dog with Exercise Intolerance

1. A heart murmur can occur anywhere in the cardiac cycle. Most heart murmurs in companion animal patients are systolic, that is, they occur between S1 and S2 like so:(1, 5, 7, 40)

   | S1 | WHOOSH | S2 | S1 | WHOOSH | S2 |
   | "Lub" | WHOOSH | "Dub" | "Lub" | WHOOSH | "Dub" |

   By contrast, diastolic murmurs are whooshing sounds that occur between S2 and S1:(1, 5, 7, 40)

   | S1 | S2 | WHOOSH | S1 | S2 | WHOOSH | S1 | S2 | WHOOSH |
   | "Lub" | "Dub" | WHOOSH | "Lub" | "Dub" | WHOOSH | "Lub" | "Dub" | WHOOSH |

2. Murmurs that occur throughout systole and diastole are called continuous.(1, 5, 7, 14)

3. Continuous murmurs sound like a washing machine in the midst of a laundry cycle.(14) Others say that it mimics wind blowing through a tunnel.(1, 14)

4. The most common cause of a continuous heart murmur in a dog or cat is PDA.(1, 5, 7, 41–43)

5. I will perform an echocardiogram to confirm my suspicion that Darby has PDA. This imaging modality will allow me to visualize the abnormal connection between Darby's aorta and pulmonary artery.

Returning to Case 39: The Dog with Exercise Intolerance

You perform an echocardiogram and confirm that Darby has PDA (see Figure 39.2).

Round Three of Questions for Case 39: The Dog with Exercise Intolerance

1. In a patient with PDA, which fetal structure persists after birth?
2. What is the purpose of the fetal structure that you identified in Question #1 (above)?

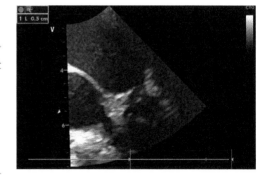

Figure 39.2 This echocardiogram is diagnostic for PDA. Courtesy of Justin Thomason, DACVIM (Cardiology; SAIM), Wildcat Cardiology, and Christy Zimmer Coyle, RVT.

3. What causes this fetal structure to close shortly after birth?
4. When should closure of this fetal structure take place relative to birth?
5. Name the two types of PDA that occur in companion animal patients.
6. Which of the two types occurs with greater frequency?
7. Describe the impact that the type of PDA you identified in Question #6 (above) has on the circulation.
8. What causes a reverse PDA?
9. Which clinical finding on physical exam is suggestive of a reverse PDA?
10. How does the body attempt to compensate for poor oxygenation in cases involving reverse PDA?
11. Which canine breeds are most affected by PDA?
12. Can PDA occur in cats?
13. How is PDA addressed?
14. Can reverse PDA be surgically repaired? Why or why not?
15. What is the prognosis if patients with reverse PDA are untreated?

Answers to Round Three of Questions for Case 39: The Dog with Exercise Intolerance

1. PDA is a congenital defect in which a fetal structure, the ductus arteriosus, persists after birth. (1, 7, 28, 30, 41–45) Rather than closing over to form the ligamentum arteriosum, the ductus arteriosus remains patent.(1, 7, 28, 30)

2. In the fetus, the ductus arteriosus connects the descending aorta to the pulmonary artery.(1) This allows fetal blood to bypass the lungs.(1, 41–44) There is no need for the fetus to pump blood through the pulmonary tree because oxygen is delivered to the fetus through the placenta.(1)

3. Upon birth, the patient takes its first breath.(1, 46) This requires the lungs to work for the very first time.(1) The lungs take over the role of oxygenation.(1) In response, the ductus arteriosus will close.(1, 46)

4. Closure of the ductus arteriosus should take place shortly after birth, typically within two to three days.(42, 44, 47, 48) Within a month of life, all that remains of the ductus arteriosus is a collection of elastic fibers, the ligamentum arteriosum.(7, 28, 30) If this structure instead remains patent, then the patient is said to have a PDA.(7)

5. There are two types of PDAs that occur in companion animal patients:(7, 41–43)

   • left-to-right
   • right-to-left.

6. Left-to-right PDAs occur with greater frequency in companion animal patients.(7, 41–44)

7. In a left-to-right PDA, the high-pressure aorta shunts blood inappropriately into the pulmonary circulation. Recall that the pulmonary circulation in health only receives blood from the pulmonary artery.(7, 41–43) When the pulmonary circulation now receives additional blood from the aorta, it becomes volume overloaded.(7, 41–43) When the pulmonary circulation pushes forward this additional blood supply, it in turn overwhelms the left atrium. Over time, volume overload of the left atrium into the left ventricle causes both chambers of the heart to dilate and hypertrophy.(7, 41–43) Without surgical correction for the left-to-right PDA, the patient is likely to develop left-sided CHF with pulmonary congestion.(7, 28, 30, 41–43)

8. A reverse or right-to-left PDA develops in response to increased pulmonary vascular resistance. (7, 28, 30, 41, 42) When pulmonary vascular resistance exceeds systemic vascular resistance, oxygen-poor blood follows the same pathway as in the fetus. That is, oxygen-poor blood is inappropriately shunted from the pulmonary artery to the aorta, distal to the brachiocephalic and left subclavian arteries.(7, 28, 30, 41, 42, 44)

   Cranial to these arteries, aortic blood is oxygen-rich and delivers its typical supply to the head and forelimbs.(44) These structures therefore receive the same quality of arterial blood that they would have, had the patient not been affected by a reversed PDA.

   Distal to the brachiocephalic and left subclavian arteries, arterial blood is diluted by oxygen-poor blood that has been shunted into systemic circulation.(7, 28, 30, 41, 42, 44) The arterial blood that reaches the caudal half of the patient contains less oxygen content.(44) Caudal tissues become significantly hypoxic.(7, 28, 30, 41, 42)

9. Patients that have reverse PDAs typically exhibit caudal cyanosis, otherwise known as differential cyanosis.(7, 28, 30, 41, 42, 49) The cranial half of the body has pink mucous membranes because tissues are adequately perfused.(7, 28, 30, 41, 42, 49) The caudal half of the body becomes cyanotic.(7, 28, 30, 41, 42, 49)

10. The body attempts to compensate through polycythemia.(42, 44, 45) However, this can only increase perfusion to tissues so much.(28, 30)

11. Canine breeds that are at increased risk of PDAs include:(7, 28, 30, 46, 50–52)

    - Bichon Frise
    - Chihuahua
    - Cocker spaniel
    - Collie
    - English springer spaniel
    - Keeshond
    - Maltese
    - Miniature poodle
    - Pomeranian
    - Shetland sheepdog
    - Shih Tzu
    - Toy poodle
    - Yorkshire terrier
    - Welsh Corgi.

12. Yes, PDA can occur in cats.(53)

13. Left-to-right PDA is surgically repaired.(1) The goal is to halt blood flow through the shunt by either tying off the patent ductus arteriosus or occluding it with a transarterial coil.

14. Reverse PDA cannot be surgically repaired.(44) Ligation of a reverse PDA would lead to life-threatening pulmonary hypertension.(44) In order for the heart to continue to pump blood, its right side would need to raise its pressure significantly to exceed that of the pulmonary vasculature. This is not sustainable.

15. Patients with reverse PDA will ultimately succumb to right-sided heart failure, hypoxemia, fatal cardiac arrhythmias, and/or thrombus formation.(44, 54)

CLINICAL PEARLS

- A basic understanding of anatomy and physiology is essential when considering cardiomyopathy. You must first understand how the heart works as a mechanical pump to push blood through the vasculature before you can understand where problems may arise.

- Understanding the heart as a pump requires you to track the flow of blood through the chambers of the heart and locate the heart valves through which blood passes.

- It is the coordinated closure of heart valves that causes normal heart sounds to be audible using a stethoscope to auscultate the chest.

- S1 and S2 are normal heart sounds that should be audible through auscultation, using the diaphragm chest piece of the stethoscope. S1 and S2 create the classic "lub-dub" sounds of the heart.

- Additional heart sounds S3 and S4 do not typically occur in normal patients. When they do, they create a characteristic gallop rhythm that is often a sign of cardiac pathology.

- In addition to having extra heart sounds, the heart can sound muffled or turbulent blood flow can lead to the development of murmurs.

- Systolic murmurs are more common than diastolic murmurs in companion animal patients.

- Continuous heart murmurs occur throughout systole and diastole and have a characteristic "washing machine" sound.

- PDA is a congenital heart condition that is classically associated with a continuous heart murmur.

- In patients with PDA, a fetal structure, the ductus arteriosus, persists after birth. PDA leads to volume overload of the heart. Without surgical correction, PDA leads to left-sided CHF.

- Reverse PDAs may also occur due to increased pulmonary vascular resistance. This is not a surgical condition. It will progress to right-sided CHF.

References

1. Englar RE. Common clinical presentations in dogs and cats. Hoboken, NJ: Wiley/Blackwell; 2019. pages cm p.
2. Cunningham JG, Klein BG. Cunningham's textbook of veterinary physiology. 5th ed. St. Louis, MO: Elsevier/Saunders; 2013.
3. Singh B, Dyce KM. Dyce, Sack, and Wensing's textbook of veterinary anatomy. 5th ed. St. Louis, MOi: Saunders; 2018.
4. Evans HE, Miller ME. Miller's anatomy of the dog. 4th ed. St. Louis, MO: Elsevier; 2013.
5. Englar RE. Performing the small animal physical examination. Hoboken, NJ: Wiley/Blackwell; 2017.
6. Dyce KM, Sack WO, Wensing CJG. Textbook of veterinary anatomy. 4th ed. St. Louis, MO: Saunders/Elsevier; 2010.
7. Englar RE. Performing the small animal physical examination. Hoboken, NJ: Wiley/Blackwell; 2017.
8. Hall JE, Guyton AC. Guyton and Hall textbook of medical physiology. 12th ed. Philadelphia, PA: Saunders/Elsevier; 2011.
9. Stokhof AA, De Rick A. Circulatory system. In: Rijnberk A, van Sluijs FJ, editors. Medical history and physical examination in companion animals. St. Louis, MO: Saunders; 2009.
10. Lorenz MC, Neer TM, DeMars P. Small animal medical diagnosis. 3rd ed. Ames, IA: Blackwell; 2009.

11. Estrada A. Cardiac physical examination. NAVC clinician's brief [Internet]. Available from: https://www.cliniciansbrief.com/article/cardiac-physical-examination.

12. DeFrancesco T. Cardiac Auscultation 1012012. Available from: https://cvm.ncsu.edu/wp-content/uploads/2015/06/DeFrancesco2012_CardiacAusculation.pdf.

13. Garcia JL. Lecture link: feline cardiology review. 2014. DVM. Available from: http://veterinarymedicine.dvm360.com/lecture-link-feline-cardiology-review.

14. Mandese WW, Estrada AH. The basic cardiology examination. NAVC Clin's Brief 2017 (May):91–7.

15. De Madron E. Pericardial diseases. In: De Madron E, Chetboul V, Bussadori C, editors. Clinical echocardiography of the dog and cat. St. Louis, MO: Elsevier; 2015.

16. Wey AC. Cardiomegaly. NAVC Clin's Brief 2005 (March):7–8.

17. Laste NJ. Canine pericardial effusion. NAVC Clin's Brief 2016 (January):65–72.

18. Hall DJ, Shofer F, Meier CK, Sleeper MM. Pericardial effusion in cats: a retrospective study of clinical findings and outcome in 146 cats. J Vet Intern Med 2007;21(5):1002–7.

19. DeFrancesco TC. Management of cardiac emergencies in small animals. Vet Clin North Am Small Anim Pract 2013;43(4):817–42.

20. Scansen BA. Interventional cardiology for the criticalist. J Vet Emerg Crit Care (San Antonio) 2011;21(2):123–36.

21. MacDonald K. Pericardial effusion: causes and clinical outcomes in dogs. DVM 360 [Internet]. 2009. Available from: http://veterinarycalendar.dvm360.com/pericardial-effusion-causes-and-clin;ical-outcomes-dogs-proceedings-0.

22. Bille C, Bomassi E, Libermann S. Muffled heart sounds in a dog. Compend Contin Educ Vet 2010 (June).

23. Estrada AH. Physiologic murmur. Clinician's brief [Internet]. Available from: https://www.cliniciansbrief.com/cardiac-library/heart-sound/physiologic-murmur.

24. Côté E, Edwards NJ, Ettinger SJ, Fuentes VL, MacDonald KA, Scansen BA, et al. Management of incidentally detected heart murmurs in dogs and cats. J Vet Cardiol 2015;17(4):245–61.

25. Garcia JL. Journal Scan: Physiological heart murmurs are more common in our veterinary patients than we may think; 2015. DVM. Available from: http://veterinarymedicine.dvm360.com/journal-scan-physiological-heart-murmurs-are-more-common-our-veterinary-patients-we-may-think.

26. Drut A, Ribas T, Floch F, Franchequin S, Freyburger L, Rannou B, et al. Prevalence of physiological heart murmurs in a population of 95 healthy young adult dogs. J Small Anim Pract 2015;56(2):112–8.

27. Wagner T, Fuentes VL, Payne JR, McDermott N, Brodbelt D. Comparison of auscultatory and echocardiographic findings in healthy adult cats. J Vet Cardiol 2010;12(3):171–82.

28. Bulmer BJ. The cardiovascular system. In: Peterson ME, Kutzler MA, editors. Small animal pediatrics: the first 12 months of life. St. Louis, MO: Saunders/Elsevier; 2011.

29. Schrope DP. Prevalence of congenital heart disease in 76,301 mixed-breed dogs and 57,025 mixed-breed cats. J Vet Cardiol Off J Eur 2015;17(3):192–202.

30. Strickland KN. Congenital heart disease. In: Tilley LP, Smith FWK, Oyama MA, Sleeper MM, editors. Manual of canine and feline cardiology. 4th ed. Philadelphia, PA: W. B. Saunders; 2008. p. 215–39.

31. MacDonald K. Murmurs in puppies and kittens. 2011. DVM. Available from: http://veterinarycalendar.dvm360.com/murmurs-puppies-and-kittens-proceedings.

32. Rishniw M. Canine heart murmur. NAVC Clin's Brief 2011 (May):49–52.

33. Oliveira P, Domenech O, Silva J, Vannini S, Bussadori R, Bussadori C. Retrospective review of congenital heart disease in 976 dogs. J Vet Intern Med 2011;25(3):477–83.

34. Buchanan JW. Prevalence of cardiovascular disorders. In: Fox PR, Sisson DD, Moize NS, editors. Textbook of canine and feline cardiology. Philadelphia, PA: W. B. Saunders; 1998. p. 457–70.

35. Baumgartner C, Glaus TM. Congenital cardiac diseases in dogs: a retrospective analysis. Schweiz Arch Tierheilkd 2003;145(11):527–33.

36. Hunt GB, Church DB, Malik R, Bellenger CR. A retrospective analysis of congenital cardiac anomalies (1977–1989). Aust Vet Pract 1990;20(2):70–5.

37. Tidholm A. Retrospective study of congenital heart defects in 151 dogs. J Small Anim Pract 1997;38(3):94–8.

38. MacDonald KA. Congenital heart diseases of puppies and kittens. Vet Clin North Am Small Anim Pract 2006;36(3):503–31.

39. Tilley LP, Smith FWK. The 5-minute veterinary consult: canine and feline. 3rd ed. Baltimore, MD: Lippincott Williams & Wilkins; 2004.

40. Gompf RE. The history and physical examination. In: Tilley LP, Smith FWK, Oyama M, Sleeper MM, editors. Manual of canine and feline cardiology. St. Louis, MO: Saunders; 2008. p. 2–23.
41. Côté E. Clinical veterinary advisor. Dogs and cats. 3rd ed. St. Louis, MO: Elsevier Mosby; 2015.
42. Tilley LP, Smith FWK, Tilley LP. Blackwell's five-minute veterinary consult: canine and feline. 4th ed. Ames, IA: Blackwell; 2007.
43. The Merck veterinary manual. Whitehouse Station, NJ: Merck & Co., Inc. 2016.
44. Arora M. Reversed patent ductus arteriosus in a dog. Can Vet J 2001;42(6):471–2.
45. Scurtu I, Pestean C, Lacatus R, Lascu M, Mircean M, Codea R, et al. Reverse PDA – less common type of patent ductus arteriosus – case report. Bull UASVM Vet Med;2106(73 (2)):351–5.
46. Broaddus K, Tillson M. Patent ductus arteriosus in dogs. Compend Contin Educ Vet 2010;32(9):E3.
47. Oliver NB. Congenital heart disease in dogs. In: Fox PR, editor. Canine and feline cardiology. New York: Churchill Livingstone; 1988. p. 360–5.
48. Nelson RW, Couto CG. Small animal internal medicine. St. Louis, MO: Mosby; 1998.
49. Houghton HE, Ware WA. Patent ductus arteriosus in dogs. Iowa State Univ Vet 1996;58(2).
50. Orton EC. Cardiac surgery. In: Slatter D, editor. Textbook of small animal surgery. Philadelphia, PA: W.B. Saunders; 2003. p. 955–9.
51. Fossum TW. Small animal surgery. St. Louis, MO: Mosby Elsevier; 2007.
52. Buchanan JW, Patterson DF. Etiology of patent ductus arteriosus in dogs. J Vet Intern Med 2003;17(2):167–71.
53. Cote E, MacDonald KA, Montgomery Meurs K, Sleeper MM. Feline cardiology. Oxford: John Wiley & Sons, Inc.; 2011.
54. Bonagura JD, Darke PG. Congenital heart disease. In: Ettinger SJ, Feldman EC, editors. Textbook of veterinary internal medicine. Philadelphia, PA: W.B. Saunders; 1989. p. 892–943.

Case 40

The Wheezing Cat

You aren't supposed to have favorite patients, but "Wellie," short for Sir Wellington, is one of yours. His visits to your practice began as early as his first week of life, when he had been labeled by his breeder as a "failure to thrive." Born into a litter of four, he was the only one who had difficulty latching onto the teat. His inability to nurse, or to at least consume enough milk for growth, led to a significant discrepancy in body weight between himself, as the runt, and the rest of his siblings. Each day that they made forward strides, his strides seemed to go backward. When he caught an upper respiratory infection (URI) on top of everything else, the breeder was certain he would not survive. But you managed to partner with her to pull him through. By switching him to a bottle and upping the number of feedings per day, he was more than able to make up for lost time. He regained his vigor and was sold at 5 months old to his current owner, Emma Briggs.

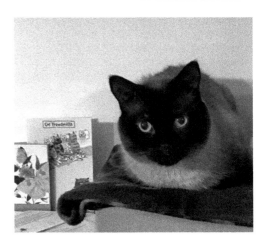

Figure 40.1 Meet your patient, Sir Wellington, a 4-year-old castrated male Siamese cat. Courtesy of Amanda Spector, DVM.

Wellie has resided exclusively with Emma until 6 weeks ago, when Emma's boyfriend, Gordon, moved into the home. Emma had been dating Gordon on and off these past 2 years, so he is not a stranger to Wellie. In fact, Wellie had grown accustomed to his weekend visits. What Wellie hadn't prepared for was a full-time, live-in roommate that monopolized Emma's time. Wellie was still feeling prickly about the whole situation.

Thankfully, Gordon has no children and no pets of his own to relocate, so it's just the three of them who now share a two-story townhome. There is plenty of space for Wellie, who has no intention of relinquishing his claim over top dollar seating – the sofa, the lounge chair, the foyer bench, and the trunk at the foot of the bed. These are his and he was here first. So far, so good. Gordon has respected his boundaries, and Wellie has been able to spend his days as planned, indoors, chasing the sun from room to room.

For a young cat, Wellie is surprisingly lazy, and although he was more of a grazer as a kitten, he has turned into quite the foodie. He is good at convincing others that he is starving and has managed to swindle Gordon out of a few bites of every meal since he arrived. So, when Wellie started to stretch out his neck and make unusual sounds as if about to upchuck, Emma convinced herself that it was related to overeating. What was strange, though, was that nothing ever came up.

These events were uncharted ground for Wellie. He'd never experienced them before Gordon's arrival, at least not in plain sight of Emma. The episodes were sporadic but seemed to be increasing in both frequency and duration. There was no apparent rhyme or reason to it.

Emma videoed one of the episodes to share with friends and elicit their perspective as to what they thought might be happening. Several agreed with her that Wellie was trying to purge something, albeit unsuccessfully. Others suggested that he might be overloaded with hairballs and having trouble expelling them. She thought about purchasing an over-the-counter remedy, but Wellie was already sullen about Gordon. She didn't want to push him over the edge by force-feeding him malt-flavored hairball paste that he hated.

Emma didn't begin to worry until a colleague at work overheard her telephone conversation over lunch in the break room. "Are you sure he's not coughing?" her co-worker asked. "That doesn't sound normal. You might want to have that checked out."

Prior to that moment, Emma had never worried all that much. The episodes had seemed benign enough. Just as surely as he launched into them, he always came out of them. But what if one day he didn't? What then? Emma agreed it was time to get to the bottom of this.

She is here now to see you with Wellie. Your technician leads them both into the first available exam room and documents Wellie's vital signs as they wait for you to initiate the consultation.

Use the following questions to guide your approach to this appointment.

Weight: 12.4 lb (5.6 kg)
BCS: 6/9
Mentation: BAR

TPR

T: 100.6°F (38.1°C)
P: 175 beats per minute
R: 27 breaths per minute

Round One of Questions for Case 40: The Wheezing Cat

1. Your technician relays Emma's concerns that Wellie might be coughing. What is a cough?
2. How does the patient initiate a cough?
3. Which cranial nerve(s) trigger(s) the coughing reflex?
4. Which upper respiratory tract diseases in cats and dogs are associated with cough?
5. Which lower respiratory tract diseases in cats and dogs are associated with cough?
6. Cough may also be triggered by cardiomyopathy. Which cardiomyopathies are most often associated with cough?
7. Explain the link between atrial enlargement and cough.
8. Explain the link(s) between heart failure and cough.
9. Esophageal disease may also lead to bouts of coughing. Explain the link between the two.
10. How does a cough differ from an expiratory wheeze?
11. What causes wheezing?
12. Which airway condition is associated with expiratory wheezing?
13. Explain the link between the condition that you named in Question #12 (above) and wheezing.
14. Can wheezes be audible without a stethoscope?
15. What are potential triggers for the condition that you identified in Question #12 (above)?
16. Give examples of how you can use both open-ended and closed-ended questions to ask about Wellie's potential exposure to these triggers in his home environment.

Answers to Round One of Questions for Case 40: The Wheezing Cat

1. A cough is the forceful expulsion of the air through the glottis.(1–3)

2. To produce a cough, the patient reflexively inspires.(1–3) The glottis then closes, raising intrathoracic pressure.(1–3) At that point, the glottis opens to allow for the cough to occur.(1–3)

3. The glossopharyngeal and vagus nerves mediate cough.(1) Fibers of the glossopharyngeal nerve are located within the pharynx itself. Fibers of the vagus nerve reside within the larynx, trachea, and large bronchi.(1, 4)

4. The following upper respiratory tract diseases in cats and dogs are associated with cough in companion animal patients:(1, 5–26)

- foreign body obstruction, partial or complete:

  - nasopharyngeal
  - laryngeal
  - tracheal

- inhalation of irritants:

  - dust particles
  - gas
  - hair
  - litter (cats)
  - pollen
  - smoke

- infectious tracheobronchitis
- laryngeal paralysis
- neoplasia:

  - nasopharyngeal
  - laryngeal
  - tracheal

- rhinitis and sinorhinitis with post-nasal drip
- tracheal collapse.

5. The following lower respiratory tract diseases in cats and dogs are associated with cough in companion animal patients:(1, 5–26)

- bronchial foreign body obstruction
- bronchitis
- feline asthma/bronchitis complex
- infectious tracheobronchitis
- neoplasia:

  - primary lung tumor
  - metastatic lung tumor

- parasitic:

  - feline heartworm-associated respiratory disease (HARD)
  - lungworms

- pleuritis or other pleural space disease:

  - pleural effusions

- pneumonia:

  - aspiration
  - bacterial
  - fungal
  - viral

- pulmonary edema, non-cardiogenic
- pulmonary embolism
- pulmonary fibrosis
- pulmonary infiltrates with eosinophils (PIE).

6. Coughing may also be triggered by cardiac pathology. The most common cardiac causes of cough include:(1, 6, 20, 27–29)

    - cardiogenic pulmonary edema
    - dilated cardiomyopathy (DCM)
    - left atrial enlargement associated with mitral regurgitation (MR)
    - left-sided congestive heart failure (CHF)
    - heartworm disease (HWD).

7. Left atrial enlargement due to MR physically compresses the bronchi, mediating cough.(30)

8. The heart is a pump.(25, 26, 31, 32). The purpose of the left ventricle is to mechanically pump blood into systemic circulation via the aorta.(33, 34) When this side of the heart fails, blood backflows from the left ventricle into the left atrium and, ultimately, the pulmonary vasculature. (33, 34)

    The lungs are said to be congested.(35) The presence of pulmonary infiltrate triggers the cough.(30)

9. Aspiration pneumonia can result from esophageal disease because affected patients exhibit regurgitation.(26, 36, 37) Regurgitation precipitates aspiration pneumonia in many patients with megaesophagus.(36–38)

10. Whereas coughs are productive at expelling air, patients that exhibit expiratory wheezing have increased resistance to airflow.(39, 40) They struggle to get air out.(26) This results in the "musical" sound of vibrations within the walls of the airway.(26, 39)

11. Wheezing typically occurs in patients that have reactive or thickened airways, as from airway inflammation.(26, 39, 40) Wheezing may also occur in patients with partially collapsed or obstructed airways due to neighboring pulmonary disease.(26, 39)

12. Feline asthma is associated with expiratory wheezing.(19, 26, 39–41)

13. Asthma is characterized by chronic inflammation of the bronchi and bronchioles.(1, 5, 26, 42) Inflammation of the respiratory mucosa increases secretions, which narrow the lumen of the airway.(1, 5, 19, 26, 42) A reduction in the diameter of the airway appreciably reduces airflow. (42) Let's consider an airway, the diameter of which has been reduced by 50%. This airway now has a 16-fold reduction in airflow.(42)

    The bronchoconstriction that occurs during an asthma attack further reduces the diameter of an already pathologically narrowed space.(1, 5, 26, 42) When the patient tries to exhale, s/he has to work harder to get air out. The resultant sound is a wheeze.(26)

14. Yes, wheezes can be audible without a stethoscope.(25, 26)

15. Potential triggers for feline asthma include:(1, 26)

    - air fresheners
    - cigarette smoke
    - dusty cat litter
    - hair spray
    - scented candles.

    Many of these are extrapolated from what is known about triggers in human asthmatics.(19)

16. You may elect to ask Emma about Wellie's exposure to these potential triggers through either closed- or open-ended questions.

Closed-ended questions are direct and to the point.(43, 44) Their intent is to get clients to respond in an abbreviated manner.(45) The answer to a closed-ended question is often "yes" or "no."(45) The utility of asking closed-ended questions in this clinical scenario is that you can directly ask about each individual trigger.

- Has Wellie been exposed to cigarette smoke? Or does anyone in the home smoke?
- Do you use air fresheners in the home?
- Do you use scented candles?
- Is Wellie's cat litter scented?

Closed-ended questions are an essential part of the consultation in that they obtain the specific data that you are most interested in.(43, 44) However, you often have a need to ask a series of closed-ended questions in order for your list to be comprehensive.

To improve efficiency of history-taking, we need to consider an alternate style of questioning, the open-ended question or statement.(43, 44)

Open-ended questions and statements invite clients to share.(43, 44, 46)

To encourage the client to expand upon their answer, open-ended statements often begin with:(45, 47–49)

- Tell me
- Help me
- Show me
- Share with me
- Describe

In this clinical case, you might simply say to Emma, "Tell me about any changes that you've made to Wellie's home environment." Alternatively, you may say, "Emma, help me to understand what, if anything, has changed in the home that may have led to the changes that you're seeing in Wellie."

These two options give the client an opportunity to share what is on her mind without restrictions. Because of this, I often choose to lead a consultation with an open-ended question or statement. The client can then relay information to me that strikes him/her as being important. I can then follow-up on what the client has shared with appropriate closed-ended questions that are necessary to refine and/or clarify data that the client has shared with me.(44)

Returning to Case 40: The Wheezing Cat

You ask Emma what, if anything, has changed in Wellie's environment as a result of Gordon moving into the home. She shares that Gordon smokes cigarettes exclusively, and although he respects her request that he not light up in the home, his clothing smells very strongly of smoke. To combat this, Emma purchased plug-in air fresheners, but they scarcely cover up the smell. If anything, the smell of artificial vanilla is worse than the smoke itself, so she is at a loss for how to overcome this strain on their relationship.

Other than the smoke and Gordon's presence, Emma assures you that there have been no other changes.

Emma picks up on the fact that you asked specifically about smoke and asks if that has caused Wellie to be ill. You share your desire to examine Wellie first before jumping to any conclusions, but yes, in all transparency, one possibility is that the smoke has triggered Wellie to have asthmatic fits.

Round Two of Questions for Case 40: The Wheezing Cat

Consider the following questions about feline asthma before you proceed with your consultation.

1. Is Wellie's age consistent with most asthmatic cats?
2. Is Wellie's breed predisposed to feline asthma?
3. If Wellie has asthma, what might you expect to find on physical exam?
4. Based upon your high index of clinical suspicion, which diagnostic test will you perform next with the hopes of confirming your presumptive diagnosis?
5. In addition to your answer for Question #4 (above), you also suggest that fecal analysis be performed. Why?
6. Which fecal test has the greatest chance of identifying that for which you are screening Wellie?

Answers to Round Two of Questions for Case 40: The Wheezing Cat

1. Yes, Wellie's age is consistent with most asthmatic cats. Cats that are diagnosed with asthma are most often young to middle-aged.(1, 19, 26)

2. Yes, Wellie's breed is predisposed to feline asthma. Siamese cats are overrepresented among feline asthmatics.(1, 19, 26)

3. If Wellie has asthma, he may appear to be clinically normal on physical exam, particularly if he is not in the midst of an asthma attack.(19, 26) What this means is that his lungs may give no indication of any form of bronchial disease. When you auscultate the chest, his lungs may sound clear. You may hear only bronchovesicular lung sounds, which are normal, and Wellie may not exhibit wheezing. This lack of any sort of clinical finding can be particularly frustrating for the client, who knows that something is "wrong" and may not understand why you are at a loss to find the problem.

    If you are fortunate, you may hear increased bronchovesicular sounds in asthmatic cats on thoracic auscultation.(19, 25, 26)

    You may also hear expiratory wheezes, with or without your stethoscope. These are supportive of the presumptive diagnosis, feline asthma.(19)

4. Diagnostic imaging in the form of thoracic radiography is the next most appropriate diagnostic test to perform to look for evidence to support your presumptive diagnosis.(26, 50–52)

5. In addition to thoracic radiographs, you also suggest that fecal analysis be performed to rule out lungworms as a cause of feline cough.(1)

6. The Baermann fecal test is the preferred test for ruling out lungworms.(1, 26, 53)

Returning to Case 40: The Wheezing Cat

Emma consents to fecal flotation and a Baermann test. No lungworms are seen. Emma also grants permission for you to proceed with two-view thoracic radiography. The right lateral view has been provided in Figures 40.2 and 40.3 for your review.

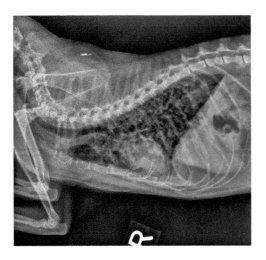

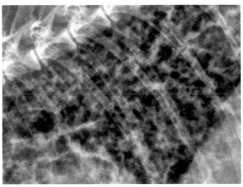

Figure 40.2 Right lateral thoracic radiograph. Courtesy of Daniel Foy, MS, DVM, DACVIM, DACVECC.

Figure 40.3 Close-up of right lateral thoracic radiograph. Courtesy of Daniel Foy, MS, DVM, DACVIM, DACVECC.

Round Three of Questions for Case 40: The Wheezing Cat

1. Assuming that Wellie is in fact negative for lungworms, what is Wellie's diagnosis?
2. What do you see on Wellie's right lateral radiograph that is conclusive?
3. How was this condition treated in the past?
4. Which potential concerns about this treatment option led to changes in recommendations for medical management?
5. Currently, which is the most appropriate treatment for Wellie's condition?
6. How is this treatment administered?
7. What might you prescribe for Emma to administer if Wellie experiences acute onset of respiratory distress due to a flare-up in his condition?
8. Do you have any other recommendations for Wellie's home environment?
9. Is Wellie's condition curable?

Answers to Round Three of Questions for Case 40: The Wheezing Cat

1. Wellie's diagnosis is feline asthma.

2. I can identify a classic "donut" bronchial pattern on Wellie's right lateral radiograph (see Figure 40.4).

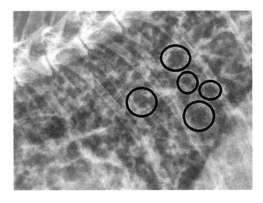

Figure 40.4 Close-up of right lateral thoracic radiograph of a cat with feline asthma, with the classic "donut" bronchial pattern identified. Courtesy of Daniel Foy, MS, DVM, DACVIM, DACVECC.

Wellie's right lateral radiograph demonstrates diffuse thickening of his bronchial walls.(1) This thickening creates the illusion of a "donut."(19, 39) Each bronchus is outlined by a thicker-than-normal circle of black.(39) This is referred to as peri-bronchial cuffing.(19) Such cuffing is indicative of airway inflammation that is consistent with feline asthma.

Note that radiographs are supportive of the diagnosis; however, they are not pathognomonic for asthma. Lungworms may result in a similar radiographic appearance.(26)

3. In the past, oral prednisolone was administered to cats with asthma.(26)

4. Long-term use of oral steroids may potentiate systemic side effects, which include:(42, 50, 54)

    - polyuria and polydipsia (PU/PD)
    - polyphagia
    - ulcerations within the gastrointestinal tract.

    Long-term administration of glucocorticoids may also increase the risk of developing diabetes mellitus.(54, 55)

5. Inhalant corticosteroids, such as fluticasone, are now preferred over oral prednisolone.(1, 42)

6. Inhalant corticosteroids are administered by fitting a metered dose inhaler into a spacer that has been outfitted with a feline-friendly facemask.(26) (See Figure 40.5.)

    The spacer is primed with the medication and the facemask is placed over the cat's mouth and nose.(26) The cat is observed to breathe 7 to 10 times before the treatment is said to be complete.(26, 42)

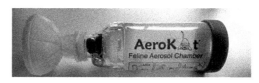

Figure 40.5 Example of a commercial device for delivery of inhalant medications to feline asthmatics.

7. I would prescribe a "rescue inhaler," such as albuterol.(19, 21, 22, 42) Albuterol is administered during an asthmatic crisis to counter bronchoconstriction.(19, 21, 22, 42) Its route of administration is the same as fluticasone's.(19, 21, 22, 42)

    Wellie will still benefit from in-clinic evaluation and monitoring through these episodes, in which case Emma should be directed to get him to any clinic urgently.

8. Certain scents can trigger asthmatic episodes. In the ideal world, I would recommend removing the following allergens from the environment:

    - smoke
    - air fresheners.

9. Asthma is a chronic condition. It is lifelong and may progress in intensity.(1) Medical management is therefore aimed at reducing the severity of clinical signs and increasing the length of time between attacks.(26)

CLINICAL PEARLS

- Wheezing is a clinical sign that suggests narrowed airways due to inflammation and/or secretions.

- Expiratory wheezes are "musical" sounds that arise as the patient struggles to expel air from the lower airways. These sounds may be audible without a stethoscope.

- Expiratory wheezes are supportive of the diagnosis, feline asthma.

- Feline asthma typically targets young to middle-aged cats. Siamese cats are overrepresented among clinical cases of feline asthma.

- Clients may report unusual episodes in which the patient hyperextends its neck to gasp. Clients may state that the cat acts like it is trying to cough or bring up a hairball.

- Episodes may be triggered by air fresheners, scented candles, smoke, pollen, dust, and dander in patients with pre-existing disease.

- Physical exam findings may reveal increased bronchovesicular sounds on thoracic auscultation +/– audible wheezes, or the patient's exam may be unremarkable.

- Thoracic radiographs are supportive of the diagnosis of feline asthma when they demonstrate a bronchial pattern with peri-bronchial cuffing. This means that each bronchus is outlined by a thicker-than-normal circle of black. This creates the illusion of "donuts" throughout the lung field.

- These "donuts" are not pathognomonic for asthma. Patients that have lungworms may have similar findings on thoracic radiographs.

- Feline asthma is managed with inhalant corticosteroids and bronchodilators, as necessary. Treatment is lifelong and aimed at reducing severity of clinical signs.

References

1. Tilley LP, Smith FWK. Blackwell's five-minute veterinary consult. Canine and feline. 6th edition. Ames, IA: John Wiley & Sons, Inc.; 2016.
2. Newhouse M, Sanchis J, Bienenstock J. Lung defense mechanisms (second of two parts). N. Engl. J. Med. 1976;295(19):1045–52.
3. Newhouse M, Sanchis J, Bienenstock J. Lung defense mechanisms (first of two parts). N. Engl. J. Med. 1976;295(18):990–8.
4. Widdicombe JG. Mechanism of cough and its regulation. Eur. J. Respir. Dis. Suppl. 1980;110:11–20.
5. Mason RA, Rand J. The coughing cat. In: Rand J, editor. Problem-based feline medicine. Philadelphia, PA: Elsevier; 2006. p. 90–108.
6. Hawkins EC. Coughing dogs: Determining why. NAVC Clin's Brief [Internet]. Available from: https://www.cliniciansbrief.com/column/category/column/capsules/coughing-dogs-determining-why.
7. Johnson LR. Chronic cough. NAVC Clin.'s Brief. 2006 (July):51–2.
8. Ellis J. Chronic cough in a puppy. NAVC Clin's Brief [Internet]. Available from: https://www.cliniciansbrief.com/article/chronic-cough-puppy.
9. Clercx C, Roels E. Exercise intolerance and chronic cough in a geriatic dog. NAVC Clin.'s Brief. 2015 (December).
10. Grobman M, Reinero C. Investigation of Neurokinin-1 receptor antagonism as a novel treatment for chronic bronchitis in dogs. J. Vet. Intern. Med. 2016;30(3):847–52.

11. Dye J. Cough in cats. NAVC Clin.'s Brief. 2008(July);17.

12. Deweese MD, Tobias KM. Tracheal collapse in dogs. NAVC Clin.'s Brief. 2014 (May):83–7.

13. Palma D. Common pulmonary diseases in dogs. NAVC Clin.'s Brief. 2016 (October):77–109.

14. Palma D. Common pulmonary diseases in cats. NAVC Clin.'s Brief. 2017 (March):107–15.

15. Fry JK, Burney DP. Canine infectious respiratory disease. NAVC Clin.'s Brief. 2012 (November):34–8.

16. Conboy G. Helminth parasites of the canine and feline respiratory tract. Vet. Clin. North Am. Small Anim. Pract. 2009;39(6):1109–26.

17. Kumrow KJ. Canine chronic bronchitis: A review and update. Today's. Vet. Pract. 2012 (November/December):12–7.

18. Carey SA, editor. Current therapy for canine chronic Bronchitis. 2018: Michigan veterinary Medical Association.

19. Padrid P. Feline asthma and bronchitis. NAVC Clin.'s Brief. 2005 (October):37–40.

20. Byers CG, Dhupa N. Feline asthma and heartworm disease – Reply. Comp Cont. Educ. Pract. 2005;27(8):573.

21. Byers CG, Dhupa N. Feline bronchial asthma: Pathophysiology and diagnosis. Comp. Cont. Educ. Pract. 2005;27(6):418.

22. Byers CG, Dhupa N. Feline bronchial asthma: Treatment. Comp Cont. Educ. Pract. 2005;27(6):426–31.

23. Little S. Coughing and wheezing cats: Diagnosis and treatment of feline asthma. DVM. 360 [Internet]; 2010. Available from: http://veterinarycalendar.dvm360.com/coughing-and-wheezing-cats-diagnosis-and-treatment-feline-asthma-proceedings.

24. Traversa D, Di Cesare A. Diagnosis and management of lungworm infections in cats: Cornerstones, dilemmas and new avenues. J. Feline Med. Surg. 2016;18(1):7–20.

25. Englar RE. Performing the small animal physical examination. Hoboken, NJ: Wiley/Blackwell; 2017.

26. Englar RE. Common clinical presentations in dogs and cats. Hoboken, NJ: Wiley/Blackwell; 2019.

27. Miller MW. Canine cough. NAVC Clin.'s Brief. 2007 (September);27.

28. Miller MW, Gordon SG. Canine congestive heart failure. NAVC Clin.'s Brief. 2007 (September):31–5.

29. Lee ACY, Kraus MS. Coughing cat: Could it be heartworm? NAVC Clin.'s Brief. 2012 (June):91–5.

30. Wray J. The coughing dog with a heart murmur2018. Available from: https://veterinary-practice.com/article/the-coughing-dog-with-a-heart-murmur.

31. Cunningham JG, Klein BG. Cunningham's textbook of veterinary physiology. 5th ed. St Louis, MO: Elsevier/Saunders; 2013.

32. Singh B, Dyce KM. Dyce, Sack, and Wensing's textbook of veterinary anatomy. St. Louis, MO: Saunders; 2018.

33. Reece WO, Erickson HH, Goff JP, Uemura EE. Dukes' physiology of domestic animals. 13th ed. Ames, IA Wiley/Blackwell; 2015.

34. Estrada A. Heart disease: Diagnosis and treatment NAVC clinician's. Brief 2014 (March):91–5.

35. Rozanski E. Pulmonary edema. DVM. 360 [Internet]; 2009. Available from: http://veterinarycalendar.dvm360.com/print/328751?page=full.

36. Sherding RG. Esophagitis and esophageal stricture. DVM. 360 [Internet]; 2011. Available from: Esophagitis and esophageal stricture.

37. Sherding RG. Regurgitation, dysphagia, and esophageal dysmotility. DVM. 360 [Internet]; 2011. Available from: http://veterinarycalendar.dvm360.com/regurgitation-dysphagia-and-esophageal-dysmotility-proceedings.

38. Bissett S. Esophagitis. NAVC Clin.'s Brief. 2012 (June):23–6.

39. Englar RE. Performing the small animal physical examination. Hoboken, NJ: Wiley; 2017.

40. Hansen B. What's that noise? Interpreting lung sounds. DVM. 360 [Internet]; 2009. Available from: http://veterinarycalendar.dvm360.com/whats-noise-interpreting-lung-sounds-proceedings.

41. Abnormal breath sounds: RnCeus Interactive™, LLC; 1996. Available from: http://www.rnceus.com/resp/respabn.html.

42. Padrid P. Diagnosing and treating feline asthma (including the use of inhalants). DVM. 360 [Internet]; 2011. Available from: http://veterinarycalendar.dvm360.com/diagnosing-and-treating-feline-asthma-including-use-inhalants-proceedings.

43. Englar R. Writing skills for veterinarians. Sheffield: 5M Publishing; 2019.

44. Englar R. A guide to oral Communication in Veterinary Medicine. Sheffield: 5M Publishing; 2020.

45. Shaw JR. Four core communication skills of highly effective practitioners. Vet. Clin. North Am. Small Anim. Pract. 2006;36(2):385–96.

46. Englar RE, Williams M, Weingand K. Applicability of the Calgary-Cambridge guide to dog and cat owners for teaching veterinary clinical communications. J. Vet. Med. Educ. 2016;43(2):143–69.

47. Kurtz SM, Silverman JD, Draper J. Teaching and learning communication skills in medicine. Grand Rapids, FL: Radcliffe 2004.

48. Adams CL, Kurtz SM. Skills for communicating in veterinary medicine. Oxford: Otmoor Press and Dewpoint Publishing; 2017.

49. Silverman J, Kurtz S, Draper J. Skills for communicating with patients. Oxford: Radcliffe Medical Press; 2008.

50. Côté E. Clinical veterinary advisor. Dogs and cats. 3rd ed. St. Louis, MO: Elsevier Mosby; 2015.

51. Thrall DE. Textbook of veterinary diagnostic radiology. 7th ed. St. Louis, MO: Elsevier; 2018.

52. Ettinger SJ, Feldman EC, Côté E. Textbook of veterinary internal medicine: diseases of the dog and the cat. 8th ed. St. Louis, MO: Elsevier; 2017.

53. Bowman DD, Georgi JR. Georgis' parasitology for veterinarians. 9th ed. St. Louis, MO: Saunders/Elsevier; 2009.

54. Plumb DC. Plumb's veterinary drug handbook. 9th ed. Hoboken, NJ: Pharma Vet, Inc.; 2018.

55. The Merck veterinary manual. Whitehouse Station, NJ: Merck & Co., Inc.; 2016.

Case 41

The Snoring Dog

Whipple is new to your practice. Her owners, Finnick and Primrose Reynolds, recently moved from upstate New York to Scottsdale, Arizona. It was a challenging cross-country move, made primarily so that Finnick could be closer to his elderly mother, whose health was failing. Primrose understood her husband's need to be near but was finding it extra challenging to leave her friends and family behind.

For the past 10 years of their marriage, Primrose had been, by her own admission, spoiled. She and Finn had never lived more than 20 minutes by car from her parents. Now they were going to be an entire country apart. Even the time zones would be an insurmountable hurdle. By the time Primrose finished her shift as a nurse at the local hospital, assuming she could find a job, her parents would be in bed.

Making the move in the middle of summer did not make the journey any more appealing. This climate was brutal. The daily high this week averaged 115°F (46.1°C). Even worse, they'd been told that this was typical summer weather.

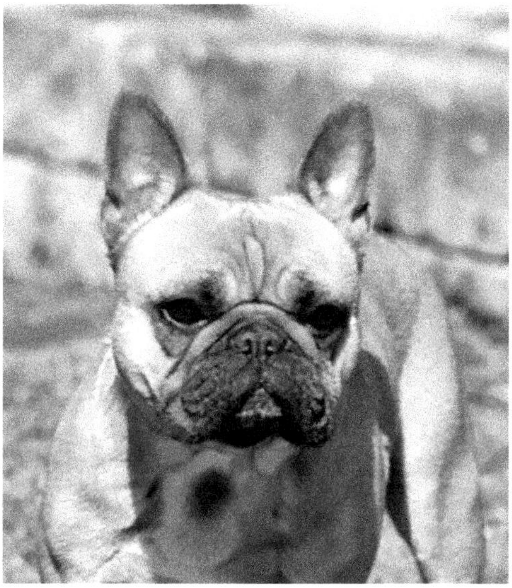

Whipple had a better attitude toward the

Figure 41.1 Meet your patient Whipple, a 1.5-year-old spayed female French Bulldog.

move than Primrose. Then again, she was of the age where everything seemed like an adventure. As long as she had her family in sight, she was content to experience life, come what may.

Whipple had been with the Reynolds since she was three months old. She had been purchased by Finn as an anniversary gift for his wife. Primrose had always wanted a Frenchie but had never owned one as a kid. She came from a family of human athletes and sporty dogs. Her parents much preferred Duck Tolling Retrievers over those with stumpy legs and spent much of their free time camping, fishing, hunting, or in the Winnebago on road trips. In fact, this cross-country trek would have been right up their alley. Primrose had tried to convince them that a Frenchie could fit that active lifestyle, but even she knew when to call it quits. A dog with a foreshortened muzzle would have been, to her family, like a fish out of water. So, she'd only ever dreamed about the Frenchie she would never own, until Finn came into her life and surprised her with one.

Whipple was an instant hit. Inquisitive and gregarious, she was exactly what Prim had hoped for. With one exception. She was loud. Not loud, as in barky. Loud, as in you could hear every breath she took.

Weight: 28.0 lb (12.7 kg)
BCS: 6/9
Mentation: BAR

TPR

T: 102.3°F (39.1°C)
P: 112 beats per minute
R: Panting

It wasn't a big deal as a pup. The fact that she snored was almost cute. Until her snores grew louder. And louder, to the point that she couldn't sleep with Prim and Finn at all. Both were light sleepers, and neither could afford to be up all night. It was becoming a real problem.

Whipple's noisy breathing has only intensified now that the trio has arrived in Arizona. They've been settling into town for three weeks now and are finally starting to get the lay of the land.

Finn and Prim are here today to have Whipple evaluated.

Work through the following questions to prepare you for Whipple's consultation.

Round One of Questions for Case 41: The Snoring Dog

1. Track the flow of air from the external environment to Whipple's lower airway. Assume that Whipple is breathing through her nose.
2. What is the primary purpose of panting in dogs?
3. Why else might a dog switch from nasal breathing to breathing through the mouth?
4. Is panting typical in cats?
5. What might cause panting in cats?
6. How can you assess nasal airflow clinically?
7. If severe enough, an obstruction to airflow may cause the mucous membranes to change color. Which change in color is most likely?
8. Airway resistance secondary to obstructive disease may result in two abnormal upper airway sounds, stertor and stridor. Describe and differentiate these sounds.
9. Are stertor and stridor purely inspiratory sounds?
10. What are the primary causes of stertor and stridor in companion animal patients?
11. Which of the causes that you identified in Question #9 (above) is Whipple predisposed to and why?
12. You can tell that Prim is very concerned about Whipple's breathing. Which communication skill might you use to encourage her to share her concerns with you? Give at least one example of what you might say to demonstrate use of this skill.

Answers to Round One of Questions for Case 41: The Snoring Dog

1. Air is funneled into Whipple's upper airway by the nasal alae, that is, the wings of rounded tissue on either side of her nares (nostrils).(1–8) Nares should be open and symmetrical, to support maximal air flow into the upper airway.(1) Air travels through paired nasal cavities that are separated by the nasal septum.(1–8) Each nasal cavity channels air through one of three passageways: the dorsal, medial, and ventral meatus.(1–8) As air passes through, it passes over highly vascularized nasal mucosa.(1, 6) The mucosa warms incoming air, and mucus that lines the passageways traps particulate matter through ciliary action.(1, 6) The cleansed, warmed air ultimately passes through the larynx and into the trachea.(9, 10) The trachea is a single tube that bifurcates into two bronchi, the left and right bronchus.(9, 10) The left bronchus supplies the left lung; the right bronchus supplies the right.(9, 10) Air travels through each bronchus and into bronchioles. Bronchioles terminate in air sacs called alveoli.(10) Alveoli are the site of gas exchange.(10) Oxygen enters to the blood here; carbon dioxide exits.(10)

2. The primary purpose of panting in dogs is to assist with thermoregulation.(11–14) Panting facilitates evaporative cooling from the respiratory tract.(11–14)

3. A dog may also choose to pant if there is a nasal or nasopharyngeal obstruction. Panting allows dogs to take in air through an alternate pathway, their mouth.

4. No, panting is not typically seen in cats, unlike dogs.(1, 15) When cats pant, they are said to exhibit open-mouth breathing.(1, 15) Open-mouth breathing is not sustainable in cats for long periods.(1, 15, 16)

5. An open-mouth breathing cat is either extremely excited, significantly stressed, or in distress from respiratory or cardiac disease.(1, 15, 17–21)

6. You can assess airflow through each nostril by placing a glass slide in front of the nose.(1, 15) The patient's breath should fog up the slide in two concentric circles: one per nare.(1, 15) If one side lacks a circle of fog on the slide, then airflow is said to be reduced through that nasal passageway.(1, 15)

   Alternatively, the clinician may hold a tuft of cotton in front of each nostril and assess for movement of the cotton.(1, 15)

7. If an airway obstruction is severe enough, then you would expect the patient to have a build-up of deoxygenated hemoglobin in circulation.(1, 22) This causes the mucous membranes to appear cyanotic, that is, purple-blue.(1, 22)

8. Stertor and stridor are both abnormal upper airway sounds that stem from airway resistance because of underlying obstructive disease.(1, 2, 15, 22–29)

   Stertor is a low-pitched snoring sound that is caused by the vibration of flaccid tissues or secretions.(1, 15, 22, 23) This snore most typically originates within the nose itself or the pharynx.(1, 15, 21–23)

   Stridor is a harsher, high-pitched sound that occurs when rigid tissues vibrate.(1, 15, 21–23) This sound may result from obstruction within the nasal cavity itself.(1, 15) More commonly, stridor is linked to laryngeal pathology, such as laryngeal paralysis, or tracheal collapse.(1, 2, 15, 21–23)

9. No, stertor and stridor are not purely inspiratory sounds.(1, 2) They may also be expiratory.(1, 2)

10. In dogs and cats, the primary causes of stertor and stridor are:(21–23, 26–28, 30–42)
    - cleft palate
    - foreign body obstruction, such as grass awns
    - infectious upper airway disease, such as chronic rhinitis and sinorhinitis
    - inflammatory upper airway disease, such as lymphoplasmacytic rhinitis
    - mechanical obstruction:
      - brachycephalic airway syndrome
      - laryngeal paralysis
      - nasopharyngeal polyp
      - tracheal collapse
    - neoplasia
    - trauma:
      - nasal fractures
      - oro-nasal fistula.

11. Whipple predisposed to brachycephalic airway syndrome because he is a French Bulldog. Frenchies are brachycephalic breeds.(1, 3, 22, 34, 43–48)

12. I can make use of the communication skill, eliciting the client's perspective, to ask Prim how she feels about Whipple's situation.(49)

Eliciting the client's perspective often takes the form of an open-ended question or statement.(49) This phrasing invites clients to share their story in greater detail.(49, 50) In this regard, open-ended questions or statements are relationship-builders.(49) They help us to know our clients better.(49) They open doors so that we hear what is weighing on our clients' minds.(49) They tell our clients that we value what they have to say and that we're interested in their thoughts.(49)

Statements that elicit the client's perspective often start with:(49)

- Tell me
- Share with me
- Describe for me
- Explain to me.

You might try out one or more of the following examples with Prim:(49)

- Tell me what about Whipple is weighing on your mind.
- Share with me your concerns about Whipple's noisy breathing.
- Describe what you are hearing when Whipple breathes.
- Explain to me what concerns you most about Whipple.

Sometimes the way that these statements are phrased sounds unnaturally forceful, like a command. If you prefer, you may soften these statements by tacking on "please" and/or "can":(49)

- Please, can you explain to me what concerns you most about Whipple?

Returning to Case 41: The Snoring Dog

You elicit Prim's perspective by asking what concerns her most. She explains that she once owned a cat with a nasopharyngeal polyp. She is concerned that Whipple may have the same condition. Prim recalls that snoring sound well and would like to surgically intervene if doing so would make for an easy fix.

You validate Prim's concerns but indicate that it is more likely for Whipple to have brachycephalic syndrome.

Round Two of Questions for Case 41: The Snoring Dog

1. What is a nasopharyngeal polyp?
2. In which patients are nasopharyngeal polyps most likely to occur?
3. Which clinical signs are likely to be associated with nasopharyngeal polyps?
4. How are nasopharyngeal polyps diagnosed?
5. Whipple is a brachycephalic breed. What does it mean to say that she is brachycephalic?
6. Which other canine breeds are brachycephalic?
7. Which feline breeds are brachycephalic?
8. In broad terms, what is brachycephalic syndrome?
9. Why does brachycephalic syndrome occur?
10. What are the components of brachycephalic syndrome?

Answers to Round Two of Questions for Case 41: The Snoring Dog

1. A nasopharyngeal polyp is a benign growth that arises from the caudal nasopharynx, auditory tube epithelium, or the middle ear.(1, 15, 51–54) It is associated with non-infectious upper airway disease.(1, 3, 53–58) Its appearance is variable in that it may be fixed or mobile, smooth

or nodular.(1, 53) Polyps frequently attach to underlying tissue by means of a stalk.(53) These polyps are said to be pedunculated and take on the appearance of a mushroom.

2. Nasopharyngeal polyps are most likely to occur in young adult cats.(1, 15, 51, 52)

3. Depending upon their location, nasopharyngeal polyps may cause upper airway obstruction during inspiration.(1, 15, 51, 52) This can precipitate stertor.(1, 15, 51, 52)

    In addition, patients with nasopharyngeal polyps may present with one or more of the following signs:(1, 51)

    • dyspnea
    • nasal discharge
    • sneezing.

    If polyps grow into the back of the throat, then the patient may present for dysphagia or gagging. (1, 51)

    When the middle and/or external ear is involved, polyps may cause unilateral otitis, head-shaking, or pawing at the ears.(1, 53, 54)

4. If the caudal nasopharynx is involved, then an oropharyngeal examination under sedation may be sufficient to make the presumptive diagnosis.(1, 15) The fleshy pink tissue should be evident dorsal to the soft palate.(51) A spay-hook is often used to facilitate examination of the soft palate where it joins the caudal nasal cavities. Advanced imaging such as computed tomography (CT) may be necessary to evaluate the extent of disease.(1, 15) A CT scan, for instance, provides exceptional detail of the upper airway sinuses and can simultaneously evaluate the patient for turbinate destruction.(55)

    If the external ear is involved, polyps may be diagnosed by otoscopy in the awake patient. (53, 59, 60) However, advanced imaging studies are often indicated to track the extent of the mass through the middle ear.(1, 53, 54)

    If the middle ear is involved, the tympanum may appear to bulge due to the build-up of fluid from otitis media.(51)

    Ultimately, histopathology of the growth itself is necessary to make a definitive diagnosis.(51)

5. Brachycephalic breeds are those that have a high cephalic index (CI).(1) CI is a ratio of skull width to length.(1, 3) Therefore, those with a high CI, such as brachycephalic dogs, have skulls that are much wider than they are long.(1, 3, 45, 46, 61–67)

    Because of this, brachycephalic breeds have distinct facial morphology.(1, 3, 15, 34) Specifically, they have a foreshortened muzzle.(1, 15) This gives them a "pushed in" or "smushed face" appearance.(1, 3, 15, 62, 63) In addition, they have shallow orbits and bulgy eyes.(1, 3) Sometimes they are said to be "bug-eyed" because the globes protrude from shallow orbits.(1, 3) Their eyes are also spaced further apart than in dolicocephalic dogs, that is, those whose skulls are longer than they are wide.(1, 3)

6. In addition to French bulldogs, common breeds of dog that are brachycephalic are:(1, 3, 15, 22, 34, 43–48)

    • Boston terriers
    • Boxers
    • Brussels griffons
    • Bull mastiffs
    • Chinese Shar-Peis
    • Dogue de Bordeaux
    • English bulldogs
    • King Charles Cavalier spaniels
    • Lhasa apsos
    • Pekingese
    • Pugs
    • Shih tzus.

7. Common brachycephalic feline breeds include:(1, 3, 15, 22)

- British shorthair
- Exotic shorthair
- Himalayans

- Persians
- Ragdolls
- Scottish folds.

8. Brachycephalic syndrome represents a constellation of structural defects that stem from the cosmetic appearance of brachycephalic breeds.(1, 15, 51, 52)

9. Although the skull length is short in brachycephalic breeds, the surrounding soft tissue structures are not proportionally reduced.(1, 22, 29, 61) This means that excessive tissue bulges into the airway lumen, precipitating airway obstruction.(22)

10. Patients with brachycephalic syndrome may have one or more of the following structural defects:(1, 3, 15, 22, 29, 43, 68–70)

- abnormal conchae
- elongated soft palate
- everted laryngeal saccules

- laryngeal collapse
- laryngeal edema
- stenotic nares.

Returning to Case 41: The Snoring Dog

You perform a physical exam on Whipple and identify the following abnormalities:

- Whipple has an elevated BCS of 6/9
- Whipple has a pronounced underbite.

In addition, you take note of her nares (see Figure 41.2).

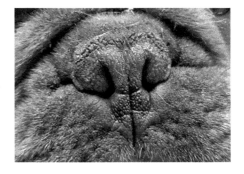

Figure 41.2 Close-up photograph of Whipple's nares.

Round Three of Questions for Case 41: The Snoring Dog

1. What is the appropriate medical terminology to describe what you are seeing in Figure 41.2?
2. What is the impact of this clinical finding on Whipple's inspiratory effort?
3. What might be the consequence of this clinical finding on surrounding soft tissue structures?
4. Which patient-specific factor(s) exacerbate(s) brachycephalic airway syndrome?
5. Which environmental factor exacerbates brachycephalic airway syndrome?
6. Which treatment option(s) do you propose for Whipple?

Answers to Round Three of Questions for Case 41: The Snoring Dog

1. Whipple has stenotic nares.(1, 15)

2. Stenotic nares require patients to work harder to take in air.(1, 15, 64) Taking in air through narrowed slits requires a significant increase in negative pressure during the inspiratory half of the respiratory cycle.(64, 71, 72)

3. The increase in negative pressure that is required for dogs with stenotic nares to take air in impacts surrounding soft tissue structures.(64) Over time, these tissues become edematous.(1, 64) In this way, stenotic nares worsen other components of brachycephalic airway syndrome.(1, 64)

Elongated soft palates may be sucked into the airway lumen due to the increased negative pressure, creating an obstruction to air flow.(64)

In addition, increases in negative pressure may cause laryngeal saccules to evert or laryngeal cartilages to weaken.(64) Any of these changes further restrict air flow by reducing the diameter of the airway.(64)

It is a vicious cycle. The patient must work harder to get air into the system, yet in order to make that happen, increased negative pressure creates additional obstacles to air flow.(64)

4. Obesity exacerbates upper respiratory obstruction caused by brachycephalic syndrome.(1, 22, 43) Although Whipple is not obese, she is currently overweight. You will need to work with Finn and Prim to keep Whipple lean.

Anxiety also intensifies the effects of brachycephalic syndrome because anxious dogs are more likely to pant.(1) Because these patients have compromised airways due to reduction in airflow, panting is inefficient at best.(1, 25, 26, 28, 33) Anxious patients with brachycephalic syndrome are therefore much more likely to overheat.(1) This will increase the chance that the patient will develop respiratory distress if anxiety persists.(1)

For the same reasons outlined above, intense bouts of exercise may exaggerate brachycephalic syndrome.(1, 29, 73) These patients are incapable of maximizing evaporative cooling through panting and so they overheat.(1, 25, 26, 28, 33)

5. Brachycephalic syndrome is exacerbated by hot, humid weather.(1, 22, 29, 73) This climate requires patients to pant more as a means of evaporative cooling, yet they are predisposed to hyperthermia because their airways are compromised.(1, 25, 26, 28, 33) Furthermore, panting is likely to worsen airway edema, thereby increasing resistance to airflow.(1, 22)

6. It is advisable that Whipple undergo surgical reconstruction of her nares to reduce their contribution to upper airway pathology.(1, 46, 65, 66, 74–76) Resection techniques are beyond the scope of this clinical case.(1) However, various wedge approaches have been described in the veterinary medical literature with successful cosmetic and functional outcomes.(1, 66, 74, 77)

It is intentionally unclear from this case description if Whipple has additional aspects of brachycephalic syndrome other than just stenotic nares. It is critical that you investigate these other potential problem areas and intervene accordingly. For instance, if Whipple has an elongated soft palate, then she may benefit from surgically trimming the excessive tissue.(1, 74) Trimming requires excising enough tissue to improve the patient's respiratory status while not taking so much as to cause rhinitis, sinusitis, or potentially even aspiration pneumonia.(1, 46, 66, 74, 76, 77)

You will also want to examine Whipple to see if she has everted laryngeal saccules. Laryngeal saccules are normal laryngeal structures in dogs that sit between the lateral larynx and the vocal folds.(1, 6, 15, 62) In health, they are hidden from view, even on a comprehensive oropharyngeal examination.(1, 64, 74) However, everted laryngeal saccules occur in approximately 50% of dogs with brachycephalic airway syndrome.(1, 48, 64, 76, 78) Eversion of laryngeal saccules occurs because these patients have established excessively negative airway pressure to overcome airway resistance.(1, 22) This forces the saccules out of their hideaways and into the airway lumen.(1)

Everted laryngeal saccules appear on oropharyngeal examination as whitish pink and shiny, convex pieces of tissue.(1, 29, 43, 48, 64, 74, 76, 77, 79, 80) These structures vibrate during the respiratory cycle and contribute to stertor.(22) If present in Whipple, these structures can be surgically excised.(74)

CLINICAL PEARLS

- Abnormal respiratory sounds may arise from structural defects in the upper airway.

- Structural defects in the upper airway may occur in any patient; however, they are common among brachycephalic breeds.

- Brachycephalic breeds have a high cephalic index. This means that their skulls are wider than they are long. Although this causes a cosmetic appearance that many find aesthetically pleasing, the surrounding tissues are not proportionally reduced. This results in excessive tissues that bulge into the airway.

- When tissues are excessive to the point that they bulge into the airway lumen, they increase resistance to airflow. The patient now must work harder to take air in. This requires increased negative pressure.

- Increased negative pressure within the airway creates additional hurdles. For instance, it may exacerbate elongated soft palates and cause everted laryngeal saccules. These are common structural issues in patients with brachycephalic syndrome.

- Patients with brachycephalic syndrome frequently present with stertor and stridor. These clinical signs worsen with environmental heat and humidity, exercise, and patient obesity.

- Patients with brachycephalic syndrome are prone to overheating because they are unable to maximize the evaporative cooling potential of panting. Instead, panting leads to edematous tissues that further narrow the airway and reduce air flow.

- Many components of brachycephalic syndrome are amenable to surgical correction.

References

1. Englar RE. Common clinical presentations in dogs and cats. Hoboken, NJ: Wiley/Blackwell; 2019.
2. Stokhof AA, Venker-van Haagen AJ. Respiratory system. In: Rijnberk A, van Sluijs FJ, editors. Medical history and physical examination in companion animals. Philadelphia, PA: Saunders Elsevier; 2009. p. 63–74.
3. Englar RE. Performing the small animal physical examination. Hoboken, NJ: Wiley; 2017.
4. Elie M, Sabo M. Basics in canine and feline rhinoscopy. Clin Tech Small Anim Pract 2006;21(2):60–3.
5. Grandage J. Functional anatomy of the respiratory system. In: Slatter DH, editor. Textbook of small animal surgery. Philadelphia, PA: Saunders; 2003. p. 763–80.
6. Singh B, Dyce KM. Dyce, Sack, and Wensing's textbook of veterinary anatomy. 5th ed. St. Louis, MO: Saunders; 2018.
7. Evans HE, Miller ME. Miller's anatomy of the dog. 3rd ed. Philadelphia, PA: W. B. Saunders; 1993.
8. Labuc R, editor. The approach to nasal discharge in the dog. The 8th Annual Vet Education International Online Veterinary Conference; 2017.
9. Singh B, Dyce KM. Dyce, Sack, and Wensing's textbook of veterinary anatomy. 5th ed. St. Louis, MO: Saunders; 2018.
10. Cunningham JG, Klein BG. Cunningham's textbook of veterinary physiology. 5th ed. St. Louis, MO: Elsevier/Saunders; 2013.
11. Crawford EC, Jr. Mechanical aspects of panting in dogs. J Appl Physiol 1962;17:249–51.
12. Schmidt-Nielsen K, Bretz WL, Taylor CR. Panting in dogs: unidirectional air flow over evaporative surfaces. Science 1970;169(3950):1102–4.
13. Blatt CM, Taylor CR, Habal MB. Thermal panting in dogs: the lateral nasal gland, a source of water for evaporative cooling. Science 1972;177(4051):804–5.

14. Goldberg MB, Langman VA, Taylor CR. Panting in dogs: paths of air flow in response to heat and exercise. Respir Physiol 1981;43(3):327–38.
15. Englar RE. Performing the small animal physical examination. Hoboken, NJ: Wiley/Blackwell; 2017.
16. Hunt GB, Foster SF. Nasopharyngeal disorders. In: Bonagura JD, Twedt DC, editors. Kirk's current veterinary therapy XIV. St. Louis, MO: Saunders Elsevier; 2009. p. 622–6.
17. Kienle RD. Feline cardiomyopathy. In: Tilley LP, Smith FWK, Oyama MA, Sleeper MM, editors. Manual of canine and feline cardiology. 4th ed. Philadelphia, PA: W. B. Saunders; 2008. p. 151–75.
18. Gompf RE. The history and physical examination. In: Tilley LP, Smith FWK, Oyama MA, Sleeper MM, editors. Manual of canine and feline cardiology. St. Louis, MO: Elsevier Saunders; 2008. p. 2–23.
19. Cote E, MacDonald KA, Meurs KM, Sleeper MM. Feline cardiology. Ames, IA: Wiley/Blackwell; 2011.
20. Allen HS, Broussard J, Noone K. Nasopharyngeal diseases in cats: a retrospective study of 53 cases (1991-1998). J Am Anim Hosp Assoc 1999;35(6):457–61.
21. Lappin MR. Feline internal medicine secrets. Philadelphia, PA: Hanley & Belfus, Inc.; 2001.
22. Tilley LP, Smith FWK. The 5-minute veterinary consult: canine and feline. 3rd edition. Baltimore, MD: Lippincott Williams & Wilkins; 2004.
23. Rand J, Mason RA. The cat with stridor or stertor. In: Rand J, editor. Problem-based feline medicine. Philadelphia, PA: Elsevier Limited; 2006. p. 32–46.
24. Defarges A. The physical examination. NAVC Clin's Brief 2015 (September):73–80.
25. Sharp CR, Rozanski EA. Physical examination of the respiratory system. Top Companion Anim Med 2013;28(3):79–85.
26. Sumner C, Rozanski E. Management of respiratory emergencies in small animals. Vet Clin North Am Small Anim Pract 2013;43(4):799–815.
27. Starybrat D, Tappin S. Approaching the dysnoeic cat in the middle of the night. Vet Irel J;6(1):37–43.
28. King L. Managing upper airway obstruction in dogs. DVM. 360 [Internet]; 2008. Available from: http://veterinarycalendar.dvm360.com/managing-upper-airway-obstruction-dogs-proceedings.
29. Fasanella FJ, Shivley JM, Wardlaw JL, Givaruangsawat S. Brachycephalic airway obstructive syndrome in dogs: 90 cases (1991–2008). J Am Vet Med Assoc 2010;237(9):1048–51.
30. Klocke E. CVC highlight: the hunt for grass awns. DVM. 360 [Internet]; 2014. Available from: http://veterinarymedicine.dvm360.com/cvc-highlight-hunt-grass-awns.
31. Ford RB, editor. Upper respiratory diseases in dogs. World Small Animal Veterinary Association World Congress Proceedings; 2005.
32. Rozanski E, Chan DL. Approach to the patient with respiratory distress. Vet Clin North Am Small Anim Pract 2005;35(2):307–17.
33. Sharp CR. Approach to respiratory distress in dogs and cats. Today's. Vet Pract 2015 (November/December):53–60.
34. Phillips H. Brachycephalic syndrome. NAVC Clin's Brief 2016 (September).
35. Linklater A. Tracheal collapse in dogs. Plumb's Ther Brief 2018 (February):46–57.
36. Mankin KT. Laryngeal paralysis diagnosis. NAVC Clin's Brief 2015 (December):67–71.
37. Mankin KT. Laryngeal paralysis surgery. NAVC Clin's Brief 2015 (December):73–9.
38. Moritz A, Schneider M, Bauer N. Management of advanced tracheal collapse in dogs using intraluminal self-expanding biliary wallstents. J Vet Intern Med 2004;18(1):31–42.
39. Hardie RJ, Gunby J, Bjorling DE. Arytenoid lateralization for treatment of laryngeal paralysis in 10 cats. Vet Surg 2009;38(4):445–51.
40. Johnson LR, Pollard RE. Tracheal collapse and bronchomalacia in dogs: 58 cases (7 /2001–1 /2008). J Vet Intern Med 2010;24(2):298–305.
41. Nelissen P, White RA. Arytenoid lateralization for management of combined laryngeal paralysis and laryngeal collapse in small dogs. Vet Surg 2012;41(2):261–5.
42. Sharp CR. Feline rhinitis and upper respiratory disease. Today's. Vet Pract 2012 (July/August):14–20.
43. Miller J, Gannon K. Perioperative management of brachycephalic dogs. NAVC Clin's Brief 2015 (April): 54–9.
44. Asher L, Diesel G, Summers JF, McGreevy PD, Collins LM. Inherited defects in pedigree dogs. Part 1: disorders related to breed standards. Vet J 2009;182(3):402–11.

45. Dupré G, Heidenreich D. Brachycephalic syndrome. Vet Clin North Am Small Anim Pract 2016;46(4):691–707.

46. Hendricks JC. Brachycephalic airway syndrome. Vet Clin North Am Small Anim Pract 1992;22(5):1145–53.

47. Meola SD. Brachycephalic airway syndrome. Top Companion Anim Med 2013;28(3):91–6.

48. Riecks TW, Birchard SJ, Stephens JA. Surgical correction of brachycephalic syndrome in dogs: 62 cases (1991–2004). J Am Vet Med Assoc 2007;230(9):1324–8.

49. Englar R. A guide to. Oral Communication in Veterinary Medicine. Sheffield: 5M Publishing; 2020.

50. Englar RE, Williams M, Weingand K. Applicability of the Calgary-Cambridge guide to dog and cat owners for teaching veterinary clinical communications. J Vet Med Educ 2016;43(2):143–69.

51. Côté E. Clinical veterinary advisor. Dogs and cats. 3rd ed. St. Louis, MO: Elsevier Mosby; 2015.

52. Ettinger SJ, Feldman EC, Côté E. Textbook of veterinary internal medicine: diseases of the dog and the cat. 8th ed. St. Louis, MO: Elsevier; 2017.

53. Lanz OI, Wood BC. Surgery of the ear and pinna. Vet Clin North Am Small Anim Pract 2004;34(2):567–99, viii, viii.

54. Kennis RA. Feline otitis: diagnosis and treatment. Vet Clin North Am Small Anim Pract 2013;43(1):51–6.

55. Quimby J, Lappin MR. The upper respiratory tract. In: Little SE, editor. The cat: clinical medicine and management. St. Louis, MO: Saunders Elsevier; 2012.

56. Henderson SM, Bradley K, Day MJ, Tasker S, Caney SM, Hotston Moore A, Gruffydd-Jones TJ. Investigation of nasal disease in the cat--a retrospective study of 77 cases. J Feline Med Surg 2004;6(4):245–57.

57. Schmidt JF, Kapatkin A. Nasopharyngeal and ear canal polyps in the cat. Feline Pract 1990;18(4):16–9.

58. Kapatkin AS, Matthiesen DT, Noone KE, Church EM. Scavelli TE, Patnaik AK. Results of surgery and long-term follow-up in 31 cats with nasopharyngeal polyps. J Am Anim Hosp Assoc 1990;26(4):387–92.

59. Cole LK. Otoscopic evaluation of the ear canal. Vet Clin North Am Small Anim Pract 2004;34(2):397–410.

60. Allyn W. Direct and indirect veterinary eye and ear examination instructions. Available from: https://www.welchallyn.com/content/dam/welchallyn/documents/sap-documents/LIT/80020/80020547LITPDF.pdf.

61. Wykes PM. Brachycephalic airway obstructive syndrome. Probl Vet Med 1991;3(2):188–97.

62. Evans HE, Miller ME. Miller's anatomy of the dog. 4th ed. St. Louis, MO: Elsevier; 2013.

63. Schuenemann R, Oechtering GU. Inside the brachycephalic nose: intranasal mucosal contact points. J Am Anim Hosp Assoc 2014;50(3):149–58.

64. Trappler M, Moore K. Canine brachycephalic airway syndrome: pathophysiology, diagnosis, and nonsurgical management. Compend Contin Educ Vet 2011;33(5):E1–4; quiz E5.

65. Hedlund CS. Brachycephalic syndrome. In: Bojrab MJ, editor. Current techniques in small animal surgery. Philadelphia, PA: Williams & Wilkins; 1998. p. 357–62.

66. Hedlund CS. Stenotic nares. In: Fossum TW, editor. Small animal surgery. St. Louis, MO: Mosby; 2002. p. 727–30.

67. Hobson HP. Brachycephalic syndrome. Semin Vet Med Surg Small Anim 1995;10(2):109–14.

68. Ginn JA, Kumar MSA, McKiernan BC, Powers BE. Nasopharyngeal turbinates in brachycephalic dogs and cats. J Am Anim Hosp Assoc 2008;44(5):243–9.

69. Koch DA, Arnold S, Hubler M, Montavon PM. Brachycephalic syndrome in dogs. Comp Cont Educ Pract 2003;25(1):48–+.

70. Findji L, Dupre G. Brachycephalic syndrome: innovative surgical techniques. NAVC Clin's Brief 2013 (June):79–85.

71. Aron DN, Crowe DT. Upper airway obstruction. General principles and selected conditions in the dog and cat. Vet Clin North Am Small Anim Pract 1985;15(5):891–917.

72. Robinson NE. Airway physiology. Vet Clin North Am Small Anim Pract 1992;22(5):1043–64.

73. Bach JF, Rozanski EA, Bedenice D, Chan DL, Freeman LM, Lofgren JL, et al. Association of expiratory airway dysfunction with marked obesity in healthy adult dogs. Am J Vet Res 2007;68(6):670–5.

74. Trappler M, Moore K. Canine brachycephalic airway syndrome: surgical management. Compend Contin Educ Vet 2011;33(5):E1–7.

75. Huck JL, Stanley BJ, Hauptman JG. Technique and outcome of nares amputation (Trader's technique) in immature shih tzus. J Am Anim Hosp Assoc 2008;44(2):82–5.

76. Poncet CM, Dupre GP, Freiche VG, Estrada MM, Poubanne YA, Bouvy BM. Prevalence of gastrointestinal tract lesions in 73 brachycephalic dogs with upper respiratory syndrome. J Small Anim Pract 2005;46(6):273–9.

77. Monnet E. Brachycephalic airway syndrome. In: Slatter D, editor. Textbook of small animal surgery. Philadelphia, PA: W.B. Saunders; 2003. p. 808–13.
78. Torrez CV, Hunt GB. Results of surgical correction of abnormalities associated with brachycephalic airway obstruction syndrome in dogs in Australia. J Small Anim Pract 2006;47(3):150–4.
79. Harvey CE. Upper airway obstruction surgery: everted laryngeal saccule surgery in brachycephalic dogs. J Am Anim Hosp Assoc 1982;18:545–7.
80. Ellison GW. Alapexy: an alternative technique for repair of stenotic nares in dogs. J Am Anim Hosp Assoc 2004;40(6):484–9.

Case 42

The Coughing Dog

Spree is new to your practice. He was adopted into his forever home 6 months ago by Katrina Schwartz. His transition from the shelter to a single-story, only pet household was not the easiest. After having been relinquished by the only person whom he had ever bonded with, Spree had trust issues. He was head shy and aloof, yet always had to have Katrina in sight. The primary problem was that Katrina worked full-time. Spree initially couldn't handle her absences and tore into the home, literally, as fully-fledged separation anxiety kicked in. The first time that Katrina came home after an 8-hour shift, the house looked as if it had been ransacked. Toilet paper had been shredded and every feather pillow, too. A fine layer of down coated the carpet and what was left of the comforter. It took the rest of the night to get the place in order, only to have the cycle repeat on day two. Katrina had contacted the shelter for support, and they came through. The director was able to connect her with a

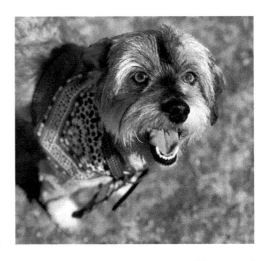

Figure 42.1 Meet Spree, a 6-year-old castrated male terrier mix. Courtesy of Keleigh Schettler.

behaviorist who came to the home for a consultation. Katrina was able to transition Spree into a crate, where he couldn't hurt himself or the home, and she hired Jon, a dog walker, to visit daily. Three days a week, she was able to enroll Spree in doggie daycare. It got his nervous energy out and helped him to socialize with the others there. Over time, he settled into the routine and realized that he was in fact home to stay.

Just when Katrina had thought that major problems had passed them by, she received a telephone call from the dog walker. Jon asked if Spree was under the weather. Jon then relayed that on their walk earlier in the day, Spree started to cough when he saw a squirrel and pulled on the leash. That seemed to launch him into a coughing fit. He sounded like a "goose."

"You may want to have him checked out," Jon said. "I'm thinking he might have picked up kennel cough from the daycare and they're not going to want him back until he's germ-free."

This cough was new. Katrina had never heard it, but then again, Spree was never leashed when he was with her. At night, they played in the fenced back yard. He hadn't seemed winded or sluggish. If anything, he was more stir crazy and rambunctious than ever before. It was as if he'd found his inner puppy.

Katrina made a mental note to keep an eye on it and tried not to worry. However, when another day passed and Jon gave the same report, she knew that she better have Spree checked out.

Spree is here today to be examined. Katrina was referred to you

Weight: 22.9 lb (10.4 kg)
BCS: 6/9
Mentation: BAR

TPR

T: 101.7°F (38.7°C)
P: 112 beats per minute
R: Panting

by one of her neighbors, who is a regular customer of the practice, and she is looking forward to the answers that undoubtedly you will provide.

Spree's vital signs are taken while they wait for you to initiate the consultation.

Use the following questions as a guide to work your way through this case.

Round One of Questions for Case 42: The Coughing Dog

1. What, in broad terms, is kennel cough?
2. What causes kennel cough?
3. What is the incubation period for kennel cough?
4. Which patients are most susceptible to kennel cough?
5. What are Spree's risk factors for contracting kennel cough?
6. How contagious is kennel cough?
7. Which clinical signs are typical of kennel cough?
8. What does kennel cough sound like?
9. How is kennel cough typically diagnosed in clinical practice?
10. If you suspected kennel cough, which additional diagnostic test(s) could you perform to obtain a definitive diagnosis?
11. What are potential disadvantages to the test(s) that you identified in Question #10 (above)?
12. Other than bacteria and viruses, what other infectious agents can cause cough?
13. Is coughing always infectious?
14. What additional clarifying questions might you want to ask Katrina to assess Spree's health relative to his chief complaint?
15. Are the clarifying questions that you asked in Question #14 (above) open-ended or closed-ended?

Answers to Round One of Questions for Case 42: The Coughing Dog

1. Kennel cough is the colloquial name for CIRD, a constellation of bacteria and viruses that individually or collectively incite airway pathology.(2–7)

2. Kennel cough, otherwise known as CIRD, is caused by:(5–9)

   - bacteria

     - *Bordetella bronchiseptica****
     - *Mycoplasma spp.*
     - *Streptococcus equi subsp. zooepidemicus*

   - viruses:

     - canine adenovirus-2 (CAV-2)
     - canine distemper virus (CDV)
     - canine herpesvirus
     - canine influenza (H3N8)
     - canine parainfluenza
     - canine respiratory coronavirus.

   Note that when most clinicians refer to "kennel cough," the bacteria, *Bordetella bronchiseptica*, is in the forefront of their minds even though many other infectious agents cause canine infectious respiratory disease (CIRD).(2, 3, 5) Likewise, when clinicians recommend that clients authorize the administration of "kennel cough" vaccines to dogs, they most often are referring to products that reduce the risk of contracting *Bordetella bronchiseptica*.

3. The incubation period depends upon the infectious agent.(6, 7) Most CIRD-associated pathogens have an incubation period that spans up to 14 days, with active shedding for approximately the same amount of time post-infection.(3, 6–11)

4. Young, stressed, and/or immunocompromized patients are most susceptible to CIRD.(3, 5, 12–14) Other risk factors for contracting CIRD include close contact with conspecifics.(3, 5, 12–14) Dogs that are housed in crowded conditions, such as kennels or shelters, are at increased risk of developing disease.(3, 5, 12–14)

5. Spree encounters other dogs three days each week at doggie day care. This close contact with conspecifics is Spree's greatest risk factor for contracting CIRD.

6. CIRD is highly contagious.(3, 6–8)

7. Common clinical signs that are associated with CIRD include:(6–9, 15)

   - cough
   - +/– lethargy
   - nasal discharge
   - +/– reduced appetite, which may be associated with a sore throat secondary to post-nasal drip
   - rhinitis
   - sneezing.

   Respiratory distress is possible, but rare.(6, 16)

8. The cough that is associated with CIRD is often described as "honking."(6, 15)

9. In clinical practice, the diagnosis of CIRD is typically presumptive, rather than definitive.(6) This presumptive diagnosis is typically made on the basis of clinical signs and history, particularly if the history reveals the patient to have been at increased risk of exposure.(5, 6)

10. If you suspected CIRD, you could swab the nose, mouth, or oropharynx for aerobic culture.(6) A better approach for reasons that will be addressed in the answer to Question #11 (below) is to sample airway secretions from transtracheal wash, endotracheal wash, or bronchoalveolar lavage.(5, 6)

11. Swabs taken from the nose, mouth, or oropharynx are poor samples for aerobic culture because these regions of the body are routinely inhabited by resident microbes.(5, 6) This makes it nearly impossible to differentiate the causative agent(s) from normal flora.(5, 6)

    For this reason, airway samples that have been collected by transtracheal aspirates, endotracheal or bronchoalveolar lavage are preferred when submitting requests for bacterial culture and susceptibility profiles.(15)

12. In addition to bacterial and viral airway infections, parasitic agents can also cause cough.(6) Of these, heartworms and lungworms are the most common culprits in companion animal practice.

    Heartworm disease (HWD) is caused by the nematode, *Dirofilaria immitis*.(6–9, 17–26) Dogs with HWD typically present for coughing, exercise intolerance, dyspnea, or syncope.(6, 8, 9, 27, 28) Cats are more likely to present for vomiting and/or be misdiagnosed with asthma due to the development of heartworm-associated respiratory disease (HARD).(6–9, 17–20, 22–24, 29)

    Lungworms can infect both dogs and cats. Among cats, *Aelurostrongylus abstrusus* is most often implicated.(30) However, other species of lungworms that are important to feline medicine include Capillaria aerophile (*Eucoleus aerophilus*) and *Paragonimus kellicotti*.(30–35)

Our patient, Spree, is not a cat; however, he can still contract lungworms of the following species:(31, 36–39)

- *Angiostrongylus vasorum*
- *Capillaria aerophila or Eucoleus aerophilus*
- *Crenosoma vulpis*
- *Eucoleus boehmi*

- *Filaroides hirthi*
- *Filaroides milksi*
- *Oslerus osleri*
- *Paragonimus kellicotti.*

Lungworm infections are indistinguishable from bronchial diseases.(30, 32) Coughing and wheezing are commonly reported with *Aelurostrongylus abstrusus* infection.(30, 32, 40, 41) Sneezing and nasal discharge are also frequent.(30, 32, 40, 41)

In addition to parasitic causes of cough, fungal pneumonia may also result in cough.(6)

13. No, coughing does not always stem from an infectious etiology.(6)

Other causes of cough in companion animal patients include:(1, 6, 8, 9, 21, 24, 29, 30, 33, 36, 42–55)

- allergic rhinitis and/or sinusitis with post-nasal drip
- aspiration pneumonia
- asthma
- bronchitis
- inhalation of irritants:

  - dust particles
  - gas
  - hair

  - litter (cats)
  - pollen
  - smoke

- laryngeal paralysis
- nasopharyngeal polyp
- nasopharyngeal, laryngeal, or tracheal foreign body obstruction
- neoplasia
- tracheal collapse.

14. I would want to ask questions about the following content areas to assess Spree's health relative to his chief complaint.

- Appetite

  - What is Spree's appetite?
  - Has Spree's appetite changed?

- Attitude

  - What is Spree's attitude or demeanor?
  - Has Spree's attitude changed?

- Cough quality

  - What is the quality of Spree's cough?

    - Is his cough wet?
    - Is his cough dry?

- Energy level

  - What is Spree's energy level?
  - Has Spree's energy level changed?

- Is Spree's cough productive?
- Is Spree demonstrating any other clinical signs (e.g. exercise intolerance, nasal discharge, respiratory distress, sneezing)?
- What exacerbates Spree's cough?

15. Note that most of the questions that I outlined in Question #14 (above) are closed-ended. That is, they direct the client to respond in an abbreviated manner.(56, 57) The answer to a closed-ended question is often "yes" or "no."(56, 57) For example: "Yes, his appetite is reduced." "Yes, his energy level has changed."

    Closed-ended questions play an important part in the veterinary consultation: there are times when we need a definite, abbreviated answer.(57) For instance: "Yes, he is sneezing." "Yes, his cough is wet."

    However, there are limitations to the use of closed-ended questions.(57) For one thing, we must ask a lot more of them to obtain an ample amount of patient-specific data.(57) There are times in the consultation when we benefit from inviting the client to share additional details with us.(57) These circumstances require us to employ a different line of questioning, the open-ended question or statement.(57)

    Open-ended questions and statements invite clients to provide an expanded answer to our questions.(57, 58) To facilitate sharing of detailed information, we often begin open-ended statements with:(56, 59–61)

- Tell me
- Help me
- Show me
- Share with me
- Describe
- Paint a picture for me

For example:

- Tell me more about Spree's cough.
- Help me to understand what Spree is experiencing when he has an episode.
- Describe Spree's coughing fit.

Returning to Case 42: The Coughing Dog

You expand upon history-taking before evaluating Spree. Katrina shares that nothing about Spree's environment has changed other than the weather outdoors. This year seemed to skip over spring, and the summer temperatures are soaring outside. It is hot. It doesn't take much activity for them both to work up a sweat. Katrina also shares that her seasonal allergies have been exceptionally bad, what with the elevation in pollen count and the flowers in the garden in full bloom, combined with the lack of rain to cleanse the patio of allergens. Katrina says that her eyes have been exceptionally watery and itchy, and she's felt congested, too. She asks if Spree could be experiencing the same thing.

According to Katrina, Spree has been eating and drinking well. There has been no change in his activity. If anything, the sunny weather has put some pep in his step and he's constantly pulling now at the leash to keep one step ahead of Katrina on walks. In fact, tugging on the leash seems to be the trigger for his cough. Although Jon was the first to notice this, now that Katrina is aware of it, she would have to agree. In retrospect, this dry, harsh cough is not necessarily new, it's just gotten worse.

Your line of questioning has jogged Katrina's memory. Now, she recalls hearing this "honk" for the very first time a few months ago. The quality of the cough hasn't changed. Spree still sounds like a goose. The frequency of cough and the duration of each coughing fit have both increased.

You examine Spree. He is mildly over-conditioned in terms of his BCS. Palpation of his trachea elicits the same cough that both Jon and Katrina appreciated. Spree's physical examination is otherwise unremarkable. He is afebrile. His submandibular, prescapular, and popliteal lymph nodes are of anticipated size and shape, bilaterally symmetrical, and non-tender to the touch. His lungs are clear on thoracic auscultation.

You tell Katrina you are not convinced that Spree's cough is infectious, particularly in light of its duration.

Round Two of Questions for Case 42: The Coughing Dog

1. Of the non-infectious causes of cough that you outlined in Answers to Round One of Questions, which is/are least likely in Spree and why?
2. Of the non-infectious causes of cough that you outlined in Answers to Round One of Questions, which is/are more likely to be possible in Spree and why?
3. Based upon your index of suspicion, which diagnostic tests are most appropriate to evaluate Spree for the differential diagnoses that you identified in Question #2 (above)?

Answers to Round Two of Questions for Case 42: The Coughing Dog

1. Of the non-infectious causes of cough, the following are LEAST likely in Spree.

    *   Allergic rhinitis and/or sinusitis with post-nasal drip – I would have expected Katrina to report sneezing and nasal discharge.
    *   Aspiration pneumonia – I would have expected Katrina to report lethargy, increased respiratory rate (RR) in the home environment, and dyspnea. Patients with aspiration pneumonia often present in respiratory distress.
    *   Asthma – I would have expected Katrina to report wheezing rather than just coughing.
    *   Inhalation of irritants – this seems less likely because the cough only seems to present itself when the patient pulls on the leash.
    *   Nasopharyngeal polyp – this condition is more likely to occur in young cats.(62–66)
    *   Nasopharyngeal, laryngeal, or tracheal foreign body obstruction – it would be unusual for this to be present and persist over the course of months unless the obstruction is partial, such as a migrating grass awn.

2. Of the non-infectious causes of cough, the following are more likely to be possible in Spree:

    *   chronic bronchitis
    *   laryngeal paralysis
    *   tracheal collapse.

    Canine bronchitis is a chronic inflammatory disease of the lower airway.(6, 49) It is persistent and progressive.(29) Over time, chronic irritation leads to airway changes that are irreversible. (6, 29) Affected patients experience cough, increased resistance to airflow and decreased ability to exhale with ease.(6, 29)

    Laryngeal paralysis describes a condition in which one or both of the laryngeal arytenoid cartilages fail to abduct during the inspiratory part of the respiratory cycle.(6, 67) Although laryngeal paralysis is inherited in certain breeds of dog, it is most often acquired later in life.(6, 67, 68) Affected patients experience faulty innervation of the abductors of the arytenoid cartilages by the recurrent laryngeal nerve.(6, 67, 69–71) If this nerve degenerates, then it no longer signals the cricoarytenoideus dorsalis muscle to contract.(6) If this muscle remains flaccid, then one or both of the arytenoid cartilages bow out into the airway lumen and obstruct air flow.(6, 67) This typically creates stridor.(6) However, affected dogs may also simply present for cough.(6)

    Tracheal collapse is a condition that is characterized by increased laxity of the trachealis muscle, which connects the dorsal aspect of the C-shaped cartilaginous rings that are responsible for keeping the lumen of the trachea open.(1, 6, 72–75) Muscle laxity may occur focally or may involve the entire length of the trachea.(1, 6) Every time the affected patient breathes, the tracheal lumen loses its shape.(6) The disease is progressive.(6) Over time the C-shaped rings lose their connection to each other and spread out.(6) The affected rings ultimately flatten and the trachea collapses.(1, 6) This can precipitate coughing or, in worst case situations, respiratory distress.(1, 6)

3. Laryngeal paralysis can be diagnosed by inspecting the larynx under a light plane of anesthesia. (67, 76) Affected patients will be unable to abduct one or both arytenoid cartilages.(6)

    Tracheal collapse is definitively diagnosed by thoracic imaging.(1) Radiographs of the cervical region and thorax are typically performed in private practice whereas fluoroscopy is more typically available in referral centers and/or teaching hospitals.(1) Either approach is effective at identifying a narrowed airway lumen at the site(s) of tracheal collapse.

    Chronic bronchitis is a diagnosis of exclusion.(6, 49, 50) Cardiac, infectious, and neoplastic causes of cough must be ruled out.(6, 49, 50) Thoracic radiographs would be an appropriate starting point to evaluate the patient for cardiomegaly through measurement of the vertebral heart score.(6) Thoracic radiographs would also allow you to rule out overt metastatic pulmonary disease, which would be rare, given Spree's age.(6) Thoracic radiographs would also rule out pneumonia, which is unlikely based upon the patient's history and physical exam findings.(6) Parasitic causes of cough could be assessed through fecal testing.(6) The Baermann fecal test is the preferred test for ruling out lungworms.(6, 25, 29)

Returning to Case 42: The Coughing Dog

Katrina consents to survey radiographs of Spree's thoracic cavity to provide a baseline assessment of his respiratory tract. You take orthogonal views. Spree's left lateral radiograph has been provided in Figure 42.2 for you to review.

Although the left lateral thoracic radiograph is diagnostic, you are employed at a university teaching hospital and feel that this would be a perfect opportunity for the students under your care to compare imaging modalities. Katrina authorizes fluoroscopy on Spree at no additional cost to her (see Figure 42.3).

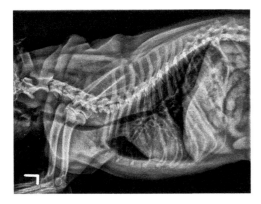

Figure 42.2 Left lateral thoracic radiograph. Courtesy of Daniel Foy, MS, DVM, DACVIM, DACVECC.

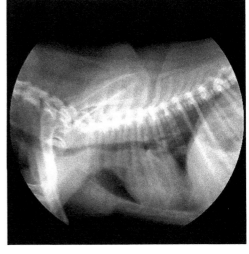

Figure 42.3 Fluoroscopy of the thorax. Courtesy of Daniel Foy, MS, DVM, DACVIM, DACVECC.

Round Three of Questions for Case 42: The Coughing Dog

1. What is Spree's diagnosis?
2. What do you see in Figures 42.2 and 42.3 that is conclusive?
3. What constitutes appropriate medical management for this condition?
4. What, if any, options are there for Spree if medical management fails?

Answers to Round Three of Questions for Case 42: The Coughing Dog

1. Spree has tracheal collapse.

2. I see diagnostic narrowing of the tracheal lumen at the level of the first rib.

3. Medical management of tracheal collapse typically involves:(77)

   - cough suppressants, such as hydroco-done, butorphanol, or codeine
   - exercise restriction, particularly in hot, humid environments in which the patient is at increased risk of overheating
   - sedatives, such as acepromazine, as needed
   - systemic steroid therapy, such as prednisone, to reduce mucosal irritation within the trachea
   - transitioning from a collar to a harness to reduce pulling on the trachea.

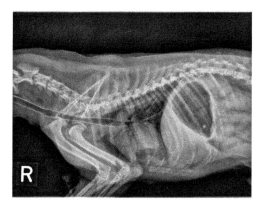

Figure 42.4 Right lateral thoracic radiograph demonstrating what a tracheal stent looks like after surgical placement in a canine patient. Courtesy of Daniel Foy, MS, DVM, DACVIM, DACVECC.

4. If medical management fails, then Spree might benefit from surgery to place extraluminal prosthetic support rings or intraluminal stents.(1, 6, 78–81) (See Figure 42.4.)

CLINICAL PEARLS

- Coughing is a common clinical sign in companion animal practice.

- Coughing is often associated with infectious airway disease.

- CIRD is caused by a myriad of bacteria and viruses, of which *B. bronchiseptica* is well known.

- Dogs are often prophylactically vaccinated against *B. bronchiseptica* as part of their preventive healthcare. Clients frequently refer to this vaccine as the "kennel cough" shot when in fact true kennel cough can be caused by several pathogens, not just *Bordetella*.

- CIRD often involves more than one infectious agent. Following primary infection, opportunistic invaders are common.

- Viral components of CIRD include:

  - canine adenovirus-2 (CAV-2)
  - canine distemper virus (CDV)

- canine influenza (H3N8)
- canine parainfluenza
- canine respiratory coronavirus.

- Kennel cough is often diagnosed presumptively based upon the patient's clinical history and physical examination findings.

- Although it is prudent to evaluate patients for respiratory infections, it is important to remember that coughing is not always a sign of infectious disease.

- Sometimes coughing results from cardiac, neoplastic, or structural disease.

- Tracheal collapse is one type of structural disease that causes a "goose honk" cough. This type of cough is exacerbated by exercise, excitement, stress, heat/humidity, and obesity.

- Small-to-toy canine breeds, such as Pomeranians, Yorkshire terriers, Chihuahuas, and Toy poodles, are overrepresented in the veterinary medical literature in terms of clinical cases of tracheal collapse.(1)

- Treatment of tracheal collapse is aimed at reducing excitement, stress, and strenuous exercise and replacing the leash with a harness to eliminate pulling on the neck.

References

1. Deweese MD, Tobias KM. Tracheal collapse in dogs. NAVC Clin's Brief 2014 (May):83–7.
2. Hurley K. Canine infectious respiratory disease complex: management and prevention in canine populations. DVM 2010;360.
3. Joffe DJ, Lelewski R, Weese JS, McGill-Worsley J, Shankel C, Mendonca S, et al. Factors associated with development of Canine Infectious Respiratory Disease Complex (CIRDC) in dogs in 5 Canadian small animal clinics. Can Vet J 2016;57(1):46–51.
4. Chalker VJ, Toomey C, Opperman S, Brooks HW, Ibuoye MA, Brownlie J, Rycroft AN. Respiratory disease in kennelled dogs: serological responses to Bordetella bronchiseptica lipopolysaccharide do not correlate with bacterial isolation or clinical respiratory symptoms. Clin Diagn Lab Immunol 2003;10(3):352–6.
5. Nafe LA. Dogs infected with Bordetella bronchiseptica and Canine influenza virus (H3N8). Today's. Vet Pract 2014 (July/August):30–6.
6. Englar RE. Common clinical presentations in dogs and cats. Hoboken, NJ: Wiley/Blackwell; 2019.
7. Weese JS, Evason M. Infectious diseases of the dog and cat: a color handbook. Boca Raton, FL: CRC Press; 2019.
8. Ettinger SJ, Feldman EC, Côté E. Textbook of veterinary internal medicine: diseases of the dog and the cat. 8th ed. St. Louis, MO: Elsevier; 2017.
9. Côté E. Clinical veterinary advisor. Dogs and cats. 3rd ed. St. Louis, MO: Elsevier Mosby.
10. Ellis JA, Krakowka GS. A review of canine parainfluenza virus infection in dogs. J Am Vet Med Assoc 2012;240(3):273–84.
11. Erles K, Toomey C, Brooks HW, Brownlie J. Detection of a group 2 coronavirus in dogs with canine infectious respiratory disease. Virology 2003;310(2):216–23.
12. Priestnall SL, Mitchell JA, Walker CA, Erles K, Brownlie J. New and emerging pathogens in canine infectious respiratory disease. Vet Pathol 2014;51(2):492–504.
13. Holt DE, Mover MR, Brown DC. Serologic prevalence of antibodies against canine influenza virus (H3N8) in dogs in a metropolitan animal shelter. J Am Vet Med Assoc 2010;237(1):71–3.
14. Radhakrishnan A, Drobatz KJ, Culp WT, King LG. Community-acquired infectious pneumonia in puppies: 65 cases (1993–2002). J Am Vet Med Assoc 2007;230(10):1493–7.
15. Ford RB. Canine infectious tracheobronchitis. In: Greene CE, editor. Infectious diseases of the dog and cat. St. Louis: Elsevier, Inc.; 2006. p. 54–63.

16. Weese JS, Stull J. Respiratory disease outbreak in a veterinary hospital associated with canine parainfluenza virus infection. Can Vet J 2013;54(1):79–82.

17. Dillon AR, Blagburn BL, Tillson M, Brawner W, Welles B, Johnson C, et al. The progression of heartworm associated respiratory disease (HARD) in SPF cats 18 months after Dirofilaria immitis infection. Parasit Vectors 2017;10(Suppl 2)(Suppl 2):533.

18. Dillon AR, Blagburn BL, Tillson M, Brawner W, Welles B, Johnson C, et al. Heartworm-associated respiratory disease (HARD) induced by immature adult Dirofilaria immitis in cats. Parasit Vectors 2017;10(Suppl 2)(Suppl 2):514.

19. Litster A, Atkins C, Atwell R. Acute death in heartworm-infected cats: unraveling the puzzle. Vet Parasitol 2008;158(3):196–203.

20. Litster AL, Atwell RB. Feline heartworm disease: a clinical review. J Feline Med Surg 2008;10(2):137–44.

21. Mason RA, Rand J. The coughing cat. In: Rand J, editor. Problem-based feline medicine. Philadelphia, PA: Elsevier Saunders; 2006. p. 90–108.

22. Nelson CT. Heartworm-associated respiratory disease in cats. NAVC Clin's Brief 2007 (May);15.

23. Lee ACY, Kraus MS. Coughing cat: could it be heartworm? NAVC Clin's Brief 2012 (June):91–5.

24. Palma D. Common pulmonary diseases in cats. NAVC Clin's Brief 2017 (March):107–15.

25. Bowman DD, Georgi JR. Georgis' parasitology for veterinarians. 9th ed. St. Louis, MO: Saunders/Elsevier; 2009.

26. Englar RE. Performing the small animal physical examination. Hoboken, NJ: Wiley/Blackwell; 2017.

27. Tams TR. Diagnosis and management of acute and chronic vomiting in dogs and cats. DVM. 360 [Internet]; 2009. Available from: http://veterinarycalendar.dvm360.com/diagnosis-and-management-acute-and-chronic-vomiting-dogs-and-cats-proceedings.

28. Tams TR. Diagnosing of acute and chronic vomiting in dogs and Cat. s2017. Available from: https://vvma.org/resources/2017%20VVC%20Notes/Tams-Vomiting%20in%20Dogs%20and%20Cats%20-%20Diagnosis.pdf.

29. Tilley LP, Smith FWK. Blackwell's five-minute veterinary consult. Canine and feline. 6th ed. Ames, IA: John Wiley & Sons, Inc.; 2016.

30. Traversa D, Di Cesare A. Diagnosis and management of lungworm infections in cats: cornerstones, dilemmas and new avenues. J Feline Med Surg 2016;18(1):7–20.

31. Pechman RD. Respiratory parasites. In: Sherding RG, editor. The cat: diseases and clinical management. New York: Churchill Livingstone; 1994. p. 613–22.

32. Traversa D, Di Cesare A. Feline lungworms: what a dilemma. Trends Parasitol 2013;29(9):423–30.

33. Conboy G. Helminth parasites of the canine and feline respiratory tract. Vet Clin North Am Small Anim Pract 2009;39(6):1109–26.

34. Brianti E, Giannetto S, Dantas-Torres F, Otranto D. Lungworms of the genus Troglostrongylus (Strongylida: Crenosomatidae): neglected parasites for domestic cats. Vet Parasitol 2014;202(3–4):104–12.

35. Bowman DD, Hendrix CM, Lindsay DS. Feline clinical parasitology. Ames, IA: Iowa State University Press; 2002.

36. Palma D. Common pulmonary diseases in dogs. NAVC Clin's Brief 2016 (October):77–109.

37. Herman LH, Helland DR. Paragonimiasis in a cat. J Am Vet Med Assoc 1966;149(6):753–7.

38. Pechman RD. Radiographic features of pulmonary paragonimiasis in dog and cat. J Am Vet Radiol Soc 1976;17(5):182–91.

39. Pechman RD. Pulmonary paragonimiasis in dogs and cats – review. J Small Anim Pract 1980;21(2):87–95.

40. Traversa D, Di Cesare A, Milillo P, Iorio R, Otranto D. Aelurostrongylus abstrusus in a feline colony from central Italy: clinical features, diagnostic procedures and molecular characterization. Parasitol Res 2008;103(5):1191–6.

41. Traversa D, Lia RP, Iorio R, Boari A, Paradies P, Capelli G, et al. Diagnosis and risk factors of Aelurostrongylus abstrusus (Nematoda, Strongylida) infection in cats from Italy. Vet Parasitol 2008;153(1–2):182–6.

42. Hawkins EC. Coughing dogs: determining why. NAVC clinician's Brief [Internet]. Available from: https://www.cliniciansbrief.com/column/category/column/capsules/coughing-dogs-determining-why.

43. Johnson LR. Chronic cough. NAVC Clin's Brief 2006 (July):51–2.

44. Ellis J. Chronic cough in a puppy. NAVC Clinician's Brief [Internet]. Available from: https://www.cliniciansbrief.com/article/chronic-cough-puppy.

45. Clercx C, Roels E. Exercise intolerance and chronic cough in a geriatic dog. NAVC Clin's Brief 2015 (December).

46. Grobman M, Reinero C. Investigation of Neurokinin-1 receptor antagonism as a novel treatment for chronic bronchitis in dogs. J Vet Intern Med 2016;30(3):847–52.

47. Dye J. Cough in cats. NAVC Clin's Brief 2008(July);17.

48. Fry JK, Burney DP. Canine infectious respiratory disease. NAVC Clin's Brief 2012 (November):34–8.

49. Kumrow KJ. Canine chronic bronchitis: a review and update. Today's. Vet Pract 2012 (November/December):12–7.

50. Carey SA, editor. Current therapy for canine chronic Bronchitis2018: Michigan veterinary Medical Association.

51. Padrid P. Feline asthma and bronchitis. NAVC Clin's Brief 2005 (October):37–40.

52. Byers CG, Dhupa N. Feline asthma and heartworm disease – Reply. Comp Cont. Educ Pract 2005;27(8):573.

53. Byers CG, Dhupa N. Feline bronchial asthma: pathophysiology and diagnosis. Comp Cont Educ Pract 2005;27(6):418.

54. Byers CG, Dhupa N. Feline bronchial asthma: Treatment. Comp Cont. Educ Pract 2005;27(6):426–31.

55. Little S. Coughing and wheezing cats: diagnosis and treatment of feline asthma. DVM. 360 [Internet]; 2010. Available from: http://veterinarycalendar.dvm360.com/coughing-and-wheezing-cats-diagnosis-and-treatment-feline-asthma-proceedings.

56. Shaw JR. Four core communication skills of highly effective practitioners. Vet Clin North Am Small Anim Pract 2006;36(2):385–96.

57. Englar R. A guide to. Oral Communication in Veterinary Medicine. Sheffield: 5M Publishing; 2020.

58. Englar RE, Williams M, Weingand K. Applicability of the Calgary-Cambridge guide to dog and cat owners for teaching veterinary clinical communications. J Vet Med Educ 2016;43(2):143–69.

59. Kurtz SM, Silverman JD, Draper J. Teaching and learning communication skills in medicine. Grand Rapids, FL: Radcliffe; 2004.

60. Adams CL, Kurtz SM. Skills for communicating in veterinary medicine. Oxford: Otmoor Press and Dewpoint Publishing; 2017.

61. Silverman J, Kurtz S, Draper J. Skills for communicating with patients. Oxford: Radcliffe Medical Press; 2008.

62. Quimby J, Lappin MR. The upper respiratory tract. In: Little SE, editor. The cat: clinical medicine and management. St. Louis, MO: Saunders Elsevier; 2012. p. 846–61.

63. Henderson SM, Bradley K, Day MJ, Tasker S, Caney SM, Hotston Moore A, Gruffydd-Jones TJ. Investigation of nasal disease in the cat--a retrospective study of 77 cases. J Feline Med Surg 2004;6(4):245–57.

64. Schmidt JF, Kapatkin A. Nasopharyngeal and ear canal polyps in the cat. Feline Pract 1990;18(4):16–9.

65. Kapatkin AS, Matthiesen DT, Noone KE, Church EM. Scavelli TE, Patnaik AK. Results of surgery and long-term follow-up in 31 cats with nasopharyngeal polyps. J Am Anim Hosp Assoc 1990;26(4):387–92.

66. Englar RE. Performing the small animal physical examination. Hoboken, NJ: Wiley; 2017.

67. Mankin KT. Laryngeal paralysis diagnosis. NAVC Clin's Brief 2015 (December):67–71.

68. Tilley LP, Smith FWK. The 5-minute veterinary consult: canine and feline. 3rd ed. Baltimore, MD: Lippincott Williams & Wilkins; 2004.

69. Thieman KM, Krahwinkel DJ, Sims MH, Shelton GD. Histopathological confirmation of polyneuropathy in 11 dogs with laryngeal paralysis. J Am Anim Hosp Assoc 2010;46(3):161–7.

70. Stanley BJ, Hauptman JG, Fritz MC, Rosenstein DS, Kinns J. Esophageal dysfunction in dogs with idiopathic laryngeal paralysis: a controlled cohort study. Vet Surg 2010;39(2):139–49.

71. Jeffery ND, Talbot CE, Smith PM, Bacon NJ. Acquired idiopathic laryngeal paralysis as a prominent feature of generalized neuromuscular disease in 39 dogs. Vet Rec 2006;158(1):17.

72. Evans HE, Miller ME. Miller's anatomy of the dog. 4th ed. St. Louis, MO: Elsevier; 2013.

73. Singh B, Dyce KM. Dyce, Sack, and Wensing's textbook of veterinary anatomy. 5th ed. St. Louis, MO: Saunders; 2018.

74. Ettinger SJ. Diseases of the trachea and upper airways. In: Ettinger SJ, Feldman EC, editors. Textbook of veterinary internal medicine. St. Louis, MO: Saunders Elsevier; 2010.

75. Sura P, Durant A. Trachea and bronchi. In: Tobias KM, Johnson SA, editors. Veterinary surgery: small animal. St. Louis, MO: Saunders Elsevier; 2012. p. 1734–50.

76. Jackson AM, Tobias K, Long C, Bartges J, Harvey R. Effects of various anesthetic agents on laryngeal motion during laryngoscopy in normal dogs. Vet Surg 2004;33(2):102–6.
77. Linklater A. Tracheal collapse in dogs. Plumb's Ther Brief 2018 (February):46–57.
78. Buback JL, Boothe HW, Hobson HP. Surgical treatment of tracheal collapse in dogs: 90 cases (1983–1993). J Am Vet Med Assoc 1996;208(3):380–4.
79. Tangner CH, Hobson HP. A retrospective study of 20 surgically managed cases of collapsed trachea. Vet Surg 1982;11(4):146–9.
80. Chisnell HK, Pardo AD. Long-term outcome, complications and disease progression in 23 dogs after placement of tracheal ring prostheses for treatment of extrathoracic tracheal collapse. Vet Surg 2015;44(1):103–13.
81. Moritz A, Schneider M, Bauer N. Management of advanced tracheal collapse in dogs using intraluminal self-expanding biliary wallstents. J Vet Intern Med 2004;18(1):31–42.

Case 43

The Snoring Cat

Biscuit is new to your practice. She was adopted one month ago into a pet-less, one-person household by Ginny Wallister. Ginny had been searching high and low for a new companion, 6 months after 18-year-old Aristocat passed away of natural causes. Aristocat was a handsome flame point Siamese male whom she had inherited from her mother. Aristocat was the perfect companion for a retiree. He was a constant companion, from sunrise tea to bedtime snacks.

Life had been lonely for Ginny since Aristocat's death. She was looking for someone new to share her life with, but the cat had to be the right "fit." She'd thought about purchasing from Aristocat's breeder, but the cattery was no longer in existence. She considered telephoning another but found it difficult to justify buying a cat when the local shelter was overrun with them. She toyed with the idea of fostering yet knew she could never give one up after bonding with the cat in her home environment. So, she kept her eyes and ears open.

It wasn't long before she stumbled across Biscuit's photo on social media. According to TonkiRescue, the organization that was respon-

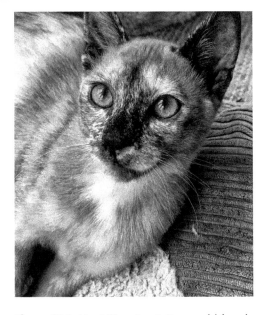

Figure 43.1 Meet Biscuit, a 1.5-year-old female spayed tortie mink Tonkinese cat. Courtesy of Allegra Loch.

sible for rehoming her, Biscuit had a back story. She had been purchased as an anniversary gift, but the marriage had not worked out. Neither party wanted to be reminded of their failed union, leaving Biscuit behind to find a new forever home. Although neither bride nor groom were willing to keep Biscuit, they did not wish to relinquish her to a shelter. Thankfully, they were able to find a local chapter of a breed-specific rescue to take on the cat and ensure her wellbeing.

When Ginny saw her striking face and those beautiful Caribbean blue-green eyes, she knew she was "The One." Biscuit was the perfect choice for Ginny. She was social and playful, inquisitive yet gentle. She brought life to Ginny's home and heart and was different enough from Aristocat so that Ginny would not forever compare the two. After all, Aristocat had big paws that were near impossible to fill.

Since coming to live with Ginny, Biscuit has been in generally good health except for nasal discharge and sneezing that just wouldn't quit. When Ginny first reported this to TonkiRescue, she was told that rehoming is a stressful event and it is not uncommon for cats to pick up a "cold." The organization told Ginny to keep an eye on it, but that symptoms ought to clear within 2 weeks. If they did not, if they worsened, and/or if Biscuit developed respiratory distress, then Ginny was instructed to seek veterinary medical care right away. Ginny was also told to keep an eye out for "pink eye" because that and upper respiratory tract infections often went hand in hand.

For the next 2 weeks, Ginny watched Biscuit like a hawk. Her eyes remained bright and clear. However, her snot continued to come and go. One day, Ginny would think it had finally flown the coop and the next, it would be back again. The nasal discharge didn't seem to bother Biscuit, but it worried Ginny, particularly when paired with a distinctive snoring sound that she'd never experienced with Aristocat. At first, Ginny attributed the sound to being congested and indeed, maybe that's all it was. But as the weeks progressed, the sound was getting worse rather than better. So, Ginny reached out to your clinic to schedule an appointment.

Ginny has just arrived with Biscuit for her consultation, and she is looking forward to finding an answer to speed resolution.

Review Biscuit's vital signs below as you prepare for this consult.

Weight: 9.6 lb (4.4 kg)
BCS: 5/9
Mentation: QAR

TPR

T: 100.3°F (37.9°C)
P: 174 beats per minute
R: 27 breaths per minute

Round One of Questions for Case 43: The Snoring Cat

1. Sneezing is an involuntary action. What is the purpose of sneezing?
2. Sneezing is often paired with nasal discharge. Which descriptors are important for us to investigate that are related to Biscuit's nasal discharge?
3. Describe what might be considered normal nasal discharge.
4. Describe what might be considered abnormal nasal discharge.
5. For each cause of abnormal nasal discharge that you identified in Question #4 (above), provide at least one plausible etiology.
6. Which additional clarifying questions might you want to ask Ginny that relates to the patient's presenting complaint, persisting sneezing?
7. In addition to what you described in Question #2, which aspects are important for you to assess on physical examination to help you further evaluate Biscuit's respiratory complaint, including her audibly loud breathing?
8. What is "pink eye?"
9. What causes "pink eye" in cats?
10. Which clinical signs are suggestive of "pink eye" in cats?
11. Which clinical condition(s) often go hand in hand with "pink eye" in cats?
12. From the patient history that you have been provided with, you know that Biscuit has not had any ocular discharge. Which follow-up questions might you want to ask Ginny to clarify if Biscuit has any additional symptoms that are suggestive of pink eye?

Answers to Round One of Questions for Case 43: The Snoring Cat

1. The purpose of sneezing is to expel irritants and particulate matter from the upper airway.(1–4)

2. Any time that a patient presents with nasal discharge, we need to clarify the following descriptors.(4)

- Distribution of nasal discharge

  - Is the nasal discharge unilateral?
  - Is the nasal discharge bilateral?

- Gross appearance of the nasal discharge

  - What is the color of the nasal discharge?
  - Is the nasal discharge transparent or opaque?

- Consistency of the nasal discharge

    - Is the nasal discharge thin and watery?
    - Is the nasal discharge thick and mucoid?

  - How, if at all, has the nasal discharge changed?

3. Small amounts of serous nasal discharge can be normal.(4–6) Serous discharge is watery and transparent.(7) Cellular content is slim to none when samples are viewed on cytological preparations.(7)

4. Excessive amounts of serous nasal discharge from one or both nostrils is abnormal.(4)
    Mucoid, purulent, and hemorrhagic nasal discharge are abnormal clinical findings in dogs and cats.(4–6, 8, 9)
    Mucoid nasal discharge appears whitish or even slightly yellow in color.(4, 7, 9) It is slimy because it has the consistency of mucus.(4, 9) There will be minimal cellular content on cytology.(4, 7)
    Purulent nasal discharge is typically yellow-green in color.(4, 9) If evaluated via microscopy, you would appreciate large populations of degenerate neutrophils and intracellular bacteria, which support a diagnosis of infectious disease.(4, 7)
    Hemorrhagic nasal discharge is bloody, as its descriptor implies.(4, 9) Patients that present with frank blood coming out of one or both nasal passageways are said to be experiencing epistaxis, that is, a nose bleed.(5, 6) There will be an abundance of erythrocytes on cytology.(4, 7)

5. Excessive amounts or serous discharge and/or or serous discharge that persists may be indicative of a brewing viral infection or early inflammation within the nasal cavity.(4, 7)
    Mucoid nasal discharge is associated with chronic inflammation.(4, 7)
    Purulent nasal discharge is associated with bacterial upper respiratory infections (URIs).(4, 7)
    Epistaxis may result from disease within the upper airway:(4, 7)

- trauma
- fungal infections
- neoplasia.

Alternatively, epistaxis may result from systemic disease, such as:(4, 7, 8, 10)

- coagulopathies
- thrombocytopenia
- vasculitis
- hypertension.

6. I would like to ask Ginny the following clarifying questions about the patient history.(4)

- What is Biscuit's environment like?

    - Is she housed in a rural, suburban, or urban environment?
    - Is she exposed to smoke?
    - Is she exposed to air fresheners, candles, or other scented items?

  - What is Biscuit's lifestyle?

    - Is she indoor-only?
    - Is she outdoor-only?
    - Is she indoor-outdoor?

  - What is Biscuit's vaccination history?
  - What is Biscuit's serologic status?

- Has she been tested for feline leukemia (FeLV) and feline immunodeficiency virus (FIV)?
- Did she test negative for FeLV?
- Did she test negative for FIV?

- Has Biscuit recently been exposed to conspecifics, particularly those that are not vaccinated?
- Has Biscuit recently been exposed to other species?
- Has Biscuit recently been to a groomer?

7. In addition to what I described in my answer to Question #2, I need to make assessments about the following features on Biscuit's physical exam.(4, 9)

- Are there erosions or other dermatologic lesions on the nasal planum?
- Is the bridge of the nose deformed?
- Is there any other facial deformity in the immediate vicinity of the nares?
- Is Biscuit open-mouth breathing?
- Is Biscuit extending her head and neck to try to take more air in?
- Is there apparent increased inspiratory effort?
- Is there apparent increased expiratory effort?
- Is there audible wheezing?
- Patency of the nares: are Biscuit's nares stenotic?
- Patency of airflow through the nasal passageways: can air flow to and from the nostrils?
- What do Biscuit's airways sound like?

  - Are her lungs clear with normal bronchovesicular sounds?
  - Are there referred upper airway sounds?
  - Are there adventitious sounds?

8. Pink eye is the colloquial term for conjunctivitis, that is, inflammation of the conjunctiva.(4, 9) The conjunctiva is a thin mucous membrane that supports the globe.(4, 9, 11, 12) In health, the conjunctiva is thin, smooth, moist, and has a characteristic light pink appearance.(6, 11, 13) Although the conjunctiva has a blood supply, the individual vessels are not typically apparent in healthy patients.(6, 14) When conjunctival tissues become inflamed, they exhibit hyperemia. (6, 11, 14, 15) This redness is the direct result of increased blood supply due to inflammation.(11, 15) For this reason, patients with conjunctivitis may appear to have bloodshot eyes.(4) Because of this, they are said to have pink eye. The conjunctiva of affected cats also takes on a billowy or "puffy" appearance due to chemosis, that is, conjunctival edema.(6, 13, 15) This is much more pronounced in cats than dogs.

9. In cats, conjunctivitis is often the result of infectious disease.(11, 16–23) The most common cause of infectious conjunctivitis in cats is feline herpesvirus type-1 (FHV-1).(16, 22, 24) Other common causes of infectious conjunctivitis in cats are:(4, 21, 25–27)

- *Chlamydophila felis*
- *Mycoplasma spp.*
- *Feline calicivirus*
- *Bordetella bronchiseptica.*

10. Clinical signs that are suggestive of "pink eye" in cats include:(4, 9, 28)

- blepharospasm, that is, squinting of the affected eye(s)
- chemosis
- hyperemia
- ocular discharge
- pawing at the eye(s)
- photophobia, that is, light sensitivity.

11. Conjunctivitis is often paired with URIs in cats. This is particularly true of FHV-1.(4, 9, 28) Sneezing, nasal discharge, generalized malaise, and decreased appetite are commonly seen in the early stages of infection, in addition to conjunctivitis.(15, 17–20, 29, 30)

12. To clarify if Biscuit has any additional symptoms that are suggestive of pink eye, I would ask Ginny the following questions specific to Biscuit's eyes.

- Does Biscuit seem to be bothered at all by her eyes?
- Have you noticed any squinting?
- Have you noticed her pawing at her eyes?

Returning to Case 43: The Snoring Cat

Ginny tells you that Biscuit's nasal discharge is bilateral and intermittent. It has always been clear and translucent. TonkiRescue had asked her to reach out if the discharge turned green-yellow or cloudy, but neither situation has presented itself thus far.

Ginny shares that Biscuit's audible breathing has been constant since adoption. She has not noticed open-mouth breathing or cyanotic mucous membranes, but there are episodes when Biscuit gags as if she has difficulty swallowing.

You examine Biscuit. You agree with Ginny that Biscuit's eyes are clear and bright. They are opened wide and alert. You do not notice any apparent photophobia or blepharospasm. There is no evidence of conjunctivitis.

Throughout the exam, Biscuit sounds congested. There is serous nasal discharge from both nares and what appears to be reduced airflow through both nasal passageways.

During the exam, Biscuit has two episodes of reverse sneezing. Ginny confirms that she has heard this sound before. When these episodes occurred at home, she thought that Biscuit was trying to clear her throat.

Biscuit's otoscopic exam is unremarkable, as is the remainder of her physical.

Round Two of Questions for Case 43: The Snoring Cat

1. What is reverse sneezing?
2. Is reverse sneezing more commonly observed in dogs or cats?
3. What are potential triggers for reverse sneezing?
4. Which of the triggers that you identified in Question #3 (above) are more likely to induce reverse sneezing episodes in cats?
5. Which is the next most appropriate step for Biscuit's diagnostic work-up to investigate the etiology/etiologies that you identified in Question #4 (above)?
6. Ginny wants to know why you examined both of Biscuit's ears. She says that "neither ear is bothering her." How might you respond?

Answers to Round Two of Questions for Case 43: The Snoring Cat

1. Reverse sneezing can be thought of as paroxysmal respiration.(4, 9) It describes a respiratory episode during which the patient exhibits repeated, rapid inspiratory attempts.(4, 9) The patient may exhibit stertor or extend its head and neck, as if having difficulty breathing.(3, 4, 9)

2. It is more common to observe reverse sneezing in dogs than cats.(3)

3. Episodes may be triggered by:(31–35)

- environmental allergens and/or particulate matter:
  - dust
  - pollen
- foreign bodies, such as grass awns
- growths associated with the nasal passageways, including nasopharyngeal polyps
- nasal parasites, such as *Capillaria boehmi.*

4. Of the triggers that I identified in Question #3 (above), nasopharyngeal polyps are the most likely culprit in cats. Nasal foreign bodies are relatively rare in dogs and cats.(4) Nasal capillariosis is more of a concern in dogs. *Capillaria boehmi* tends to inhabit the sinuses of North American and European foxes and wolves.(33, 36–39) When this nematode occurs in dogs, it induces rhinitis, nasal discharge, and reverse sneezing.(33–35)

5. The next most appropriate step in Biscuit's diagnostic work-up is to perform an oropharyngeal examination under sedation. You may be able to unearth a previously hidden nasopharyngeal polyp when you gently manipulate the soft palate.

6. I would share with Ginny that, based upon Biscuit's history and physical exam findings, I am suspicious that the cat has a nasopharyngeal polyp. These classically cause airway obstruction during the inspiratory part of the respiratory cycle, which could account for the snoring sound that Ginny has reported.(4) However, nasopharyngeal polyps can also invade the middle or external ear.(4, 40) Although I might have expected for Ginny to report head-shaking, pawing at the affected ear(s) and/or other evidence of otic pruritus, these are inconsistent findings.(4, 40, 41) To be thorough, an exam of both external ear canals is warranted.(4) Some polyps are large enough to be visualized in the external ear canal of an awake patient.(40) Many require more thorough exams under anesthesia to identify the polyp. If the polyp is in the middle ear, then computed tomography (CT) would be indicated.

Returning to Case 43: The Snoring Cat

You admit Biscuit to the clinic to perform an oropharyngeal exam under sedation after pre-anesthetic screening bloodwork and urinalysis are unremarkable.

Your exam of Biscuit's oropharynx is diagnostic (see Figure 43.2).

Round Three of Questions for Case 43: The Snoring Cat

1. Although it will need to be confirmed histologically, what is Biscuit's diagnosis?
2. Assuming that your diagnosis is correct, is this a benign lesion or a malignancy?
3. Where does this tissue come from?
4. Which patients are most susceptible?
5. What is the treatment of choice for this lesion in its current location, in Biscuit?

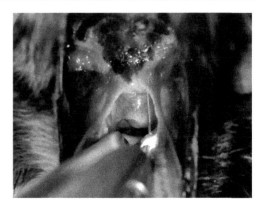

Figure 43.2 Oropharyngeal exam under sedation in a cat. Courtesy of Rodolfo Oliveira Leal, DVM (Portugal), PhD, Dipl. ECVIM-CA (Internal Medicine).

6. What is the treatment of choice for this lesion if it were instead located in the middle ear?
7. What is a potential consequence of the treatment option that you selected in your answer to Question #6 (above)?

Answers to Round Three of Questions for Case 43: The Snoring Cat

1. Biscuit has a nasopharyngeal polyp.

2. Nasopharyngeal polyps are benign.(4, 40, 41)

3. Nasopharyngeal polyps originate from the mucosa of the nasopharynx, auditory tube, or eardrum.(4, 40, 41)

4. Young adult cats are the most common age group to be diagnosed with nasopharyngeal polyps. (4, 6, 40–45)

5. If the ear were involved, I might have expected for Ginny to report head-shaking, pawing at the affected ear(s) and/or other evidence of otic pruritus, these are inconsistent findings.(4, 40, 41)

6. The treatment of choice for this lesion is surgical extraction.(4) Because of their stalk-like attachment, they are relatively easy to pluck from the pharynx of an anesthetized cat.(4) However, they are likely to regrow if the stalk is inadvertently not fully removed.(40)

7. Surgical extraction is more complicated when the middle ear is involved. In these clinical circumstances, a ventral bulla osteotomy is one of several typical approaches.(46–49) This procedure involves entering into the middle ear to scoop out the polyp.(46–49)

8. Sympathetic nerve fibers pass through the tympanic bulla in the cat. Surgical extraction of a middle ear polyp is likely to disrupt these fibers. As a result, a transient Horner's syndrome is a common adverse effect in the post-operative period.(4, 50) Horner's syndrome describes the clinical features that result from sympathetic denervation. Common features include:(4, 28, 51, 52)

   - enophthalmos
   - miosis (constriction) of the affected pupil
   - prominent third eyelid or nictitans membrane
   - ptosis (droopiness) of the upper eyelid.

CLINICAL PEARLS

- Sneezing and nasal discharge are frequently associated with URIs in cats.

- Cats that present with URIs often have concurrent conjunctivitis. FHV-1 is the most common cause of conjunctivitis in cats. Cats that are stressed are particularly prone to infection and/or recrudescence of the virus, if they have been previously exposed.

- When cats present for sneezing or nasal discharge, it is important to take a comprehensive history to establish laterality, discharge color and consistency, duration of symptoms and whether symptoms have progressed.

- It is important to recognize that persistent sneezing and chronic nasal discharge, when associated with noisy breathing, may not have an infectious origin.

- Young cats that are presented for snoring or otherwise audible breathing may have stenotic nares or they may have a nasopharyngeal polyp.

- Nasopharyngeal polyps are benign masses that arise from the nasopharynx, auditory tube, or eardrum.

- When nasopharyngeal polyps grow into the back of the throat, they may cause gagging.

- Nasopharyngeal polyps are handled surgically. Stalks can be grasped and plucked if they are pharyngeal. Middle ear involvement typically requires a ventral bulla osteotomy.

References

1. Tilley LP, Smith FWK. Blackwell's five-minute veterinary consult. Canine and feline. 6th ed. Ames, IA: John Wiley & Sons, Inc.; 2016.
2. Reece WO, ed. Dukes' physiology of domestic animals. 12th ed. Ithaca, NY: Cornell University Press; 2012.
3. Stokhof AA, v Haagen V. Respiratory system. In: Rijnberk A, van Sluijs FJ, editors. Medical history and physical examination in companion animals. Philadelphia, PA: Saunders Elsevier; 2012. p. 63–74.
4. Englar RE. Common clinical presentations in dogs and cats. Hoboken, NJ: Wiley/Blackwell; 2019.
5. Stokhof AA, Venker-van Haagen AJ. Respiratory system. In: Rijnberk A, van Sluijs FJ, editors. Medical history and physical examination in companion animals. Philadephia, PA: Saunders Elsevier; 2009. p. 63–74.
6. Englar RE. Performing the small animal physical examination. Hoboken, NJ: Wiley; 2017.
7. Gordon J. Clinical approach to nasal discharge. DVM. 360 [Internet]; 2011. Available from: http://veterinary-calendar.dvm360.com/clinical-approach-nasal-discharge-proceedings.
8. Cohn LA. Canine nasal disease. Vet Clin North Am Small Anim Pract 2014;44(1):75–89.
9. Englar RE. Performing the small animal physical examination. Hoboken, NJ: Wiley/Blackwell; 2017.
10. Chartier M. Canine primary (idiopathic) immune-mediated thrombocytopenia. NAVC Clin's Brief 2015 (September):82–6.
11. Heinrich C. Assessing canine conjunctivitis. Vet. Times [Internet]; 2015. Available from: https://www.vettimes.co.uk/app/uploads/wp-post-to-pdf-enhanced-cache/1/assessing-canine-conjunctivitis.pdf.
12. Ofri R. Conjunctivitis in dogs. NAVC Clin's Brief 2017 (April):89–93.
13. Lim CC. Conjunctiva. In: Small animal ophthalmic atlas and guide. Oxford: Wiley; 2015. p. 16–19.
14. Dyce KM, Sack WO, Wensing CJG. Textbook of veterinary anatomy. 4th ed. St. Louis, MO: Saunders/Elsevier; 2010.
15. Smith RIE. The cat with ocular discharge or changed conjunctival appearance. In: Rand J, editor. Problem-based feline medicine. Edinburgh. New York: Saunders; 2006. p. 1207–32.
16. Lim CC, Maggs DJ. Ophthalmology. In: Little SE, editor. The cat: Clinical medicine and management. St. Louis, MO: Saunders Elsevier; 2012. p. 807–45.
17. Ofri R. Conjunctivitis in cats. NAVC Clin's Brief 2017 (April):95–100.
18. Maggs DJ. Conjunctiva. In: Maggs DJ, Miller PE, Ofri R, editors. Slatter's fundamentals of veterinary opthalmology. St. Louis, MO: Elsevier; 2013. p. 140–58.
19. Aroch I, Ofri R, Sutton G. Ocular manifestations of systemic diseases. In: Maggs DJ, Miller PE, Ofri R, editors. Slatter's fundamentals of veterinary ophthalmology. St. Louis, MO: Elsevier; 2013. p. 184–219.
20. Stiles J. Feline ophthalmology. In: Gelatt KN, Gilger BC, Kern TJ, editors. Veterinary ophthalmology. Ames, IA: Wiley/Blackwell; 2013. p. 1477–559.
21. Mitchell N. Feline ophthalmology Part 2: Clinical presentation and aetiology of common ocular conditions. Ir Vet J 2006;59(4):223.
22. Chandler EA, Gaskell RM, Gaskell CJ. Feline medicine and therapeutics. Ames, IA: John Wiley & Sons; 2008.

23. Hartmann K, Levy J. Feline infectious diseases: Self-assessment color review (veterinary self-assessment color review series). Boca Raton, FL: Taylor & Francis; 2011.

24. Reinstein S, editor. The squinting cat: herpes until proven otherwise. Michigan VMA. MI; 2017.

25. Millichamp NJ. Ocular diseases unique to the feline patient. DVM. 360 [Internet]; 2010. Available from: http://veterinarycalendar.dvm360.com/ocular-diseases-unique-feline-patient-proceedings.

26. Heinrich C. Assessing conjunctivitis in cats. Vet. Times [Internet]; 2015. Available from: https://www.vettimes.co.uk/app/uploads/wp-post-to-pdf-enhanced-cache/1/assessing-conjunctivitis-in-cats.pdf.

27. Millichamp NJ. Ocular diseases unique to the feline patient (Proceedings). DVM. 360 [Internet]; 2010. Available from: http://veterinarycalendar.dvm360.com/ocular-diseases-unique-feline-patient-proceedings.

28. Côté E. Clinical veterinary advisor. Dogs and cats. 3rd ed. St. Louis, MO: Elsevier Mosby; 2015.

29. Maggs DJ. Update on pathogenesis, diagnosis, and treatment of feline herpesvirus type 1. Clin Tech Small Anim Pract 2005;20(2):94–101.

30. Nasisse MP, Guy JS, Stevens JB, English RV, Davidson MG. Clinical and laboratory findings in chronic conjunctivitis in cats: 91 Cases (1983–1991). J Am Vet Med Assoc 1993;203(6):834–7.

31. Primm K. The essence of a reverse sneeze. DVM 360 [Internet]. Available from: http://www.dvm360.com/sites/default/files/images/pdfs-for-alfresco-articles/Reverse_sneeze_handout.pdf.

32. Holt DE, Goldschmidt MH. Nasal polyps in dogs: Five cases (2005 to 2011). J Small Anim Pract 2011;52(12):660–3.

33. Veronesi F, Morganti G, Di Cesare A, Schaper R, Traversa D. A pilot trial evaluating the efficacy of a 10% Imidacloprid/2.5% moxidectin spot-on formulation in the treatment of natural nasal capillariosis in dogs. Vet Parasitol 2014;200(1–2):133–8.

34. Adolph C. Treating nasal capillariasis in dogs. NAVC Clin's Brief 2014(October);38.

35. Adolph C. No sneezing matter: Capillaria boehmi. NAVC Clin's Brief 2015(February);50.

36. Sréter T, Széll Z, Marucci G, Pozio E, Varga I. Extraintestinal nematode infections of red foxes (Vulpes vulpes) in Hungary. Vet Parasitol 2003;115(4):329–34.

37. Schoning P, Dryden MW, Gabbert NH. Identification of a nasal nematode (Eucoleus boehmi) in greyhounds. Vet Res Commun 1993;17(4):277–81.

38. Baan M, Kidder AC, Johnson SE, Sherding RG. Rhinoscopic diagnosis of Eucoleus boehmi infection in a dog. J Am Anim Hosp Assoc 2011;47(1):60–3.

39. Campbell BG, Little MD. Identification of the eggs of a nematode (Eucoleus boehmi) from the nasal mucosa of North American dogs. J Am Vet Med Assoc 1991;198(9):1520–3.

40. Lanz OI, Wood BC. Surgery of the ear and pinna. Vet Clin North Am Small Anim Pract 2004;34(2):567–99.

41. Kennis RA. Feline otitis: Diagnosis and treatment. Vet Clin North Am Small Anim Pract 2013;43(1):51–6.

42. Quimby J, Lappin MR. The upper respiratory tract. In: Little SE, editor. The cat: Clinical medicine and management. St. Louis, MO: Saunders Elsevier; 2012. p. 846–61.

43. Henderson SM, Bradley K, Day MJ, Tasker S, Caney SM, Hotston Moore A, Gruffydd-Jones TJ. Investigation of nasal disease in the cat – a retrospective study of 77 cases. J Feline Med Surg 2004;6(4):245–57.

44. Schmidt JF, Kapatkin A. Nasopharyngeal and ear canal polyps in the cat. Feline Pract 1990;18(4):16–9.

45. Kapatkin AS, Matthiesen DT, Noone KE, Church EM. Scavelli TE, Patnaik AK. Results of surgery and long-term follow-up in 31 cats with nasopharyngeal polyps. J Am Anim Hosp Assoc 1990;26(4):387–92.

46. White RA. Middle ear. In: Slatter DH, editor. Textbook of small animal surgery. Philadelphia, PA: W.B. Saunders; 2003. p. 1760–7.

47. Trevor PB, Martin RA. Tympanic bulla osteotomy for treatment of middle-ear disease in cats: 19 Cases (1984–1991). J Am Vet Med Assoc 1993;202(1):123–8.

48. Pope ER. Feline respiratory tract polyps. In: Bonagura J, editor. Kirk's current veterinary therapy. XIII. Philadelphia, PA: W.B. Saunders; 2000. p. 794–6.

49. Faulkner JE, Budsberg SC. Results of ventral bulla osteotomy for treatment of middle-ear polyps in cats. J Am Anim Hosp Assoc 1990;26(5):496–9.

50. Baines SJ. Pharynx. In: Langley-Hobbs SJ, Demetriou J, Ladlow JF, editors. Feline soft tissue and general surgery. New York: Saunders/Elsevier; 2014.

51. Penderis J. Diagnosis of Horner's syndrome in dogs and cats. Pract 2015;37(3):107–19.

52. Ettinger SJ, Feldman EC, Côté E. Textbook of veterinary internal medicine: Diseases of the dog and the cat. 8th ed. St. Louis, MO: Elsevier; 2017.

Case 44

The Lame Cat

Twix is a regular at your practice. He is an indoor/outdoor cat that has resided with Tess Peterson since he stumbled across her property at approximately 1 year old. According to Tess, he has always been a bit of a scrapper. Although he has never picked a fight with Tess, she describes him as a territorial guard cat. He is constantly on the move, walking the lay of the land to be certain that no one else is considering horning in on his landscape.

In his 9 years of life, Twix has had more rabies vaccinations than Tess can count on her own two hands. He's scrapped with two foxes, a coyote, three ground hogs, a porcupine, a stray dog here and there, and a medley of feral cats. Thanks to him, Tess's property is not overrun by freeloaders. Even so, she's becoming weary of his growing list of battle scars. For a while there, every week it seemed to be something else.

Just when she'd been fortunate enough to have a 6-week reprieve from veterinary care, Twix came down with a new injury. He had stayed outside the night before. This was not unusual for him. Although Tess preferred that he stay inside, his midnight forays were more

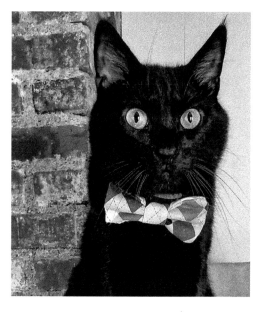

Figure 44.1 Meet Twix, a 9-year-old castrated male domestic shorthaired (DSH) cat. Courtesy of Tim Gregory.

acceptable than his marking the home with urine if she refused to allow him to come and go at will.

When Tess awoke this morning, she found Twix on the front porch. He looked somewhat disheveled and unkempt. For a cat that prided himself on good grooming, he had fallen short. When Tess opened the door, he did not sprint in as usual. Instead, he got up stiffly and awkwardly like an old man.

"Come on, slowpoke," Tess even joked, until she saw Twix's altered gait. He was observed toe-touching his right thoracic limb, but that was the extent to which he was willing to use the affected leg.

"Who beat you up this time?" she said, shaking her head. "Here we go again." Tess scooped him up and headed to the emergency clinic three blocks away.

She is here now with Twix. Review his vital signs as you consider your approach to this consultation.

Weight: 11.2 lb (5.1 kg)
BCS: 5/9
Mentation: QAR

TPR

T: 103.3°F (39.6°C)
P: 196 beats per minute
R: 32 breaths per minute

Round One of Questions for Case 44: The Lame Cat

1. Twix's chief complaint is lameness. Define lameness.
2. Assume that you have not yet heard the patient's history. What information do you need to elicit from Tess to better understand Twix's chief complaint? In other words, what do you need to know about his lameness?
3. Why is it challenging to perform a lameness exam on cats?
4. What can you do to encourage gait analysis in cats?
5. If you still cannot visualize the cat's gait after trying the tools that you outlined in Question #4 (above), what can you instruct the owner to do?
6. A thorough physical exam is an essential approach to any patient that presents for lameness. When you palpate the thoracic limb, what are you feeling for?
7. Twix has presented for right-sided thoracic limb lameness. Why is it essential for you to examine his left thoracic limb, too?
8. Identify broad causes of forelimb lameness in dogs and cats.
9. Which of the differential diagnoses in your answer to Question #8 (above) are LEAST likely given Twix's past pertinent case history, which was provided to you by way of the case vignette?
10. Which of the differential diagnoses in your answer to Question #8 (above) are MORE likely given Twix's past pertinent case history, which was provided to you by way of the case vignette?
11. Which of these differential diagnoses is most concerning from a zoonotic potential?
12. What is your diagnostic approach to forelimb lameness?

Answers to Round One of Questions for Case 44: The Lame Cat

1. Lameness refers to an abnormal gait.(1, 2)

2. To better understand Twix's lameness, it is important to ask the client the following questions. (1–5)

    - When did the lameness start?
    - What, if anything, may have triggered the lameness?
    - How, if at all, has the lameness progressed?
    - Is the patient's lameness a new finding or a recurrent one?
    - Which limb(s) appear(s) to be affected?
    - Does the lameness "jump" from one leg to another? In other words, is there shifting leg lameness?
    - Is the patient able to bear weight on the affected limb(s)?
    - Is the lameness persistent or does it wax and wane?
    - How does the lameness change after periods of inactivity?
    - How does the lameness change after periods of exercise or activity?
    - Is the lameness improved at faster gaits, i.e. when the patient runs versus walks?
    - Does the patient have a difficult time getting up or sitting down?
    - Does the patient have any draining tracts or wounds?
    - Has the patient injured the affected limb(s) before?
    - Has the patient had any form of surgical repair on the affected limb(s) in the past?

3. It is challenging to perform a lameness exam in most cats because few cats will actually be bold enough to walk around in an examination room when they are feeling healthy, let alone when they are lame.(1, 2) Cats often need to be coaxed into demonstrating their gait. (1, 2, 5, 6) In my clinical experience, they are more likely to freeze, hide, or hunch over than walk.

4. You can encourage the cat to move in an examination room by placing the patient at the opposite end of the room from its carrier or owner.(2) Doing so may motivate the cat to walk across the room.(2)

> Food-motivated cats may also be encouraged to walk if you offer a trail of treats.(2)
> Laser pointers may also entice a playful cat to move across the room.(2)

5. If you are unsuccessful at trying to coax the cat into walking in the exam room, you can ask the client to take a video of the cat in its home environment.(2) Many clients have a smart phone that allows them to videotape abnormal gaits and other behaviors that can be witnessed at home.(2, 7, 8)

6. When you palpate the thoracic limb, you are feeling for the following structures:(1–3, 9)

   - body and spine of both scapulae
   - the supraspinatus muscle dorsal to the spine of the scapula
   - the infraspinous muscle ventral to the spine of the scapula
   - the shoulder joint, formed by the articulation of the scapula and the proximal humerus
   - the greater tubercle of the proximal humerus, where the supraspinatus muscle inserts
   - body of humerus
   - the medial and lateral epicondyles at the distal humerus
   - the elbow joint, formed by the articulation between the humerus, radius, and ulna
   - the olecranon, which serves as a lever for the extensor muscles of the elbow
   - the radius, which is the primary weight-bearing agent of the antebrachium
   - the ulna
   - the radiocarpal joint, which consists of the articulation between the radius and carpus
   - the carpus, which consists of seven bones arranged in two rows
   - the metacarpal bones and phalanges:

     - the first metacarpal bone, located medially, bears only two phalanges(9)
     - the second through fifth metacarpal bones each bear three phalanges to form the second through fifth digits.

   Note that it is difficult to identify the individual bones of the carpus through palpation alone. (1, 2) Imaging at this location is often necessary to improve accuracy in formulating diagnostic assessments.(1, 2)

7. Even though Twix presented for right-sided thoracic limb lameness, it is still essential to examine his left thoracic limb, too. This is because the left side will provide an essential comparison. We need to examine both limbs for symmetry.(6, 7)

   - Symmetry between the forelimbs in terms of bone contour:

     - Is their continuity of bone or are fractures grossly or palpably apparent?

   - Symmetry between the forelimbs in terms of muscle mass:

     - Are muscles such as the supraspinatus, infraspinatus, triceps, antebrachial flexors and antebrachial extensors developed?
     - Has one side (or both!) atrophied?

   - Symmetry between the forelimbs in terms of joints:

     - Is there joint effusion?
     - Is there heat at each joint?

8. Broad causes of forelimb lameness in dogs and cats include:(1, 2, 10, 11)

- arthritis
- congenital or developmental defects (i.e. elbow dysplasia in young dogs):
    - fragmented medial coronoid process (fmcp)
    - ununited anconeal process (UAP)
- immune-mediated disease
- infectious disease
- neoplasia (i.e. osteosarcoma)
- neurologic disease (i.e. cervical spinal cord or nerve root)
- nutritional issue (i.e. secondary hyperparathyroidism or Vitamin D deficiency)
- traumatic injuries:(1, 2, 6, 10)
    - bite wounds and associated infections
    - chemical injury
    - fractures
    - gunshot wounds
    - luxations and subluxations
    - surgical interventions, such as onychectomy (i.e. declawing) in those parts of the united states where it is legal
    - tendon and ligament sprains, strains, and tears
    - thermal injury
    - vehicular trauma and other high-impact collisions.

9. Congenital and developmental defects are LEAST likely given Twix's age.

    Vehicular trauma can be ruled out because Twix does not have any open wounds or road rash, which he would be expected to if he had been hit by a car.

    Nutritional deficiencies that lead to metabolic disease can be ruled out if we take a diet history and discover that Twix consumes a commercial diet formulated for his life stage.

10. Traumatic injury, such as a bite wound abscess, is MOST likely given his history. However, the firmness of the swelling makes me concerned about the potential for primary bone disease.

11. Bite wounds are a potential means by which zoonotic disease spreads. Bite wounds involve saliva, which can transmit rabies virus to people. In any case where a bite wound is possible, any and all members of the veterinary team should don exam gloves.

12. My diagnostic approach to Twix's forelimb lameness is as follows.

    - I will try to motivate Twix to ambulate in the examination room so that I can assess his gait.
    - I will then perform a physical examination, keeping in mind that his right thoracic limb may be tender. To maximize his tolerance of the exam, I will likely examine his affected limb last. If I do so, it is important that I verbalize my reasoning aloud for the benefit of Tess so that she is aware I am intentionally saving the painful limb for last.
    - If I find swelling(s), then I might be inclined to shave the fur at the affected site(s) to look for puncture wounds.
    - I will also advise Tess that survey radiographs of the right forelimb are indicated to evaluate the structural integrity of the leg. At this point, I'm not sure where the problem is on the right thoracic limb because I have yet to complete my exam. Once my exam is finished, I may have a better understanding of where to concentrate the radiographic beam so as not to radiograph the entire leg.

Returning to Case 44: The Lame Cat

Twix refuses to walk in your presence and instead remains hunched over, as is typical of most feline patients when you need to perform a lameness exam. When you pick him up to put him on the exam room table, your right hand discerns a 3 × 3 cm firm, warm swelling over his proximal right brachium. The swelling is tender to the touch. You feel the vibration of his growl beneath your touch.

Although a bite wound remains high on your list of differentials, you are concerned about the texture and consistency of the swelling. It is hard and irregular. You advise Tess that orthogonal radiographs should be taken to rule out skeletal trauma, including but not limited to closed fractures. The lateral view has been provided in Figure 44.2 for you to evaluate.

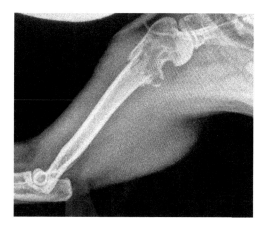

Figure 44.2 Radiograph of the patient's right brachium, lateral view. Courtesy of Allison Ward.

Round Two of Questions for Case 44: The Lame Cat

1. What specifically do you see on the radiograph that is abnormal?
2. What are your top differential diagnoses?
3. How likely is it that Twix just has a bite wound?

Answers to Round Two of Questions for Case 44: The Lame Cat

1. The radiograph demonstrates an aggressive, proliferative bone lesion that involves the proximal humerus. There is evidence of cortical lysis. There is also extensive soft tissue swelling adjacent to the primary bone lesion. The lesion does not appear to cross articular cartilage at the gleno-humeral joint.

2. My top two differential diagnoses are osteosarcoma and fungal osteomyelitis.(1, 2) Other primary bone tumors (i.e. chondrosarcoma, hemangiosarcoma, and fibrosarcoma) are possible, but much less common.(12)

3. It is unlikely that Twix just has a bite wound based upon the presence and extensiveness of the bone lesion.

Returning to Case 44: The Lame Cat

You review the radiographs with Tess and explain that Twix has an osteolytic lesion that is associated with the proximal humerus. You are concerned about primary bone cancer as well as fungal disease. You recommend that you perform a fine-needle aspirate (FNA) to narrow the diagnosis. Tess authorizes you to proceed.

Your cytological interpretation is that the mass contains bundles of spindle-shaped cells. Based upon the results of FNA, you prioritize the differential diagnosis of osteosarcoma.

Round Three of Questions for Case 44: The Lame Cat

1. What is osteosarcoma?
2. Which events may precipitate osteosarcoma, that is, make development of osteosarcoma more likely to occur?
3. Where on the skeleton can osteosarcoma develop?
4. Of those sites that you listed in Question #3 above, where does osteosarcoma prefer to target cats?
5. Of those sites that you listed in Question #3 above, where does osteosarcoma prefer to target dogs?
6. Where on the limbs does osteosarcoma prefer to target in cats and dogs?
7. Can osteosarcoma occur at extraskeletal sites in cats and dogs?
8. Where can osteosarcoma metastasize to?
9. What is the metastatic potential of osteosarcoma in dogs?
10. What is the metastatic potential of osteosarcoma in cats?
11. Outline treatment options for Twix.

Answers to Round Three of Questions for Case 44: The Lame Cat

1. Osteosarcoma is a primary bone tumor.[1, 2, 13–18]

2. Fractures have been associated with the development of osteosarcoma years after the traumatic event.[13, 19–23]

   One case report also appears in the veterinary medical literature that describes the development of osteosarcoma in a fragment of the first digit that was left behind in a declawed cat.[16] It is thought that skeletal trauma may have precipitated this event.

3. Osteosarcoma may target axial or appendicular skeletal structures.[1, 2, 24]

   - The axial skeleton consists largely of the cranium, the maxilla, mandible, ribcage, and the vertebral column.
   - The appendicular skeleton consists of the thoracic and pelvic girdles and their associated limbs.

4. In the cat, axial and appendicular osteosarcoma occur with equal frequency.[13, 25] When it occurs in the limbs of cats, osteosarcoma is more likely to occur in the pelvic limb than the forelimb.[15, 18, 26]

5. In the dog, appendicular osteosarcoma represents 75% of the clinical cases.[12]

   When it occurs in the limbs of dogs, osteosarcoma is more likely to occur in the forelimb than the pelvic limb.[12]

6. Osteosarcoma tends to originate near the knee or away from the elbow. This means that the following sites are more likely to be affected:[2, 13, 25, 27]

   - distal femur
   - distal radius
   - proximal humerus
   - proximal tibia.

7. Yes, osteosarcoma can occur at extraskeletal sites. Although rare in occurrence, osteosarcoma in cats may target injection sites.[28] In dogs, osteosarcoma has also been reported at the following extraskeletal sites:[12, 29–32]

- bowel
- liver
- mammary tissue
- spleen

- subcutaneous tissue
- testicle
- vagina.

8. Osteosarcoma metastasizes to the lungs.(12) Although dogs may not exhibit respiratory signs at the time that osteosarcoma is diagnosed, many already have evidence of metastatic pulmonary lesions on thoracic radiographs.(12)

9. Metastasis of osteosarcoma to the lungs in dogs is a frequent occurrence.(12–15, 28, 33)

10. Metastasis of osteosarcoma in cats is possible, but less likely, particularly if osteosarcoma is of appendicular origin.(14, 28)

11. Amputation of Twix's right forelimb offers a much better prognosis than if he had been diagnosed with axial osteosarcoma.(12) Axial osteosarcoma is much more difficult to resect, whereas spread of disease is easier to achieve through limb amputation, particularly since osteosarcoma does not tend to cross articular cartilage, thus sparing joints.(12)

    Depending upon which study is referenced, median survival for cats with appendicular osteosarcoma ranges from 24–44 months if amputation of the limb is the only intervention. (12, 14, 18) In some cases, limb amputation is curative, particularly if there is no evidence of metastatic lesions on thoracic radiographs.(12) This is in stark contrast to osteosarcoma of dogs, in whom limb amputation is strictly palliative.(12)

    If Tess consents to amputation, Twix should be evaluated for metastatic disease prior to surgery. Even though metastatic disease occurs with less frequency in the cat than in the dog, radiographs of the thoracic cavity are still indicated to equip Tess with the knowledge that she needs to make the best decision for Twix.

    Limb-sparing surgery or limb-shortening limb salvage (LSLS) are rarely performed in private practice, yet these are reasonable alternatives to amputation.(12, 15)

CLINICAL PEARLS

- Lameness refers to an abnormal gait.

- Patients may present with weight-bearing lameness or non-weight-bearing lameness. On occasion, patients may exhibit shifting leg lameness, which is beyond the scope of this case. Borreliosis is well known for clinical presentations involving shifting leg lameness.

- Clients need to be questioned thoroughly when they present a patient with the chief complaint of lameness. Clients need to be queried about which limb, when lameness first occurred, whether lameness has progressed, and how lameness is impacted both by activity as well as rest.

- A thorough physical examination is also essential to identify concurrent issues, such as bite wounds, that require cautious intervention because of the potential for transmission of zoonotic disease, such as rabies, through the saliva.

- There are both orthopedic and neurologic causes of lameness, so attention to detail on the physical exam is warranted to discern which type the patient most likely has.

- When examining a patient for lameness, I tend to evaluate the affected limb(s) LAST. This allows me to gain a sense of what is typical range of motion in the other limb(s), which provides a helpful comparison.

- If you do examine the affected limb(s) LAST, then client communication, specifically trans-parency, is critical. Explain why you are holding off on examining the painful limb(s) until the end of the visit. Tell the client that if you examine the painful limb(s) first, then the patient is unlikely to let you proceed with the rest of the exam, which is necessary to gain a complete clinical picture.

- Client videos augment exam findings. Patients are more likely to exhibit gait abnormalities in their home environment. It is rare to get cats to walk in the consult room.

- Radiographs are necessary to evaluate skeletal integrity and can also demonstrate the extent of soft tissue swelling. Aggressive bone lesions with cortical lysis are supportive of primary bone tumors, of which osteosarcoma is most common. Osteosarcoma can occur in cats as well as dogs.

- The feline prognosis for appendicular osteosarcoma is more favorable than in dogs.

References

1. Englar RE. Performing the small animal physical examination. Hoboken, NJ: Wiley/Blackwell; 2017.
2. Englar RE. Common clinical presentations in dogs and cats. Hoboken, NJ: Wiley; 2019.
3. Hazewinkel HAW, Meij BP, Theyse LFH, van Rijssen B. Locomotor system. In: Rijnberk A, van Sluijs FJ, editors. Medical history and physical examination in companion animals. St. Louis, MO: Saunders Elsevier; 2009.
4. Voss K, Steffen F. Patient assessment. In: Montavon PM, Voss K, Langley-Hobbs SJ, editors. Feline orthopedic surgery and musculoskeletal disease. St. Louis, MO: Saunders Elsevier; 2009.
5. Englar RE. Performing the small animal physical examination. Hoboken, NJ: Wiley/Blackwell; 2017.
6. Chandler JC, Beale BS. Feline orthopedics. Clin Tech Small Anim Pract 2002;17(4):190–203.
7. Kerwin S. Orthopedic examination in the cat: clinical tips for ruling in/out common musculoskeletal disease. J Feline Med Surg 2012;14(1):6–12.
8. Leonard CA, Tillson M. Feline lameness. Vet Clin North Am Small Anim Pract 2001;31(1):143–63.
9. Evans HE. The skeleton. In: Evans HE, Miller ME, editors. Miller's anatomy of the dog. 3rd ed. Philadelphia, PA: W. B. Saunders; 1993. p. 122–218.
10. Cook JL. Forelimb lameness in the young patient. Vet Clin North Am Small Anim Pract 2001;31(1):55–83.
11. Michelsen J. Canine elbow dysplasia: aetiopathogenesis and current treatment recommendations. Vet J 2013;196(1):12–9.
12. Dernell WS, Ehrhart NP, Straw RC, Vail DM. Tumors of the skeletal system. In: Withrow SJ, Vail DM, editors. Withrow and MacEwen's small animal clinical oncology. 4th ed. St. Louis, MO: Saunders Elsevier; 2007.
13. Baum JI, Skinner OT, Boston SE. Fracture-associated osteosarcoma of the femur in a cat. Can Vet J 2018;59(10):1096–8.
14. Bitetto WV, Patnaik AK, Schrader SC, Mooney SC. Osteosarcoma in cats: 22 cases (1974–1984). J Am Vet Med Assoc 1987;190(1):91–3.
15. Boylan MT, Boston SE, Townsend S, Cavalcanti JVJ. Limb-shortening limb salvage (LSLS) in a cat with meta-tarsal osteosarcoma. Can Vet J 2019;60(7):757–61.
16. Breitreiter K. Late-onset osteosarcoma after onychectomy in a cat. JFMS Open Rep 2019:5(1):2055116919842394.
17. Côté E. Clinical veterinary advisor. Dogs and cats. 3rd ed. St. Louis, MO: Elsevier Mosby; 2015.
18. Turrel JM, Pool RR. Primary bone tumors in the cat: A retrospective study of 15 cats and a literature review. Vet Rad 1982;23(4):152–66.
19. Stevenson S. Fracture-associated sarcomas. Vet Clin North Am Small Anim Pract 1991;21(4):859–72.

20. Sinibaldi KR, Pugh J, Rosen H, Liu SK. Osteomyelitis and neoplasia associated with use of the Jonas intramedullary splint in small animals. J Am Vet Med Assoc 1982;181(9):885–90.
21. Sonnenschein B, Dickomeit MJ, Bali MS. Late-onset fracture-associated osteosarcoma in a cat. Vet Comp Orthop Traumatol 2012;25(5):418–20.
22. Bennett D, Campbell JR, Brown P. Osteosarcoma associated with healed fractures. J Small Anim Pract 1979;20(1):13–8.
23. Fry PD, Jukes HF. Fracture associated sarcoma in the cat. J Small Anim Pract 1995;36(3):124–6.
24. Thrall DE. Textbook of veterinary diagnostic radiology. 7th ed. St. Louis, MO: Elsevier; 2018.
25. Boston S. Musculoskeletal neoplasia and limb-sparing surgery. In: Tobias KM, Johnston SA, editors. Veterinary surgery: small animal. St. Louis, MO: Elsevier Saunders; 2012. p. 1159–77.
26. Liu SK, Dorfman HD, Patnaik AK. Primary and secondary bone tumours in the cat. J Small Anim Pract 1974;15(3):141–56.
27. Schulz KS. Forelimb lameness in the adult patient. Vet Clin North Am Small Anim Pract 2001;31(1):85–99, vi.
28. Heldmann E, Anderson MA, Wagner-Mann C. Feline osteosarcoma: 145 cases (1990–1995). J Am Anim Hosp Assoc 2000;36(6):518–21.
29. Kuntz CA, Dernell WS, Powers BE, Withrow S. Extraskeletal osteosarcomas in dogs: 14 cases. J Am Anim Hosp Assoc 1998;34(1):26–30.
30. Langenbach A, Anderson MA, Dambach DM, Sorenmo KU, Shofer FD. Extraskeletal osteosarcomas in dogs: a retrospective study of 169 cases (1986–1996). J Am Anim Hosp Assoc 1998;34(2):113–20.
31. Patnaik AK. Canine extraskeletal osteosarcoma and chondrosarcoma: a clinicopathologic study of 14 cases. Vet Pathol 1990;27(1):46–55.
32. Patnaik AK, Liu S, Johnson GF. Extraskeletal osteosarcoma of the liver in a dog. J Small Anim Pract 1976;17(6):365–70.
33. Garzotto C, berg J. Oncology. In: Slatter D, editor. Textbook of small animal surgery. Philadelphia, PA: Saunders; 2003. p. 2460–74.

Case 45

The Lame Dog

It's the end of a long holiday weekend. Your practice is closed, but you've been the only doctor on call for the past 3 days. The last 72 hours have been a revolving door of legitimate problems mixed with "emergencies." The "emergency" kennel cough vaccine and the "emergency" flea infestation were your personal favorites. Only the cesarean section truly couldn't wait. You're literally just getting into your car in the front parking lot, dreaming about the nice long interrupted nap that you are going to take, when you hear a dreaded sound – a car skidding – followed by honking and a scream. You pop out of your car just in time to see commotion about a block or so away. Just as you're trying to make sense of the situation in your fog of sleep-deprivation, you see a figure race toward you, with a fuzzy gray body in his arms.

"Please help!"

You recognize the man, Jim Munson, your mechanic, right away. You didn't realize he lived around here, but that makes sense. He's always walked Teddy to the clinic whenever he's had an appointment.

You scoop Teddy's limp body out of Jim's arms to triage the patient. You breathe a sigh of relief when you see the dog blink back at you and start to whine. You see his chest rise, then fall, rise, then fall – and it occurs to you just how lucky this dog is to be alive.

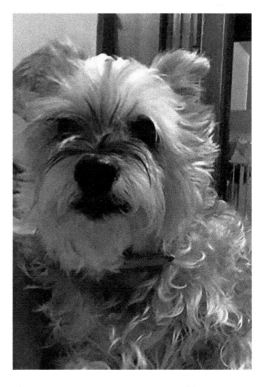

Figure 45.1 Meet your patient Teddy, a 6-year-old male intact Schnauzer cross. Courtesy of Maki RCHS.

As you continue to look Teddy over, Jim emerges from his shell-shocked state to describe what happened. It turns out that he and his son had been playing ball with Teddy in the front yard. It was Sunday just before dusk and traffic was light. In all the years that Jim owned Teddy, the dog had never once run into the street. It never occurred to Jim that Teddy would prove him wrong.

Jim's son, Jacob, was 16 years young and had been practicing his curveballs. He was the pitcher for a youth league in town and was always trying to perfect his art. He was throwing just fine until that last pitch. Something distracted him from his game and when he released the ball, it ended up rolling into the street. As Teddy went racing after it, deaf to the shouts all around him ("No, Teddy! No!"), a car came speeding toward their home. Jim saw the scene unfold before his eyes, knowing there was nothing he could do. The car was easily going 50 in a 25 mph zone. Thankfully the driver caught a glimpse of Teddy from the corner of his eye and slammed on his brakes. The car skidded and there was a sickening thud before everything went quiet. Teddy had been hit. The wind was knocked out of him and for a moment he couldn't breathe. The next thing Teddy remembered was coming to in your arms in the treatment area of the clinic. He tried to get away from the oxygen mask that was plastered to his face, but he couldn't seem to get his bearings and plant his right pelvic limb solidly beneath him. No matter how hard he tried to right himself, the leg wouldn't support his weight. It also hurt worse than anything he'd ever experienced.

As Teddy comes to, you assess and document an abbreviated set of vital signs.

Work through the following questions to prepare you for Teddy's care.

Mentation: Disoriented

TPR

T: 101.2°F (38.4°C)
P: 156 beats per minute
R: Panting

Round One of Questions for Case 45: The Lame Dog

1. Which skeletal components of the hind limb should be assessed during an orthopedic examination?
2. The hind limbs are paired structures of the appendicular skeleton that attach to the pelvic girdle. What is the pelvic girdle?
3. Which aspects of the pelvic girdle should be palpable on physical exam in a normal healthy dog?
4. Through which joint does each hind limb attach to the pelvic girdle?
5. What type of joint is the one that you identified in Question #4 (above)?
6. Specifically, which structures make up the joint that you named in Question #4 (above)?
7. To which skeletal landmarks does the joint capsule attach to when considering the joint that you named in Question #4 (above)?
8. Which muscles facilitate hip extension, abduction, and medial rotation of the pelvic limb and where do they attach?
9. Which muscles facilitate lateral rotation of the hip and where do they attach?
10. Which muscle is the primary hip flexor and where does it attach?
11. Which clinical presentations most likely result from vehicular trauma to the pelvic girdle and the surrounding structures?
12. Walk me through how you can diagnose the problem(s) that you identified in Question #11 (above).
13. Could the problem(s) that you identified in Question #11 (above) explain Teddy's apparent inability to bear weight on his right pelvic limb?

Answers to Round One of Questions for Case 45: The Lame Dog

1. The skeletal components of the hind limb that should be evaluated on every orthopedic examination include the femur, tibia, fibular, tarsus ("ankle"), metatarsus, and the phalanges.(1–5)

2. The ilium, ischium, pubis, and acetabulum comprise the pelvic girdle.(1–6)

3. The wings of both ilia and the ischiatic tuberosities should be palpable on physical exam in a normal healthy dog.(1–7) (See Figures 45.2 and 45.3.)

4. The coxofemoral joint bridges the hind limb and the pelvic girdle.(1–7)

5. The coxofemoral joint is a ball and socket joint.(1–7)

6. The coxofemoral joint consists of the femoral head and the acetabulum.(1–7) The articulating surface of the femoral head is lined by hyaline cartilage.(6) An exception is at the fovea capitis,

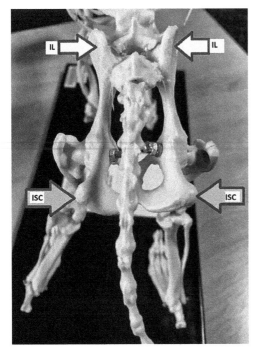

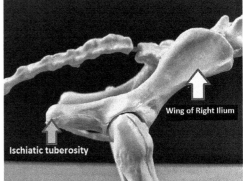

Figure 45.2 End-on-view of pelvis in a model of a canine skeleton. Note the location of the wings of the ilia, which have been labeled "IL," and the ischiatic tuberosities, which have been labeled "ISC."

Figure 45.3 Lateral view of pelvis in a model of a canine skeleton. The wing of the right ilium and the right ischiatic tuberosity have been labeled.

a depression along the medial aspect of the proximal epiphysis.(6) This site is where the ligament of the head of the femur attaches to anchor the femur to the ventral acetabulum.(6)

7. The joint capsule attaches to the circumference of the femoral neck, which is immediately distal to the femoral head, and also to the rim of the acetabulum.(1–7)

8. The middle gluteal, deep gluteal, and piriformis muscles initiate hip extension, abduction, and medial rotation of the pelvic limb.(1, 2, 6, 8, 9) These muscles attach to the greater trochanter of the femur.(1, 2, 6, 8, 9)

9. The internal and external obturator and gemelli muscles facilitate lateral rotation of the hip.(1, 2, 6, 8, 9) These attach to the trochanteric fossa, a depression in the femur that is located medial to the greater trochanter.(1, 2, 6, 8, 9)

10. The iliopsoas is the primary flexor of the hip.(1, 2, 6, 8, 9) It attaches to the lesser trochanter of the femur, which is located distal and caudomedial to the femoral neck.(1, 2, 6, 8, 9)

11. Vehicular trauma to the pelvic girdle and the surrounding structures routinely results in one or more of the following clinical presentations:(3, 6, 10–12)

    • coxofemoral luxations – 90% of these in dogs occur in a craniodorsal direction(13, 14)
    • pelvic fracture(s) and associated nerve damage, for example, sacral fracture-associated

nerve damage may cause hind limb dysfunction, urinary retention, urinary or fecal incontinence (10, 15, 16)

- uroabdomen (17–22)

12. Veterinarians can diagnose coxofemoral luxations on physical exam.(3, 6) In a normal dog, the left wing of the ilium, the left ischiatic tuberosity, and the left greater trochanter should form a triangle.(3) This triangle should mirror that which is formed by the right wing of the ilium, the right ischiatic tuberosity, and the right greater trochanter.(3) (See **Plate 49**.)

When a craniodorsal coxofemoral luxation is sustained by the patient, the greater trochanter of the affected limb migrates craniodorsally, thereby disrupting this triangle. This can be appreciated on palpation, and confirmed via radiographic examination(7, 23) (see Figure 45.4).

Another way to evaluate the patient for craniodorsal coxofemoral luxation is to support the patient in a standing position. (3) Curl your hands around the outer aspect of both upper thighs.(3) Gently lift both hind limbs up and extend them caudally. (3) Leg length is compared by assessing the location of the right and left calcanei.(3) In cases involving cranio-dorsal coxofemoral luxation, the affected side will appear to have the shorter leg because the femur has migrated craniodorsally rather than staying seated in the acetabulum.(3, 7)

Yet another approach to evaluating patients with presumptive craniodorsal coxofemoral luxations is to place your thumb caudal to the greater trochanter while externally rotating the femur.(24) In a dog with this condition, you will not feel as though your thumb is being compressed or displaced.(24)

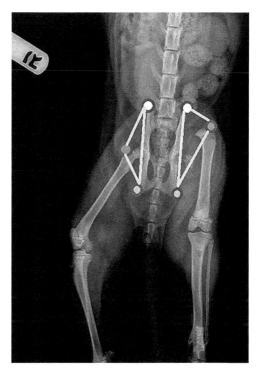

Figure 45.4 Note how the imaginary triangle that is formed by the left wing of the ilium (identified by top most circle), the left ischiatic tuberosity (identified by the middle), and the left greater trochanter (identified by bottom most circle) is shifted in a craniodorsal direction due to coxofemoral luxation of the left femur.

Pelvic fractures can be diagnosed radiographically.(3, 6, 23)

Uroabdomen can be diagnosed by positive-contrast cystourethrography.(25) Uroabdomen can also be diagnosed by tapping the abdomen through abdominocentesis to obtain a sample of fluid.(25) If the creatinine level in this sample of fluid is two to four times greater than serum levels, then the patient is said to have a uroabdomen.(25)

13. Both pelvic fracture(s) and coxofemoral luxation could explain Teddy's apparent inability to bear weight on the right pelvic limb.

Returning to Case 45: The Lame Dog

After administering analgesia to address Teddy's pain, you brief Jim about your clinical findings. Teddy is fortunate to be alive, with minimal external wounds other than road rash. However, you share that you are particularly concerned about the impact the vehicle may have had on Teddy's right hip and supporting structures. You recommend survey radiographs of the pelvis and proximal femur to evaluate skeletal stability in the hind end. Jim consents to the imaging study. Both views have been provided for you in Figures 45.5 and 45.6 to review.

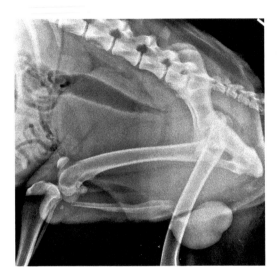 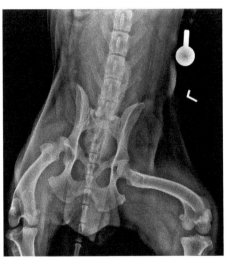

Figure 45.5 Lateral radiograph of canine pelvis. Courtesy of Michael Jaffe, DVM, MS, CCRP, and Diplomate, American College of Veterinary Surgeons.

Figure 45.6 Ventrodorsal radiograph of canine pelvis. Courtesy of Michael Jaffe, DVM, MS, CCRP, and Diplomate, American College of Veterinary Surgeons.

Round Two of Questions for Case 45: The Lame Dog

1. What is your diagnosis?
2. For this condition to occur, what must have happened to Teddy as a result of vehicular trauma?
3. Prior to radiographic confirmation, you were fairly certain of this diagnosis. Why was it still important that you image Teddy's pelvis?
4. Which is the most important aspect of your treatment plan?
5. Which additional diagnostic tests should you perform, based upon your answer to Question #4 (above)?

Answers to Round Two of Questions for Case 45: The Lame Dog

1. Teddy's diagnosis is right craniodorsal coxofemoral luxation.

2. In order for a coxofemoral luxation to occur, there must have been a tear in the joint capsule and a ruptured ligament of the head of the femur.(24)

3. Even if you suspect craniodorsal coxofemoral luxation, it is essential that you radiograph your patient's pelvis because you need to assess it for any of the following changes:(24)

- femoral fractures, particularly fractures of the:

  - femoral head
  - femoral neck
  - greater trochanter

- pelvic fractures, especially those involving the acetabulum
- presence of concurrent hip disease, such as avascular necrosis of the femoral head or hip dysplasia
- presence of osteoarthritis.

Closed reduction is contraindicated in the presence of any of the aforementioned changes.(24)

4. The most important aspect of your treatment plan is to stabilize Teddy.(24) Teddy has just sustained major trauma. He may have life-threatening injuries that are more critical than his pelvic limb.

5. If you haven't already done so, it is critical that you perform survey radiographs of the chest to evaluate Teddy for potential thoracic trauma.(24) In particular, you should assess Teddy's films for the following abnormalities:(24)

- diaphragmatic hernia
- pneumothorax
- pulmonary contusions
- rib fracture(s).

Returning to Case 45: The Lame Dog

Teddy's thoracic radiographs are unremarkable. Although you recognize that pulmonary contusions can worsen over the 24 hours that follow a traumatic event, you believe that Teddy is stable enough to undergo reduction.

Round Three of Questions for Case 45: The Lame Dog

1. Which options of reduction are available to Teddy?
2. Which option will you try first?
3. What does this option involve?
4. What is the success rate of the technique that you selected for Question #2 (above)?
5. What is the most common complication of the technique that you described in Question #2 (above)?
6. How do you propose to lessen the chance of this complication?
7. What is the patient's prognosis following your method of reduction?
8. Let's rewind this case for a moment. If Teddy had not had a history of vehicular trauma and simply had presented for evaluation of hind limb lameness, which broad categories for differential diagnoses would you have considered?

Answers to Round Three of Questions for Case 45: The Lame Dog

1. Closed and open reduction methods are both appropriate ways of managing coxofemoral luxation.(24)

2. Because Teddy does not have any apparent fractures of the femoral head, acetabulum, or femur and because the luxation just occurred, I will start with closed reduction.(24)

3. Closed reduction involves manually replacing the femoral head within the coxofemoral joint with the patient under heavy sedation or anesthesia.(24) Because Teddy's right pelvic limb is affected, he would be placed in left lateral recumbency.(24) Using a towel under the right pelvic limb, I would distract the affected limb and lift it away from the body.(24) At that point, you internally rotate the affected limb to guide the femoral head into the acetabulum.(24)

4. The success rate of closed reduction approximates 50:50.(24)

5. The most common complication of closed reduction is that coxofemoral luxation recurs.(24)

6. Following reduction, the patient should be placed in an Ehmer sling for one to two weeks to reduce the chance of recurrence.(24)

7. If after three weeks following closed reduction the hip remains in place, then the prognosis for return to function is good.(24) Lameness in the affected limb may be present due to traumatic injury of soft tissue and cartilage; however, it is typically mild when it occurs.(24)

8. Had Teddy not had a history of vehicular trauma, then I would have considered the following broad categories of differential diagnoses:

    - developmental issues, such as hip dysplasia(26–28)
    - degenerative disease, such as osteoarthritis(29)
    - immune-mediated(30–32)
    - infectious:

        - bacterial:

            - Lyme disease(33, 34)
            - rickettsial diseases(35, 36)

        - fungal:

            - coccidioidomycosis, the causative agent of valley fever(37, 38)

    - nutritional issues, including nutritional secondary hyperparathyroidism(39–44)
    - patellar luxation(3, 6)
    - primary neoplastic disease, such as osteosarcoma(45, 46) or digital squamous cell carcinoma (SCC)(47)
    - metastatic disease, as from canine prostatic adenocarcinoma(48)
    - plantar surface discomfort, as from digital paw pad laceration,(49) interdigital cysts(50) or interdigital dermatitis
    - sprain/strain of affected limb
    - other.

CLINICAL PEARLS

- Vehicular trauma to the hind end often results in pelvic fracture(s) and/or coxofemoral luxations.

- The pelvis is a box. If one side of the box fractures, then it is likely that the patient will sustain an additional fracture at another site of the box.

- Ilial fractures are commonly reported.

- Acetabular fractures carry a guarded prognosis because the acetabulum contributes to and stabilizes the coxofemoral joint.

- The coxofemoral joint can also be de-stabilized through coxofemoral luxation.

- When coxofemoral luxations occur, they are typically craniodorsal in orientation.

- The affected leg may appear shorter than the contralateral limb.

- The affected foot may also appear to be externally rotated.

- Craniodorsal coxofemoral luxations can be diagnosed on physical exam; however, radiographic confirmation is essential.

- Radiographs of the pelvis facilitate forward planning in terms of whether the patient is a candidate for closed reduction.

- Closed reduction is manually replacing the femoral head within the acetabulum with the patient under heavy sedation or anesthesia.

- Closed reduction is contraindicated if the patient has sustained pelvic or femoral fractures, and/or has any other form of hip instability.

- Closed reduction requires exercise restriction in the short-term and an Ehmer sling.

- Recurrence of coxofemoral luxation is possible.

References

1. Evans HE. The skeleton. In: Evans HE, Miller ME, editors. Miller's anatomy of the dog. 3rd ed. Philadelphia, PA: W. B. Saunders; 1993. p. 122–218.
2. Gilbert SG. Pictorial anatomy of the cat. Seattle, WA: University of Washington Press; 1989.
3. Englar RE. Performing the small animal physical examination. Hoboken, NJ: Wiley/Blackwell; 2017.
4. Evans HE, Miller ME. Miller's anatomy of the dog. 4th ed. St. Louis, MO: Elsevier; 2013.
5. Singh B, Dyce KM. Dyce, Sack, and Wensing's textbook of veterinary anatomy. 5th ed. St. Louis, MO: Saunders; 2018.
6. Englar RE. Common clinical presentations in dogs and cats. Hoboken, NJ: Wiley/Blackwell; 2019.
7. Hazewinkel HAW, Meij BP, Theyse LFH, van Rijssen B. Locomotor system. In: Rijnberk A, van Sluijs FJ, editors. Medical history and physical examination in companion animals. St. Louis, MO: Saunders Elsevier; 2009.
8. Sebastiani AM, Fishbeck DW. Mammalian anatomy: the cat. Englewood, CO: Morton Publishing; 1998.
9. Guiot LP, Demianiuk RM, Dejardin LM. Fractures of the femur. In: Tobias KM, Johnston SA, editors. Veterinary surgery small Animal One. St. Louis, MO: Saunders Elsevier; 2012. p. 865–905.
10. Stieger-Vanegas SM, Senthirajah SK, Nemanic S, Baltzer W, Warnock J, Bobe G. Evaluation of the diagnostic accuracy of four-view radiography and conventional computed tomography analysing sacral and pelvic fractures in dogs. Veterinary and Comparative Orthopaedics and Traumatology 2015;28(3):155–63.

11. Harasen G. Pelvic fractures. The Canadian Veterinary Journal = la Revue Veterinaire Canadienne 2007;48(4):427–8.
12. Draffan D, Clements D, Farrell M, Heller J, Bennett D, Carmichael S. The role of computed tomography in the classification and management of pelvic fractures. Veterinary and Comparative Orthopaedics and Traumatology 2009;22(3):190–7.
13. Fry PD. Observations on the surgical treatment of hip dislocation in the dog and cat. J Small Anim Pract 1974;15(11):661–70.
14. Christopher SA, Punke JP, Cowan W, Cook JL. What is your diagnosis? Craniodorsal luxation. J Am Vet Med Assoc 2011;239(3):301–2.
15. Lee K, Heng HG, Jeong J, Naughton JF, Rohleder JJ. Feasibility of computed tomography in awake dogs with traumatic pelvic fracture. Veterinary Radiology and Ultrasound: the Official Journal of the American College of Veterinary Radiology and the International Veterinary Radiology Association 2012;53(4):412–6.
16. Anderson A, Coughlan AR. Sacral fractures in dogs and cats: a classification scheme and review of 51 cases. J Small Anim Pract 1997;38(9):404–9.
17. Hoffberg JE, Koenigshof AM, Guiot LP. Retrospective evaluation of concurrent intra-abdominal injuries in dogs with traumatic pelvic fractures: 83 cases (2008–2013). J Vet Emerg Crit Care 2016;26(2):288–94.
18. Boysen SR, Rozanski EA, Tidwell AS, Holm JL, Shaw SP, Rush JE. Evaluation of a focused assessment with sonography for trauma protocol to detect free abdominal fluid in dogs involved in motor vehicle accidents. J Am Vet Med Assoc 2004;225(8):1198–204.
19. Simpson SA, Syring R, Otto CM. Severe blunt trauma in dogs: 235 cases (1997–2003). J Vet Emerg Crit Care (San Antonio). 2009;19(6):588–602.
20. Streeter EM, Rozanski EA, Laforcade-Buress Ad, Freeman LM, Rush JE. Evaluation of vehicular trauma in dogs: 239 cases (January–December 2001). J Am Vet Med Assoc 2009;235(4):405–8.
21. Stafford JR, Bartges JW. A clinical review of pathophysiology, diagnosis, and treatment of uroabdomen in the dog and cat. J Vet Emerg Crit Care (San Antonio). 2013;23(2):216–29.
22. Kolata RJ, Johnston DE. Motor vehicle accidents in urban dogs: a study of 600 cases. J Am Vet Med Assoc 1975;167(10):938–41.
23. Thrall DE. Textbook of veterinary diagnostic radiology. 7th ed. St. Louis, MO: Elsevier; 2018.
24. Bergh MS. Managing traumatic hip luxations. VetFolio [Internet]; 2019. Available from: https://www.vetfolio.com/learn/article/managing-traumatic-hip-luxations.
25. Gannon KM, Moses L. Uroabdomen in dogs and cats. Compend Vet Contin Educ Pract Vet. 2002;24:604–12.
26. Ginja MM, Silvestre AM, Gonzalo-Orden JM, Ferreira AJ. Diagnosis, genetic control and preventive management of canine hip dysplasia: a review. Veterinary Journal 2010;184(3):269–76.
27. Wilson B, Nicholas FW, Thomson PC. Selection against canine hip dysplasia: success or failure? Veterinary Journal 2011;189(2):160–8.
28. Woolliams JA, Lewis TW, Blott SC. Canine hip and elbow dysplasia in UK Labrador retrievers. Veterinary Journal.2011;189(2):169–76.
29. Kunst CM, Pease AP, Nelson NC, Habing G, Ballegeer EA. Computed tomographic identification of dysplasia and progression of osteoarthritis in dog elbows previously assigned ofa Grades 0 and 1. Vet Radiol Ultrasoun 2014;55(5):511–20.
30. Foster JD, Sample S, Kohler R, Watson K, Muir P, Trepanier LA. Serum biomarkers of clinical and cytologic response in dogs with idiopathic immune-mediated polyarthropathy. J Vet Intern Med 2014;28(3):905–11.
31. Johnson KC, Mackin A. Canine immune-mediated polyarthritis: Part 1: pathophysiology. J Am Anim Hosp Assoc 2012;48(1):12–7.
32. Johnson KC, Mackin A. Canine immune-mediated polyarthritis: Part 2: diagnosis and treatment. J Am Anim Hosp Assoc 2012;48(2):71–82.
33. Chomel B. Lyme disease. Revue scientifique et technique 2015;34(2):569–76.
34. Krupka I, Straubinger RK. Lyme borreliosis in dogs and cats: background, diagnosis, treatment and prevention of infections with Borrelia burgdorferi sensu stricto. Vet Clin N Am Small 2010;40(6):1103–19+.
35. Solano-Gallego L, Caprì A, Pennisi MG, Caldin M, Furlanello T, Trotta M. Acute febrile illness is associated with Rickettsia spp infection in dogs. Parasite Vector 2015;8:216.

36. Mazepa AW, Kidd LB, Young KM, Trepanier LA. Clinical presentation of 26 Anaplasma phagocytophilum-seropositive dogs residing in an endemic area. J Am Anim Hosp Assoc 2010;46(6):405–12.

37. Graupmann-Kuzma A, Valentine BA, Shubitz LF, Dial SM, Watrous B, Tornquist SJ. Coccidioidomycosis in dogs and cats: a review. J Am Anim Hosp Assoc 2008;44(5):226–35.

38. Johnson LR, Herrgesell EJ, Davidson AP, Pappagianis D. Clinical, clinicopathologic, and radiographic findings in dogs with coccidioidomycosis: 24 cases (1995–2000). J Am Anim Hosp Assoc 2003;222(4):461–6.

39. Stogdale L. Foreleg lameness in rapidly growing-dogs. J S Afr Vet Assoc 1979;50(3):193–200.

40. Bennett D. Nutrition and bone disease in the dog and cat. The Veterinary Record 1976;98(16):313–21.

41. Krook L, Whalen JP. Nutritional secondary hyperparathyroidism in the animal kingdom: report of two cases. Clinical Imaging 2010;34(6):458–61.

42. de Fornel-Thibaud P, Blanchard G, Escoffier-Chateau L, Segond S, Guetta F, Begon D, et al. Unusual case of osteopenia associated with nutritional calcium and vitamin D deficiency in an adult dog. J Am Anim Hosp Assoc 2007;43(1):52–60.

43. Taylor MB, Geiger DA, Saker KE, Larson MM. Diffuse osteopenia and myelopathy in a puppy fed a diet composed of an organic premix and raw ground beef. Journal of the American Veterinary Medical Association 2009;234(8):1041–8.

44. Lourens DC. [Nutritional or secondary hyperparathyroidism in a German Shepherd litter]. J S Afr Vet Assoc 1980;51(2):121–3.

45. Sivacolundhu RK, Runge JJ, Donovan TA, Barber LG, Saba CE, Clifford CA, et al. Ulnar osteosarcoma in dogs: 30 cases. Javma – J Am Vet Med A 2013;243(1):96–101.

46. Gasch EG, Rivier P, Bardet JF. Free proximal cortical ulnar autograft for the treatment of distal radial osteosarcoma in a dog. Canadian Veterinary Journal = la Revue Veterinaire Canadienne 2013;54(2):162–6.

47. Henry CJ, Brewer WG, Whitley EM, Tyler JW, Ogilvie GK, Norris A, et al. Canine digital tumors: A veterinary cooperative oncology group retrospective study of 64 dogs. J Vet Intern Med 2005;19(5):720–4.

48. Shafiee R, Shariat A, Khalili S, Malayeri HZ, Mokarizadeh A, Anissian A, et al. Diagnostic investigations of canine prostatitis incidence together with benign prostate hyperplasia, prostate malignancies, and biochemical recurrence in high-risk prostate cancer as a model for human study. Tumor Biol 2015;36(4):2437–45.

49. Duffy AL, Hackett TB. Canine pedal injury resulting from metal landscape edging. J Vet Emerg Crit Car 2010;20(5):533–6.

50. Duclos DD, Hargis AM, Hanley PW. Pathogenesis of canine interdigital palmar and plantar comedones and follicular cysts, and their response to laser surgery. Vet Dermatol 2008;19(3):134–41.

Case 46

The Recumbent Dog

Freckles is new to your practice. She is presenting to the emergency service for acutely collapsing in her hind end on a Sunday afternoon after a midday romp through a field. Freckles is a well-conditioned athlete and agility champion. She literally just won a championship two weekends ago and her favorite pastime is catching frisbees in mid-air. Her owner, Paula Priskett, can't believe that after all the cumulative torque on her spine over the course of the past six years, it's a mere run that has stopped her mid-stride. She is looking to you and your team for guidance.

Your triage team takes Freckles' vital signs and reports these immediately to you.

Work through the following questions to guide your thought process as you approach this clinical case.

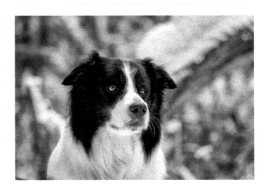

Figure 46.1 Meet your patient, Freckles, a 6-year-old female spayed Border Collie. Courtesy of Pamela Mueller, DVM.

Weight: 34.6 lb (15.7 kg)
BCS: 4/9
Mentation: QAR

TPR

T: 100.9°F (38.3°C)
P: 112 beats per minute
R: Panting

Round One of Questions for Case 46: The Recumbent Dog

1. When you hear that your patient is acutely down in the hind end, which body systems might be involved?
2. Which clarifying questions might you wish to ask the client to expand upon the patient's history?
3. Which of those same clarifying questions might you wish to ask the technician who loaded the patient into the examination room?
4. In addition to those that you outlined in Question #3 (above), what else might you want to ask the technician who loaded the patient into the examination room?
5. Based upon the abbreviated clinical history, you know that you want to examine this patient's nervous system. What are the two components of the mammalian nervous system?
6. Neurons are the messengers of the nervous system. Which neurons in particular are responsible for making connections between the nervous system and effector organs?
7. What are the two sub-types of the neurons that you identified in Question #6 (above)?
8. Neuromuscular dysfunction can occur at any point along the pathway. Explain what you would expect to see if either sub-type of neurons that you named in Question #7 (above) became dysfunctional?
9. Many clinical presentations of neuromuscular disease look alike. Which groups of spinal cord segments or nerves are beneficial to lump together to help you localize neuromuscular disease?

10. Explain what you might expect to see in your patient if each group of spinal cord segments or nerves that you identified in Question #9 (above) became dysfunctional?
11. Outline the broad components of the neurological exam that you will perform on Freckles.

Answers to Round One of Questions for Case 46: The Recumbent Dog

1. When a patient presents that is acutely down in the hind end, I am concerned about the following organ systems.(1, 2)

   - Cardiovascular system – i.e. has a thrombus occluded the vasculature, as in cases of aortic thromboembolism?
   - Musculoskeletal system – i.e. has the skeletal stability of the pelvis been compromised, preventing the limbs from being load-bearing structures?
   - Nervous system – i.e. has the spinal cord been compressed in such a way as to impede message signaling downstream of the injury?

2. I might wish to ask the client one or more of the following clarifying questions.(3)

   - Does the patient's mentation appear normal?
   - Did the patient vocalize at any point – before, during, or after the episode?
   - This episode appears to have occurred out of the blue. Looking back in time, has the patient ever before experienced something like this?
   - Can the patient stand or support her weight at all?
   - Is the patient able to move her pelvic limbs? In other words, do they appear to be paralyzed or do they just seem weak?
   - Are both hind limbs involved or does there appear to be unilateral involvement?
   - Is/are the affected limb(s) flaccid or rigid?
   - Does there appear to be any front limb involvement?
   - The client rushed the patient here, so not much time has passed between the episode and the patient's arrival at the clinic. Even so, has the owner noticed any progression in terms of the patient's status?
   - How has the patient's general health been here of late? Are there any signs of systemic illness that the client has noticed? (I.e. changes in appetite, vomiting/diarrhea, coughing/sneezing, changes in activity level, changes in attitude?)
   - Is the client familiar with the patient's lineage?
   - Does the patient have a familial history of back disease?
   - Has the client medicated the patient with anything between the incident occurring and their arrival at the clinic?
   - What, if any, medical issues or concerns has the patient had in the past?
   - What, if any, ongoing medical issues or concerns does the patient currently have?
   - What, if any, medication is the patient currently receiving, including prescription medications and those that are over-the-counter. These are especially important from the standpoint of drug interactions, i.e. if the patient is receiving non-steroidal anti-inflammatory medications, then you will not want to administer steroids or another non-steroidal anti-inflammatory drug without a proper washout period.

3. I might want to ask the technician some of the same questions that I outlined in Question #2 (above) to gain his/her medical insight as to the following.

   - Can the patient stand or support her weight at all?
   - Is the patient able to move her pelvic limbs? In other words, do they appear to be paralyzed or do they just seem weak?

- Are both hind limbs involved or does there appear to be unilateral involvement?
- Is/are the affected limb(s) flaccid or rigid?
- Does there appear to be any front limb involvement?

4. In addition, I would want to ask the technician if the patient seemed painful. I might also ask if s/he had felt the hind limbs to appreciate whether either felt cool to the touch as compared to the patient's forelimbs. Although this is somewhat of a subjective assessment, it may help to guide us in terms of the circulatory status of the pelvic limbs. Review Case #38 to recall that patients with the saddle thrombus form of aortic thromboembolism typically present with palpably cool hind limbs.(2) These patients are also likely to have cyanotic digital and metatarsal pads, as well as cyanotic nail beds.(2, 4, 5) They typically lack voluntary motor function and deep pain sensation in the affected limbs.(2)

5. The two components of the mammalian nervous system are the central nervous system (CNS) and the peripheral nervous system (PNS).(1, 2, 6–9)
    The CNS includes the brain, which is protected by the skull, and the spinal cord, which is protected by the vertebral column.(1, 2, 6–9)
    The PNS includes the autonomic and somatic nervous systems.(1, 2, 6–9)

6. Motor neurons are responsible for making connections between the nervous system and effector organs.(1, 2, 6)

7. There are two main types of motor neurons: upper (UMNs) and lower (LMNs).(6, 9)
    UMNs arise from the CNS and make connections between the brain and spinal cord segments in order to regulate posture and muscle tone, and modulate gait.(6, 9)
    UMNs use LMNs as intermediaries in the transmission of electrical impulses to muscle fibers and glands.(6) UMN axons may synapse directly onto LMNs or they may synapse onto one or more interneurons that pass the electrical signal onto LMNs.(6, 8, 9)
    LMNs carry signals from UMNs to effectors.(6) When effectors are muscles, their response is to contract.(6)

8. Neuromuscular dysfunction can result from a break at any point in the pathway that was described in the answer to Question #7 (above).(1, 2, 6, 9) Depending upon which aspect of the pathway is broken, the patient may be said to have UMN or LMN disease.(1, 2, 6)
    UMN dysfunction is characterized by hyperreflexia.(1, 2, 9–12) This is because UMNs are primarily inhibitory.(2, 9) When they become dysfunctional, inhibition is released, allowing for unregulated excessive tone.(2, 13) Affected patients will present with limb spasticity, that is, affected legs are stiff and rigid.(2, 9–12)
    Affected patients with lesions cranial to L4 may also develop a so-called UMN bladder.(2) Because there is a loss of inhibition to the urinary bladder, the urethral sphincters are excessively toned.(2) The urinary bladder will fill to the point that it overflows, but it will be difficult to express.(2)
    LMN dysfunction is characterized by hyporeflexia.(1, 2, 9–12) Affected patients will present with flaccidity of posture due to loss of muscle tone.(2) They may also exhibit muscular weakness.(2) Over time, muscles that are disengaged will atrophy.(2)
    Affected patients with lesions caudal to L4 may also develop a so-called LMN bladder.(2) Because the urethral sphincters lack tone, the urinary bladder will continuously dribble.(2) The urinary bladder is easy to express and will only partially fill.(2)

9. The following groupings are beneficial in helping you to localize neuromuscular disease:

- forebrain and brainstem
- C1–C5
- C6–T2
- T3–L3
- L4–L6
- L7–S3.

10. Lesions in the forebrain or brainstem may alter the patient's mentation or awareness of its surroundings.(9) Clients may report one or more of the following clinical signs:(1, 2, 9)

    • aggression
    • compulsive behaviors: circling, head-pressing, pacing
    • disorientation
    • unusual or persistent vocalization.

    Patients with C1-C5 lesions develop UMN signs in all four limbs.(11, 12)

    Patients with C6-T2 lesions develop LMN signs in the thoracic limbs and UMN signs in the pelvic limbs.(11, 12) These patients look very different in the front half of the body versus the back half, so much so that they are sometimes said to have a two-engine gait.(1, 2)

    Patients with T3-L3 lesions have unaffected thoracic limbs and UMN signs in the pelvic limbs.(1, 2, 11, 12)

    Patients with L4-L6 lesions have unaffected thoracic limbs and LMN signs in the pelvic limbs. (1, 2, 11, 12)

    Patients with L7-S3 lesions develop LMN signs that are restricted to the tail and perineum. (1, 2, 11, 12)

11. The main components of the neurological exam include assessment of the following.(1–3, 14, 15)

    • Mentation(1, 2, 9, 16–18)

        • Is the patient alert?
        • Is the patient depressed?
        • Is the patient obtunded?
        • Is the patient stuporous?
        • Is the patient comatose?

    • Posture

        • Does the patient have a head tilt?
        • Does the patient have a whole-body lean?
        • Is the patient exhibiting extension of all limbs in recumbency, with or without head and neck dorsiflexion (opisthotonus)? This is characteristic of a brain stem lesion and is referred to as decerebrate rigidity
        • Is the patient exhibiting thoracic limb extension with hip flexion and opisthotonos? This is characteristic of acute cerebellar injury and is termed decerebellate rigidity

    • Gait and coordination

        • Can the patient generate a gait?
        • What is the quality of the gait?

            • Is the gait smooth, strong, and even?

        • Is forelimb stride equivalent to hindlimb stride?
        • Is the patient experiencing cerebellar ataxia?

            • Does the patient exhibit a "toy soldier" gait?
            • Is the gait stilted, high-stepping, and over-reaching, with exaggerated flexion and force of movement?(19)

        • Is the patient experiencing vestibular ataxia?

            • Is the patient drifting or falling to one side?
            • Is the patient reluctant to move?
            • Is the patient keeping low to the ground and swaying its head from side to side like a pendulum?(17, 20)

- Is the patient experiencing proprioceptive or sensory ataxia?

  - Does the patient know where its feet are in space relative to its body?(17, 20)
  - Is foot placement solid?

- Is any component of the gait associated with weakness?

  - If so, is weakness generalized or localized?
  - Does weakness appear to be linked to activity or exercise?

- Is the patient experiencing any form of paralysis that precludes gait generation?

Note that subtle gait changes are most easily detected when the handler leads the patient to make tight turns.(2, 17, 19)

- Postural reactions

  - Proprioceptive positioning or the knuckling-over reflex:(16–19, 21)

    - Each foot must be evaluated separately, and the patient must be supported throughout the process.
    - With the patient standing and supported, grasp one paw at a time.
    - Position the paw so that its dorsal surface meets the ground.
    - A patient with normal proprioception will "recognize" that this is inappropriate and will fix its paw position so the palmar/plantar aspect contacts the floor.(18, 19)
    - A patient with normal proprioception may even refuse to allow its paw to be misplaced on the floor.(16, 18, 19)
    - A patient with abnormal proprioception will remain knuckled over onto the dorsal aspect of its affected paw(s).(18, 19)
    - Hopping
    - The patient is lifted off the ground and supported, except for the limb of interest.
    - The limb of interest is brought into contact with the floor.
    - The clinician directs the patient's weight to fall to the side.
    - This sideways motion displaces the patient's center of gravity, causing the patient to "fall" to the side. This creates a "hopping" motion in the normal patient.(16–19, 22)
    - Abnormal patients will stumble because they lose their foot placement or they will knuckle.(19)

  - Hemi-hopping or hemi-walking

    - A variation of the hopping test that allows ipsilateral limbs to be tested concurrently.
    - To test the patient's left forelimb and left hind limb, the patient's right forelimb and right hind limb are lifted off the ground as the patient is pushed to the left. To test the patient's right forelimb and right hind limb, the patient's left forelimb and left hind limb are lifted off the ground as the patient is pushed to the right.(17–20, 22)
    - Abnormal patients will stumble because they lose their foot placement or they will knuckle.(19)

  - Wheel-barrowing

    - Tests both forelimbs or both hind limbs concurrently.(16–19)
    - To test both forelimbs, the patient is supported under the abdomen.
    - Without the hind limbs meeting the ground, the patient is coaxed to move forward. In a normal patient, the forelimbs will alternate movements.
    - To test both hind limbs, the patient is supported under each axillary region with its thoracic end raised so that the forelimbs do not meet the ground.
    - With the patient standing, in effect, upright on both hind limbs, the patient is

encouraged to move backward. In a normal patient, the hind limbs will alternate movements.

- Abnormal patients will stumble because they lose their foot placement or they will knuckle.(19)

- Spinal reflexes

  - A solid understanding of the pathway of each reflex is required and what a "normal" reflex looks like so that exaggerated, weak, or absent reflexes can be noted.(16–18)
  - The two most reliable spinal reflexes that can be performed in the dog are:(9)

    - The patellar reflex:

      - Evaluates whether the femoral nerve and the associated L4-L6 segments of the spinal cord are intact.
      - With the patient restrained in lateral recumbency, the clinician uses one hand to support the limb that is "up" by seating this hand under the medial thigh.
      - The stifle of the "up" limb is positioned so that it is partially flexed.
      - The clinician then uses his other hand to swing the plexor firmly and smoothly to make contact with the patellar ligament.
      - The stifle should respond by automatically extending.(9, 17, 18, 22)
      - If the patellar reflex is weak or absent, then a lesion is likely to be present within the femoral nerve itself or within the L4–L6 spinal segments.
      - If the patellar reflex is exaggerated in combination with other gait and postural deficits, then these findings are suggestive of a UMN lesion cranial to L4.(9)
      - The patellar reflex may also appear to be exaggerated if the flexor muscles of the stifle, those that typically counteract stifle extension that is elicited in the reflex arc, have decreased tone as from a lesion within the sciatic nerve or spinal cord segments caudal to L6.(9)

    - The withdrawal or flexor reflex:

      - Evaluates the C6–T2 spinal cord segments as well as the musculocutaneous, axillary, median, ulnar, and radial nerves, when performed in the thoracic limb.(9, 17, 18, 22)
      - Evaluates the L7–S1 segments and the sciatic nerve, when performed in the pelvic limb.(9, 17, 18, 22)
      - With the patient restrained in lateral recumbency, the clinician pinches interdigital skin on each limb, one limb at a time, with the limb being tested held in extension.
      - When the thoracic limb is tested, the patient should automatically respond by flexing the shoulder, elbow, and carpus to pull the limb away from the clinician.
      - When the pelvic limb is tested, the patient should automatically respond by flexing the hip, stifle and hock to pull the limb away from the clinician.
      - The contralateral limb should be unaffected, meaning that if the right hind limb is evaluated for the withdrawal reflex, the left hind limb should not respond.
      - If the contralateral limb extends when the opposite limb is being tested for the withdrawal reflex, an abnormal crossed-extensor reflex is present and requires further investigation.(9, 17, 18, 22)

- Cranial nerves

  - There are 12 pairs.
  - These pairs are numbered in the order in which they arise from the brain, from cranial to caudal:(18)

- CN I: the olfactory nerve
- CN II: the optic nerve
- CN III: the oculomotor nerve
- CN IV: the trochlear nerve
- CN V: the trigeminal nerve
- CN VI: the abducens nerve
- CN VII: the facial nerve
- CN VIII: the vestibulocochlear nerve
- CN IX: the glossopharyngeal nerve
- CN X: the vagus nerve
- CN XI: the accessory nerve
- CN XII: the hypoglossal nerve

Refer to *Performing the Small Animal Physical Examination*(1) or *Common Clinical Presentations in Dogs and Cats*(2) for additional information concerning CN function.

Returning to Case 46: The Recumbent Dog

In response to your line of questioning, Paula expands upon the clinical history. She shares that Freckles yelped mid-stride before she fell over. By the time that Paula reached her, Freckles was panting and whining. She seemed to be in pain.

When Paula called out to her, Freckles tried to stand but her hind end seemed unable to support her weight and she sunk back to the ground. Freckles could only stand if Paula supported her hind end, and even then, she seemed to be unaware of the limbs beneath her. Paula noticed that the tops of Freckles' hind paws scuffed against the ground. Her hind legs also seemed rigid and stiff.

It was at that point that Paula lifted Freckles into her arms, carried her to the car, and drove straight here.

Round Two of Questions for Case 46: The Recumbent Dog

1. Based upon Paula's description, is Freckles likely to be exhibiting LMN or UMN signs in her pelvic limbs? Explain your answer.
2. If Freckle's forequarters are normal, then where would you expect to localize her lesions based upon the type of signs that the clinical history suggests?
3. What is the next appropriate step in case management?

Answers to Round Two of Questions for Case 46: The Recumbent Dog

1. Based upon the description, it is unclear. You need to examine the dog. If the dog's pelvic limbs are rigid and stiff, then Freckles likely has UMN signs.

2. If Freckle's forequarters are normal, then I would expect her lesion to be somewhere between T3 and L3.

3. The next appropriate step in case management is to perform a physical exam.(1) Up to this point, all of the information that you have considered has stemmed from the client's and/or technician's observations. It is critical that you also put your hands on the patient in order to confirm your suspicions and guide your diagnostic plan.

Returning to Case 46: The Recumbent Dog

You examine the patient.

Freckles is QAR. Mentation is normal. She seems aware of her surroundings and responds favorably to her owner's voice and touch.

Freckles has no CN deficits.

Freckles is non-ambulatory and paraparetic. She is reactive to palpation of the thoracolumbar spine. You suspect spinal hyperesthesia.

Freckles' forelimbs are normal, but both hind legs are rigid and stiff. Patellar and withdrawal reflexes are exaggerated. Nociception is intact.

Round Three of Questions for Case 46: The Recumbent Dog

1. Were you correct about whether Freckles' hind limbs are exhibiting LMN or UMN signs?
2. Has your exam of Freckles reinforced or refuted your anticipated lesion localization?
3. Based upon your current knowledge of clinical medicine, which differential diagnoses will you prioritize?
4. What are intervertebral discs?
5. What is the purpose of intervertebral discs?
6. What is intervertebral disc disease (IVDD)?
7. Differentiate Hansen Type I IVDD from Hansen Type II.
8. Which is the next appropriate step in the diagnostic process?

Answers to Round Three of Questions for Case 46: The Recumbent Dog

1. My original suspicions were correct: Freckles' hind limbs are demonstrating UMN signs.

2. Freckles' neurologic exam has reinforced my suspicion that her lesion is located between T3–L3.

3. Based upon my current knowledge of clinical medicine, I would prioritize the following differential diagnoses:(1, 2, 14, 15, 23–26)

    *   acute non-compressive nucleus pulposus extrusion (ANNPE)
    *   fibrocartilaginous embolic myelopathy (FCEM)(27)
    *   intradural/intramedullary intervertebral disc extrusion (IIVDE)
    *   ischemic injury as from a cerebrovascular accident(28–30) or infarct(31)
    *   other forms of vertebral canal compression, causing impingement of the spinal cord, such as a space-occupying lesion (cyst or tumor).

4. Intervertebral discs are cushions of cartilage (the gelatinous nucleus pulposus) surrounded by fibrous tissue (the annulus fibrosus) that sit between adjacent vertebrae.(32, 33)

5. Intervertebral discs allow for the spine to be flexible. In addition, they support the spine during high-impact activities, such as running and jumping.(32, 33)

6. IVDD is a condition in which there is one or more slipped or bulging discs.(1, 2, 32, 33)

7. Hansen Type I IVDD involves one or more slipped discs. These occur when the nucleus degenerates, meaning that it loses water content and calcifies.(2, 34, 35) This degeneration is part of

a normal aging process in all dogs.(32, 36, 37) However, this process occurs sooner in life in chondrodystrophic dogs, such as dachshunds.(34, 35, 37–40) Problems arise when this calcified material herniates dorsally toward the vertebral canal.(1, 2) This so-called disc extrusion impinges upon the spinal cord and precipitates signs of neurologic dysfunction that depend ultimately upon where in the spinal column impingement occurred. Dachshunds are predisposed, representing 45–73% of cases.(37, 41–44) Sixty-two percent of certain lineages are expected to develop IVDD at some point in their lifetime (42, 43). The Pekingese, Beagle, and Cocker spaniel are also predisposed.(45)

Hansen Type 2 IVDD involves one or more discs in which the outer annulus fibrosus bulges outwards and puts pressure on the spinal cord.(1, 2) This condition can be thought of as disc protrusion rather than extrusion, and more commonly occurs in middle-aged to older large-breed dogs.(1, 2, 32, 35, 37)

8. The next appropriate step in the diagnostic process is to perform advanced imaging of the spinal cord. Magnetic resonance imaging (MRI) is commonly employed for this purpose.

Returning to Case 46: The Recumbent Dog

You discuss your top differentials with Paula, who agrees that Freckles should be referred to a neurology practice that offers MRI. As is typical of referral scenarios, you are not present for the imaging study or for the clinical conversation that transpired between Paula and the neurologist. However, within 48 hours, you are faxed the clinical report, which provides a diagnostic image along with the diagnosis, ANNPE between L2–L3 (see Figure 46.2).

ANNPE is sometimes referred to as high velocity-low volume disc extrusion or Hansen type III in the veterinary medical literature.(24)

After briefing yourself on the condition, you telephone Paula to check in on Freckles. The past few days have been a whirlwind and it's clearly a lot for Paula to process. Paula has several questions for you about the condition. She was going to reach out to the neurologist, but seeing as how you're on the telephone . . .

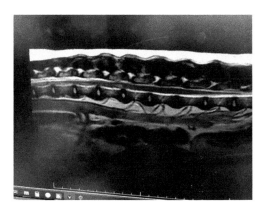

Figure 46.2 MRI of the affected portion of the patient's spine. Courtesy of Pamela Mueller, DVM.

Round Four of Questions for Case 46: The Recumbent Dog

1. What causes this condition to occur?
2. Which breeds are predisposed to this condition?
3. Between which spinal segments is ANNPE most likely to occur?
4. What is the proposed treatment for this condition?
5. What is the prognosis?

Answers to Round Four of Questions for Case 46:
The Recumbent Dog

1. Strenuous exercise or trauma are frequently implicated in cases of ANNPE.(24–26, 46–49)

2. Mixed-bred dogs are overrepresented in clinical cases of ANNPE.(25) Among pure-bred dogs, Staffordshire bull terriers, Labrador retrievers, Border Collies, greyhounds, and whippets seem predisposed.(24, 25)

3. ANNPE most frequently occurs between T3–L3.(26) In particular, the spaces between T12 and L2 are overrepresented.(26, 46, 48, 50–56) This has been attributed to the thoracolumbar junction being a site of contrasting mobility, between the relatively static thoracic spine and the mobile lumbar spine.(26)

4. Treatment for ANNPE is largely supportive.(26, 46, 48) Nursing care and physical therapy are the staples of therapy.(26, 46, 48) Analgesia is indicated in patients, such as Freckles, who experience spinal hyperalgesia.(48)

   Alternative, complementary therapies may be available at referral or specialty practices. Although more comprehensive studies of these therapies are essential to round out the current veterinary medical literature, the following treatment options offer potential hope:

   - acupuncture
   - hyperbaric oxygen therapy
   - laser treatments.

   (See Figures 46.3 and 46.4.)

5. The prognosis is variable.(25) Recovery may be complete, partial, or non-existent. Clinicians need to be transparent with owners that recovery, if it occurs, will take time. Clinicians need to solicit and address client expectations so that clients are able to freely communicate their needs and clinicians can appropriately respond.

   Patients with T3–L3 lesions may experience persistent urinary and/or fecal incontinence.(25) Impaired continence may challenge the human–animal bond.

   Patients with severe neurologic dysfunction may be euthanized, particularly if clients do not recognize clinical improvement or trends in the right direction, or if the patient's impaired status prevents it from performing tasks independently.(25)

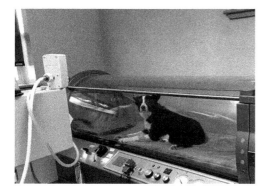

Figure 46.3 Canine patient in hyperbaric chamber. Courtesy of Pamela Mueller, DVM.

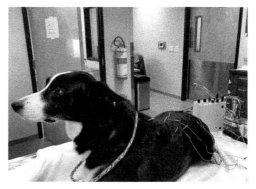

Figure 46.4 Acupuncture in a canine patient. Courtesy of Pamela Mueller, DVM.

CLINICAL PEARLS

- Neurologic dysfunction is common in companion animal practice.

- Neurologic lesions may arise within the CNS or PNS, within cranial or spinal nerves, or in the signaling pathways between nerves and their effector organs, such as muscle.

- Although advanced imaging modalities, such as MRI, are essential for diagnosis, there is no replacement for thorough history-taking and a comprehensive physical exam.

- The history and physical exam findings can collectively assist you with narrowing your scope of imaging as well as your list of prioritized differentials.

- Chunking the nervous system into segments facilitates lesion localization:

  - forebrain and brainstem
  - C1–C5
  - C6–T2

  - T3–L3
  - L4–L6
  - L7–S3.

- Pairing lesion localization with a solid understanding of UMN and LMN function is key to understanding the kinds of pathology that can go wrong and why certain clinical presentations look a certain way. For instance, understanding that patients with C6–T2 lesions develop LMN signs in the thoracic limbs and UMN signs in the pelvic limbs explains why patients present with a "two-engine gait."

- In most neurological cases, you will still need to rely upon advanced imaging to make a definitive diagnosis. However, lesion localization prevents you from having to imagine the whole dog.

- Lesion localization also helps you to predict which differential is most likely in which patient, which facilitates treatment planning when diagnostic tools are cost prohibitive.

References

1. Englar RE. Performing the small animal physical examination. Hoboken, NJ: Wiley/Blackwell; 2017.
2. Englar RE. Common clinical presentations in dogs and cats. Hoboken, NJ: Wiley/Blackwell; 2019. pages cm p.
3. Parent J. Clinical approach and lesion localization in patients with spinal diseases. Vet Clin North Am Small Anim Pract 2010;40(5):733–53.
4. Luis Fuentes VL. Arterial thromboembolism: risks, realities and a rational first-line approach. J Feline Med Surg 2012;14(7):459–70.
5. Smith SA, Tobias AH. Feline arterial thromboembolism: an update. Vet Clin North Am Small Anim Pract 2004;34(5):1245–71.
6. Molenaar GJ. The nervous system. In: Dyce KM, Sack WO, Wensing CJG, editors. Textbook of veterinary anatomy. 2nd ed. Philadelphia, PA: W. B. Saunders Company; 1996. p. 259–324.
7. Behan M. Organization of the nervous system. In: Reece WO, editor. Dukes' physiology of domestic animals. 12th ed. Ithaca, NY: Comstock Publishing Associates; 2004. p. 757–69.
8. Kitchell RL. Introduction to the nervous system. In: Evans HE, editor. Miller's anatomy of the dog. 3rd ed. Philadelphia: Saunders. p. 758–75.
9. Garosi L. Neurological examination of the cat. How to get started. J Feline Med Surg 2009;11(5):340–8.
10. Schubert. Physical and neurologic examinations. Meck veterinary manual [Internet]; 2018. Available from: https://www.merckvetmanual.com/nervous-system/nervous-system-introduction/physical-and-neurologic-examinations.

11. Millis DL, Mankin J. Orthopedic and neurologic evaluation. In: Millis DL, Levine D, editors. Canine rehabilitation and physical therapy. 2nd ed. Philadelphia, PA: Elsevier; 2014. p. 180–200.
12. DeLahunta A, Glass E, Kent M. Veterinary neuroanatomy and clinical neurology. 4th ed. St. Louis, MO: Elsevier; 2015.
13. Brashear A. Spasticity. In: LeDoux M, editor. Animal models of movement disorders. London: Elsevier Academic Press; 2005. p. 679–86.
14. DeLahunta A, Glass E, Kent M. Veterinary neuroanatomy and clinical neurology. 4th ed.St. Louis, MO: Elsevier; 2015.
15. Dewey CW, Da Costa RC. Practical guide to canine and feline neurology. 3rd ed. Chichester: Wiley/Blackwell; 2016.
16. van Nes JJ, Meij BP, van Ham L. Nervous system. In: Rijnberk A, van Sluijs FJ, editors. Medical history and physical examination in companion animals. 2nd ed. St. Louis, MO: Saunders Elsevier; 2009. p. 160–74.
17. Thomas WB. Initial assessment of patients with neurologic dysfunction. Vet Clin North Am Small Anim Pract 2000;30(1):1–24.
18. Thomas WB, Dewey CW. Performing the neurologic examination. In: Dewey CW, editor. A practical guide to canine and feline neurology. 2nd ed. Ames, IA: Wiley/Blackwell; 2008. p. 53–74.
19. Averill DR, Jr. The neurologic examination. Vet Clin North Am Small Anim Pract 1981;11(3):511–21.
20. Parent JM. The cat with a head tilt, vestibular ataxia, or nystagmus. In: Rand J, editor. Problem-based feline medicine. Edinburgh. New York: Saunders; 2006. p. 835–51.
21. Chrisman CL. The neurologic examination. NAVC Clin's Brief 2006:11–6.
22. de Lahunta A, Glass E. The neurologic examination. In: de Lahunta A, Glass E, editors. Veterinary neuroanatomy and clinical neurology. St. Louis, MO: Saunders Elsevier; 2009. p. 487–501.
23. De Risio L, Platt SR. Fibrocartilaginous embolic myelopathy in small animals. Vet Clin North Am Small Anim Pract 2010;40(5):859–69.
24. Fenn J, Drees R, Volk HA, De Decker S. Comparison of clinical signs and outcomes between dogs with presumptive ischemic myelopathy and dogs with acute noncompressive nucleus pulposus extrusion. J Am Vet Med Assoc 2016;249(7):767–75.
25. Mari L, Behr S, Shea A, Dominguez E, Johnson PJ, Ekiri A, De Risio L. Outcome comparison in dogs with a presumptive diagnosis of thoracolumbar fibrocartilaginous embolic myelopathy and acute non-compressive nucleus pulposus extrusion. Vet Rec 2017;181(11):293.
26. De Risio L. A review of fibrocartilaginous embolic myelopathy and different types of peracute non-compressive intervertebral disk extrusions in dogs and cats. Front Vet Sci 2015;2:24.
27. Cook JR. Fibrocartilaginous embolism. Vet Clin N Am Small 1988;18(3):581–92.
28. Thomsen B, Garosi L, Skerritt G, Rusbridge C, Sparrow T, Berendt M, Gredal H. Neurological signs in 23 dogs with suspected rostral cerebellar ischaemic stroke. Acta vet scand 2016;58(1):40.
29. Joseph RJ, Greenlee PG, Carrillo JM, Kay WJ. Canine cerebrovascular-disease – clinical and pathological findings in 17 cases. J Am Anim Hosp Assoc 1988;24(5):569–76.
30. Wessmann A, Chandler K, Garosi L. Ischaemic and haemorrhagic stroke in the dog. Vet J 2009;180(3):290–303.
31. Gonçalves R, Carrera I, Garosi L, Smith PM, Fraser McConnell JF, Penderis J. Clinical and topographic magnetic resonance imaging characteristics of suspected thalamic infarcts in 16 dogs. Vet J 2011;188(1):39–43.
32. Brisson BA. Intervertebral disc disease in dogs. Vet Clin N Am Small 2010;40(5):829.
33. King AS, Smith RN. A comparison of the anatomy of the intervertebral disc in dog and man: with reference to herniation of the nucleus pulposus. Br Vet J 1955;3:135–49.
34. Ghosh P, Taylor TK, Braund KG. The variation of the glycosaminoglycans of the canine intervertebral disc with ageing. I. Chondrodystrophoid breed. Gerontology 1977;23(2):87–98.
35. Hansen HJ. Comparative views of the pathology of disk degeneration in animals. Lab Investig J Tech Methods Pathol 1959;8:1242–65.
36. Modic MT, Masaryk TJ, Ross JS, Carter JR. Imaging of degenerative disk disease. Radiology 1988;168(1):177–86.
37. Hansen HJ. A pathologic-anatomical study on disc degeneration in dog, with special reference to the so-called enchondrosis intervertebralis. Acta orthop scand Suppl 1952;11:1–117.
38. Ghosh P, Taylor TK, Braund KG, Larsen LH. A comparative chemical and histochemical study of the chondrodystrophoid and nonchondrodystrophoid canine intervertebral disc. Vet Pathol 1976;13(6):414–27.

39. Ghosh P, Taylor TK, Braund KG, Larsen LH. The collagenous and non-collagenous protein of the canine intervertebral disc and their variation with age, spinal level and breed. Gerontology 1976;22(3):124–34.
40. Ghosh P, Taylor TK, Braund KG. Variation of the glycosaminoglycans of the intervertebral disc with ageing. II. Non-chondrodystrophoid breed. Gerontology 1977;23(2):99–109.
41. Gage ED. Incidence of clinical disc disease in the dog. J Am Anim Hosp Assoc 1975;11:135–8.
42. Ball MU, Mcguire JA, Swaim SF, Hoerlein BF. Patterns of occurrence of disk disease among registered dachshunds. J Am Vet Med Assoc 1982;180(5):519–22.
43. Priester WA. Canine intervertebral disc disease – occurrence by age, breed, and sex among 8,117 cases. Theriogenology 1976;6(2–3):(293–303).
44. Brown NO, Helphrey ML, Prata RG. Thoracolumbar disk disease in the dog: a retrospective analysis of 187 cases. J Am Anim Hosp Assoc 1977;13:665–72.
45. Goggin JE, Li AS, Franti CE. Canine intervertebral disk disease: characterization by age, sex, breed, and anatomic site of involvement. Am J Vet Res 1970;31(9):1687–92.
46. De Risio L, Adams V, Dennis R, McConnell FJ. Association of clinical and magnetic resonance imaging findings with outcome in dogs with presumptive acute noncompressive nucleus pulposus extrusion: 42 cases (2000–2007). J Am Vet Med Assoc 2009;234(4):495–504.
47. Chang Y, Dennis R, Platt SR, Penderis J. Magnetic resonance imaging of traumatic intervertebral disc extrusion in dogs. Vet Rec 2007;160(23):795–9.
48. McKee WM, Downes CJ, Pink JJ, Gemmill TJ. Presumptive exercise-associated peracute thoracolumbar disc extrusion in 48 dogs. Vet Rec 2010;166(17):523–8.
49. Henke D, Gorgas D, Flegel T, Vandevelde M, Lang J, Doherr MG, Forterre F. Magnetic resonance imaging findings in dogs with traumatic intervertebral disk extrusion with or without spinal cord compression: 31 cases (2006–2010). J Am Vet Med Assoc 2013;242(2):217–22.
50. Montavon PM, Weber U, Guscetti F, Suter PF. What is your diagnosis? Swelling of spinal cord associated with dural tear between segments T13 and L1. J Am Vet Med Assoc 1990;196(5):783–4.
51. Roush JK, Douglass JP, Hertzke D, Kennedy GA. Traumatic dural laceration in a racing greyhound. Vet Radiol Ultrasound 1992;33(1):22–4.
52. Hay CW, Muir P. Tearing of the dura mater in three dogs. Vet Rec 2000;146(10):279–82.
53. Yarrow TG, Jeffery ND. Dura mater laceration associated with acute paraplegia in three dogs. Vet Rec 2000;146(5):138–9.
54. Liptak JM, Allan GS, Krockenberger MB, Davis PE, Malik R. Radiographic diagnosis: intramedullary extrusion of an intervertebral disc. Vet Radiol Ultrasound 2002;43(3):272–4.
55. Kent M, Holmes S, Cohen E, Sakals S, Roach W, Platt S, et al. Imaging diagnosis-CT myelography in a dog with intramedullary intervertebral disc herniation. Vet Radiol Ultrasound 2011;52(2):185–7.
56. Kitagawa M, Okada M, Kanayama K, Sakai T. Identification of ventrolateral intramedullary intervertebral disc herniation in a dog. J S Afr Vet Assoc 2012;83(1):103.

Case 47

The Dog with Perineal Discharge

Pipsqueak has lived with her owners, Geo and Astrid Haverty, for the past 9 years, but she is new to your practice. The couple, along with their 8- and 6-year-old sons, recently moved to the area as a result of Astrid being promoted at work. They were exceptionally busy getting their bearings and had yet to select a veterinarian for Pipsqueak when she unexpectedly took ill.

She's always been a hardy dog with a stomach of steel. In fact, they often joked that Pipsqueak was a cat in dog's clothes because she seemed to have (and use up!) all her nine lives. Although Pipsqueak has slowed down at 11 years young and has put on some weight, the Havertys still see the spark of life in her, like the way, for instance, she perks up when she hears a bag of treats open from two rooms away. It doesn't matter how sound asleep she is, her ears will prick up. Then like, clockwork, they'll hear the pitter patter of her feet going click, click, click with her nails on the tile until she finds the treat-holder.

She's had a full life. In her heyday, she loved to wrestle with the boys, but through every adventure, she was always in control enough to keep everyone safe. She may not have looked tough, but she was the perfect guard dog. Protective of

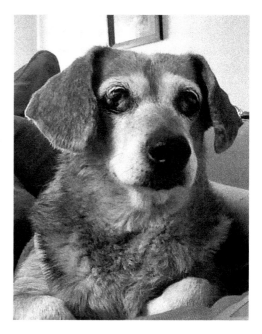

Figure 47.1 Meet Pipsqueak, an 11-year-old female Beagle mix.

those she loved most, she was willing to fight for her home and her family, especially the kids. No one came between her and them. They were her life.

Three days ago, Geo noticed that Pipsqueak seemed to be paying a bit more attention to her bottom. She didn't seem particularly bothered by anything. She was just unusually fussy about grooming.

It wasn't until Pipsqueak started asking to go outside more that Geo wondered if she was having an issue. Pipsqueak's bladder had never been weak. Although they hated to make her do so, she could hold her urine for up to 12 hours at a time. It was out of the ordinary for her to request bathroom breaks every 2 to 4 hours. There also seemed to be an urgency about it. Last night, when Pipsqueak asked to go outside, her request was overlooked. Astrid had seen her standing by the door. She had even heard her paw once, gently, at the barrier between her and the outside world. But Astrid had been tied up on a work call and before she could make it over to her, Pipsqueak squatted on the welcome mat.

Astrid had scolded her for having an accident. This took Pipsqueak by surprise. She was not used to being yelled at and she leaned herself away from Astrid until her rump hit the floor. When she finally scurried away, Astrid noticed what appeared to be brown discharge on the floor where Pipsqueak had been seated. The discharge had an odd odor. She assumed that Pipsqueak had released her anal glands.

About an hour later, Pipsqueak vomited. The vomitus was relatively undigested dinner. Astrid blamed herself for stressing Pipsqueak out. She knew she shouldn't have yelled. Deep down, Astrid blamed herself for not listening to Pipsqueak. The move and Astrid's work had just ramped her up and life was moving too quickly for her to catch her breath. She vowed to pay better attention to Pipsqueak and the family. After all, they were the only support she had, and they had turned their lives upside down for her to be here.

This morning, Pipsqueak turned up her nose at breakfast. Pipsqueak is the prototypical Beagle. She has never refused any meal any day in her life. This, combined with her vomiting last night, raised a red flag. Geo agreed to have her evaluated. He telephoned your clinic because it was the first one in the area to pop up when he googled "vets near me" and was able to be fit into the schedule for later that afternoon.

Geo drove Pipsqueak to the clinic. When Pipsqueak got out of the car, he noticed that she soiled the car seat. With what, he can't be sure. It's not feces, but clearly there's a stain where she was sitting.

When Geo checks Pipsqueak in at the receptionist desk, he mentions that she might have something going on "under her tail" and "could the vet check it out?"

The technician adds this to Pipsqueak's list of presenting complaints before loading her into an empty examination room to take her vital signs.

Use the following questions to guide your review of this clinical case.

Weight: 28.9 lb (13.1 kg)
BCS: 6/9
Mentation: QAR

TPR

T: 103.8°F (39.9°C)
P: 106 beats per minute
R: 30 breaths per minute

Round One of Questions for Case 47:
The Dog with Perineal Discharge

1. Pipsqueak has reportedly been paying extra attention to her rear end. Which structures are perineal?
2. What, in broad terms, could cause Pipsqueak to be paying excess attention to her perineum?
3. Which clarifying questions do you want to ask Geo about Pipsqueak when you take a comprehensive patient history?
4. After taking Pipsqueak's history, what is the next appropriate step in the diagnostic process?

Answers to Round One of Questions for Case 47:
The Dog with Perineal Discharge

1. The perineum spans the region of Pipsqueak's body from the pubic symphysis to coccyx and includes the following structures:(1–4)

   - fur
   - skin
   - soft tissue
   - underlying musculature
   - nerves
   - opening to the digestive tract:

- anus:
  - at the four o'clock and eight o'clock positions, on either side of the anus, sit the anal sacs, deep to the skin and not typically visible to the naked eye
- opening to the urinary tract:
  - urethra
- opening to the reproductive tract:
  - vulvar lips
  - vulva
  - vagina.

2. Any of the following problems could cause Pipsqueak to be paying excess attention to her perineum:(1, 2, 5, 6)

- potential digestive tract issues:
  - anal sac abscess
  - anal sac impaction
  - anal sac tumor
  - foreign body protruding from the anus
  - rectal prolapse
- potential urogenital tract issues:
  - urinary incontinence / urine dribbling
  - peri-vulvar dermatitis
  - pyometra
- potential "other" issues:
  - fecolith
  - matted fur
  - perineal hernia
  - perineal wound.

3. Based upon the limited history that I was provided with in clinical vignette, I would want to ask Geo the following clarifying questions.

- Tell me about Pipsqueak's reproductive status.
  - Is Pipsqueak intact or has she been spayed?
  - If Pipsqueak is intact:
    - Has she ever been bred before? If so, when?
    - Has she ever delivered pups before? If so, when?
    - Has she ever experienced complications related to breeding?
    - Has she ever experienced complications related to parturition?
  - If Pipsqueak is intact, ask Geo to describe her last estrous cycle.
    - When did it occur?
    - How long did it last?
    - What did you notice?
    - Was this cycle typical of others that you have witnessed?
- Describe Pipsqueak's lifestyle:

- Indoor?
- Outdoor?
- Unsupervised access outdoors?

- Does Pipsqueak have exposure to conspecifics?
- Does Pipsqueak have exposure to other animals?
- Tell me more about what you have observed when you see Pipsqueak grooming excessively at her hind end.

  - Is she chewing or biting?
  - Is she licking?

- Is Pipsqueak scooting?
- Has Pipsqueak ever had anal gland issues before?
- Has Geo ever smelled anal glands before?
- Does the discharge that he and his wife have observed smell like anal glands?
- What does the discharge that he and his wife have observed smell like?
- Has Geo noticed any unusual swelling in the perineal region?
- Has Geo looked under Pipsqueak's tail to see where the discharge is coming from?
- For how long has the discharge been there?
- Has the discharge changed in terms of odor?
- Has the discharge changed in terms of color?
- Has the discharge changed in terms of consistency? (i.e. serous to mucopurulent)
- Has the discharge changed in terms of amount/volume?
- Are Pipsqueak's urinary frequency and urgency still present?
- Does Pipsqueak exhibit any of the following urinary signs: dysuria, hematuria, or stranguria?
- Has Pipsqueak ever had a urinary tract infection (UTI)?
- How are Pipsqueak's bowels?
- Does Pipsqueak exhibit any of the following bowel-related signs: diarrhea, dyschezia, hematochezia, or tenesmus?
- Has Pipsqueak's diet changed?
- Has Pipsqueak's thirst changed?
- Could Pipsqueak have gotten into anything?
- Has Pipsqueak vomited again since last night?
- Has Pipsqueak ever had skin conditions, including peri-vulvar dermatitis?
- How is Pipsqueak's attitude now relative to what it has been before?
- Is Pipsqueak currently taking any medications, including prescription preventatives and over-the-counter supplements?

Note that these questions represent a combination of open- and closed-ended questions and statements.(7) These questions are designed to flush out additional details concerning Pipsqueak's clinical signs to facilitate pattern recognition and to guide our approach to case management. Although Pipsqueak will benefit from and receive a comprehensive physical examination, Geo's answers to the questions (above) will provide clues as to which organ system(s) may require additional investigation. For example, if we were to unearth that the patient has a history of UTIs, then we may be more suspicious that an infection has recurred. It does not mean that we cut corners and ignore everything else. We still need to comprehensively examine the patient. However, pattern recognition can highlight problem areas that we are likely to discover if we go searching for them.

4. After taking Pipsqueak's history, the next appropriate step in the diagnostic process is to perform a physical exam.(1)

Returning to Case 47: The Dog with Perineal Discharge

When you ask Geo to expand upon the patient's history, he shares that Pipsqueak has not been spayed. He had inherited Pipsqueak from his mother after her untimely passing. For 6 months after her death, Geo was in a mental and emotional fog. It was all he could do to keep one foot moving in front of the other. He hadn't even realized that Pipsqueak was overdue on vaccines or that she was still intact until one day she came into heat. He recalled taking her in to the clinic to discuss getting her spayed after that cycle. But then Astrid had gotten pregnant with their oldest son, Sol, and life never slowed down. Geo maintained Pipsqueak's vaccinations, but never followed through with the spay. After that visit, no one ever asked again and you know what they say, "out of sight, out of mind."

Pipsqueak has never been bred. Her last heat cycle was just before they moved, so, maybe 6 or 8 weeks ago.

Geo also shares that Pipsqueak seems depressed. He can't quite put his finger on why. Initially he chalked it up to the move, but now he is not convinced. Maybe there's something more going on with her. She just seems sick. For the past few days, she has been quieter. Calmer, even. And while that's been a nice change from her being underfoot, Geo is now wondering if her change in demeanor is something more. You confirm that Pipsqueak has a fever, and that might explain her subdued attitude and lack of activity.

You examine Pipsqueak and make note of the following findings:

- BCS: 7/9
- bilateral cherry eye
- nuclear sclerosis OU
- diffuse gingivitis with thick calculus deposition throughout all dental arcades
- tucked-up vulvar conformation
- vulvar discharge (see Figure 47.2).

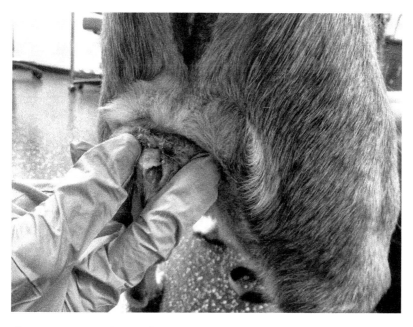

Figure 47.2 Perineal view of the patient. Note that there is significant peri-vulvar crusting and that when you part the vulvar lips, the mucosa appears redder than normal. You also note a brown-red opaque and malodorous discharge.

Round Two of Questions for Case 47: The Dog with Perineal Discharge

1. What is cherry eye?
2. What is nuclear sclerosis?
3. What is a tucked-up vulvar conformation?
4. What might this vulvar conformation predispose Pipsqueak to?
5. Is vulvar discharge normal in dogs? If so, when?
6. Is vulvar discharge normal in cats? If so, when?
7. What else could cause vulvar discharge?
8. Based upon the history and your experience with clinical medicine, what is your top differential diagnosis?
9. How will you confirm your top differential diagnosis?

Answers to Round Two of Questions for Case 47: The Dog with Perineal Discharge

1. Cherry eyes is the colloquial term for a prolapsed nictitans, the nictitating membrane or third eyelid.(2)

    Recall from Case #27 that the nictitans typically rests hidden, out of sight, in the ventro-medial orbit.(1, 2) Its position in the orbit is maintained by the sympathetic tone of the orbital smooth muscles.(8)

    The purpose of the nictitans is to produce and spread tear film across the surface of the eye. (1, 2, 8–10) The nictitans is typically pink and shiny because its surfaces are lined with moist conjunctiva.(1, 2) When the nictitans prolapses, it dries out.(8, 11, 12) This is why Pipsqueak's cherry eyes appear dull and crusty rather than shiny.(1, 2)

2. Nuclear sclerosis refers to the normal aging process of the lens of the eye.(13–15) As the patient ages, new cells are produced within the cortical lens, forcing the older cells inward.(16) This makes the nucleus more compact.(13, 15–17) This denseness scatters light, creating a haze that is visible to the observer.(16) The eyes of a patient with nuclear sclerosis appear cloudy. It can be difficult to differentiate cataracts from nuclear sclerosis on physical exam. Cataracts are pathologic opacities of the lens or lens capsule.(13, 14, 17–19) Refer to Case #29 for additional information.

3. A tucked-up conformation refers to a common clinical presentation in which a hypoplastic vulva appears to be hidden or recessed.(1, 2) This conformation tends to be exaggerated in overweight and obese dogs, which tend to develop excessive peri-vulvar skin folds.(1, 2, 20)

4. The tucked-up or recessed vulvar conformation predisposes patients to peri-vulvar dermatitis and chronic and/or recurrent UTIs.(2, 18)

5. Vulvovaginal discharge is normal during certain phases of the estrous cycle in both dogs and cats.

    During anestrus, the canine vulva is small and there is minimal to no vulvar discharge.(21) If discharge is present, it is mucoid in the healthy female dog.(2)

    During pro-estrus, the canine vulva swells and serosanguinous vulvar discharge develops. (2) This discharge arises from the uterus. (2, 22, 23)

    Vulvar discharge persists through estrus and is hemorrhagic.(2, 18)

    As estrus progresses, vulvar discharge reduces in amount and lightens in color from red to light pink or straw-colored.(2, 18)

During early diestrus, the patient may have milky, odorless vulvar discharge.(2, 18) This discharge should resolve as diestrus progresses. (2, 22, 23)

6. Cats are very different from dogs in that the feline estrous cycle involves minimal vulvar discharge.(2, 18, 24, 25) Pro-estrus cats may develop a mucoid plug at the vulva.(22, 26, 27) Cats in estrus may have serous to mucoid vulvar discharge.(18, 27) At no point throughout the estrous cycle do cats have hemorrhagic vulvar discharge.(18)

7. The most common causes of abnormal vulvovaginal discharge in the dog and cat include:(20, 24, 27–36)

    •   reproductive tract disease:

        •   endometritis   •   ovarian remnant syndrome (ORS)
        •   metritis   •   pyometra
        •   mucometra   •   vaginal foreign body
        •   neoplasia   •   vaginitis

    •   urinary tract disease:

        •   neoplasia
        •   urinary incontinence
        •   UTI.

    In addition, vulvovaginal discharge may develop as a result of systemic dysfunction or infection. (20) Consider, for example, atopy-associated peri-vulvar dermatitis.

8. Based upon the patient's signalment (intact female), clinical history (discharge coming from the back end, presenting six to eight weeks after being in estrus, associated with changes in attitude/appetite/ urination frequency, and vomiting), and vital signs (fever), I will prioritize the differential diagnosis of pyometra.

9. Although it is possible to palpate a tubular, distended uterus on abdominal palpation in some patients with pyometra, abdominal imaging is most often used to confirm the diagnosis.(1, 2, 18) Abdominal radiographs and abdominal ultrasound are both diagnostic for pyometra.(1, 2, 18, 37)

Returning to Case 47: The Dog with Perineal Discharge

You share your concerns with Geo that Pipsqueak has an open pyometra, which you confirm by taking two-view abdominal radiographs (see Figure 47.3 and **Plate 50**).

After discussing the diagnosis and your proposed treatment plan, Geo is onboard with taking Pipsqueak to surgery. You direct your team to draw blood for pre-anesthetic screening. Your technician in training calls your attention to Pipsqueak's blood smear (see Figures 47.4 and 47.5).

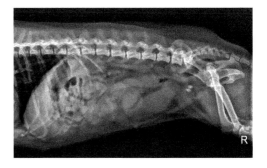

Figure 47.3 Right lateral abdominal radiograph demonstrating canine pyometra in a different patient. Note that this patient also had an incidental finding of bladder stones, which Pipsqueak did not have.

627

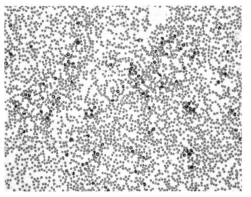

Figure 47.4 Canine blood smear using 20x objective. Courtesy of Nora Springer, DVM, DACVP.

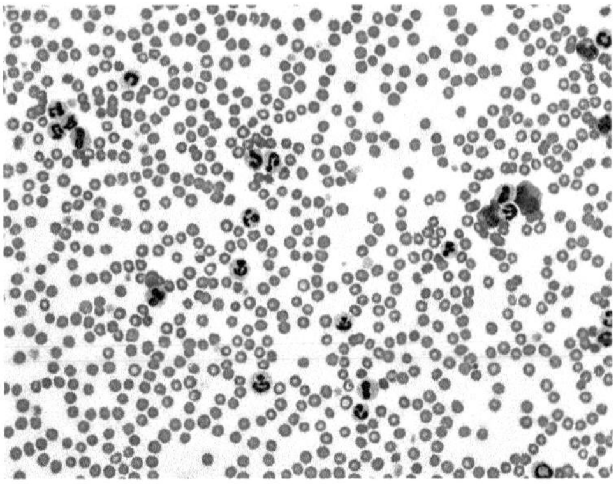

Figure 47.5 Canine blood smear using 40x objective. Courtesy of Nora Springer, DVM, DACVP.

Round Three of Questions for Case 47: The Dog with Perineal Discharge

1. What is pyometra?
2. What is an open pyometra?
3. How does an open pyometra compare with a closed pyometra?
4. With which systemic signs of illness do patients with pyometra typically present?
5. Which patient tends to be sicker on presentation, the one with an open pyometra or the one with a closed pyometra?
6. What are risk factors for development of pyometra?
7. Can pyometra also occur in cats?
8. What is the link between pyometra and increased urination?
9. What is the treatment of choice for pyometra?
10. If the patient is intended to be used for future breeding, then what potentially could you do to medically manage pyometra?
11. Why is the treatment plan that you outlined in Question #10 (above) contraindicated if the patient has a closed pyometra?
12. In addition to erythrocytes, which cell population is most prominent on Pipsqueak's blood smear?
13. Some of the cells of the type that you identified in Question #6 are immature. What do we call these cells?
14. Why are these cells present?
15. Fill in the blank: when these cells are present on a blood smear, we say that the patient has a
_____ _____ .

Answers to Round Three of Questions for Case 47: The Dog with Perineal Discharge

1. Pyometra is a uterine infection in which the uterus distends with pus.(1, 2, 18, 38)

2. The cervix remains open in an open pyometra.(1, 2, 18) Uterine contents trickle down the female reproductive tract, producing vulvovaginal drainage.(18) Gross inspection of the vulva typically reveals sanguinous to mucopurulent discharge.(29, 38–40)

3. The cervix is closed in a closed pyometra.(1, 2, 18) In a closed pyometra, uterine contents are retained. The patient does not present with vulvovaginal discharge.(18) Instead, the uterus continues to "store" the pus. The uterus may distend to the point that it ruptures.(18)

4. Patients with pyometra often present with one or more of the following signs of systemic illness: (2, 38, 41)

- anorexia
- depression
- diarrhea
- fever

- lethargy
- polydipsia
- polyuria
- vomiting.

5. Because pus is trapped within the body with no place to go, patients with closed pyometras often appear to be sicker at initial presentation.(38)

6. The following are risk factors for the development of pyometra:(1, 2, 38, 41–44)

- being in estrus within the past 12 weeks
- being nulliparous
- prior hormonal therapy with estrogens or progestins
- prior pregnancy termination.

7. Yes, pyometra can also occur in cats.(2) However, feline pyometra occurs with less frequency. (18) Pyometra occurs in 2.2% of intact queens by the time they reach 13 years of age. Siamese, Korat, Ocicat, and Bengal cats may present for pyometra earlier in life than the general feline population.(45)

8. Many cases of pyometra involve *Escherichia coli*.(29, 31, 46) Toxins that are associated with *Escherichia coli* interfere with the nephron's ability to reabsorb sodium.(47) This results in polyuria.

9. The treatment of choice for pyometra is ovariohysterectomy.(27, 29, 31)

10. If the patient is intended to be used for future breeding, then you can potentially administer injectable prostaglandin F2α to facilitate expulsion of uterine contents.(27, 29, 30)

11. If the patient has a closed pyometra, then administration of injectable prostaglandin F2α is ill-advised because uterine rupture is possible.(2, 29, 31) This would lead to peritonitis.(2, 29, 31)

12. In addition to erythrocytes, leukocytes are the most prominent cell type on Pipsqueak's blood smear. Specifically, I see an abundance of neutrophils.

13. The immature leukocytes that I see are referred to as band neutrophils. Their nuclei are much less segmented than mature neutrophils. Band neutrophils often have "C" or "S" shaped nuclei.

14. Band neutrophils represent a small fraction of peripheral leukocytes; however, their numbers increase in infectious and inflammatory conditions.(48)

15. When these cells are present on a blood smear, we say that the patient has a left shift.(48)

Returning to Case 47: The Dog with Perineal Discharge

You take Pipsqueak to surgery and perform an ovariohysterectomy (see Figures 47.6 and 47.7).

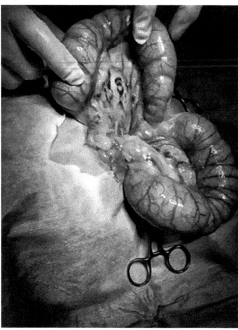

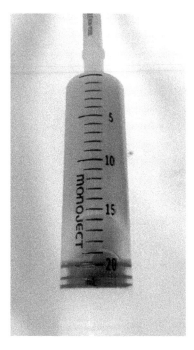

Figure 47.6 Canine pyometra visualized at surgery. Courtesy of Patricia MacCabe, DVM.

Figure 47.7 Fluid that has been aspirated from the uterus following ovariohysterectomy. Courtesy of Patricia MacCabe, DVM.

Round Four of Questions for Case 47: The Dog with Perineal Discharge

1. What is a potential intraoperative complication during ovariohysterectomy to address pyometra?
2. Why did you aspirate the fluid from the uterus after removing it during ovariohysterectomy?

Answers to Round Four of Questions for Case 47: The Dog with Perineal Discharge

1. A potential intraoperative complication during ovariohysterectomy to address pyometra is uterine rupture.

2. Fluid is often aspirated from the uterus after removing the organ during ovariohysterectomy to submit for bacterial culture and a susceptibility profile.
    Escherichia coli is commonly implicated in cases of pyometra.(29, 31, 46)

Other common bacteria include:(27, 31)

- *Kleibsiella* spp.
- *Proteus* spp.
- *Staphylococcus* spp.
- *Streptococcus* spp.

Bacterial culture and a susceptibility profile facilitate case management involving antibiotic selection.

CLINICAL PEARLS

- Signalment is an important part of the consultation.

- We may take it for granted that most of our patients are spayed or castrated. This means that we do not often have to consider reproductive problems on our list of differential diagnoses.

- However, we do and will encounter intact patients in clinical practice.

- It is essential to identify and document sexual status for any patient that we examine so that we do not lose sight of potentially obvious and easy-to-diagnose medical problems.

- Pyometra is a uterine infection that occurs with frequency in dogs. It much less commonly occurs in cats.

- Dogs with pyometra often present with signs of systemic illness, including, but not limited to changes in attitude or appetite, vomiting, diarrhea, and change in urinary habits or urination frequency.

- Dogs with open pyometra will present with vulvar discharge that may range in color from bloody to purulent.

- Dogs with closed pyometra will not present with vulvar discharge. These patients tend to be sicker on presentation because the uterus continues to distend with pus that has nowhere to go. If untreated, the uterus may rupture.

- The uterus of a non-pregnant healthy patient is not typically palpable on abdominal palpation. However, a patient with pyometra may have a palpably enlarged uterus.

- Pyometra is typically diagnosed either through abdominal palpation or imaging, by way of radiographs or ultrasound.

- Pyometras are typically managed surgically through ovariohysterectomy. Bacterial culture and susceptibility of uterine contents is encouraged to facilitate antibiotic selection.

- Breeders may inquire about options involving medical rather than surgical management.

- Open pyometras may be successfully managed through concurrent administration of antibiotics and prostaglandin F2α to expel uterine contents.

References

1. Englar RE. Performing the small animal physical examination. Hoboken, NJ: Wiley/Blackwell; 2017.
2. Englar RE. Common clinical presentations in dogs and cats. Hoboken, NJ: Wiley/Blackwell; 2019.
3. Evans HE, Miller ME. Miller's anatomy of the dog. 4th ed. St. Louis, MO: Elsevier; 2013.
4. Singh B, Dyce KM. Dyce, Sack, and Wensing's textbook of veterinary anatomy. 5th ed. St. Louis, MO: Saunders; 2018.

5. Côté E. Clinical veterinary advisor. Dogs and cats. 3rd ed. St. Louis, MO: Elsevier Mosby; 2015.

6. Ettinger SJ, Feldman EC, Côté E. Textbook of veterinary internal medicine: diseases of the dog and the cat. 8th ed. St. Louis, MO: Elsevier; 2017.

7. Englar RE. A guide to oral communication in veterinary medicine. Sheffield: 5M Publishing; 2020.

8. Maggs DJ. Third eyelid. In: Maggs DJ, Miller PE, Ofri R, Slatter DH, editors. Slatter's fundamentals of veterinary ophthalmology. 5th ed. St. Louis, MO: Elsevier; 2013. p. 151–6.

9. Brooks DE. Removal of the third eyelid. NAVC Clin's Brief 2005(January):47–9.

10. Gómez JB. Repairing nictitans gland prolapse in dogs. Vet Rec 2012;171(10):244–5.

11. Hendrix DVH. Canine conjunctiva and nictitating membrane. In: Gelatt KS, editor. Veterinary ophthalmology. Oxford: Blackwell; 2007. p. 662–89.

12. Mazzucchelli S, Vaillant MD, Wéverberg F, Arnold-Tavernier H, Honegger N, Payen G, et al. Retrospective study of 155 cases of prolapse of the nictitating membrane gland in dogs. Vet Rec 2012;170(17):443.

13. Sapienza JS. Feline lens disorders. Clin Tech Small Anim Pract 2005;20(2):102–7.

14. Boeve MH. Stades FC, Djajadningrat-Laanen. Eyes. In: Rijnberk A, van Sluijs FJ, editors. Medical history and physical examination in companion animals. Oxford: Elsevier; 2009. p. 175–201.

15. Tobias G, Tobias TA, Abood SK. Estimating age in dogs and cats using ocular lens examination. Comp Cont Educ Pract 2000;22(12):1085–91.

16. Giresi JC. Cataracts: How to uncover the imposter lenticular sclerosis. DVM. 360 [Internet]; 2005. Available from: http://veterinarynews.dvm360.com/cataracts-how-uncover-imposter-lenticular-sclerosis.

17. La Croix NL. Cataracts: when to refer. Top Companion Anim Med 2008;23(1):46–50.

18. Englar RE. Performing the small animal physical examination. Hoboken, NJ: Wiley; 2017.

19. Singh B, Dyce KM. Dyce, Sack, and Wensing's textbook of veterinary anatomy. 5th ed. St. Louis, MO: Saunders; 2018.

20. Root Kustritz MV. Vaginitis in dogs: A simple approach to a complex condition. DVM. 360 [Internet]; 2008. Available from: http://veterinarymedicine.dvm360.com/vaginitis-dogs-simple-approach-complex-condition.

21. Davidson AP. Breeding management of the bitch. Available from: http://www.vetmed.ucdavis.edu/vmth/local_resources/pdfs/repro_pdfs/ceBM.pdf.

22. Schaefers-Okkens AC, Kooistra HS. Female reproductive tract. In: Rijnberk A, van Sluijs FJ, editors. Medical history and physical examination in companion animals. St. Louis, MO: Saunders Elsevier; 2009.

23. Root Kustritz MV. Clinical canine and feline reproduction: Evidence-based answers. Ames, IA: Wiley/Blackwell; 2010.

24. Nicastro A, Walshaw R. Chronic vaginitis associated with vaginal foreign bodies in a cat. J Am Anim Hosp Assoc 2007;43(6):352–5.

25. Johnson CA. Vulvar discharges. Kirk's Current Veterinary Therapy X: Small Animal Practice. Philadelphia, PA: W.B. Saunders; 1989.

26. Little SE. Female reproduction. In: Little SE, editor. The cat: Clinical medicine and management. St. Louis, MO: Saunders Elsevier; 2012.

27. Pelsue D. Pyometra and vaginal discharges. In: Lappin MR, editor. Feline internal medicine secrets. Philadelphia, PA: Hanley & Belfus; 2001. p. 295–8.

28. Memon MA. Vaginitis in small animals. Merck Vet Man 2018. Available from: https://www.merckvetmanual.com/reproductive-system/reproductive-diseases-of-the-female-small-animal/vaginitis-in-small-animals.

29. Norsworthy GD, Restine LM Hoboken NJ, ed. The feline patient. 5th edition. Chichester: Wiley; 2018.

30. Nak D, Nak Y, Tuna B. Follow-up examinations after medical treatment of pyometra in cats with the progesterone-antagonist aglepristone. J Feline Med Surg 2009;11(6):499–502.

31. Hollinshead F, Krekeler N. Pyometra in the queen: To spay or not to spay? J Feline Med Surg 2016;18(1):21–33.

32. Johnson CA. Diagnosis and treatment of chronic vaginitis in the bitch. Vet Clin North Am Small Anim Pract 1991;21(3):523–31.

33. Davidson AP. Vulvar discharge in the bitch. NAVC Clin's Brief 2012 (January):70–4.

34. Demirel MA, Acar DB. Ovarian remnant syndrome and uterine stump pyometra in three queens. J Feline Med Surg 2012;14(12):913–8.

35. Hagman R. Canine pyometra: What is new? Reprod Domest Anim 2017;52;Suppl 2:288–92.

632

36. Johnstone IP. The cat with vaginal discharge. In: Rand J, editor. Problem-based feline medicine. New York: Saunders; 2006. p. 1160–4.
37. Thrall DE. Textbook of veterinary diagnostic radiology. 7th ed. St. Louis, MO: Elsevier; 2018
38. Pretzer SD. Clinical presentation of canine pyometra and mucometra: a review. Theriogenology 2008;70(3):359–63.
39. Feldman EC, Nelson RW. Cystic endometrial hyperplasia/pyometra complex. In: Kersey R, editor. Canine and feline endocrinology and reproduction. Philadelphia, PA: W.B. Saunders; 2004. p. 852–67.
40. Renton JP, Boyd JS, Harvey MJ. Observations on the treatment and diagnosis of open pyometra in the bitch (Canis familiaris). J Reprod Fertil Suppl 1993;47:465–9.
41. Wheaton LG, Johnson AL, Parker AJ, Kneller SK. Results and complications of surgical-treatment of pyometra – A review of 80 cases. J Am Anim Hosp Assoc 1989;25(5):563–8.
42. Bowen RA, Olson PN, Behrendt MD, Wheeler SL, Husted PW, Nett TM. Efficacy and toxicity of estrogens commonly used to terminate canine pregnancy. J Am Vet Med Assoc 1985;186(8):783–8.
43. Sutton DJ, Geary MR, Bergman JGHE. Prevention of pregnancy in bitches following unwanted mating: A clinical trial using low dose doseoestradiol benzoate. J Reprod Fertil 1997:239–43.
44. Dow C. The cystic hyperplasia--Pyometra complex in the bitch. The Veterinary record 1957;69:1409–15.
45. Hagman R, Ström Holst B, Möller L, Egenvall A. Incidence of pyometra in Swedish insured cats. Theriogenology 2014;82(1):114–20.
46. Arora N, Sandford J, Browning GF, Sandy JR, Wright PJ. A model for cystic endometrial hyperplasia/pyometra complex in the bitch. Theriogenology 2006;66(6–7):1530–6.
47. Bruyette DS. Diagnostic approach to polyuria and polydipsia. DVM. 360 [Internet]; 2008. Available from: http://veterinarycalendar.dvm360.com/diagnostic-approach-polyuria-and-polydipsia-proceedings-0.
48. Thrall MA. Veterinary hematology and clinical chemistry. 2nd ed. Ames, IA: Wiley/Blackwell; 2012.

Case 48

The Dog with the Unusual Attraction

Daquiri and his owner, Florence Gallagher, are long-term clients of yours. You have known "Daq" since he was a pup. At that time, Florence had intended on establishing herself as a Schnauzer breeder. She had never bred dogs before but had always been a fan of genetics at the university level and thought this was an opportunity to contribute to a breed that had long ago stolen her heart.

Although just a novice, Florence was not blind to the challenges of the road ahead. From shadowing other breeders, she was aware that this was often an uphill battle and a costly pursuit. At the advice of her mentor, she decided it would be a smart move to ease her way into the field by owning the stud first before transitioning to work with the dams.

Daq was supposed to be her first sire. Unfortunately, he never made the cut. On two different occasions, he was called upon to service bitches, yet seemed to have little to no interest in procreation.

Florence blamed the first failure on inexperience. Daq had misinterpreted his reason for being there. He looked at the bitch as a new playmate and was a little put out when she refused to return his play bow. On the second occasion, the bitch snapped at him when he approached her flank. He was just being inquisitive, but her reaction sent him running for cover behind Florence's legs. Florence tried to coax him out of hiding, but as far as Daq was concerned, his precarious friendship with the other dog was over.

Over the weeks and months that followed, Florence enrolled Daq in a slew of training classes, hoping that exposure to conspecifics would teach him how to interact with other dogs. In the process, Florence made two discoveries (1) Daq was a sensitive soul – it didn't take much

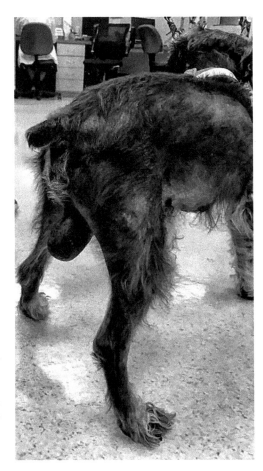

Figure 48.1 Meet Daquiri, a 9-year-old intact male miniature Schnauzer. Courtesy of Beki Cohen Regan.

to break his spirit; and (2) Daq wasn't very successful at reading canine body language. In fact, he could be quite oblivious at times. His obtuseness was a giant strike against his prospective career as a stud. His clear preference was to interact with other people rather than dogs. Florence soon realized that she would never have the breeding empire that she envisioned, at least not with Daq at the helm.

By the time Florence came to this realization, she was attached to Daq despite his deficiencies. Not wanting to start over again with another pup, she relinquished her dreams of becoming a famous breeder and settled for keeping him as a dutiful companion.

Florence never neutered Daq. By the time she gave up on his breeding career, he was 2.5 years young and had never given her a reason to. Most of her friends owned neutered male dogs and had them castrated young to reduce marking behaviors. Daq had never marked once. Not in the house. Not on her furniture. Not even on an outside scrub. Instead, when he urinated, he squatted.

It didn't seem necessary to put him through a procedure to curb behaviors that weren't even there. And so Daq remained intact, healthy, and happy. He was a lively, good-spirited dog with a gentle nature. Over the past 9 years, Daq had been in generally good health. It wasn't until the past 6 weeks that Florence became concerned.

Six weeks ago, Daq's coat began to thin. Initially, it was only along the sides where he had been known to itch sporadically. This served as a reminder to Florence to restart the topical flea preventative, with which she had been lax. Despite applying this product, Daq's coat continued to thin. Each day, his skin seemed to peek through the thinning coat a bit more prominently. The thinness extended down his ventrolateral abdomen, bilaterally, over his rump, and along his caudal thighs. At the same time, the skin beneath seemed to darken in terms of pigment.

Daq did not seem particularly bothered by this change in his coat. What concerned him was when he started to attract the attention of the male dog next door. Florence had been outside with Daq, tending to her garden, when she heard an uncharacteristic growl. She turned to find that the neighbor's dog had jumped the fence and was trying to mount Daq. Daq was having none of this. He escaped and ran for cover. Florence managed to shoo the other dog from her yard, but the effect on Daq was scarring. Florence decided to schedule an appointment for Daq to be evaluated, both for his hair coat and for his increasingly timid demeanor.

Florence has just now arrived at the clinic with Daq in tow. Your technician documents his vital signs as follows.

Use the following questions to guide your review of this clinical case.

Weight: 23.2 lb (10.5 kg)
BCS: 5/9
Mentation: BAR

TPR

T: 101.2°F (38.4°C)
P: 102 beats per minute
R: Panting

Round One of Questions for Case 48: The Dog with the Unusual Attraction

1. What is the appropriate medical jargon that signifies "thinning of the fur?"
2. What is the appropriate medical jargon that signifies "complete hair loss?"
3. Which clarifying details might we ask Florence about to obtain additional information about Daq's loss of fur?
4. What are major differential diagnoses for thinning and/or loss of fur? Develop a comprehensive list.
5. Of the differential diagnoses that you outlined in Question #4, which broad categories are LEAST likely in this patient given the patient's signalment and health history? Explain your reasoning for each category that you are effectively ruling out.
6. Of the differential diagnoses that you outlined in Question #4, which broad categories seem MOST likely in this patient given the patient's signalment and health history?

7. If Daq does have one or more of the differential diagnoses that you outlined in Question #6 (above), what other clinical findings might you expect to see?
8. Other than clarifying the patient's history, which is the next most appropriate step in the diagnostic process?

Answers to Round One of Questions for Case 48: The Dog with the Unusual Attraction

1. Hypotrichosis is the appropriate medical term to describe "thinning of the fur."(1–6)

2. Alopecia is the appropriate medical term to describe "complete hair loss."(1–6)

3. When we describe fur thinning or fur loss, we should consider asking Florence about the following details.

- Is hypotrichosis/alopecia focal or generalized?
- What is the pattern of distribution of the hypotrichosis/alopecia?

    - Is it truncal?
    - Is it symmetrical?
    - Is it normal for the species?
    - Is it normal for the breed?

- Where specifically on the body is there hypotrichosis/alopecia?
- Did something specifically occur at the site(s) of hypotrichosis/alopecia? For example:

    - Was a vaccine administered at that location?
    - Was a topical product applied to that location?

- Has the patient been observed to be grooming the site(s) of hypotrichosis/alopecia?

    - Does the patient appear to be overgrooming the location(s)?

- Is the hypotrichosis/alopecia paired with other primary or secondary dermatologic lesions?

    - Primary skin lesions include:(5, 7)

        - papules: small elevations of the skin
        - nodules: large papules
        - tumors: large nodules
        - pustules: pus-filled papules (so-called pimples)
        - vesicles: fluid-filled elevations that do not contain pus
        - bullae: large vesicles
        - wheals: pruritic, circumscribed areas of solid tissue that are raised in appearance due to dermal edema
        - plaques: thickened or raised circumscribed areas of solid tissue with flat tops that are not associated with dermal edema.

    - Secondary skin lesions include:(5, 7)

        - scales: loose flakes of skin; so-called dandruff
        - collarettes: circular lesions that are rimmed with scale; essentially what is left after pustules rupture
        - crusts consist of dried exudate and keratin, as opposed to scabs, which are dried plugs of fibrin and platelets that cover the surface of a wound during the healing process, as a new layer of skin begins to form(5)

- comedones: plugs of oil and dead skin cells; so-called blackheads
- lichenification: thickened, leathery skin that develops as a response to chronic skin irritation or inflammation
- hyperpigmentation: dark grey-black discoloration of the skin that develops as a response to chronic skin irritation and inflammation.(5)

- How long has the hypotrichosis/alopecia been present?
- Is the hypotrichosis/alopecia progressing?
- Is the hypotrichosis/alopecia seasonal?

These clarifying details help seasoned clinicians to narrow down their list of differential diagnoses.

4. The major differential diagnoses for thinning of and/or loss of fur include:(5–9)

- species-specific alopecia, e.g. feline peri-aural (pre-auricular) alopecia
- tardive hypotrichosis or alopecia: patients are born with normal coats; however, the coats thin as they age:

  - pattern baldness:

    - pinnal alopecia: dogs (especially dachshunds) > cats
    - bald thigh syndrome: dogs (especially greyhounds)

  - black hair follicular dysplasia: abnormalities in hair shafts and follicles leads to loss of black fur only
  - color dilution alopecia: typically targets those with blue, red, and fawn coats

- non-color-linked, cyclical follicular dysplasias, e.g. seasonal flank alopecia
- non-color-linked, non-cyclical follicular dysplasias, e.g. alopecia X: typically targets Nordic breeds and others with plush coats
- non-endocrine, non-inflammatory hair loss:

  - congenital hypotrichosis and alopecia:

    - canine:(10)
    - Mexican hairless or xoloitzcuintli
    - Chinese crested
    - Inca hairless
    - Peruvian Inca orchid
    - Feline:
    - Sphynx
    - Donskoy
    - the elf cat: a hybrid of the American Curl cat and the Sphynx
    - the Ukranian Levkoy: a hybrid of the Scottish Fold cat and the Sphynx
    - the Bambino: a hybrid of the Munchkin and the Sphynx

- endocrine, non-inflammatory hair loss:

  - hyperadrenocorticism
  - hyperestrogenism
  - hypothyroidism
  - exposure to human topical hormone replacement therapy

- non-endocrine, inflammatory hair loss:

  - bacterial pyoderma
  - dermatophytosis
  - mange

- hepatocutaneous syndrome
- chemotherapy
- radiation therapy
- alopecia associated with topical medications
- non-medical causes of hair loss, e.g. pressure alopecia
- nutritional causes of alopecia, e.g. zinc deficiency or deficiency in linoleic acid
- environmental cause of alopecia
- compulsive and/or displacement disorders:

    - acral lick dermatitis
    - flank sucking
    - fur mowing.

5. Of the differential diagnoses that have been outlined in the answer to Question #4 (above), the following broad categories are LEAST likely in this patient given the patient's signalment and health history:

- species-specific alopecia – Daq is a dog, not a cat
- tardive hypotrichosis – Daq is not a breed of dog that is known for pattern baldness
- non-color-linked, non-cyclical follicular dysplasias – Daq is not a Nordic breed
- congenital hypotrichosis and alopecia – Daq is presenting at 9 years old and fur thinning/ loss is a new complaint
- chemotherapy – you are Daq's primary care doctor. You have not prescribed chemotherapy
- radiation therapy – you are Daq's primary care doctor. You have not prescribed radiation therapy
- alopecia associated with topical medications – you are Daq's primary care doctor and you have not prescribed topical medications (you will need to follow-up to be sure that the client is not self-medicating)
- pressure alopecia – the location of fur loss as described is not in a typical site for pressure alopecia. Pressure alopecia typically occurs at elbows, which in turn develop calluses.

6. Given the patient's signalment and health history, the following broad categories for fur thinning or hair loss seem MOST likely:

- endocrine, non-inflammatory hair loss:

    - hyperadrenocorticism
    - hyperestrogenism
    - hypothyroidism

- non-endocrine, inflammatory hair loss:

    - bacterial pyoderma
    - dermatophytosis
    - mange.

7. If Daq has hyperadrenocorticism, then I might expect to find:(5, 6, 8, 9, 11)

- bilaterally symmetrical truncal alopecia
- calcinosus cutis, that is, deposits of calcium within the dermis (12)
- comedones
- excessive appetite (polyphagia – PP)
- excessive panting(12, 13)
- excessive thirst (polydipsia – PD)
- excessive urination (polyuria – PU)

THE DOG WITH THE UNUSUAL ATTRACTION

- hyperpigmentation of the skin
- increased ease with which bruising occurs due to dermal vessel fragility(12)
- muscle atrophy, especially around the head and face
- pot-bellied appearance secondary to hepatomegaly, a glucocorticoid-induced catabolic state, and fat redistribution
- secondary bacterial or fungal infections
- thin skin along the ventral abdominal wall.(11, 12)

If Daq has hyperestrogenism, then I might expect to find:(5, 6, 14–21)

- atrophy of the non-neoplastic testicle
- bilaterally symmetrical flank alopecia with hyperpigmentation
- gynecomastia, or enlargement of the mammary glands
- linear preputial dermatosis. This is a strip of redness and scaling between the prepuce and the scrotum along the ventral midline(12, 22)
- pendulous prepuce
- penile atrophy
- sexual attraction of other males
- squamous metaplasia of the prostate
- testicular tumor(s)
- thinning of the epidermis.

If Daq has hypothyroidism, then I might expect to find:(5, 6, 12)

- alopecia over pressure points in addition to bilaterally symmetrical truncal alopecia(12)
- cardiovascular system dysfunction, e.g. bradycardia
- central nervous system (CNS) dysfunction, e.g. ataxia, head tilt, and seizure disorders or dull mentation
- cold or exercise intolerance
- musculoskeletal system dysfunction, e.g. muscle weakness or slow, stiff gait
- peripheral nervous system (PNS) dysfunction, e.g. knuckling
- "ring around the collar", meaning that there is an alopecic patch outlining the neck, and/ or "rat tail"
- secondary bacterial or fungal infections
- weight gain without increased caloric intake.

The following changes are possible in hypothyroid dogs; however, these occur with less frequency:(5, 6, 12)

- gastrointestinal system, e.g. constipation
- special senses, e.g. anterior uveitis or corneal lipid deposits
- urogenital system, e.g. testicular atrophy and infertility

If Daq has bacterial pyoderma, then I might expect to find:(5, 6, 23)

- crusts
- epidermal collarettes
- papules
- pustules.

If Daq has dermatophytosis, then I might expect to find:(5, 6)

- circular alopecia
- crusting
- kerion formation.

If Daq has generalized demodectic mange, then I might expect to find:(24–26)

- erythema
- face, muzzle, and forelimbs affected first
- fever
- folliculitis
- furunculosis
- hypotrichosis or alopecic patches with or without a papulopustular rash
- lymphadenopathy
- paronychia
- pododermatitis
- scale.

If Daq has sarcoptic mange, then I might expect to find:

- lesions on the head, pinnae, elbows, and hocks(27, 28)
- pinnal-pedal reflex
- severe pruritus.

8. Other than clarifying the patient's history, the next most appropriate step in the diagnostic process is to perform a physical exam.(5)

Returning to Case 48: The Dog with the Unusual Attraction

When you ask Florence to expand upon the patient's clinical history, she shares that Daq has not had any changes in attitude, appetite, or weight. He is consuming the same over-the-counter, commercially available dry food that is marketed for use in adult dogs. He receives topical flea/tick preventative once per month, year-round (when Florence remembers!) and oral heartworm medication year-round (which Daq never lets her forget!). Daq has not been to any other veterinarian for care, so no other medications have been prescribed since the last time you saw him, over 6 months ago. Daq also does not have any exposure to human topical medications, as from skin-to-skin contact with Florence. Florence does not use topical hormone replacement therapy and Daq has only been around Florence here of late.

Florence has not noticed any skin lesions other than thinning of the fur, which is bilaterally symmetrical and along the flank line. In particular, she says that she has not noticed any pimples or rashes. Daq also does not appear to be pruritic.

Florence is embarrassed about the incident with the neighbor's dog. She didn't want to bring it up but explains that this act was what prompted today's visit. It occurred yesterday and something like that has never happened before. It seemed to petrify Daq, who is already shy and reserved. Now he seems reluctant to hang out in the yard unattended.

You ask if anything else seems amiss. Florence says that Daq's nipples seem to be larger than she recalls. She doesn't want you to think she's odd for pointing that odd. It just seems like he's more developed than he used to be and more developed than what he ought to be. She can't chalk it up to weight gain because he's the same weight that he was at the last visit.

Round Two of Questions for Case 48: The Dog with the Unusual Attraction

1. Based upon the extended history and Florence's description of Daq's clinical signs, which differential diagnosis do you want to prioritize?
2. Which aspect of the physical exam are you most interested in investigating to confirm or refute your suspicion?

Answers to Round Two of Questions for Case 48: The Dog with the Unusual Attraction

1. Based upon the extended history and Florence's description of Daq's clinical signs, I will prioritize the differential diagnosis of hyperestrogenism.

2. Based upon the presumptive diagnosis of hyperestrogenism, I will need to perform a testicular exam to confirm or refute my suspicion.(5, 6)

Returning to Case 48: The Dog with the Unusual Attraction

Having completed a thorough history, you turn your attention now to Daq's physical exam. In addition to bilaterally symmetrical truncal alopecia, you make note of the following abnormalities:

- hyperpigmentation of the skin in the regions of hypotrichosis and alopecia
- generalized gynecomastia
- palpably enlarged right testicle:

    - heterogeneous consistency
    - possible central mass – tissue feels firmer than normal and lobulated

- palpably small left testicle
- penile atrophy.

Round Three of Questions for Case 48: The Dog with the Unusual Attraction

1. When you examine both testicles through palpation of the scrotum, which testicular features are you taking into consideration?
2. If one or both testicles are missing from the scrotum, then the patient is said to be what? (Note that Daq has two descended/scrotal testicles so this question is just for your consideration.)
3. How is it possible for one or both testicles to be missing from the scrotum? (Hint: where do the testicles arise from in embryonic life?) (Note that Daq has two descended/scrotal testicles so this question is just for your consideration.)
4. Is the condition whereby one or both testicles are missing from the scrotum thought to be inherited? (Note that Daq has two descended/scrotal testicles so this question is just for your consideration.)
5. Are patients with bilaterally abdominal testicles capable of achieving erection? (Note that Daq has two descended/scrotal testicles so this question is just for your consideration.)
6. Are patients with bilaterally abdominal testicles fertile? Explain your answer. (Note that Daq has two descended/scrotal testicles so this question is just for your consideration.)
7. What is the epididymis?
8. What is the texture of the epididymis relative to the rest of the testicle?
9. Should you be able to palpate the epididymis in health?
10. You palpated an enlarged right testicle in Daq. What are the three main types of testicular tumors in dogs?
11. Which testicular tumor is associated with excessive testosterone production?
12. Which might this excess in testosterone production lead to?
13. Which testicular tumor is associated with excessive estrogen production?
14. Which might this excess in estrogen production result in?

15. Can dogs have more than one type of testicular tumor?
16. Is testicular asymmetry commonly appreciated in dogs in which only one testicle has a tumor?
17. Based upon your suspicion that Daq has hyperestrogenism, which testicular tumor type is most likely?
18. Can the diagnostic tool, ultrasound, definitively diagnose which testicular tumor type Daq has?
19. Why might you want to perform testicular imaging?
20. Why might you want to perform abdominal ultrasound?
21. Why might you want to perform three-view thoracic radiographs?
22. If Daq does indeed have hyperestrogenism, then which changes might you expect to see on his CBC?
23. Why do these changes occur?
24. Are these changes reversible?
25. What is your recommendation for Daq's case management?
26. When do you suspect that Daq's feminization will dissipate relative to initiating treatment?

Answers to Round Three of Questions for Case 48: The Dog with the Unusual Attraction

1. The following testicular features should be appreciated by palpation through the scrotum:(5, 6, 29, 30)

   - presence of scrotal testicles (as opposed to inguinal or intraabdominal testicles)
   - presence or absence of pain – normal testicles should be non-tender to the touch and non-tender to palpate(29)
   - shape of testicles – normal canine testicles are ovoid in shape
   - size of testicles relative to one another – normal testicles should be relatively similar in size to one another. it is not uncommon for one to be slightly larger, but there should not be significant size discrepancies between the two
   - texture or consistency of testicles:

     - normal testicles should have a smooth surface
     - normal testicles should feel homogenously firm, yet semi-compressible, like a shell-less hardboiled egg or a semi-ripe plum.

2. If one or both testicles are missing from the scrotum, then the patient is said to be cryptorchid. (5, 6)

3. Canine and feline testes do not originate from the scrotum.(29–31) In embryonic life, the testes develop within the abdomen, near the caudal pole of each kidney.(30–32) The testes must migrate from this location within the abdomen to the scrotum through the inguinal canal before the canal closures, between 4 and 6 months of age.(29–36) The inguinal canal is a passageway through the abdominal wall that is located in the groin.(31) Failure of testicular descent to the scrotum, cryptorchidism, is a common presentation among companion animal patients.(29–33, 35, 37–42)

4. Yes, cryptorchidism is thought to be inherited.

5. Most bilaterally cryptorchid patients can achieve erection.(32, 42, 43)

6. Bilaterally cryptorchid patients are infertile.(31, 32, 39, 43) While most can achieve intromission, many do not ejaculate.(32, 42, 43) Those that do may not ejaculate live sperm.(32, 43)

If they do, progressive motility of sperm is often impaired due to the thermal stress of having spermatogenesis occur within the abdomen as opposed to the scrotal sac.(32, 43)

7. The epididymis is a tubular structure that connects each testicle to the vas deferens, the conduit through which sperm pass into the urethra.(31)

8. The epididymis is firmer than the testis itself.(29, 31) The epididymis, including its tail, should feel somewhat rubbery.(29)

9. Yes, you should be able to palpate the epididymis in health along the dorsolateral surface of each canine testis, and the craniolateral surface of each feline testis.(5, 6)

10. The three most common types of testicular tumors in dogs are:(15, 21, 44–48)

    • interstitial or Leydig cell
    • seminoma
    • Sertoli cell.

11. Interstitial or Leydig cell tumors are associated with testosterone production.(21) These tumors are soft and cystic.(15, 49) On cross-section, they appear yellow-orange.(15, 49) They rarely metastasize, and affected patients are rarely ill at time of presentation.(15, 21, 45) Most are incidental findings.(6)

12. The increased production of testosterone by interstitial or Leydig cell tumors may result in:(21, 45, 48, 50, 51)

    • perianal adenoma   • perineal hernia
    • perianal gland hyperplasia   • prostatomegaly.

13. Sertoli cell tumors are associated with excessive estrogen production.(14, 15, 17) These tumors are firm.(15, 49) On cross-section, they are white-grey in color and may feel greasy.(15, 49)

14. The increased production of estrogen by Sertoli cell tumors may result in feminization, which is evident on physical examination.(14–16, 21, 52–56) Findings that are suggestive of hyperestrogenism include:(14–21)

    • atrophy of the non-neoplastic testicle
    • bilaterally symmetrical flank alopecia with hyperpigmentation
    • galactorrhea, or milk production
    • gynecomastia, or enlargement of the mammary glands
    • pendulous prepuce
    • penile atrophy
    • sexual attraction of other males
    • squamous metaplasia of the prostate
    • thinning of the epidermis.

15. Yes, dogs can have more than one type of testicular tumor.(16, 57–61)

16. Yes, testicular asymmetry is commonly appreciated in dogs in which only one testicle has a tumor. The neoplastic testicle enlarges whereas the unaffected testicle atrophies.(15)

17. Based upon your suspicion that Daq has hyperestrogenism, a Sertoli cell testicular tumor is most likely.

18. No, ultrasound cannot definitively diagnose which testicular tumor type Daq has.(15)

19. You may want to perform testicular imaging in order to perform ultrasound-guided FNA of the testicular mass.(62–64)

20. You may want to perform abdominal ultrasound to rule out metastasis.

   - Leydig cell tumors rarely metastasize.(15, 21, 45)
   - Fewer than 15% of seminomas metastasize.(15, 21, 45, 50, 65–68) Those that do spread primarily to regional lymph nodes.(15, 21, 45, 50, 65–68)
   - Fewer than 15% of Sertoli cell tumors metastasize.(15) Those that do metastasize to regional lymph nodes, the kidneys, pancreas, liver, spleen, and the lung.(6, 21, 50)

21. You may want to perform three-view thoracic radiographs to rule out metastatic pulmonary disease.(6) Sertoli cell tumors have been known to metastasize to the lung.(6, 21, 50)

22. If Daq does indeed have hyperestrogenism, then I might expect to see the following changes on his CBC:(6, 15, 21, 55, 69)

   - neutropenia
   - nonregenerative anemia
   - thrombocytopenia.

23. Excessive estrogen suppresses bone marrow function.(6, 15, 55, 69)

24. These changes to Daq's CBC may not be reversible.(6, 15, 55, 69)

25. I propose that Daq undergo staging as follows:(6, 15)

   - CBC
   - chemistry panel
   - urinalysis
   - three-view thoracic radiographs
   - abdominal ultrasonography.

   Following staging, I propose that Daq undergo bilateral orchiectomy.(6) The bilateral nature of this procedure is considered standard of care, even if only one testicle appears to be involved based upon physical exam findings.(6) As many as 50% of dogs have tumors in the contralateral testicle at time of diagnosis.(15, 70)

   If Florence is amenable to proceeding with bilateral castration, then there is no advantage to pre-operative testicular imaging for ultrasound-guided FNA because the entire testicle can be submitted for histopathology.

26. Assuming that there are no hormonally active areas of metastasis, Daq's feminization should resolve within 1 to 3 months following castration.(6, 15, 53, 71, 72)

CLINICAL PEARLS

- Testicular exams should be performed in any intact male dog.

- Testicular descent into the scrotum typically occurs after birth in the dog and cat.

- Testicles originate near the caudal pole of each kidney in embryonic life. They then must descend through the inguinal canal into the scrotum.

- The inguinal canal closes between four and six months of age. If one or both testicles have not entered into the scrotum after the inguinal canal closes, then the patient is said to be cryptorchid.

- Every intact male patient should have their testicles palpated to confirm their scrotal presence as well as to appreciate their shape, size, and consistency.

- Testicular masses are routinely diagnosed as incidental findings on physical exam.

- Interstitial or Leydig cell tumors are associated with production of testosterone, whereas Sertoli cell tumors are associated with hyperestogenism.

- Hyperestrogenism is likely to cause feminization of the patient. The patient may develop mammary tissue and may attract attention from other male dogs.

- Excess estrogen may also result in blood dyscrasias, which may or may not be reversible after surgical excision of the testicular tumor.

- Bilateral orchiectomy is considered the standard of care for patients with testicular tumors.

References

1. Moriello KA. Dermatology. In: Little SE, editor. The cat: clinical medicine and management. St. Louis, MO: Elsevier Saunders; 2012. p. 371–424.
2. Breathnach RMS, Shipstone M. The cat with alopecia. In: Rand J, editor. Problem-based feline medicine. Toronto: Elsevier Saunders; 2006. p. 1052–66.
3. Kennis RA. Disorders causing focal alopecia. In: Morgan RV, editor. Handbook of small animal practice. 5th ed. St. Louis, MO: Saunders/Elsevier; 2008. p. 834–40.
4. Ghubash RM. Disorders causing symmetrical alopecia. In: Morgan RV, editor. Handbook of small animal practice. 4th ed. Philadelphia, PA: Saunders; 2003. p. 841–9.
5. Englar RE. Performing the small animal physical examination. Hoboken, NJ: Wiley/Blackwell; 2017.
6. Englar RE. Common clinical presentations in dogs and cats. Hoboken, NJ: Wiley/Blackwell; 2019.
7. Englar RE. Common clinical presentations in dogs and cats. Hoboken, NJ: Wiley/Blackwell; 2019.
8. Côté E. Clinical veterinary advisor. Dogs and cats. 3rd ed. St. Louis, MO: Elsevier Mosby; 2015.
9. Ettinger SJ, Feldman EC, Côté E. Textbook of veterinary internal medicine: diseases of the dog and the cat. 8th ed. St. Louis, MO: Elsevier; 2017.
10. Mecklenburg L. An overview on congenital alopecia in domestic animals. Vet Dermatol 2006;17(6):393–410.
11. Zur G, White SD. Hyperadrenocorticism in 10 dogs with skin lesions as the only presenting clinical signs. J Am Anim Hosp Assoc 2011;47(6):419–27.
12. Frank LA. Comparative dermatology--canine endocrine dermatoses. Clin Dermatol 2006;24(4):317–25.
13. Feldman EC, Nelson RW. Canine and feline endocrinology and reproduction. St. Louis, MO: W. B. Saunders; 2004.
14. Hoskins JD. Testicular cancer remains easily preventable disease. DVM. 360 [Internet]; 2004. Available from: http://veterinarynews.dvm360.com/testicular-cancer-remains-easilypreventable-disease.

15. Lawrence JA, Saba CF. Tumors of the male reproductive system. In: Withrow SJ, Vail DM, Page RL, editors. Withrow and MacEwen's small animal clinical oncology. 5th ed. St. Louis, MO: Elsevier; 2013. p. 557–71.

16. Lipowitz AJ, Schwartz A, Wilson GP, Ebert JW. Testicular neoplasms and concomitant clinical changes in the dog. J Am Vet Med Assoc 1973;163(12):1364–8.

17. Huggins C, Moulder PV. Estrogen production by Sertoli cell tumors of the testis. Cancer Res 1945;5(9):510-and.

18. Zuckerman S, Groome JR. The ætiology of benign enlargement of the prostate in the dog. J Pathol 1937;44(1):113–24.

19. Zuckerman S, McKeown T. The canine prostate in relation to normal and abnormal testicular changes. J Pathol 1938;46(1):7–19.

20. Greulich WW, Burford TH. Testicular tumors associated with mammary, prostatic, and other changes in cryptorchid dogs. Am J Cancer 1936;28(3):496–511.

21. Paepe D, Hebbelinck L, Kitshoff A, Vandenabeele S. Feminization and severe pancytopenia caused by testicular neoplasia in a cryptorchid dog. Vlaams Diergen Tijds 2016;85(4):197–205.

22. Rosychuk RAW. Cutaneous manifestations of endocrine disease in dogs. Comp Cont Educ Pract 1998;20(3):287–+.

23. Craig M. Lesion morphology in veterinary dermatology. Companion Animal 2009;14(3):54–60.

24. Mueller RS, Bensignor E, Ferrer L, Holm B, Lemarie S, Paradis M, et al. Treatment of demodicosis in dogs: 2011 clinical practice guidelines. Vet Dermatol 2012;23(2):86–96.

25. Rouben C. Claw and claw bed diseases. Clin's Brief 2016 (April):35–40.

26. Manning TO. Cutaneous diseases of the paw. Clin Dermatol 1983;1(1):131–42.

27. Pin D, Bensignor E, Carlotti DN, Cadiergues MC. Localised sarcoptic mange in dogs: a retrospective study of 10 cases. J Small Anim Pract 2006;47(10):611–4.

28. Scott DW, Miller WH, Griffin CE. Parasitic skin diseases. Muller and Kirk's Small Animal dermatology. Philadelphia, PA: W. B. Saunders; 2001.

29. de Gier J, van Sluijs FJ. Male reproductive tract. In: Rijnberk A, Sluijs FJv, editors. Medical history and physical examination in companion animals. 2nd ed. New York: Saunders/Elsevier; 2009. p. 117–22.

30. Englar RE. Performing the small animal physical examination. Hoboken, NJ: Wiley; 2017.

31. Evans HE, Christensen GC. The urogenital system. In: Evans HE, Miller ME, editors. Miller's anatomy of the dog. 3rd ed. Philadelphia, PA: W. B. Saunders; 1993. p. 494–558.

32. Romagnoli SE. Canine cryptorchidism. Vet Clin North Am Small Anim Pract 1991;21(3):533–44.

33. Veronesi MC, Riccardi E, Rota A, Grieco V. Characteristics of cryptic/ectopic and contralateral scrotal testes in dogs between 1 and 2 years of age. Theriogenology 2009;72(7):969–77.

34. Yates D, Hayes G, Heffernan M, Beynon R. Incidence of cryptorchidism in dogs and cats. Vet Rec 2003;152(16):502–4.

35. Amann RP, Veeramachaneni DN. Cryptorchidism in common eutherian mammals. Reproduction 2007;133(3):541–61.

36. Bushby PA. Cryptorchid surgery and simple ophthalmic procedures. DVM. 360 [Internet]; 2010. Available from: http://veterinarycalendar.dvm360.com/cryptorchid-surgery-and-simple-ophthalmic-procedures-proceedings.

37. Wolff A. Castration, cryptorchidism, and cryptorchidectomy in dogs and cats. Vet Med Small Anim Clin 1981;76(12):1739–41.

38. Osterhoff DR. Canine cryptorchidism. J Am Vet Med Assoc 1978;172:333.

39. Birchard SJ, Nappier M. Cryptorchidism. Compend Contin Educ Vet 2008;30(6):325–36; quiz 36–7.

40. Hannan MA, Kawate N, Kubo Y, Pathirana IN, Büllesbach EE, Hatoya S, et al. Expression analyses of insulin-like peptide 3, RXFP2, LH receptor, and 3beta-hydroxysteroid dehydrogenase in testes of normal and cryptorchid dogs. Theriogenology 2015;84(7):1176–84.

41. Pathirana IN, Yamasaki H, Kawate N, Tsuji M, Büllesbach EE, Takahashi M, et al. Plasma insulin-like peptide 3 and testosterone concentrations in male dogs: changes with age and effects of cryptorchidism. Theriogenology 2012;77(3):550–7.

42. Davidson AP. Canine cryptorchidism. NAVC Clin's Brief 2014 (January):102–4.

43. Kawakami E, Tsutsui T, Yamada Y, Yamauchi M. Cryptorchidism in the dog: occurrence of cryptorchidism and semen quality in the cryptorchid dog. Nihon Juigaku Zasshi 1984;46(3):303–8.

44. von Bomhard D, Pukkavesa C, Haenichen T. The ultrastructure of testicular tumours in the dog: I. Germinal cells and seminomas. J Comp Pathol 1978;88(1):49–57.

45. Lopate C. Clinical approach to conditions of the male. In: England GCW, Von Heimendahl A, editors. BSAVA manual of canine and feline reproduction and neonatology. Gloucester: British Small Animal Veterinary Association; 2010. p. 191–211.

46. Kim O, Kim KS. Seminoma with hyperesterogenemia in a Yorkshire Terrier. J Vet Med Sci 2005;67(1): 121–3.

47. Kang SC, Yang HS, Jung JY, Jung EH, Lee HC. Malignant Sertoli cell tumor in shuh tzu dog. Korean J Vet Res 2011;51:171–5.

48. Grieco V, Riccardi E, Greppi GF, Teruzzi F, Iermanò V, Finazzi M. Canine testicular tumours: a study on 232 dogs. J Comp Pathol 2008;138(2–3):86–9.

49. McEntee MC. Reproductive oncology. Clin Tech Small Anim Pract 2002;17(3):133–49.

50. Johnston SD, Root Kustritz MV, Olson PNS. Disorders of canine testes and epididymes. Canine and feline theriogenology. Philadelphia, PA: W.B. Saunders; 2001. p. 312–32.

51. Sanpera N, Masot N, Janer M, Romeo C, de Pedro R. Oestrogen-induced bone marrow aplasia in a dog with a Sertoli cell tumour. J Small Anim Pract 2002;43(8):365–9.

52. Weaver AD. Survey with follow-up of 67 dogs with testicular Sertoli-cell tumors. Vet Rec 1983;113(5):105–7.

53. Brodey RS, Martin JE. Sertoli cell neoplasms in the dog; the clinicopathological and endocrinological findings in thirtyseven dogs. J Am Vet Med Assoc 1958;133(5):249–57.

54. Mischke R, Meurer D, Hoppen HO, Ueberschär S, Hewicker-Trautwein M. Blood plasma concentrations of oestradiol-17 beta, testosterone and testosterone/oestradiol ratio in dogs with neoplastic and degenerative testicular diseases. Res Vet Sci 2002;73(3):267–72.

55. Morgan RV. Blood dyscrasias associated with testicular-tumors in the dog. J Am Anim Hosp Assoc 1982;18(6):970–5.

56. Peters MAJ, de Jong FH, Teerds KJ, de Rooij DG, Dieleman SJ, van Sluijs FJ. Ageing, testicular tumours and the pituitary-testis axis in dogs. J Endocrinol 2000;166(1):153–61.

57. Hayes HM, Jr., Pendergrass TW. Canine testicular tumors: epidemiologic features of 410 dogs. Int J Cancer 1976;18(4):482–7.

58. Peters MAJ, de Rooij DG, Teerds KJ, van der Gaag I, van Sluijs FJ. Spermatogenesis and testicular tumours in ageing dogs. J Reprod Fertil 2000;120(2):443–52.

59. Scully RE, Coffin DL. Canine testicular tumors – with special reference to their histogenesis, comparative morphology, and endocrinology. Cancer 1952;5(3):592–605.

60. Kennedy PC, Cullen JM, Edwards JF, editors. Histological classifications of tumors of the genital system of domestic animals. World Health Organization international histological classification of tumors of domestic animals; 1998. American Registry of Pathology.

61. Nødtvedt A, Gamlem H, Gunnes G, Grotmol T, Indrebø A, Moe L. Breed differences in the proportional morbidity of testicular tumours and distribution of histopathologic types in a population-based canine cancer registry. Vet Comp Oncol 2011;9(1):45–54.

62. Johnston GR, Feeney DA, Johnston SD, O'Brien TD. Ultrasonographic features of testicular neoplasia in dogs: 16 cases (1980–1988). J Am Vet Med Assoc 1991;198(10):1779–84.

63. Pugh CR, Konde LJ. Sonographic evaluation of canine testicular and scrotal abnormalities – a review of 26 case-histories. Vet Rad 1991;32(5):243–50.

64. Eilts BE, Pechman RD, Hedlund CS, Kreeger JM. Use of ultrasonography to diagnose Sertoli-cell neoplasia and cryptorchidism in a dog. J Am Vet Med Assoc 1988;192(4):533–4.

65. Ciaputa R, Nowak M, Kiełbowicz M, Antończyk A, Błasiak K, Madej JA. Seminoma, Sertolioma, and Leydigoma in dogs: clinical and morphological correlations. B Vet Pulawy 2012;56(3):361–7.

66. Gawlik-Jakubczak T, Krajka K. A case of non-seminomatous testis tumor. Przegl Lek 2004;61(5):528–30.

67. Restucci B, Maiolino P, Paciello O, Martano M, De Vico G, Papparella S. Evaluation of angiogenesis in canine seminomas by quantitative immunohistochemistry. J Comp Pathol 2003;128(4):252–9.

68. Slatter DH. Textbook of small animal surgery. Philadelphia, PA: W. B. Saunders; 1985.

69. Sherding RG, Wilson GP, 3rd, Kociba GJ. Bone marrow hypoplasia in eight dogs with Sertoli cell tumor. J Am Vet Med Assoc 1981;178(5):497–501.

70. Reif JS, Maguire TG, Kenney RM, Brodey RS. A cohort study of canine testicular neoplasia. J Am Vet Med Assoc 1979;175(7):719–23.

71. Hogenesch H, Whiteley HE, Vicini DS, Helper LC. Seminoma with metastases in the eyes and the brain in a dog. Vet Pathol 1987;24(3):278–80.

72. Gopinath D, Draffan D, Philbey AW, Bell R. Use of intralesional oestradiol concentration to identify a functional pulmonary metastasis of canine Sertoli cell tumour. J Small Anim Pract 2009;50(4):198–200.

Case 49

The Dog with Priapism

K.C. is new to your practice. He is presenting for priapism of less than 24 hours duration (see **Plate 51**).

K.C. had recently been adopted by Ronald and Tricia Stiltz after the couple stumbled across his photograph on a social media profile of a friend of a friend. Tricia had always had a soft spot in her heart for puggles, and this was the perfect chance to add to her collection without having to struggle through housetraining and the other "joys" of puppyhood.

There was only one catch. K.C. was not neutered. Neither was their 6-year-old female Puggle, Posey.

Posey had the most incredible temperament of any dog that Tricia had ever known, so much so that Tricia had dreams of breeding her to carry her personality into the next generation. Whereas Tricia was a dreamer, Ronald was a realist. He had done enough research to realize that he and his wife were completely out of their element. Breeding dogs may not have been rocket science but obtaining the desired outcome – a healthy bitch and litter – wasn't necessarily a cake walk. Ronald had read up on caesarian sections, the cost as well as the potential risk to Posey. At the end of the day, her life wasn't something he was willing to bet on.

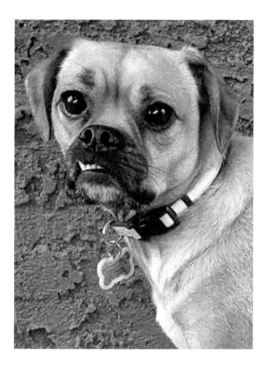

Figure 49.1 Meet your Patient, K.C., a 3-year-old intact male Puggle dog. Courtesy of Kara Jones.

Ronald agreed that they could adopt K.C. with one provision. He had to be neutered right away. Tricia reluctantly agreed, but a deal was a deal. Unfortunately, timing wasn't on their side. Posey's heat cycle was delayed such that she was just coming out of estrus when K.C. arrived home. The plan was still to neuter K.C., but his surgery could not be scheduled until the following week.

Although Posey was not receptive to K.C. and her growls kept him more than an arm's length away, her scent enticed him, and he developed an intermittent erection through the weekend. Otherwise, there were no surprises to K.C.'s adjustment to his new surroundings, and because he did not seem to be in any danger or distress, neither dog was kept apart.

When Ronald and Tricia awoke on Monday morning, they found K.C. pacing in the living room. When they drew near, they saw that K.C.'s penis was unsheathed from his prepuce. It was

Weight: 36.8 lb (16.7 kg)
BCS: 7/9
Mentation: BAR

TPR

T: 103.3°F (39.6°C)
P: 166 beats per minute
R: Panting

erect and starting to change color from the shiny pink that it had been to an angry sort of dried out red. K.C. was whining and clearly uncomfortable. It was at that point that the couple recognized an emergent need to have K.C. evaluated.

They have just arrived at your clinic as a walk-in emergency. Your technician has greeted them and taken K.C.'s vital signs while they wait for you to initiate the consultation.

Use the following questions to guide your approach to K.C.'s care.

Round One of Questions for Case 49: The Dog with Priapism

1. Describe erectile physiology.
2. Which nerve(s) and/or muscle contraction(s) mediate erection?
3. What is the purpose of the so-called copulatory tie?
4. Which innervation triggers ejaculation?
5. What is priapism?
6. How does priapism differ from paraphimosis?
7. What causes paraphimosis?
8. Why is paraphimosis detrimental to the health of the penis?
9. What does conservative treatment for paraphimosis involve?
10. How might surgery be of use in correcting paraphimosis?
11. What causes priapism?
12. Why is priapism a medical emergency?
13. How might mild cases of priapism be managed through conservative treatment?

Answers to Round One of Questions for Case 49: The Dog with Priapism

1. The canine penis is a vascular structure.(2–6) During arousal, penile smooth muscle relaxes to allow columns of erectile tissue within the penis to rapidly fill with arterial blood.(2, 3, 7–11) This causes the penis to lengthen, which unsheathes it from the prepuce in anticipation of mating.(2, 3, 7) Outflow of blood is occluded during erection because blood filling the sinusoidal system has compressed the venous channels.(1)

2. Erection is a function of several nerves, working in concert. Erection begins with parasympathetic innervation to the pelvic nerve, which arises from S1-S2.(1, 3) This initiates erection through dilation of the penile arteries.(3) Arterial blood is preferentially shunted to the cavernous bodies. (3) At the same time, venous drainage is inhibited, increasing penile blood pressure (BP).(3) The penis becomes erect.(3)

   During intromission, the female's constrictor vulvae and vestibuli muscles contract.(3) This triggers the male's ischiourethralis muscle to reflexively contract, shunting venous blood flow from the cavernous spaces to the bulbis glandis, a structure at the base of the glans penis.(3) As this structure fills with blood, it creates a ring around the penile base.(5, 9) This so-called knot is what creates the characteristic copulatory tie.(5)

   Sensory and somatic input from the pudendal nerve also contributes to maintenance of erection, as does sympathetic innervation by the hypogastric nerve.(1, 3) The hypogastric nerve facilitates prostatic secretions in anticipation of ejaculation.

3. The tie is a process that locks the male inside of the female during intromission.(2, 3, 5, 12) As the tie persists, the male turns his body around so that he faces the direct opposite from the female. They stand rear-to-rear for the remainder of the tie. This requires the erect penis to rotate

180 degrees just caudal to the bulbus glandis.(9) The os penis functions to maintain patency of the urethral opening during this twist so that ultimately ejaculation can transfer semen from the male to the female.(9)

4. Sympathetic innervation triggers ejaculation.(1, 3)

5. Priapism refers to pathologically prolonged erections that exceed four hours' duration.(13–19) Such erections persist long after sexual arousal has ceased, and are exceedingly painful.(13, 14, 16–19)

6. Paraphimosis also involves the penis being unsheathed from the prepuce. However, the penis of a patient with paraphimosis is non-erect and simply cannot retract back into the prepuce.(20–26)
   Priapism may be confused with paraphimosis.(17, 27) However, they are grossly distinguishable from one another. The penis is flaccid in cases of paraphimosis, as compared to priapism, in which the penis is erect.(13, 14)

7. Paraphimosis may be idiopathic (20, 21, 28) or may result from:(5, 20–25, 29–38)
   - acquired narrowing of the preputial opening:
     - foreign body:
       - foxtails
       - long fur
       - the patient mates as expected
       - in the process of mating, preputial fur creates a ring around the preputial opening and/or the base of the penis
       - when the patient dismounts and the glans undergoes detumescence, the penis itself is unable to retract back into its sheath
       - the penis becomes strangulated by the fur ring
       - the penis swells
     - scarring from past penile trauma
   - arousal without erection
   - balanoposthitis
   - congenitally abnormal, narrowed preputial opening
   - exposure to a female in estrus
   - excessive licking at the prepuce and/or penis by the patient
   - fractured os penis
   - increased sexual activity
   - ineffective preputial muscles
   - masturbation
   - neoplasia, e.g. transmissible venereal tumor (TVT)
   - neuropathology
   - penile swelling secondary to trauma.

8. It might seem that paraphimosis should be harmless to the patient because the penis is not erect and therefore not under sustained extreme pressure. However, the viability of the tissue is compromised by having the penis exposed for long periods of time.(13, 14) When the penis is trapped outside of its sheath, its tissues desiccate.(21, 22, 24)

9. Treatment for paraphimosis is aimed at replacing the penis within its sheath. Mild cases can be managed conservatively, by lubricating the penis with water-soluble gel in an attempt to digitally replace it within the prepuce.(21, 24, 39) Following manual replacement, the patient may benefit from placing a temporary purse-string suture at the opening of the prepuce.(25, 32, 36, 38)

10. When the preputial opening is too small for the extruded penis to be replaced within its sheath, surgical correction may be undertaken to increase the diameter of the preputial opening.(29)

    Another approach is to surgically advance the prepuce; however, there are limits to the extent to which this is possible.(5) In general, the prepuce cannot be advanced beyond one to one-and-a-half centimeters, so this technique will only work if penile exposure is minimal.(5, 29) If penile exposure is extensive, then advanced surgical techniques may be indicated to shorten the preputial muscles.(22, 25, 29, 30, 37)

11. Priapism may be due to:(5, 13–16, 21, 23, 29, 40–45)

    - lower urinary tract disease:

        - urethritis
        - urinary tract infection (UTI)

    - overstimulation of parasympathetic pathways via the pelvic nerve:

        - infectious neuropathy

            - canine distemper virus (CDV)
            - rabies (rabies-associated priapism has been documented in people only)(46, 47)

        - mechanical compression of the pelvic nerve:

            - constipation
            - obstipation
            - sublumbar mass

        - pharmacologic agents:

            - acepromazine
            - amphetamine
            - sildenafil

        - spinal cord trauma

    - penile trauma that was sustained during mating
    - reduced venous outflow from the penis:

        - pelvic mass occluding circulation
        - penile thromboembolism
        - post-castration in cats (16, 48, 49)

    - vasculitis, feline infectious peritonitis (FIP).(15, 16)

12. Like paraphimosis, priapism also involves prolonged exposure of the penis to life outside of its sheath, which causes the tissues to dry out and become irritated.(13, 14, 21, 22, 24)

    However, in cases of priapism, there is the added concern that the penis, which is now erect, is under extreme pressure. "Old" blood is unable to exit the erect penis and fresh blood is unable to enter. This leads to vascular stasis with the potential for blood clots to form within the cavernous sinuses.(1, 15, 42) In addition, endothelial and smooth muscle cells are damaged and penile tissues become ischemic.(1, 15, 42) Ischemia precipitates necrosis.

    If uncorrected, priapism not only leads to structural damage of the penis, it may also compromise the patient's ability to breed in the future. It has been reported in the human medical literature that people with priapism are at great risk of developing erectile dysfunction.(50) Veterinary patients are equally at risk of sustaining permanent damage to erectile tissue that could lead to erectile dysfunction.(15)

13. Conservative management of priapism mirrors what is typically attempted in mild cases involving paraphimosis: topical lubrication of the penis to rehydrate the glans.(13, 21, 23–25, 39, 49, 51)

In addition, hygroscopic agents may be applied topically to draw water out of the penis. (23, 24) The hope is that this action will reduce penile girth so that the organ can more easily be replaced within its sheath.(23) Sugar, honey, various salts, and 50% dextrose have been used for this purpose.(1, 13, 23–25)

Intracavernosal injections of phenylephrine have been attempted in people to restore blood flow to the penis.(17) This intervention may also be attempted in veterinary patients.(17)

Unfortunately, ischemic damage to the penis is often advanced by the time most veterinary patients present for evaluation.(5) In these cases, the patient is unlikely to respond to conservative therapy.(5)

Returning to Case 49: The Dog with Priapism

You demonstrate positive regard and transparency throughout the consultation. You explain to Ronald and Tricia that they did the right thing by bringing K.C. in so quickly. However, K.C.'s prognosis for complete return to function is unknown.

You express concern that K.C. may have been in this state all night. K.C.'s penis is starting to develop signs of necrosis, and that process is likely to progress. If it does, surgery will be indicated.

Ronald and Tricia beg you to try anything you can to spare K.C. from surgery. After an honest discussion about the various interventions that are available to them, Ronald and Tricia consent only to conservative therapy. They understand your reservations because the pharmacologic plan that you propose has not been validated in the veterinary medical literature. They appreciate your willingness to try, even though you've made it clear you worry that the odds are against them.

You administer pain medication to reduce K.C.'s discomfort. You then apply a liberal amount of 50% dextrose, lubricant, and topical combination antibacterial/steroid ointment to K.C.'s extruded penis.

You prescribe oral cefadroxil, benztropine mesylate, and terbutaline sulfate and send K.C. home with his owners. You discharge K.C. with an Elizabethan collar.

You ask Ronald and Tricia to cleanse K.C.'s penis tonight with chlorhexidine solution if his penis is still unsheathed and to present K.C. for a recheck examination tomorrow. They agree to the prescribed plan.

Round Two of Questions for Case 49: The Dog with Priapism

1. What is the purpose of initiating antibiotic therapy?
2. What is the purpose of prescribing benztropine?
3. If you do not have access to benztropine, which drug combination might you administer?
4. What kind of drug is terbutaline sulfate?
5. What is the purpose of prescribing terbutaline sulfate?
6. Why should you send K.C. home with an Elizabethan collar?

Answers to Round Two of Questions for Case 49: The Dog with Priapism

1. K.C.'s penile tissue has been compromised. Its surface is dried out and irritated. The tissue is no longer healthy, and it has been exposed to the environment for a prolonged period of time. Secondary opportunistic infections are likely. Antibiotic use is prophylactic, to guard against impending infection.

2.   Benztropine mesylate contains atropine and diphenhydramine.(1) It has been primarily admin-istered in horses and people with priapism with success attributed to its central anticholinergic effects.(1, 52) Its use has also recently been described in a canine patient.(1)

3.   If you do not have access to benztropine mesylate, then you might consider the administration of atropine sulfate and antihistamines (diphenhydramine +/– chlorpheniramine) to achieve a similar effect.(1)

4.   Terbutaline sulfate is a β-2-adrenergic agonist.(1, 53) Although its primary role in clinical medi-cine is to initiate smooth muscle relaxation in the bronchioles to treat asthma, it has been used successfully to medically manage human patients with priapism.(1, 53–56) The mechanism by which this occurs is unknown, but may have something to do with sympathetic stimulation.(1) Recall from erectile physiology that parasympathetic innervation is responsible for initiating and maintaining erection, while sympathetic innervation is responsible for ceasing erection and hastening ejaculation.

5.   You should send K.C. home with an Elizabethan collar to prevent self-trauma.

Returning to Case 49: The Dog with Priapism

Unfortunately, when K.C. returns the following day, it is apparent that necrosis has progressed to the point that it has nearly overtaken his entire penis. You recommend phallectomy.

Round Three of Questions for Case 49: The Dog with Priapism

1.   Ronald and Tricia would prefer that you take a less extreme approach. They ask you if castration would be an effective alternative to resolving K.C.'s priapism. How do you respond?
2.   Define phallectomy.
3.   If you proceed with phallectomy, Ronald and Tricia ask you how K.C. will be able to urinate following surgery. Which procedure will you need to perform concurrently with phallectomy to allow K.C. to urinate?
4.   What are potential complications of the procedure that you outlined in Question #3 (above)?

Answers to Round Three of Questions for Case 49: The Dog with Priapism

1.   I would share that unfortunately priapism is not mediated by testosterone.(57) Therefore, castra-tion will not hasten resolution.(57)

2.   Phallectomy is surgical amputation of the penis.(5, 17)

3.   K.C. will be able to urinate following surgical amputation of the penis if we concurrently perform a urethrostomy.(58) This creates a permanent opening in the urethra at an alternate location, which is necessary because the urethra will no longer tract through the penis.(58) Scrotal ure-throstomy is preferred. This procedure requires scrotal ablation and neutering.

4.   Urethral stricture is possible.(58) However, this is unlikely because of the width of the urethra at this level.

CLINICAL PEARLS

- Priapism and paraphimosis are rare clinical presentations in the canine and feline patient.

- Because both presentations involve the penis becoming trapped outside of its sheath, clinicians may mistake one condition for the other.

- Both conditions should be relatively easy to distinguish based upon gross observation.

- In cases of priapism, the penis is erect, whereas in paraphimosis, the penis is flaccid.

- In both cases, exteriorization of the penis for prolonged periods of times leads to desiccation of the tissues. The penis dries out and is susceptible to secondary opportunistic infections.

- Patients with priapism experience additional complications. Persistent erection causes the penis to experience sustained elevations in pressure. Persistent erection means that blood flow into the penis and blood flow out of the penis does not occur.

- Vascular stasis sets the stage for clot formation within the cavernous sinuses of the penis.

- Vascular stasis also precipitates ischemic necrosis.

- Conservative management of priapism involves lubrication of the penis and the topical application of hygroscopic agents to reduce edema.

- Administration of benztropine mesylate and terbutaline have shown promise in human medical reports. Recently, a combination of atropine sulfate and antihistamine plus terbulaline were found to be effective at resolving canine priapism.(1)

- Unfortunately, by the time that most patients present, ischemic necrosis of the penis necessitates phallectomy with urethrostomy.

References

1. Cassutto BH. Using drug therapy to treat priapism in two dogs. DVM360 [Internet]; 2012. Available from: https://www.dvm360.com/view/using-drug-therapy-treat-priapism-two-dogs.
2. The urogenital apparatus. In: Dyce KM, Sack WO, Wensing CJG, editors. Textbook of veterinary anatomy. 2nd ed. Philadelphia, PA: Saunders; 1996.
3. Evans HE, Christensen GC. The urogenital system. In: Evans HE, Miller ME, editors. Miller's anatomy of the dog. 3rd ed. Philadelphia, PA: W. B. Saunders; 1993. p. 494–554.
4. Englar RE. Performing the small animal physical examination. Hoboken, NJ: Wiley/Blackwell; 2017.
5. Englar RE. Common clinical presentations in dogs and cats. Hoboken, NJ: Wiley/Blackwell; 2019.
6. Evans HE, Miller ME. Miller's anatomy of the dog. 4th ed. St. Louis, MO: Elsevier; 2013.
7. Englar RE. Performing the small animal physical examination. Hoboken, NJ: Wiley; 2017.
8. Goericke-Pesch S, Hölscher C, Failing K, Wehrend A. Functional anatomy and ultrasound examination of the canine penis. Theriogenology 2013;80(1):24–33.
9. Kutzler MA. Semen collection in the dog. Theriogenology 2005;64(3):747–54.
10. Dorr LD, Brody MJ. Hemodynamic mechanisms of erection in the canine penis. Am J Physiol 1967;213(6):1526–31.
11. Christensen GC. Angioarchitecture of the canine penis and the process of erection. Am J Anat 1954;95(2): 227–61.
12. Hart BL. The action of extrinsic penile muscles during copulation in the male dog. Anat Rec 1972;173(1):1–5.

13. Tilley LP, Smith FWK. The 5-minute veterinary consult: canine and feline. 3rd ed. Baltimore, MD: Lippincott Williams & Wilkins; 2004.
14. Côté E. Clinical veterinary advisor. Dogs and cats. 3rd ed. St. Louis, MO: Elsevier Mosby; 2015.
15. Rota A, Paltrinieri S, Jussich S, Ubertalli G, Appino S. Priapism in a castrated cat associated with feline infectious peritonitis. J Feline Med Surg 2008;10(2):181–4.
16. Gunn-Moore DA, Brown PJ, Holt PE, Gruffydd-Jones TJ. Priapism in seven cats. J Small Anim Pract 1995;36(6):262–6.
17. Lavely JA. Priapism in dogs. Top Companion Anim Med 2009;24(2):49–54.
18. Burnett AL, Bivalacqua TJ. Priapism: current principles and practice. Urol Clin North Am 2007;34(4): 631–42.
19. Yuan J, Desouza R, Westney OL, Wang R. Insights of priapism mechanism and rationale treatment for recurrent priapism. Asian J Androl 2008;10(1):88–101.
20. Boothe HW. Diseases of the external male genitalia. In: Morgan RV, editor. Handbook of small animal practice. 5th ed. St. Louis, MO: Saunders/Elsevier; 2008. p. 587–92.
21. Kustritz MVR. Disorders of the canine penis. Vet Clin N Am. Small 2001;31(2):247–+.
22. Papazoglou LG. Idiopathic chronic penile protrusion in the dog: a report of six cases. J Small Anim Pract 2001;42(10):510–3.
23. Coomer AR. Male reproductive and penile surgery. World Congress Proceedings [Internet]; 2013. Available from: https://www.vin.com/apputil/content/defaultadv1.aspx?pId=11372andmeta=genericandcatId=35320a ndid=5709894andind=282andobjTypeID=17.
24. Pavletic MM. Management of Canine Paraphimosis2005; (September): [6–10 pp.]. Available from: http://www.hungarovet.com/wp-content/uploads/2008/07/management-of-canine-paraphimosis-2005.pdf.
25. Somerville ME, Anderson SM. Phallopexy for treatment of paraphimosis in the dog. J Am Anim Hosp Assoc 2001;37(4):397–400.
26. Wasik SM, Wallace AM. Combined preputial advancement and phallopexy as a revision technique for treating paraphimosis in a dog. Aust Vet J 2014;92(11):433–6.
27. Kustritz MVR, Olson PN. Theriogenology question of the month. Priapism or paraphimosis. J Am Vet Med Assoc 1999;214(10):1483–4.
28. Fowler JD. Preputial reconstruction. In: Bojrab MJ, editor. Current techniques in small animal surgery. Baltimore, MD: Williams & Wilkins; 1998. p. 534–7.
29. Papazoglou LG. Diseases and surgery of the canine penis and prepuce. World Congress Proceedings [Internet]; 2004. Available from: https://www.vin.com/apputil/content/defaultadv1.aspx?pId=11181andmeta=generican dcatId=30097andid=3852322andprint=1.
30. Chaffee VW, Knecht CD. Canine paraphimosis: sequel to inefficient preputial muscles. Vet Med Small Anim Clin 1975;70(12):1418–20.
31. Johnston DE. Repairing lesions of the canine penis and prepuce. Mod Vet Pract 1965;46:39.
32. Elkins AD. Canine paraphimosis of unknown etiology – a case-report. Vet Med Sm Anim Clin 1984;79(5):638–9.
33. Boothe HW. Penis, prepuce, and scrotum. In: Slatter D, editor. Textbook of small animal surgery. Philadelphia, PA: W.B. Saunders; 2002. p. 1531–42.
34. Johnston SE. Disorders of the external genitalia of the male. In: Ettinger SJ, editor. Textbook of veterinary internal medicine. Philadelphia, PA: W. B. Saunders; 1989. p. 1881–9.
35. Feldman EC, Nelson RW. Disorders of the penis and prepuce. Philadelphia: W. B. Saunders; 1996.
36. Ndiritu CG. Lesions of the canine penis and prepuce. Mod Vet Pract 1979;60(9):712–5.
37. Fossum SJ. Surgery of the reproductive and genital systems. In: Fossum SJ, editor. Small animal surgery. St. Louis, MO: Mosby; 1997. p. 565–72.
38. Soderbergh SF. Diseases of the penis and prepuce. In: Birchard SJ, Sherding RG, editors. Saunders manual of small animal practice. Philadelphia, PA: W. B. Saunders; 1994. p. 886–91.
39. Nelson RW, Couto CG. Small animal internal medicine. 5th ed. St. Louis, MO: Elsevier/Mosby; 2014.
40. Winter CC, Mcdowell G. Experience with 105 patients with priapism – update review of all aspects. J Urol 1988;140(5):980–3.
41. Guilford WG, Shaw DP, O'Brien DP, Maxwell VD. Fecal incontinence, urinary incontinence, and priapism associated with multifocal distemper encephalomyelitis in a dog. J Am Vet Med Assoc 1990;197(1):90–2.

42. Bivalacqua TJ, Burnett AL. Priapism: new concepts in the pathophysiology and new treatment strategies. Curr Urol Rep 2006;7(6):497–502.
43. Rochat MC. Priapism: a review. Theriogenology 2001;56(5):713–22.
44. Johnston DE, Archibald J. Male genital system. In: Archibald J, editor. Canine surgery. California: American Veterinary Publications; 1974. p. 703–49.
45. Graves TK. Diseases of the penis and prepuce. In: Birchard SJ, Sherding RG, editors. Saunders manual of small animal practice. 3rd ed. St. Louis, MO: Saunders Elsevier; 2006.
46. Depani S, Molyneux EM. Case Report: an unusual case of priapism. Malawi Med J 2012;24(1):17–8.
47. Dutta JK. Rabies presenting with priapism. J Assoc Phys India 1994;42(5):430.
48. Orima H, Tsutsui T, Waki T, Kawakami E, Ogasa A. Surgical treatment of priapism observed in a dog and a cat. Nihon Juigaku Zasshi 1989;51(6):1227–9.
49. Swalec KM, Smeak DD. Priapism after castration in a cat. J Am Vet Med Assoc 1989;195(7):963–4.
50. Levey HR, Segal RL, Bivalacqua TJ. Management of priapism: an update for clinicians. Ther Adv Urol 2014;6(6):230–44.
51. Pearson H, Weaver BM. Priapism after sedation, neuroleptanalgesia and anaesthesia in the horse. Equine Vet J 1978;10(2):85–90.
52. Wilson DV, Nickels FA, Williams MA. Pharmacologic treatment of priapism in two horses. J Am Vet Med Assoc 1991;199(9):1183–4.
53. Plumb DC. Plumb's veterinary drug handbook. 9th ed. Hoboken, NJ: Pharma Vet Inc.; 2018.
54. Lowe FC, Jarow JP. Placebo-controlled study of oral terbutaline and pseudoephedrine in management of prostaglandin E1-induced prolonged erections. Urology 1993;42(1):51–3.
55. Priyadarshi S. Oral terbutaline in the management of pharmacologically induced prolonged erection. Int J Impot Res 2004;16(5):424–6.
56. Shantha TR, Finnerty DP, Rodriquez AP. Treatment of persistent penile erection and priapism using terbutaline. J Urol 1989;141(6):1427–9.
57. Davidson AP. Priapism in small animals. Merck veterinary manual [Internet]. Available from: https://www.merckvetmanual.com/reproductive-system/reproductive-diseases-of-the-male-small-animal/priapism-in-small-animals.
58. Hedlund CS. Surgery of the reproductive and genital systems. In: Fossum TW, Duprey LP, O'Connor D, editors. Small animal surgery. 3rd ed. Boston, MA: Elsevier; 2007.

Case 50

The Last Goodbye

Nina is a new patient of yours. Her owner, Ryane Englar, is an associate professor at an established college of veterinary medicine.

Nina was purchased from a Maryland breeder when she was 11 weeks old, along with 12-week old Bailey, from a separate litter. Nina has been an Englar for nearly half of Ryane's life. They have been together through every milestone, starting with the summer before Ryane matriculated into Cornell University College of Veterinary Medicine. Nina has seen her through the highs and lows of her formal education, postgraduate professional employment, and personal life. For those who aren't familiar with Tonks, they are among the most engaging, interacting breed of cat that one could ever meet. They are gregarious and chatty, and some might even suggest – dare I say it – doglike. Nina was no exception to the rule. She was an incredible constant amidst the sea of change that is life. She was always there, always in the way, yet forever trying to "help." Nina may not have been the sharpest crayon in the box, but her lack of common sense was more than made up for by her empathy. Nina and Ryane had a connection that transcended time and space. Nina was the one who, at the end of a hard day, could melt away stress and right a wrong.

Ryane, Nina, and Bailey together journeyed from Maryland to upstate New York to Arizona and, ultimately, Kansas. The trio was about to return "home" to Arizona to start a new chapter when Nina took ill.

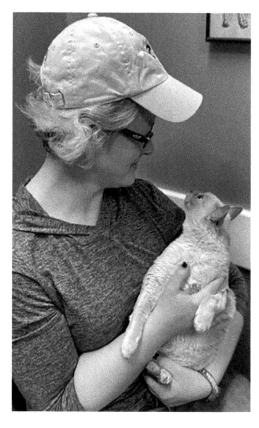

Figure 50.1 Meet your patient, Nina, a 16-year-old spayed female Tonkinese cat.

Other than having International Renal Interest Society (IRIS) Stage 2 chronic kidney disease (CKD) that was managed by a prescription diet, Nina had been in generally good health. It was a shock for all who knew her to see her health tank in a span of 72 hours.

What started as subtle yellow undertones in her peri-aural region transformed overnight into full-fledged icterus (see Figures 50.2 and 50.3).

In addition to her icteric undertones, Nina became clinically ill. She went off food altogether and vomited six times within a 24-hour period. She grew lethargic and weak. Her mentation rapidly declined from being bright, alert, and responsive to depressed to stuporous to borderline obtunded.

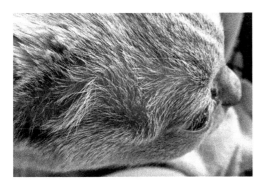

Figure 50.2 Peri-aural icterus.

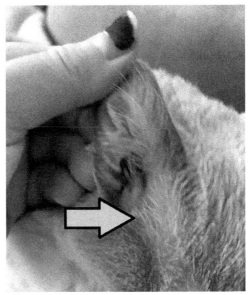

Figure 50.3 Progressing peri-aural icterus.

In-house bloodwork confirmed hepatopathy with cholestasis. Diagnostic imaging revealed a mass effect in the cranial abdomen, adjacent to the liver and continuous with the biliary tract. Findings obtained by abdominal ultrasonography were consistent with extrahepatic biliary obstruction. Neoplasia was suspected, both because of the cranial abdominal mass and because thoracic radiographs identified pulmonary nodules. A presumptive diagnosis of hepatobiliary malignancy with metastasis was made. Although exploratory laparotomy was discussed to further explore Nina's clinical presentation, Ryane elected not to pursue additional diagnostic tests. She planned to spend one last night with Nina in the comfort of their own home before returning with Nina for humane euthanasia.

When Ryane returns this morning to facilitate Nina's passing, she is told that Nina's doctor had unexpectedly called off today. You are the relief veterinarian who has agreed to take on Nina's care. You review the results of Nina's diagnostic work-up but find that Nina's medical records are otherwise scant. There is minimal documentation about yesterday's consultation and no real outline of the agreed-to plan for Nina.

Your technician assumes that Nina is here for humane euthanasia, but did not clarify if this is true. From what you gather from your team, as well as your review of the diagnostic test results, euthanasia would be an appropriate patient outcome. However, having never met Ryane or Nina, you know you need to approach this case gingerly.

Your technician takes Nina's vital signs as you consider how you will approach this situation.

Weight: 11.2 lb (5.1 kg)
BCS: 6/9
Mentation: Depressed

TPR

T: 99.1°F (37.3°C)
P: 138 beats per minute
R: 18 breaths per minute

Round One of Questions for Case 50: The Last Goodbye

1. Client communication is an essential part of end-of-life case management. Give examples of open-ended statements that you might use at the start of your consultation to elicit Ryane's perspective.
2. Why is it essential that you elicit Ryane's perspective?

3. A significant part of clinical communication is non-verbal. Which aspects of our own body language communicate a message to our clients?
4. We also need to tap into our ability to read clients' body language. Which features might Ryane demonstrate if she is feeling uncomfortable and wants to disengage from conversation?
5. Why is it important that we face Ryane during this difficult conversation?
6. What are potential physical barriers that may get in between us and our client in the examination room?
7. What else might you do to eliminate physical barriers between you and Ryane as you discuss her reason for presenting Nina today?
8. Empathy plays an essential role in end-of-life discussions. What is empathy? Differentiate cognitive empathy from emotional empathy.
9. Give examples of empathetic statements that you might use to improve your connection to Ryane.
10. What are potential challenges for the clinician that are associated with empathetic displays?
11. Empathy is not easy for some people to demonstrate through words. Give examples of empathetic actions that you could take in the examination room to improve your connection to Ryane.

Answers to Round One of Questions for Case 50: The Last Goodbye

1. The following open-ended statements might be appropriate for use at the start of the consultation to elicit Ryane's perspective.

   • Tell me how Nina managed last night.
   • Share with me how last night went for both of you.
   • Walk me through how these past few days have been for you.
   • Take me through how you are holding up through this.
   • Tell me how I can help you best.

   These phrases may be softened with, "Please," or "Can you . . . .(1) For example:

   • Can you tell me how Nina managed last night?
   • Please share with me how last night went for both of you.
   • Can you walk me through how these past few days have been for you?
   • Please take me through how you are holding up through this.
   • Please tell me how I can help you best.

2. Eliciting the client's perspective gives Ryane an opportunity to express her expectations for today's visit.(1, 2) This communication skill opens the door to a difficult conversation about end-of-life. Eliciting the client's perspective in this case allows Ryane to share the details of how Nina has progressed since her last visit to the clinic, and what about her interactions with Nina last night reinforced her decision to euthanize Nina today.

   If Ryane is given the opportunity to share what transpired last night, she will likely provide her rationale for euthanasia. She may share, for instance, that Nina continued to decline mentally and that, by morning, she was hardly aware of her surroundings. She may share that she is at peace with her decision today because she had an opportunity for closure last night. Or she may share that she is having second thoughts and wants to be sure that she is doing the "right" thing for Nina.

   Eliciting the client's perspective is an essential component of end-of-life visits because it invites Ryane to share what is on her mind and how she is processing those thoughts. Eliciting the client's perspective invites Ryane to share her reasoning with the veterinary team as to why she has made the decisions that she has and if there are any areas that she still needs help to work through.

3. The following aspects of body language collectively communicate a message to our clients: (1, 3–12)

- body position in space, e.g. forward versus backwards lean
- body posture, e.g. open versus closed body posture
- whole-body movement
- body part isolations and movements
- body tension
- eye contact
- facial expressions
- gestures
- touch.(7, 13–17)

4. If Ryane feels uncomfortable during this consultation, she may non-verbally communicate her desire to disengage from conversation through one or more of the following cues.(1, 3)

- She may lean away.
- She may increase personal space.
- She may place physical barriers in the way, e.g. she may retreat to the opposite side of the examination room table.
- She may exhibit a closed-off posture by crossing her arms or legs.
- She may break eye contact.
- She may turn her head and look away.
- She may cling to the patient.

5. When we face our clients, we convey our interest in what they have to say.(1) This is especially important during end-of-life consultations because clients need to feel heard, respected, and not rushed.

   If we do not face our clients, for instance, if we have our back to them, as we may be apt to do when typing patient notes into the medical record, then our clients may feel unheard, unwelcome to share, and/or unappreciated.(1)

   Clients that are in the process of deciding whether to euthanize or not need to feel heard and supported. They need to feel as if their time with you is valued. If we choose to look or walk away from them during a time when they need our support most, then clients may get the sense that we are distant, cold, or unfeeling. This may damage the professional relationship that we share with them, moving forward, and/or make them second guess their decision to euthanize today.

6. Consultation rooms contain many physical barriers between us and our client. These may include:(1, 3, 4, 18, 19)

- the medical record
- the patient
- the patient's carrier or crate
- seating, including benches, that are built into consultation room walls and corners
- the examination room table
- consulting room computer(s) and/or television monitor(s)
- watches, pagers, and/or cellular phones – the client's and/or the veterinarian's.

7. To eliminate physical barriers between me and Ryane as we discuss her reason for presenting Nina today, I could do one or more of the following.(1)

- Put down the medical record.
- Stop taking notes.
- Step away from the exam room computer.

661

- Silence my pager or cellular phone.
- Alter my position in the room relative to the client so that the exam room table is not wedged between us.
- Position myself at the end of the consult table.(5) This allows me to create an "L" shape with my client.(5) This shape is thought to facilitate conversation by leveling the playing field and reducing the spatially perceived position of authority.(5)
- Stand at my client's side, shoulder-to-shoulder.(5) This positioning demonstrates an active attempt at partnership.(5)

8. At a most basic level, being empathetic at a cognitive level simply means that you have connected to another individual such that you can identify with him/her.(1, 20) You may or may not agree with this individual's perspective or insight, but you can appreciate his/ her thought process.(1) You cognitively understand why s/he thinks the way s/he does about certain scenarios or events.(1, 21) This form of empathy is purely cerebral.(1)

   Cognitive empathy allows the veterinary team to view the situation from the perspective of the client, whether the client's perspective is accurate.(1, 20) This connectivity between provider and client helps the veterinarian to acknowledge and address the client's concerns so that there is mutual understanding.(1) That kind of common ground plays a critical role in decision making in clinical practice.(1) Clients need to feel heard and understood if they are to commit to diagnostic and/or treatment options.(1)

   Cognitive empathy provides a solid foundation for the veterinary team to establish a connection with the client.(1) Emotional empathy takes that connection a step further.(1) Emotional empathy implies that we can put ourselves in the shoes of another being and feel what it is that they feel to the extent to which it is humanly possible.(1, 4, 20–25)

   In this respect, emotional empathy humanizes medicine.(1) It removes the titles of both parties to equalize the conversation.(1) It replaces the relationship of veterinarian-client with human-human to convey the following message. (1)

- I get you.
- I feel you.
- I am there for you.

- I can relate to you.
- Your pain is my pain.

9. It is appropriate to make use of empathetic statements to improve your connection to Ryane. Empathetic phrases may include statements of acknowledgement.(1)

- I see that you care very deeply about Nina.
- I can see how hard it is for you to make this decision.
- I can tell that Nina's illness is really weighing on your mind.
- I know that you would do anything in your power to take away Nina's pain.
- I appreciate that you are putting her needs first and that you do not want Nina to suffer.
- You two have been through so much together. Saying goodbye to Nina today must feel like losing family.

Empathetic statements of acknowledgement may mirror reflective listening.(1, 20)

- It sounds like your greatest concern is . . .
- I hear that you are worried most about . . .
- I'm hearing you say that you cannot bear to see Nina like this anymore.
- I'm hearing that quality of life is most important to you as we consider what is best for Nina.
- What you're saying is that Nina acts like she's in pain and that is distressing to you.
- What you're telling me is that you don't want Nina to suffer.

Empathetic phrases may also include statements that normalize and/or validate the client's expressed emotion.(1, 20)

- It must be so difficult for you to make this decision.
- It must have been so scary to see Nina go downhill so fast.
- It must be stressful to feel like you have to make this decision all by yourself.
- You're right, it's so overwhelming to have to make this decision for Nina.
- It's understandable that you would worry about making the right decision.
- It's normal to second guess yourself.

Empathetic phrases may include connectivity statements that express shared experiences.(1, 20)

- I share your same concern.
- When my own cat developed the same condition, I asked myself many of the same questions you find yourself working through today.
- I know what it's like to have to make this decision. It isn't easy.

If, on the other hand, you have never experienced the same situation, then full disclosure is important and may take the form of an empathetic statement.(1)

- I can only imagine what you are going through.
- I can't begin to understand the depth of your pain.

10. Clinicians may struggle to find the "right" words to share with their clients. They may worry about saying the "wrong" thing or they may stress over sharing the "right" words at the "wrong" time.

    Empathy does not come easily to everyone. Some clinicians may struggle to find words that come across as sincere and genuine.

    Clinicians may find that their own empathy varies depending upon the clinical scenario and associated circumstances. If they have previously experienced a similar situation in their own lives, they may be able to tap into that experience and more easily connect to their clients' emotions. Or they may find themselves shutting down in those circumstances as a self-protective measure so that they do not have to relive the experience all over again.

    Clinicians may struggle with empathetic displays depending upon the client's emotions and how s/he is reacting to the situation. For example, some clinicians may struggle with clients who cry. They may feel paralyzed at the sight of tears.

    The following barriers may complicate the clinician's ability to demonstrate empathy:(1)

- the clinician not agreeing with the client's decision to euthanize
- the clinician not agreeing with the client's decision not to euthanize
- stress
- time constraints
- burn-out
- compassion fatigue
- what else has happened that day on the job:
    - if I have had to euthanize 25 patients before coming into my 26th exam room of the day to discuss quality of life, then I may be emotionally exhausted
    - for self-preservation, I may not want to put myself in my client's shoes
    - in that case, I need to learn how to lean on other communication tools to support my client
- what else is going on in the clinician's personal life matters greatly in terms of whether or not the clinician is capable of expressing empathy in the moment
    - if the clinician is grieving an unrelated loss, then it may be that much harder to provide empathy to someone else when the clinician is also hurting and is in just as much need of support.

11. Empathy is not easy for some people to demonstrate through words, in which case it may be easier to demonstrate empathy through actions.(1) Empathetic actions include the following.

- Making eye contact.(20, 23)
- Maintaining eye contact when a client is expressing an emotion.(20, 23)
- Mirroring the client's posture, that is, if the client is seated, seat yourself.(3, 20, 23, 25)
- Angling your body at a 5–10 degree angle from the horizontal line between you and the client.(25)
- Avoiding towering above the client, if you are standing.
- Sitting on the floor, with your eye level below the client's, can be a nice gesture to put the patient at ease and to reduce feelings of vulnerability that the client may have.(3, 26)
- Decreasing the distance between you and the client, i.e. bringing one's chair nearer to the client or sitting beside the client on an examination room bench.
- Talking slowly to allow the client to process details.(23)
- Using a moment of silence.(23)
- Using touch appropriately at one of the following locations: the client's shoulder, upper arm, forearm, or top of the hand to console.(27)
- Touching the patient, particularly if the clinician is uncomfortable with touching the client.(26)
- Providing a box of tissues to a grieving or crying client.

Note that clients may respond differently to being handed a box of tissues.(1) Many clients feel comforted.(1) Some may feel like you're communicating that you're uncomfortable with tears, so here, let's dry them up.(1) For this reason, many clinicians choose to make tissues readily available in the consultation room, rather than directly handing them to the client, so that the client can partake of them if s/he feels the need.

Returning to Case 50: The Last Goodbye

During the consultation, Ryane expresses guilt that she should have noticed Nina's poor health sooner. After all, she is a veterinarian. Perhaps had she not been so occupied with her work, she would have recognized the problem earlier, when surgical intervention may have carried a better prognosis. Ryane is clearly beating herself up for not taking better care of Nina or bringing her in to the clinic more quickly.

Round Two of Questions for Case 50: The Last Goodbye

1. What is active listening?
2. What is another term for active listening?
3. How might you make use of the communication skill, reflective listening, to address what Ryane has shared?
4. What is unconditional positive regard?
5. How might you make use of the communication skill, unconditional positive regard, to help Ryane work through her feelings?
6. Describe the term, transparency, in human healthcare as it relates to medical mistakes.
7. How does the term, transparency, apply to veterinary medicine as it relates to medical errors?
8. Other than medical errors, what might we choose to be transparent about in clinical practice?
9. How might you make use of the communication skill, transparency, to help Ryane work through her feelings?
10. What is partnership?
11. Why are partnership statements particularly valuable during consultations about end-of-life and end-of-life planning?
12. How might you make use of the communication skill, partnership, to help Ryane through this difficult time?

Answers to Round Two of Questions for Case 50: The Last Goodbye

1. Active listening in the medical field refers to a humanistic approach to reframing clinic consultations as dialogues between two individuals, with the listener concentrating on hearing the message that the speaker wants to convey.(1, 21, 23, 24, 28–34)

    If they are successful in hearing what has been shared, then active listeners will be able to answer the following questions at the end of every conversation.(1, 35)

    - Did I hear the message that my client wanted to share?
    - I know what my client said, but what exactly did s/he mean?
    - How do I know that I heard the message correctly?

    Answering these questions requires the following three elements.(1, 28, 31, 32, 36, 37)

    - The listener needs to communicate non-verbally that the speaker has undivided attention.

        - This usually involves head-nods or facial expressions.
        - The listener may also provide minimal feedback responses to convey attentiveness, such as "hmh", "uh-huh", "yeah", "ok", and "sure" or "right."

    - The listener needs to paraphrase, restate, or otherwise reflect back what the speaker shared to check for clarity and accuracy of understanding.
    - The listener needs to invite the speaker to elaborate on what s/he has shared.

2. Another term for active listening is reflective listening.(1) They are synonymous.

3. I might make use of the following phrases to demonstrate to Ryane that I am actively listening: (1)

• It sounds like . . .	• It seems to me that . . .
• It sounds to me as if . . .	• I get the impression that . . .
• It sounds to me that . . .	• I sense that . . .
• What I'm hearing you say is . . .	• You are wondering if . . .
• What I think you're saying is . . .	• So you are concerned about . . .
• So if I understand this correctly . . .	• So you aren't sure if . . .
• So you're saying that . . .	• So your primary concern is . . .
• If I have this correct, then . . .	• So you are worried that . . .

    Unconditional positive regard is a concept that was initially coined by Carl Rogers, a leader in the field of human mental health.(38) Although it is most typically used to describe the work of clinicians in psychiatry, social work, counseling, and psychology, unconditional positive regard can be ascribed to all health professionals. The practice of unconditional positive regard suggests that the clinician approaches each patient as an individual deserving of respect.(39) Patients are to be valued, rather than judged, and to be accepted for who they are rather than to be held to standards that they are incapable of meeting.(39) Even patients that are so-called "difficult" should not be labeled as such. Rather than focusing on good versus bad qualities, the clinician should focus on shared common ground: that is, what do both patient and provider wish to achieve and how can they work together to achieve it?(40)

    Unconditional positive regard presents a challenge to many because judgment is intrinsic to human nature. It is relatively easy to ascribe labels to people, including clients. It is relatively easy to judge their beliefs or mistakes. As a result, it can be difficult to imagine how to demonstrate unconditional positive regard, particularly if the clinician disagrees with the patient. In such circumstances, it is important to remember that "individual practitioners do not have to morally agree with an individual's behavior, nor should we avoid counseling for fear of intruding on individual values, but we must never view the individual as unworthy of conscientious care."(41)

Judgments about people and circumstances are not unique to human healthcare. The veterinary team is not immune to the tendency to judge clients, their beliefs, and/or their actions.

Veterinary clients fear those judgments. This fear may handicap them from participating in frank dialogue about patient care. They may worry about full disclosure, particularly if they feel that their actions are being judged.

In a focus group study that my colleagues and I conducted, dog- and cat-owners expressed their desire to be respected rather than judged by their actions.(39) In particular, cat-owners wanted to be understood as being well-intentioned, even if their actions were improper or inadequate.(39)

One participant expressed the use of unconditional positive regard at its best: "Have you ever done something stupid with your cat and you've got to go tell the vet you did something stupid? [Vets] don't look at you like you're crazy. They understand that we make mistakes."(39)

Another gave an example of dietary indiscretion to demonstrate the use of unconditional positive regard: "[When] the cat [eats] a cardboard box and [swallows] it, [vets] don't say, 'Why on earth did you let him eat the cardboard box?'"(39)

4. To help Ryane work through her feelings of guilt, I could make use of the following statements that are consistent with a display of unconditional positive regard.

   - What you're feeling is completely normal. Hindsight is 20:20. We often wish we could have done better. You did the best you could in the moment.
   - Although it may not feel this way right now, you did right by Nina. It's clear that you put her needs first.
   - I know you wished you had brought Nina in sooner. What's most important is that you're here now. You did the best you could.
   - Your approach to Nina's care was reasonable.
   - You did exactly as I would have done were I in your shoes.
   - Through all of this, you have only put Nina first.
   - It's very apparent to me how much you care about Nina.
   - It's clear to me that you made every decision you did for Nina's benefit.
   - How would you have known how quickly Nina would go downhill?
   - You responded as quickly as you could.

5. Transparency is a buzzword in human healthcare that emerged nearly two decades ago, when in 1999 the Institute of Medicine released a controversial report. The report, "To Err is Human," estimated that 44,000–98,000 people die every year in the US because of preventable medical errors.(42) These errors included delays in diagnosis or treatment; procedural errors; equipment failure; pharmaceutical mistakes including miscalculations in dosing, or the accidental administration of the wrong medication; lost follow-up; and failure to communicate.(42) This publication hoped to shed light on the fact that the practice of medicine is imperfect, but can be improved when dialogue is initiated about how to reduce errors.

6. Medical mistakes are not unique to human healthcare. Although incidence reports in the literature are infrequent, one study in the UK confirmed that veterinary errors are relatively common: 78% of graduates admitted to making a mistake that adversely impacted patient care.(43, 44) When such errors occur, veterinarians are increasingly encouraged to disclose what happened and why, the impact on the patient, and how the error will be prevented in the future.(44)

7. Medical mistakes are not the only circumstance in which transparency may be warranted or desired.

   A focus group study by my colleagues and I confirmed that veterinary clients expect the veterinary team to be transparent about patient illness. In particular, dog-owners did not want facts withheld, even when such details conveyed bad news such as a cancer diagnosis.(39)

One participant captured this perspective best: "Don't beat around the bush. I already know it's cancer. I know what that means. So get to the point of what needs to be done. We know what needs to be done. We just need to hear you say it."(39)

Directness was prized by dog-owners: "Get right to it. Don't soften things up. I want to know exactly what's happening with the dog and what the worst outcome could be."(39)

When information is withheld either about prognosis or terminal diagnosis, dog-owning participants felt offended. To these individuals, failure to disclose such information implied that the veterinary team did not feel they could handle the facts. Dog-owners also felt denied the opportunity to make informed decisions about their pet's care because they lacked the details that would have facilitated decision making.(39)

Directness was also prized by cat owners, who felt that it was equally important for the veterinary team to be honest about what it didn't know: "I want them to say, 'No, I really don't know.' The test for [diagnosing this condition] is $300, the medicine is $100, let's just give the medicine and see what happens. And if it doesn't work, we'll move on to something else. Be open to saying, 'I don't know, but this is the best course to try.'"(39)

In addition to directness about diseases and ongoing disease processes, clients appreciated frank discussion about finances – what is covered by insurance, for example, versus what is not – as well as openness regarding how the veterinarian would proceed if the pet were his/her very own. Hearing that this is what s/he would do facilitates decision making and directs dialogue during difficult conversations about patient care.(39)

8. Transparency might be of benefit in this situation if I have not experienced what Ryane has. I might share the following.

- I don't know what you're going through.
- I can only imagine how hard this is for you.
- I don't know what it's like to be you right now or to have to make this difficult decision.
- I don't know what I can say to make this any better.
- I am at a loss for words myself. I can't begin to know the pain you are feeling.
- I don't know how best to help you know that you are making the best choice for Nina.

Transparency might also be of benefit in addressing the reality of the situation, that is, you are powerless to cure Nina and you both can only provide palliative care:

- Nina is very ill.
- Nina has a mass in her abdomen that is most likely cancer.
- Nina's condition is serious.
- Even if we did everything – meaning surgery – I am doubtful that we could pull her through.
- Surgery might give you more time with her, but if this mass is what we think it is, then it is not something we can cure.
- I wish I could fix Nina, but I can't.
- I wish this were fixable.
- I wish that she hadn't declined so fast.
- I wish you had more time with her.
- Nina's body is starting to shut down and let go. She's making the decision for us.
- We are going to have to make some really difficult decisions sooner than we both had anticipated.
- We need to decide what's best for her, even though that may not be what's best for us.

9. Partnership in healthcare refers to a conscious commitment to include the human patient or veterinary client in decision making.(1) This aspect of relationship-centered care communicates to the client that s/he is part of the veterinary team and that his/her contributions matter.(1) In order for partnership to be effective, the veterinary team may adopt the following strategies. (21, 45–49)

- Consider the client part of the healthcare team.
- Demonstrate respect for the client.
- Demonstrate respect for the patient.
- Recognize the role of the patient in the client's life.
- Acknowledge and validate the client's concerns.
- Be responsive and receptive to client concerns.

10. Partnership statements are particularly valuable during end-of-life visits and end-of-life planning because of the strength of the human–animal bond. Each patient has a different connection to each client, and this connection needs to be acknowledged. Partnership statements are a way to include the client in these final moments with the patient. For example, we might ask the client the following.

- How can we be of help to you?
- How can we help you to make the best decision for Nina?
- Do you need us to contact anyone on your behalf?
- What do you need from us to help with decision making?
- What can we do to support you through this difficult time?
- What are your preferences during this challenging time?
- Do you want us to give you time alone with Nina?

The client is the patient's best advocate. The client knows best what that patient needs and how best to address those needs. Partnership statements are about respect. They help the veterinary team acknowledge the important role that a client plays in the patient's life, particularly at time of death. For instance, we might ask the client the folllwing.

- What can we do to make you more comfortable?
- What can we do to make Nina more comfortable?
- Would it help Nina if . . .?

Partnership statements are also a way to reinforce that the client is not alone. Although s/he may feel like s/he is making this difficult decision to euthanize on one's own, s/he is supported by the veterinary team.

- We are here for you.
- We support you.

11. There are many ways that I can demonstrate partnership with Ryane. Above all, remember the old adage, "There is no I in team."(1) This means that we replace "I" statements with "we" statements and actually mean them.(1)
    For example, instead of saying, "I want to make Nina comfortable," consider rewording your statement as such: "We both want Nina to be as comfortable during this process as possible."(1)
    Other examples of "we" statements include the following.(1)

- We are going to get through this together.
- We are both here for Nina and are going to do everything we can to keep her comfortable.

Partnership statements might also make use of the phrase, let us, or the contraction, let's.(1)

- Let's consider what we can do to make this process as pain-free as possible for Nina.
- Let's decide how best to proceed so that we can keep Nina comfortable.

Sometimes, the additional word, together, is tacked onto the statement to further emphasize partnership.

- Let's see what we can do together to make this process as pain-free as possible for Nina.
- Let's decide together how best to proceed so that we can keep Nina comfortable.

Other inclusive language includes the words ours and us.(2) Using inclusive language helps us to establish and reinforce a team approach to case management.(2)

Returning to Case 50: The Last Goodbye

After an emotional discussion about Nina's health and quality of life, Ryane makes the most difficult decision in Nina's best interest. Ryane elects to have Nina humanely euthanized.

Round Three of Questions for Case 50: The Last Goodbye

1. Which questions are essential for you to ask of any client before you proceed with euthanasia?
2. Because of Ryane's credentials (DVM), you assume that she has practiced as a veterinarian and has had to euthanize patients in the past. What are potential problems with making this assumption?
3. Which communication skill(s) can you draw upon to discover Ryane's knowledge base rather than making assumptions?
4. Which communication skill(s) can you draw upon to determine if Ryane has any concerns about the process of euthanasia or what to expect?
5. What can you do during the process of euthanasia to facilitate a smooth transition from life to death?
6. Some practices offer clay paws or a clipping of fur as a form of pet memorial. Why is it important that you ask Ryane first before you provide her with one of these mementos?

Answers to Round Three of Questions for Case 50: The Last Goodbye

1. The following questions are essential for you to ask of any client before you proceed with euthanasia.

- Do you want time alone with Nina before we proceed?
- Are you ready to proceed?
- Do you want to be present for the euthanasia?
    - If yes, have you ever witnessed euthanasia before?
        - If not, may I share with you how the process works so that you know what to expect?
- Do others want to be present for the euthanasia?
- Do you need to get a hold of anyone else before we proceed?
- Does anyone else want to see Nina or say goodbye before we proceed?
- Would you like us to call anyone so that they can be here with you?
- Is it okay if we borrow Nina so that we can place an intravenous IV catheter in preparation for euthanasia?
- After Nina has passed, do you know how you would like us to handle her body? In other words, do you have a plan for her aftercare?
    - At-home burial
    - Group cremation
        - Ashes are not returned to the client
    - Individual cremation
        - Ashes are returned to the client

2. Your assumptions may or may not be correct.

There are many roles that DVMs may have outside of clinical practice. Not all DVMs practice clinical medicine and not all DVMs routinely perform euthanasia. Moreover, not all DVMs treat the same species. A DVM who is involved in laboratory medicine, for instance, is likely to be familiar with how to euthanize those species with which s/he works, but s/he may not be familiar with the process in cats.

If you assume that Ryane has practiced companion animal medicine and has euthanized patients in the past, then you may be tempted to skip over key details about the euthanasia process that she may value in her role as client.

Even if Ryane knows the process of euthanasia, she may not be familiar with how your clinic operates. For instance, some clinics routinely place intravenous (IV) catheters; others almost never do. Rather than assume she knows how your practice operates, it is best to both ask for permission to share your protocol and be transparent about the process.

Another faulty assumption may be that Ryane knows options for how Nina's body can be handled after euthanasia. If Ryane has practiced in clinical medicine, then she may be familiar with options that have historically been available to her, as a clinician. These options may or may not be available to her as a client of your practice. Moreover, in the United States, pet burial laws may vary between states and potentially different cities. If Ryane previously practiced in a state where at-home burial was legal, but she is now living in a state where it is not, she may or may not be familiar with local regulations and statutes that may preclude her aftercare wishes.

3. Instead of making assumptions about what Ryane knows about the euthanasia process, you can assess her knowledge directly.

- What has your experience been concerning euthanasia in cats?
- What do you know about the euthanasia process in cats?
- Have you ever had to euthanize a cat here at our practice?

You can then address Ryane's responses by asking permission to provide clarification on the process if there are discrepancies that need to be addressed.

- Would it be okay if I walked you through the euthanasia process here at our clinic?
- Would it be okay if I outlined how euthanasia is performed at our practice so that you know what to expect?

4. You can elicit Ryane's perspective by asking one or more of the following.
- Do you have any questions about the process?
- Do you have any concerns about the process?
- What concerns you most?
- What are you most worried about?
- What is most important for us to know about Nina moving forward?
- What do you need from us as we go through this process?
- How can we best support you during this process?
- How can we best support Nina as we go through this process together?

5. To facilitate the transition between life and death, you can prepare the client for what to expect. For instance:

- You may prepare the client by reviewing the process through signposting:

  - I am going to first inject a sedative.
  - I will then administer the euthanasia solution.

- You may prepare the client that the patient will not likely close his/her eyes after passing
- You may prepare the client that the patient may take several deep breaths at or after passing.

- You may prepare the client that the patient may experience some twitches at or after passing:

  - That is the patient's stored energy letting go. Nina will not be in any pain or distress. She will not even be aware that this is even happening.

- You may prepare the client that the patient may lose control over his/her bladder or bowels.
- You may announce the administration of each medication.

  - I am now going to administer the sedative that is going to help Nina drift off into a peaceful sleep.
  - I am now going to administer the euthanasia solution.

- You should listen to the patient's chest after euthanasia to confirm that the heartbeat has stopped.
- You should announce aloud that the patient has passed to help assist with closure.

  - Nina's heart has stopped beating.
  - Nina is no longer with us.

- You should express your condolences to the client.
- You should offer to give the client privacy and/or space if s/he would like some time alone with the patient's body.
- You should do your best to leave judgment at the door.

  - Some of our clients choose not to be present during euthanasia.
  - We need to respect that not everyone chooses to be present.
  - We may not always understand why our clients make the choices we do, but we need to do our best to accept and support them.

6. The way in which we process grief is unique. We all have own needs, expectations, and desires concerning how we mourn (and choose to remember) the loss of a loved one. Even when individuals share love for the same person or pet, their relationship with the deceased individual is uniquely distinct. We honor the human–animal bond best when we ask our clients directly what they need from us and whether a certain memorial item would be beneficial to them. It is always better to ask if a client would like a fur clipping and be turned down, then to assume that s/he wants one and to have that gesture backfire. Euthanasia is often an emotionally challenging clinical experience for all involved. We do not want to make it worse by making assumptions that are proven wrong. When possible, ask what the client wants and needs, and do all you can to respect those boundaries.

CLINICAL PEARLS

- End-of-life consultations are an emotionally taxing time for both veterinary clients and veterinary teams.

- Patients may present with acute or chronic conditions, some of which can be medically or surgically treated. Other patients only qualify for palliative care.

- The practice of veterinary medicine allows for quality of life to be a guiding principle in terms of whether to facilitate the patient's transition from life to death.

- Euthanasia is an acceptable treatment outcome.

- When clients consent to humane euthanasia, it is a critical procedure that must be performed with as much respect and care for the patient and the human–animal bond as is possible.

- Clinical communication plays an essential role in straddling this transition from life to death.

- When communication is effective, clients feel heard, valued, and supported.

- When communication is poor, clients may feel disrespected or that the veterinary team, simply put, didn't care.

- Communication skills that may facilitate consultations about euthanasia include the use of open-ended questions, active (reflective) listening, appropriate non-verbal cues, empathetic actions and/or statements, eliciting the client's perspective, assessing the client's knowledge, offering partnership, asking permission, being transparent, and demonstrating unconditional positive regard.

- Be honest. If you've never experienced what the client is facing, then do not pretend to understand. Become comfortable with uncertainty and with expressing that "I don't know what it feels like to be you" or "I can't even begin to imagine what you're going through." These statements are powerful and validate the client's experience.

- When in doubt, ask the client what s/he needs, wants, or expects from you and your team.

- Don't assume that all clients grieve the same way. Customize your approach to meet clients' needs and expectations.

References

1. Englar RE. A guide to oral communication in veterinary medicine. Sheffield: 5M Publishing; 2020.
2. Hunter LJ, Shaw JR. How to exceed – Not merely meet – Client expectations. March: Veterinary Team Brief:19–22; 2018.
3. Carson CA. Nonverbal communication in veterinary practice. Vet Clin North Am Small Anim Pract 2007;37(1):49–63.
4. Shaw JR. Four core communication skills of highly effective practitioners. Vet Clin North Am Small Anim Pract 2006;36(2):385–96.
5. Myers WS. Nonverbal communication speaks volumes: Building better client relationships. Exceptional Veterinary Team. 2009 (November):3–5.
6. Roter DL, Frankel RM, Hall JA, Sluyter D. The expression of emotion through nonverbal behavior in medical visits. Mechanisms and outcomes. J Gen Intern Med 2006;21(Suppl 1):S28–34.
7. Caris-Verhallen WM, Kerkstra A, Bensing JM. Non-verbal behaviour in nurse-elderly patient communication. J Adv Nurs 1999;29(4):808–18.
8. Marcinowicz L, Konstantynowicz J, Godlewski C. Patients' perceptions of GP non-verbal communication: A qualitative study. Br J Gen Pract 2010;60(571):83–7.
9. Verderber RF, Verderber KS. Inter-Act: Using interpersonal communication skills. Belmont, Wadsworth, CA; 1980.
10. Gabbott M, Hogg G. The role of non-verbal communication in service encounters: A conceptual framework. J Mark Manag 2001;17(1–2):5–26.
11. Duggan P, Parrott L. Physicians' nonverbal rapport building and patients' talk about the subjective component of illness. Hum Commun Res 2001;27(2):299–311.
12. Endres J, Laidlaw A. Micro-expression recognition training in medical students: A pilot study. BMC Med Educ 2009;9:47.

13. Cocksedge S, George B, Renwick S, Chew-Graham CA. Touch in primary care consultations: Qualitative investigation of doctors' and patients' perceptions. Br J Gen Pract 2013;63(609):e283–90.
14. Peloquin SM. Helping through touch: The embodiment of caring. J Relig Health 1989;28(4):299–322.
15. Edwards SC. An anthropological interpretation of nurses' and patients' perceptions of the use of space and touch. J Adv Nurs 1998;28(4):809–17.
16. Estabrooks CA, Morse JM. Toward a theory of touch – The touching process and acquiring a touching style. J Adv Nurs 1992;17(4):448–56.
17. Connor A, Howett M. A conceptual model of intentional comfort touch. J Holist Nurs 2009;27(2):127–35.
18. Argyle M. Spatial behavior. Bodily communication. 2nd ed. Madison, CT: International Universities Press; 1988.
19. Hall E. Space speaks. The Silent Language. Garden City, NY: Anchor Press; 1973:162–85.
20. McMurray J, Boysen S. Communicating empathy in veterinary practice. Vet Irel J 2017;7(4):199–205.
21. Adams CL, Kurtz SM. Skills for communicating in veterinary medicine. Oxford: Otmoor Press and Dewpoint Publishing; 2017.
22. Preusche I, Lamm C. Reflections on empathy in medical education: What can we learn from social neurosciences? Adv Health Sci Educ Theor Pract 2016;21(1):235–49.
23. Silverman J, Kurtz S, Draper J. Skills for communicating with patients. Oxford, UK.K. Radcliffe Medical Press; 2008.
24. Kurtz SM, Silverman JD, Draper J. Teaching and learning communication skills in medicine. Grand Rapids. Radcliffe; 2004.
25. Shea SC. Psychiatric interviewing: The art of understanding. 2nd ed. Philadelphia, PA: W.B. Saunders Company; 1998.
26. Morrisey JK, Voiland B. Difficult interactions with veterinary clients: Working in the challenge zone. Vet Clin North Am Small Anim Pract 2007;37(1):65–77; abstract viii:abstract viii.
27. Bateman SW. Communication in the veterinary emergency setting. Vet Clin North Am Small Anim Pract 2007;37(1):109–21.
28. Weger H, Castle GR, Emmett MC. Active listening in peer interviews: The influence of message paraphrasing on perceptions of listening skill. Int J Listening 2010;24(1):34–49.
29. Adler RB, Rosenfeld LB, Proctor RF. Interplay: The process of interpersonal communication. Oxford: Oxford University Press; 2006.
30. Canary DJ, Cody MJ, Manusov VL. Interpersonal communication: A Goals-Based Approach. Bedford, NY: St Martin's; 2003.
31. Devito JA. The interpersonal communication book. New York: Pearson; 2007.
32. Trenholm S, Jensen A. Interpersonal communication. Oxford: Oxford University Press; 2004.
33. Verderber KS, Verderber RF. Inter-Act: Interpersonal communication concepts, skills, and contexts. Oxford: Oxford University Press; 2004.
34. Wood JT. Interpersonal communication: everyday encounters. New York: Wadsworth; 1998.
35. van Dulmen S. Listen: When words don't come easy. Patient Educ Couns 2017;100(11):1975–8.
36. Levitt DH. Active listening and counselor self-efficacy: Emphasis on one micro-skill in beginning counselor training. Clin Superv 2002;20(2):101–15.
37. Simon C. The functions of active listening responses. Behav Processes 2018;157:47–53.
38. Amadi C. Clinician, society and suicide mountain: Reading Rogerian doctrine of unconditional positive regard (UPR). Psychol Thought 2013;6(1):75–89.
39. Englar RE, Williams M, Weingand K. Applicability of the Calgary-Cambridge guide to dog and cat owners for teaching veterinary clinical communications. J Vet Med Educ 2016;43(2):143–69.
40. Gibson S. On judgment and judgmentalism: how counselling can make people better. J Med Eth 2005;31(10):575–7.
41. Larkin GL, Iserson K, Kassutto Z, Freas G, Delaney K, Krimm J, et al. Virtue in emergency medicine. Acad Emerg Med 2009;16(1):51–5.
42. Kohn LT, Corrigan JM, Donaldson MS, editors, Institute of Medicine (US) Committee on Quality of Health Care in America. To err is human: building a safer health system. Washington, DC: National Academies Press; 2000.

43. Mellanby RJ, Herrtage ME. Survey of mistakes made by recent veterinary graduates. Vet Rec 2004;155(24):761–5.

44. Bonvicini KA, O'Connell D, Cornell KK. Disclosing medical errors: restoring client trust. Compend Contin Educ Vet 2009;31(3):E5.

45. Küper AM, Merle R. Being nice is not enough-exploring relationship-centered veterinary care with structural equation modeling. A quantitative study on German pet owners' perception. Front Vet Sci 2019;6:56.

46. Donovan JL. Patient decision making. The missing ingredient in compliance research. Int J Technol Assess Health Care 1995;11(3):443–55.

47. Donovan JL, Blake DR. Patient non-compliance: deviance or reasoned decision-making? Soc Sci Med 1992;34(5):507–13.

48. Abood SK. Increasing adherence in practice: making your clients partners in care. Vet Clin North Am Small Anim Pract 2007;37(1):151–64.

49. Kanji N, Coe JB, Adams CL, Shaw JR. Effect of veterinarian-client-patient interactions on client adherence to dentistry and surgery recommendations in companion-animal practice. J Am Vet Med Assoc 2012;240(4):427–36.

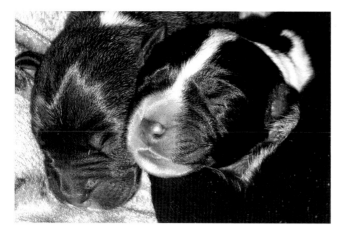

Plate 1 Although this image is of a 1-day-old pup instead of a kitten, you can appreciate the strikingly pink color of the neonate's muzzle. This is considered normal. This color would deepen to dark pink or red with dehydration; however, that is a subjective measure. Courtesy of Tara Beugel.

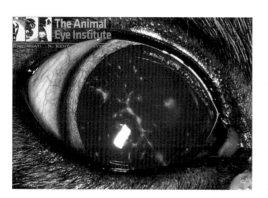

Plate 2 The classic FHV-1 induced corneal ulcer. Courtesy of DJ Haeussler Jr BS MS DVM DACVO and The Animal Eye Institute.

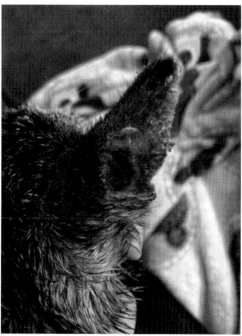

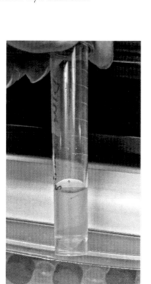

Plate 3 Circular alopecia along the external aspect of the right pinna. Courtesy of Colleen Cook.

Plate 4 Well-concentrated urine. First catch of the day. Courtesy of Brynn Zittle.

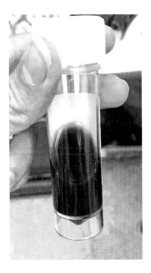

Plate 5a Myoglobinuria.
Courtesy of Holly Elvans.

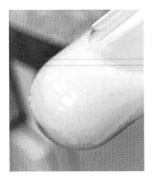

Plate 5b Milky urine due
to extreme pyuria, the
presence of leukocytes in
urine.

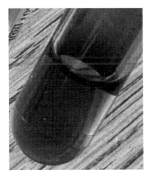

Plate 5c Orange
urine due to extreme
dehydration.

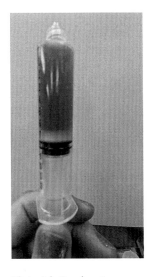

Plate 5d Peach urine.
Courtesy of Lori Kruse.

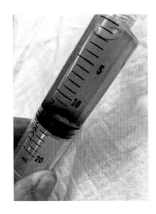

Plate 5e Pink urine.
Courtesy of Lori Danelle
Capobianco.

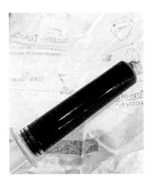

Plate 5f Red urine.
Courtesy of Alexis
Hendrix.

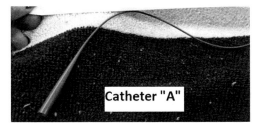

Plate 6a Urinary catheter option "A."

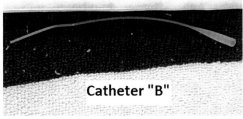

Plate 6b Urinary catheter option "B."

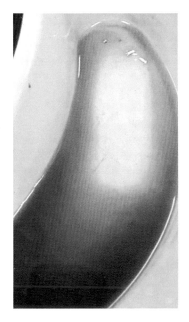

Plate 7 Photographic evidence of house-soiling. Note that this urine sample demonstrates hematuria.

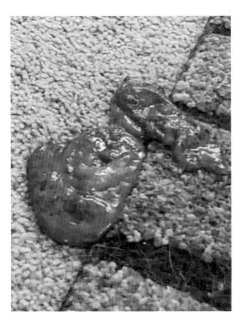

Plate 8 Gelatinous diarrhea. Courtesy of Monica Runge.

Plate 9 Adult dog exhibiting tenesmus and hematochezia. Courtesy of Danelle Capobianco.

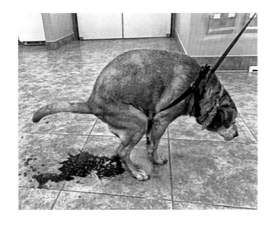

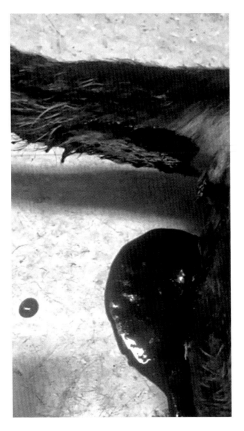

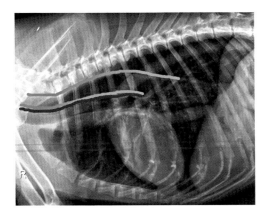

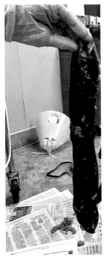

Plate 11 Same right lateral thoracic radiograph as in Figure 24.2. The borders of the esophagus have been outlined in blue. The classic "tracheal stripe" sign is present as the summation of the dorsal tracheal wall with the ventral wall of the esophagus. This "stripe" has been drawn in, in the color red.

Plate 10 Example of melena that has just been passed by a laterally recumbent patient. Only the patient's tail is visible in this photograph. Courtesy of Chloe Bush.

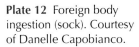

Plate 12 Foreign body ingestion (sock). Courtesy of Danelle Capobianco.

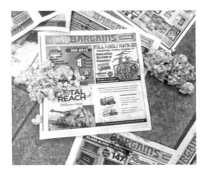

Plate 13 Foreign body ingestion (corn cobs). Courtesy of Danelle Capobianco.

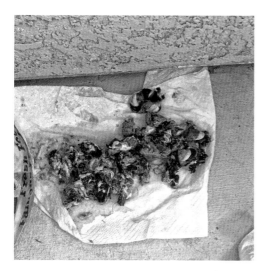

Plate 14 Foreign body ingestion (dog toy). Courtesy of Kim Wallitsch.

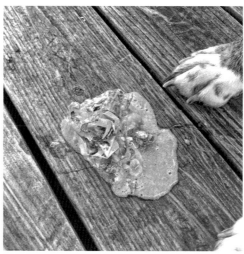

Plate 15 Chocolate candy ingestion. Courtesy of Rachel Sahrbeck.

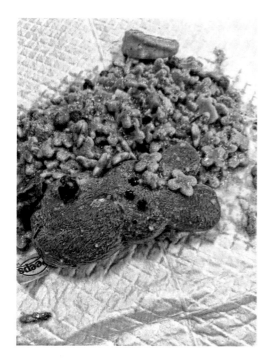

Plate 16 Easter candy ingestion, including sugar-free items. Courtesy of Deb Moray.

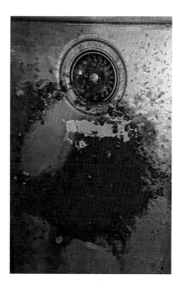

Plate 17 Snail bait ingestion. Courtesy of Whitney Rouse.

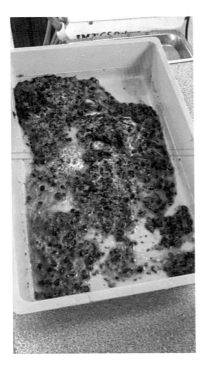

Plate 18 Raisin ingestion. Courtesy of Holly Elvans.

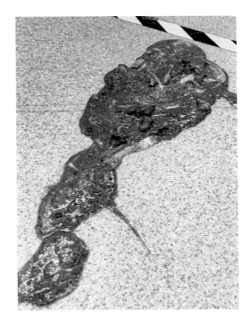

Plate 19 Rat bait-containing vomitus induced by apomorphine. Courtesy of Ethel Koh.

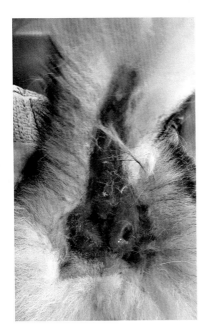

Plate 20 Feline perineum. Courtesy of Lori Stillmaker.

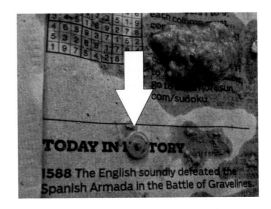

Plate 21 Roundworm in feline vomitus. Courtesy of Cassandra Corkell.

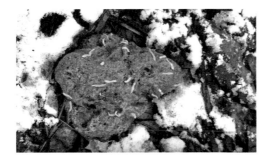

Plate 22 Tapeworm proglottids. Courtesy of Michelle Lugones, DVM.

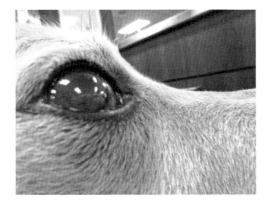

Plate 23 "Red eye" in a canine patient with glaucoma. Courtesy of Patricia Bennett, DVM.

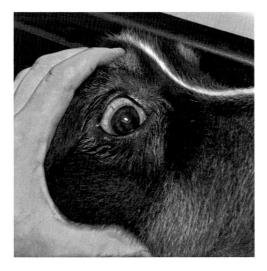

Plate 24 Conjunctivitis in a canine patient. Courtesy of Kimberly Wallitsch.

Plate 25 Blepharitis in a feline patient.

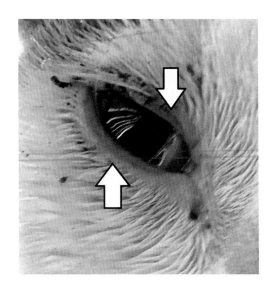

Plate 26 Gross appearance of one of Pico de Gato's eyes. Only one eye has been shown here, but both eyes appear the same. Courtesy of D.J. Haeussler, Jr., BS, MS, DVM, DACVO.

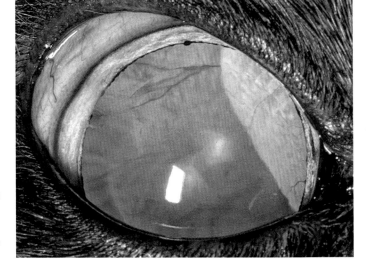

Plate 27 Fundic appearance of one of Pico de Gato's eyes. Only one eye has been shown here, but both eyes appear the same. Courtesy of D.J. Haeussler, Jr., BS, MS, DVM, DACVO.

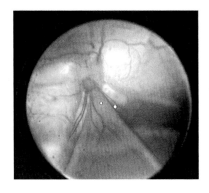

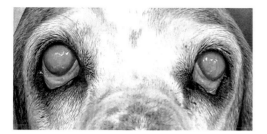

Plate 28 Corneal edema in a canine patient. Note that the eyes take on a characteristic blue color.

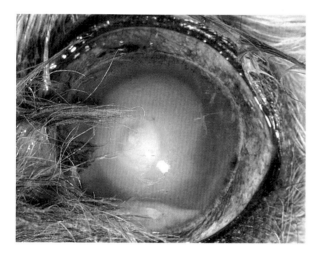

Plate 29 Infiltration of the cornea with inflammatory cells causes the stroma to take on a yellow-green appearance. Courtesy of D.J. Haeussler, Jr., BS, MS, DVM, DACVO.

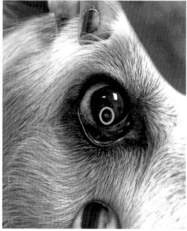

Plate 30 Focal lipid deposit in a canine patient. The result is a silvery or white opacity. Mineral deposits result in the same opacity, but are typically due to calcium.

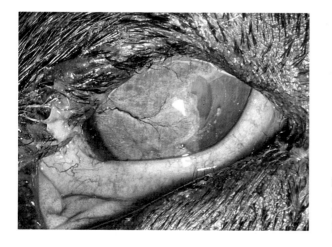

Plate 31 Corneal neovascularization in a canine patient. Courtesy of D.J. Haeussler, Jr., BS, MS, DVM, DACVO.

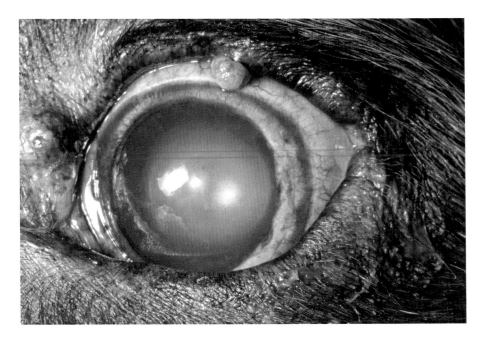

Plate 32 Nuclear sclerosis in a canine patient. This age-related process confer a hazy appearance to the lens. Note the unrelated, incidental finding of a papilloma associated with the upper eyelid. Courtesy of D.J. Haeussler Jr., BS, MS, DVM, DACVO.

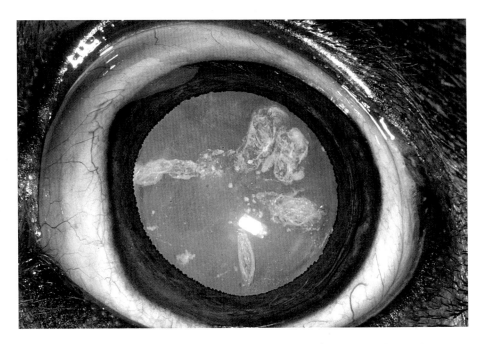

Plate 33 Incipient cataract in a dog. Courtesy of D.J. Haeussler Jr., BS, MS, DVM, DACVO.

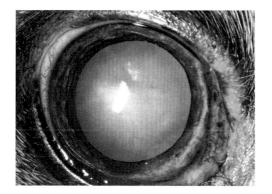

Plate 34 Mature cataract in a dog. Courtesy of
D.J. Haeussler Jr., BS, MS, DVM, DACVO.

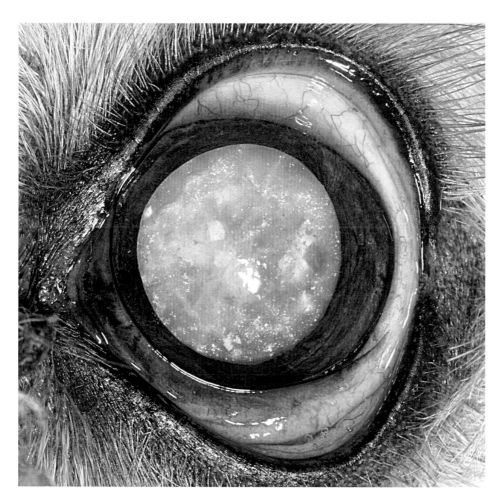

Plate 35 Hypermature cataract in a dog. Courtesy of D.J. Haeussler Jr., BS, MS, DVM, DACVO.

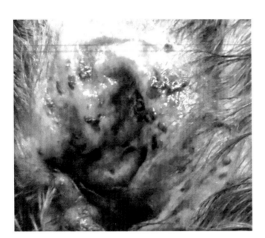

Plate 36 Aural debris prior to ear cleaning.

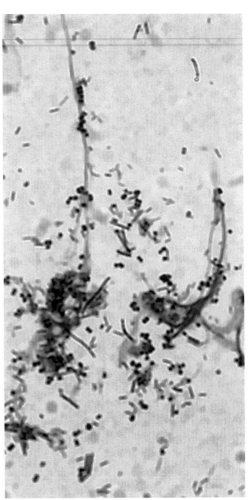

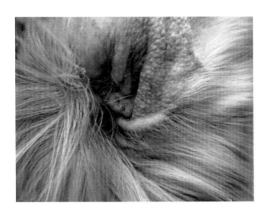

Plate 37 Entrance to external ear canal after ear cleaning.

Plate 38 Low power ear cytology.

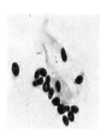

Plate 39 High power ear cytology. Note that this is only one field of vision.

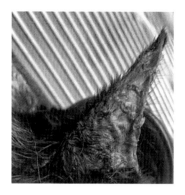

Plate 40 Caudodorsal aspect of right pinna. Note that the left ear bears the same appearance. Courtesy of Lauren Bessert, DVM.

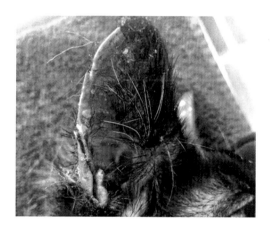

Plate 41 Rostral aspect of right pinna, when viewed head-on. Note that the left ear bears the same appearance. Courtesy of Lauren Bessert, DVM.

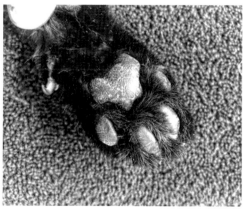

Plate 42 Hyperkeratosis of the foot pads. Courtesy of Lauren Bessert, DVM.

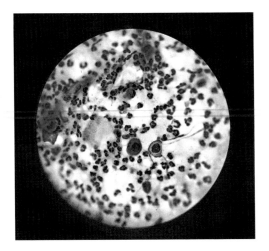

Plate 43 Caudodorsal aspect of right pinna. Note that the left ear bears the same appearance. Courtesy of Lauren Bessert, DVM.

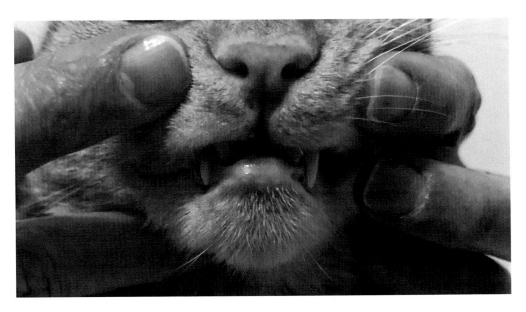

Plate 44 Facial swelling in a cat. Courtesy of Michael Edgar.

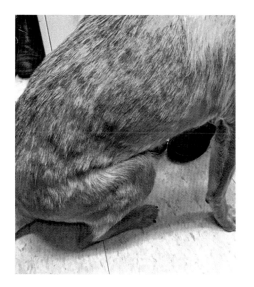

Plate 45 Caudolateral view of the patient's right side. The lesions that you see here are also present on the patient's left side. Courtesy of Georgia Hymmen.

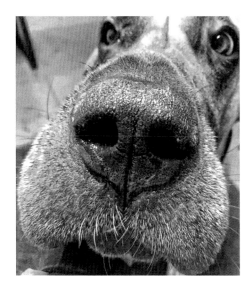

Plate 46 Head-on view of the patient's muzzle. Courtesy of Georgia Hymmen.

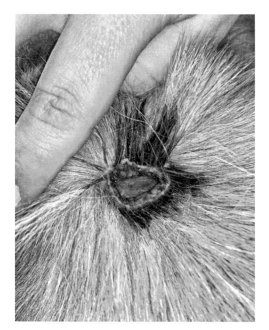

Plate 47 Laceration between shoulder blades, sustained during dog fight. Courtesy of Katherine Anne Crocco.

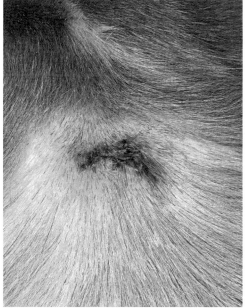

Plate 48 Surgical wound closure with suture. Courtesy of Katherine Anne Crocco.

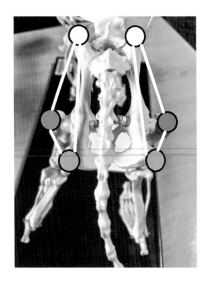

Plate 49 Note the imaginary triangles that are formed by the wings of the ilia (identified by circles filled in with white), the ischiatic tuberosities (identified by circles filled in with pink), and the greater trochanters (identified by circles filled in with blue).

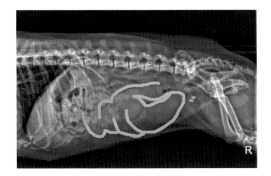

Plate 50 Right lateral abdominal radiograph demonstrating canine pyometra in a different patient, with the uterus outlined in blue. Again, ignore the incidental finding of bladder stones, which were in a different patient, not Pipsqueak.

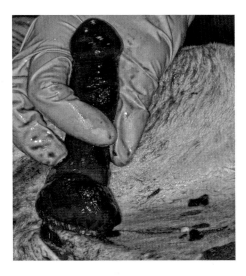

Plate 51 Priapism in a canine patient. Courtesy of Laura Polerecky, LVT.

Index